BDJ Clinician's Guides

This series enables clinicians at all stages of their careers to remain well informed and up to date on key topics across all fields of clinical dentistry. Each volume is superbly illustrated and provides concise, highly practical guidance and solutions. The authors are recognised experts in the subjects that they address. The *BDJ Clinician's Guides* are trusted companions, designed to meet the needs of a wide readership. Like the *British Dental Journal* itself, they offer support for undergraduates and newly qualified, while serving as refreshers for more experienced clinicians. In addition they are valued as excellent learning aids for postgraduate students.

The BDJ Clinicians' Guides are produced in collaboration with the British Dental Association, the UK's trade union and professional association for dentists.

Winston Chee • Saj Jivraj
Editors

Treatment Planning In Implant Dentistry

Second Edition

Springer

Editors
Winston Chee
Advanced Prosthodontics, Herman Ostrow School of Dentistry
University of Southern California
Los Angeles, CA, USA

Saj Jivraj
Private Practice
Anacapa Dental Art Institute
Oxnard, CA, USA

ISSN 2523-3327 ISSN 2523-3335 (electronic)
BDJ Clinician's Guides
ISBN 978-3-031-68725-9 ISBN 978-3-031-68726-6 (eBook)
https://doi.org/10.1007/978-3-031-68726-6

This Springer imprint is published by the registered company Springer Nature Switzerland AG
The registered company address is: Gewerbestrasse 11, 6330 Cham, Switzerland

Foreword

In 1982, the historic Branemark Conference on osseointegration was held in Toronto, Canada, and forever changed the course of restorative dentistry. The conference highlighted long-term data on multiple splinted titanium root-form implants inserted with a detailed surgical protocol. The implants were placed in the anterior mandible and supported hybrid prostheses opposing a maxillary complete denture. The outcomes were astounding, and clinicians worldwide scrambled to avail themselves with this amazing new technology.

In the initial few years of osseointegration, only one company was approved for use and sold in the United States. The sale of the surgical and restorative components from this company was restricted to surgical and restorative specialists (oral and maxillofacial surgeons, periodontists and prosthodontists) who had attended a certified course on the topic. This was likely a wise decision, and while limiting commercial sales, it tilted the odds of successful outcomes of therapy because of the quality and calibration of the providers.

In subsequent years, multiple manufacturers entered the market, and implants and their components became available to anyone who wanted them. Amidst this chaos, peer-reviewed research and case reports began to explore how and when clinicians could stray from the original Branemark protocol and still sustain high levels of clinical success. Clinicians also explored the use of implants in different types of bone, in partially dentulous cases, in the aesthetic zone and as anchorage of orthodontic movement. In this period, private practitioners, and dental schools, including the University of Southern California School of Dentistry (USCSD), contemplated the optimal process for incorporating this new technology into their practices and/or curriculum.

As Chair of the Department of Restorative Dentistry and Director of the Advanced Education in Prosthodontics Program at USCSD, understanding that implementing an implant dentistry programme at USCSD was essential, I made two critical decisions. The first was to appoint Dr. Winston Chee as the Director of Implant Dentistry, which was not centred in one department, but crossed multiple disciplines. Dr. Chee possessed the knowledge, clinical skills and personal courage to integrate this emerging technology into an already crowded and complex curriculum. The second, made in concert with Dr. Chee, was that implant dentistry was a restorative, rather than surgically driven, discipline.

The implant dentistry programme at USCSD has always been centred in the traditional periodontal-prosthetics treatment planning seminar, attended by residents and faculty from most of the specialty programmes for 2 h every week. The strength of the seminar was the presence of many highly qualified full- and part-time faculty in all clinical disciplines who had widely divergent philosophies regarding the optimum treatment approach for patients with complex periodontal and restorative needs. This inevitably resulted in detailed, passionate discussions regarding almost every patient presented in the seminar; however, consensus was eventually developed, and patient treatment initiated. In the early years, all implant-related treatment was completed in the specialty programmes. In the early 1990s, it was expanded to allow pre-doctoral students to restore implants that were placed in the advanced periodontics programme, with the students participating in the diagnosis and treatment planning phase under the supervision of a prosthodontist. The students would also assist in the implant placement appointment. Eventually, the advanced prosthodontics residents began placing implants under the supervision of advanced periodontics faculty.

Another key player in USCSD's implant programme was Dr. Sajid Jivraj who joined the faculty after graduating from the Advanced Education in Prosthodontics Program. Drs. Jivraj and Chee, along with other specialists from USCSD, teamed together to author numerous articles on a wide variety of topics related to implant dentistry that were published in the British Dental Journal.

These articles formed the core of the first edition of this textbook, and subjects covered included screw-retained versus cement-retained restorations, immediate implant placement, biomechanics and occlusion, treatment planning in the aesthetic zone, edentulous maxilla and mandible and many others.

The authors based the articles on evidence-based information, and all possessed high ethical standards and excellent clinical skills and made recommendations using a patient-centred approach.

Drs. Chee and Jivraj, and the other contributing authors, are to be congratulated for compiling a contemporary, comprehensive text to help guide clinicians and residents in various specialty programmes entering the world of complex interdisciplinary dental treatment of patients using dental implants.

Professor (Retired), The University of North Carolina at Chapel Hill
Chapel Hill, NC, USA

Terry Donovan

Preface

Dr. Jivraj and I co-authored the first edition of Treatment Planning in Implant Dentistry in 2007; many things have changed since then, and many things have not; these "things" would include decision-making, effects of systemic health, effects of medications, new materials and new methods, and the list goes on.

It remains that dental implants are one of the most significant developments in replacing missing teeth; when osseointegrated implants were introduced to North America in 1982 at the Toronto Conference, a strict protocol was presented and adhered to.

Since then, there have been many deviations to the early days of delivering dental implants; in the beginning, osseointegrated dental implant providers were limited to oral and maxillofacial surgeons, periodontists and prosthodontists; initially, most of these disciplines obtained training from continuing education programmes and then developed their own skills and pathways. Soon, dental implants were incorporated into the respective postgraduate programmes where all graduates were trained with the usage of dental implants. At present, dental schools have included dental implants into their curriculum, and replacing teeth with dental implants is accepted as a norm. In some dental schools, implant placement is taught to all students as routine, not to make them experts but to introduce them to the mode of treatment for patients.

With time, many innovations were implemented by clinicians, better delivery systems were developed, newer materials were introduced for clinical procedures and outcomes of treatment provided the profession with more information.

Most of the continuing education and publications that are available are focused on techniques and materials. There are in general three phases of treatment: first (1) data collection, diagnosis and then development of a treatment plan; (2) executing the treatment plan with suitable outcomes; and (3) maintenance and care of the patients.

This second edition of the book will focus on the first phase which is diagnosis and treatment planning; each chapter of the book with feature element of providing dental implants attempts to help clinicians make the best choice for their patients.

All the contributors to the book chapters are alumni of the Ostrow School of Dentistry of the University of Southern California; the chapter authors are periodontists and prosthodontists; our programme meets every Thursday for 2 h in treatment planning sessions—we have all the residents attend and many faculty in attendance.

Each resident in turn will collect data of patients that will be treated; the resident will present the data collected with images and then develop a course of treatment. Every resident from the time that I was a resident would be asking "why is the patient here", what is the "biologic price" and "if you do not know where you are going, you never get lost".

Why is the patient here—what are the patient's wants and needs, and what are the patient's complaints? For the clinician's thoughts, what is our diagnosis? How will management be for this patient?

What is the biologic price? What is the least invasive path towards a good outcome.

If you do not know where you are going, you never get lost: this is a paraphrase of a saying by Henry Kissinger, "if you don't know where you are going, every road will get you nowhere". One clear example of this would be some facilities which seem to have almost all their patients have the same treatment protocol. Wouldn't a proper diagnosis dictate differing treatment? Would some clinicians be "lost"?

Our alumni do not graduate as clones—based on the treatment planning programme, we all develop differently, but we consider all the factors that drive our treatment plans. It is the most important phase that we try to inculcate to our residents.

Readers of this book will clearly be able to develop a customized treatment plan that will lead to predictable and favourable outcomes for their patients. In more complex care where patients may require more tooth replacement with time, decisions to use implants already placed to support future restorations can be very helpful. Dr. Jivraj and I have had an association for over 30 years; it has been a pleasure to see him grow in stature in our profession and become a leader in clinical practice and education. It is my privilege to co-edit and co-author this book with Dr. Jivraj and help all clinicians with decision-making for their implant-related patient treatments.

Los Angeles, CA, USA Winston Chee

Acknowledgements

Acknowledgements by Winston Chee

There is nothing impossible to him who will try—Alexander the Great

From the first edition of Treatment Planning in Implant Dentistry to now, the task to update this edition was much more tedious than I thought.

To My Family

I want to thank my wife, Dr. Tina Siu, for being supportive of me in all facets. I would and could not have a great professional and academic journey; she has given me the time, the encouragement and any help that I would ask for. She was also responsible for raising my two children to adulthood; my daughter, Michelle, is a neurologist and my son, Daniel, an orthodontist. I cannot be more blessed with my beloved wife and family.

To My Mentors

Dr. Chong Lin Chew was an influential professor that I had from my dental school in Singapore; he was trained in the University of Indiana as a prosthodontist and dental materialist. He was stern as a teacher and encouraged me to get into an advanced prosthodontics programme to improve my professional career. From my relationship to him as a student, we are good friends and colleagues. My other mentor is Terry Donovan, who is an alumnus of our Advanced Education in Prosthodontics; he offered me a job as a faculty member at the University of Southern California and was very supportive. We have published many articles together. He had appointed me as his Co-director of the Advanced Prosthodontics Program and then later the Director of the Program. He also tasked me to initiate the implant dentistry programme at the dental school. It was a great journey for me, and along the way, I learnt much about dentistry and much about people. To my two mentors, I am thankful and indebted.

To My Alumni

I am so pleased to see you all gain stature in your professions, some in academics, some as researchers and many as clinicians. We have also had meetings in different continents, and we have all gathered to meet. We congregate to learn and to rekindle our friendships. Interestingly, we have many of our alumni meet each other for the first time—where they think and discuss issues about prosthodontics—and there is a strong commonality that develops.

I want to especially thank our alumni who contributed chapters to this book and those who shared their images with us.

To Saj

He was the one who coaxed me into editing this book, and it is only now that we have finished it that I am thankful—Saj you can edit the next one.

Acknowledgements by Saj Jivraj

> Don't fear the difficult times in life. They are the best way to prove to yourself that you can do difficult things—Matthew Hussey

As the years pass, the things that become important really come into perspective. It is to these important aspects of my life that I wish to dedicate this book.

To My Family

First and foremost, and without hesitation, I would like to thank my beautiful wife, Dilaz. She is my life, my inspiration and a wonderful mother to my two beautiful children, Sara and Zain. You said "yes" to everything which should have been "no"; you allowed me the time to become professionally what I dreamed about as a young graduate. You persevered when times got tough and gave up everything moving with me to the United States. You supported me through school and spent countless evenings on your own while I was preparing for the next day. For the countless hours I did not spend with you and the kids and for the unconditional love, friendship and unwavering support, I thank you. To Sara and Zain, words cannot express the profound love I have for you. You have taught me to appreciate life in ways I thought were not possible; the little things you do and say make me a better person, husband and father. I will always be by your side to support you in anything you do. Work hard and dream big and believe in the impossible. You can do what you set your mind to, and do not let anybody else tell you otherwise.

I would also like to dedicate this book to the memory of two exceptional women: Mrs Amina and Rukiya Jivraj who were taken from this world far too early. Not a day goes by when I do not think of you. I feel your presence in all the important decisions that I make. I miss you both dearly and wish we could have created more memories together. When people say, "Life is too short", I now understand what that means. I do know that we will meet again, and it is that day to which I look forward. I would also like to acknowledge Mrs. Zarina Parekh who became a second mother to me and who always inspired me to be and do my best and to never give up. Thanks also goes to Mehboob Jivraj, my eldest brother, who from a young age gave me the confidence and belief that I could do anything I set my mind to.

To My Colleagues

I would like to thank Drs. Winston Chee, Terry Donovan and George Cho, who believed in me and who provided me with the opportunity to complete my education in prosthodontics at the Herman Ostrow USC School of Dentistry. Thank you is not enough. I want you to know that I will be forever grateful and that opportunity changed my life.

Dr. Robert Schneider is also acknowledged, who opened doors and believed that one day I would realize my potential at a time I was being told otherwise. I learned that believing in yourself is important. Your voice is important, and your dreams are important, because there is one you and you are worth it. I learned that even if people stand in your way as an obstacle, you must find a way to overcome it.

I would like to acknowledge all the students and faculty involved with the Advanced Prosthodontics and Periodontics Program at Herman Ostrow USC School of Dentistry from whom I have learnt so much and continue to do so.

I would be remiss if I did not thank my team at Anacapa Dental Art Institute: Laura Castellanos RDA who has assisted me for the last 10 years and has been instrumental in implementing protocols we use on a day-to-day basis—she is someone who always works with a smile on her face and makes a complex day go very smoothly; Sonia Escamilla for her positive demeanour, amazing leadership and ability to bring the best out of people; Ale Prado for keeping everything light when the day gets tough and willingness to do whatever it takes; Maricel Estoque for her excellent patient management skills and warm and caring attitude towards everyone she meets; Erika Simental for her kindness and professionalism; Amber Padilla RDH who started the journey with me as my assistant and progressed to becoming a wonderful hygienist; and Darlene Herrera RDH who has assisted me in the maintenance of these patients and whose attention to detail is exceptional. I cannot forget Karina Gutierrez, Yomaly Gutierrez, Ashley Gutierrez, Vanessa Murillo, Nancy Lara, Griselda Barraza Adriana Perez, Elain Carrera, Chelsea Benavidez and Alexa Ayala. My whole team is amazing. They make coming into work each day enjoyable and always go the extra mile for our patients. Their dedication and commitment are second to none, and I want to let you know that I appreciate everything you do. Special thanks to Octavio Guerra who behind the scenes makes our practice better every day.

I would like to thank the team at Digital Dental Arts Laboratory in Ventura for their exceptional work ethic and the ability to get the job done: Artem Avanesov, Raffi Rshtuni and Yvette Mistajo. Without a great laboratory partner, we cannot do what we do for patients.

To My Patients

Thanks to my patients who make each day enjoyable for me. Thank you for allowing me to compile these clinical photographs. It is caring for these patients that makes my profession so rewarding and makes me look forward to the next day.

To God

Thanks to God who has made everything possible. His guidance has allowed me to pursue my dreams and realize them.

Fight On

Contents

1 Rationale for Dental Implants

Winston Chee and Saj Jivraj

1.1 Non-replacement of Missing Teeth

At about 18 years of age, we have a full complement of teeth; we have 32 teeth that make 16 opposing tooth units. More often than not, many of us have our third molars removed and consider 28 teeth to be accepted as the norm. As time passes by, we observe that the occlusal system does not remain stable, and physiological and pathologic changes take place. Teeth shift, teeth wear, caries and periodontal disease cause tooth loss.

A dogma that many dental textbooks and many teachings at dental schools purport is that a full complement of teeth is required to have a healthy masticatory system that will satisfy oral health and function. For those that peruse the literature, the evidence leans toward the concept that a full complement of teeth is not necessary.

DeVan stated, "Our objective should be the perpetual preservation of what remains rather than the meticulous restoration of what is missing" [1].

Ramfjord stated, "Satisfactory function and occlusion as well as neuromuscular stability usually can be established if all the anterior teeth and bicuspids are present and the diet of modern man does not require an intact dentition to meet functional demands" [2].

Waerhaug stated, "Since the construction or a bridge or denture may have deleterious effects on periodontal health, this view should be re-examined. It is suggested that many patients would be better off if bridges or partial dentures were not constructed" [3].

W. Chee (✉)
Advanced Prosthodontics, Herman Ostrow School of Dentistry, University of Southern California, Los Angeles, CA, USA

S. Jivraj
Private Practice, Anacapa Dental Art Institute, Oxnard, CA, USA

W. Chee, S. Jivraj (eds.), *Treatment Planning In Implant Dentistry*, BDJ Clinician's Guides, https://doi.org/10.1007/978-3-031-68726-6_1

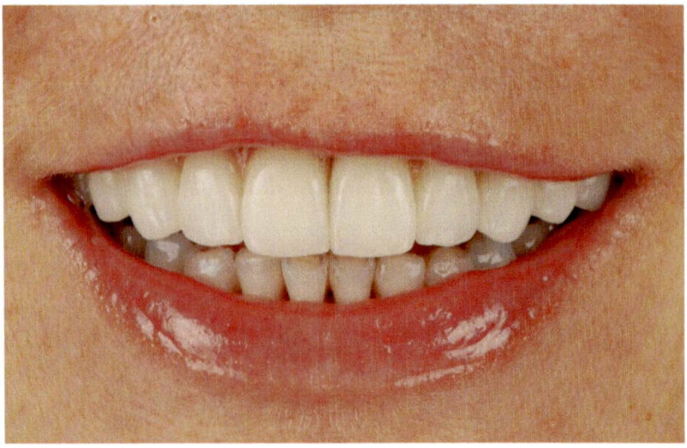

Fig. 1.1 Image of a patient with shortened dental arch; number of teeth is sufficient to fill buccal corridors and function adequately. (Figs. 1.1–1.4 courtesy of Dr. Sangho Byun)

In many cultures, the appearance of missing anterior teeth may not be acceptable and will demand replacement by patients to allow social interaction; more will be discussed with tooth replacement and aesthetics in this book (Chaps. 13 and 14). Patients with missing posterior teeth are less likely to ask for replacement but might be more motivated by clinicians to have them replaced (Chap. 12).

When suitable, our profession should offer the shortened dental arch (SDA) as an option for treatment. The shortened dental arch is a concept where most patients can function with fewer tooth pairs (opposing teeth) than full complements of teeth, with the SDA patients that can be satisfied with fewer teeth. It is our goal in dental care to ensure maintenance of a functional dentition throughout life. Having self-esteem, aesthetics, function and oral comfort would satisfy most patients; they may be satisfied with less than 14 occluding tooth pairs; limiting treatment goals may help to prolong dentitions [4–8] (Figs. 1.1, 1.2, 1.3 and 1.4).

1.2 Removable Prostheses

This section refers to removable prostheses without the use of dental implants. Removable prostheses do need to be provided when there are limitations due to finances for use of dental implants and when systemic health conditions preclude the use of dental implants.

Bite forces with complete dentures are about 20% of a dentate patient; this is largely due to pain on biting when mucosa is pinched between the denture base and underlying bone [9]. Other reasons that compromise function and comfort are instability, a gag reflex, xerostomia and psychological inability to accept removing the prostheses [9–12].

Even though there are patients who are satisfied with complete denture prostheses, these patients suffer continued bone loss over time. With age, changes that include a reduced saliva flow can cause poor retention and discomfort when using complete dentures. These factors can reduce satisfaction of the prostheses [13] (Figs. 1.5 and 1.6).

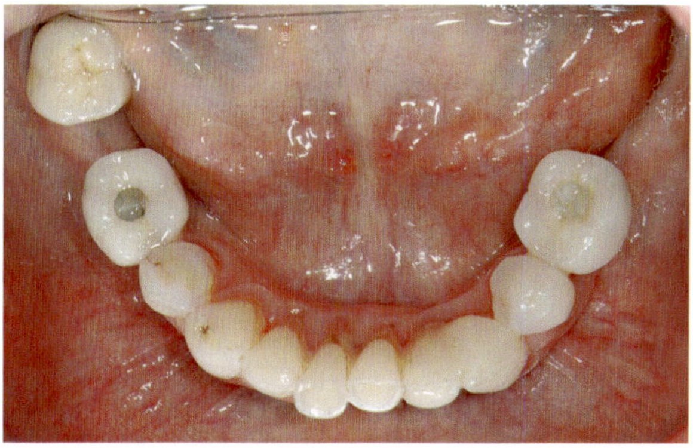

Fig. 1.2 Occlusal view of shortened dental arch maxilla with 10 units; all units are implant supported

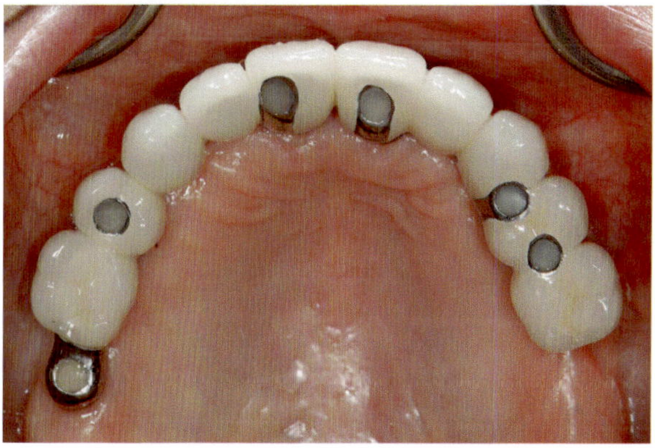

Fig. 1.3 Occlusal view of shortened dental arch mandible with 10 functional units; two distal units are implant supported

For patients who present with complete dentures, they should be introduced to the benefits of incorporating dental implants for their betterment. Patients who may present with a terminal dentition likewise should be presented with the option of dental implants [14]. With the use of complete dentures, stability of the prostheses can be compromised with bone resorption, reduced saliva flow and reduced neuromuscular control. In addition, pain and discomfort are also manifested due to occluding forces being directed to the oral mucosa as mucosa is not meant to support occlusal forces.

With placement of implants, several types of restorations for edentulous patients can be offered, overdentures that are implant retained and tissue supported, overdentures that are implant retained and supported and fixed prostheses supported by implants. These restorations will be described in more detail in other chapters (Chaps. 15 and 16). When implants are placed, they will prevent continued resorption of bone in proximity; they will add to stability and retention and provide support for the restorations (Fig. 1.7).

For removable partial dentures (RPDs), their indications should be considered with care; the use of RPDs has been shown to shift the ecology of the oral cavity toward decay and periodontal disease. Literature has been presented that clearly

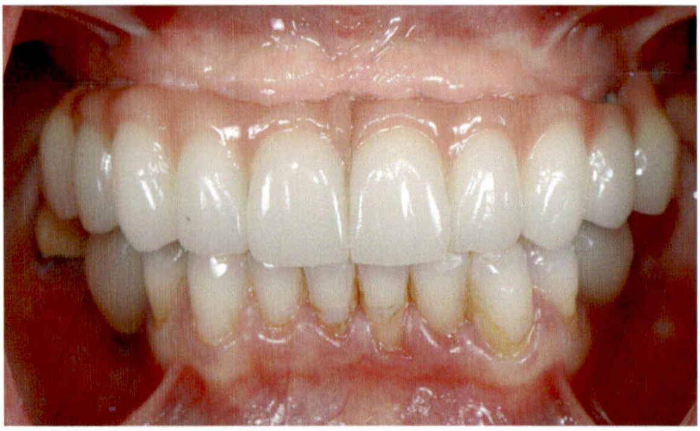

Fig. 1.4 Anterior view of both arches in occlusion

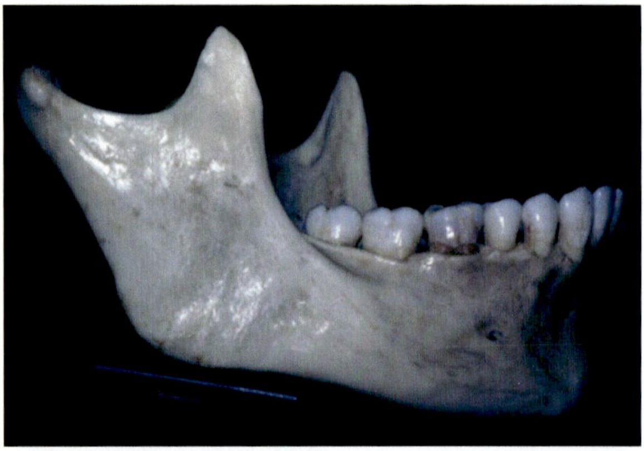

Fig. 1.5 Retained teeth preserve bone due to function

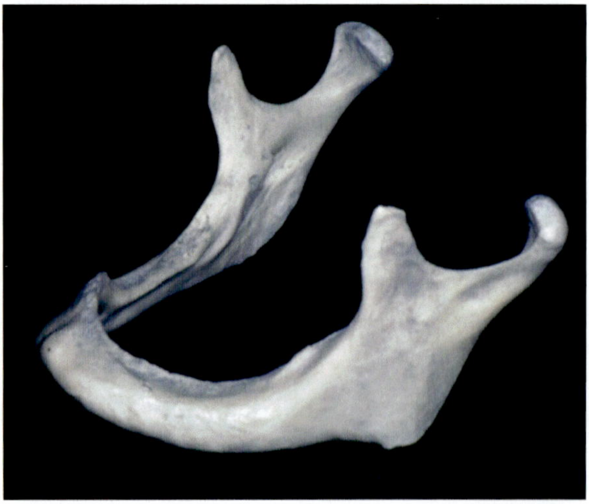

Fig. 1.6 Edentulous ridge with no stimulation to bone

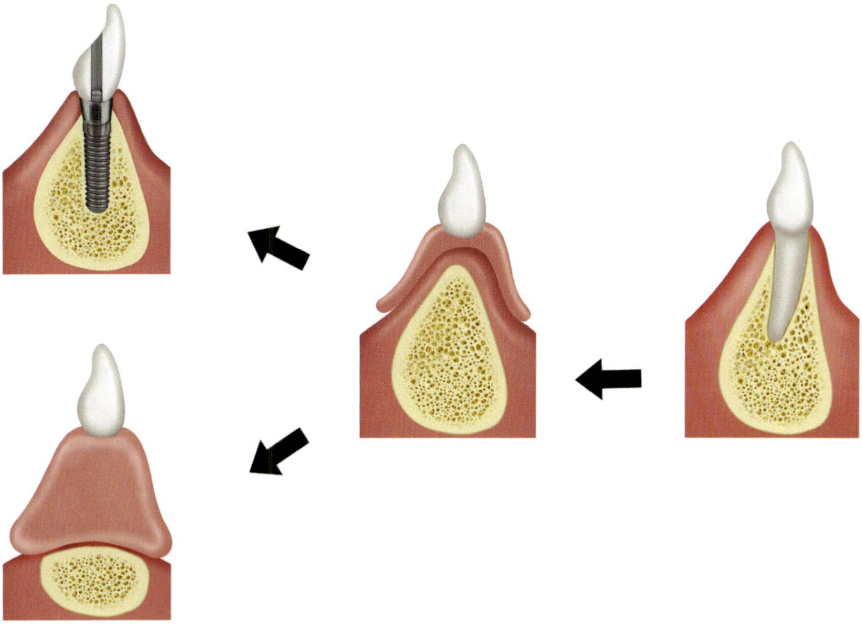

Fig. 1.7 Retention of bone with implant placed compared to the use of a removable prosthesis over time

demonstrates that teeth related to a partial denture develop decay more than teeth that are unrelated to the RPD [15]. Similarly, increased mobility and attachment loss occur at higher rates to teeth that are related to the removable prostheses [16]. With distal extension, RPD support for the missing teeth depends on mucosal support; lateral forces applied to the abutment teeth lead to forces that are detrimental to the abutment teeth [17]. In addition, in areas of mucosal support, the underlying bone is resorbed due to occlusal forces directed to the distal extension areas.

In addition, much of the dogma about clasp designs and altered cast impressions is not supported by the more current literature. For example, there are no differences to abutment tooth mobility with differing clasping assemblies though some design methods have been proposed in which they are able to prevent increased mobility to abutment teeth [18, 19]. Many studies indicate that the shortened dental arch can satisfy functional needs of many patients; avoiding the use of removable partial dentures would be a better option than using RPDs to replace missing posterior teeth [20–23]. When consulting with a patient, they should be informed that implant-supported restorations can replace distal extension partial dentures, and they can be told that a shortened dental arch can provide function without the use of an RPD but there can be some wear of the remaining teeth and shifting of the remaining teeth that can develop diastema. Alternatively, implant-supported restorations will be able to distribute forces to the dentition and will reduce any tooth migration.

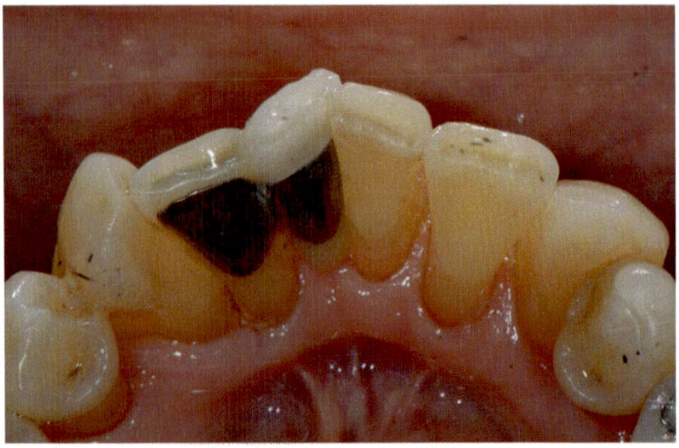

Fig. 1.8 Adhesive-bonded fixed partial denture with support by one abutment

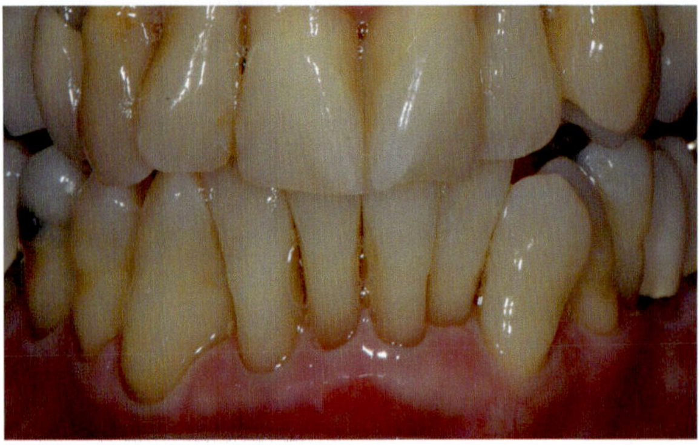

Fig. 1.9 Anterior view of restoration of mandibular right lateral incisor forces is minimal in this site

1.3 Fixed Partial Dentures Supported by Teeth

Adhesive-type fixed partial dentures are a category of fixed partial dentures where pontics are supported by being adhesively attached to abutment teeth; they can be indicated for use in short spans and are more efficacious in anterior teeth where less forces are applied. Survival rates after 10 years are reported to be about 89%, but many have been re-cemented at intervals, and additionally, chipping of ceramic layering occurs often over periods. Counter-intuitively, bonding to a single abutment will have fewer failures of bonding and will have longer periods of being attached compared to multiple abutment teeth [24, 25] (Figs. 1.8 and 1.9).

Conventional fixed partial dentures (FPDs) have been considered the standard of care prior to the advent of implant therapy. When preparing teeth to support pontics, a significant amount of tooth structure needs to be removed for an aesthetic outcome (Figs. 1.10, 1.11 and 1.12). This removal of tooth structure compromises the longevity of the tooth and can in some instances result in endodontic, periodontal and mechanical complications [26–29]. The long-term survival of fixed partial dentures has been reported to be 69% at 15 years and 46% at 20 years. Factors that predispose to failure included non-vital abutments and longer span prostheses [30–32]. The most common causes of failures are fracture of abutments and caries. With the

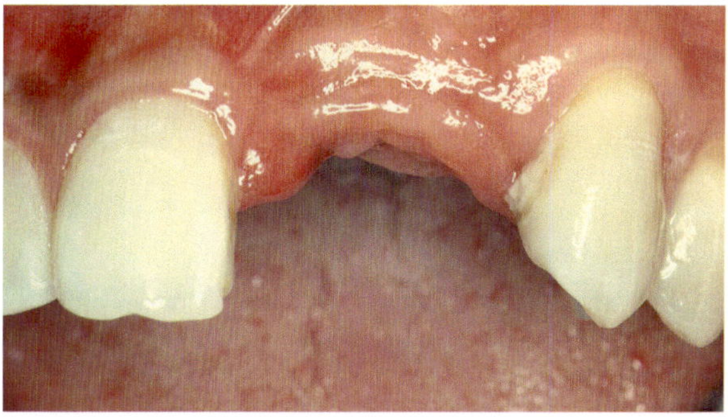

Fig. 1.10 Patient was using a removable partial denture; note the plaque accumulation; teeth are unrestored; before the advent of implants, these teeth were prepared

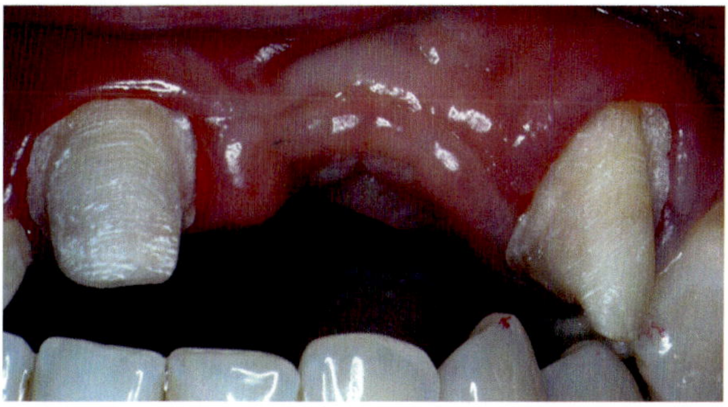

Fig. 1.11 A significant amount of healthy tooth structure was removed to accommodate the restoration

longer the span of an FPD, there is more difficulty to have abutments that do not fit as well due to distortions of materials—some materials used expand and some contract, leading to less precise fit causing cement wash-out and decay. Figures 1.13, 1.14 and 1.15 illustrate a fixed partial denture spanning #2–5 with #2 and #5 as abutments (maxillary right second molar to maxillary right #5 first premolar). The patient presents with the FPD displaced; intraorally, the images will show that the distal abutment #2 has been decemented for a period of time; the discoloration is visible, and some decay on the occlusal surface of the tooth preparation is evident; after this, decementation and mobility of the prosthesis cause the anterior abutment #5 to fracture.

1.4 Dental Implant Placement

It is required today that the use of dental implants is taught by all dental schools in North America; most of the schools incorporate patient treatment as part of the clinical experience for all pre-doctoral students. Several of the dental schools provide an opportunity for pre-doctoral students to place implants. In both aspects, restoration of implants and surgical placement of the implants will introduce the future dental professionals to the benefits and risks of providing dental implants.

In comparison to the other methods that have been described above, replacing teeth with osseointegrated implants is a significant advancement when replacing

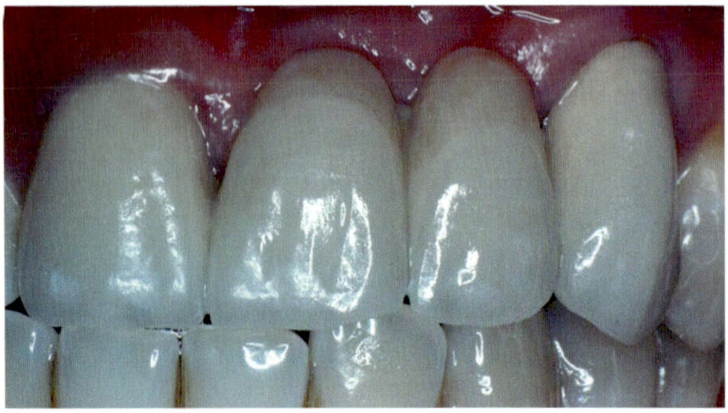

Fig. 1.12 A metal ceramic fixed partial denture restored the two missing teeth

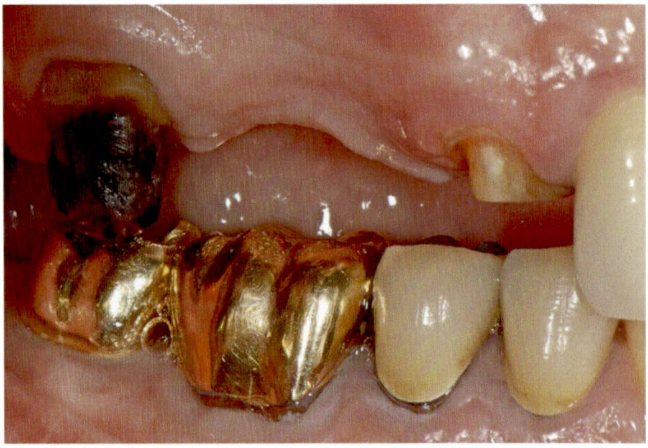

Fig. 1.13 Lateral view of fixed partial denture with fracture of anterior abutment and decay on posterior abutment due to cement wash-out

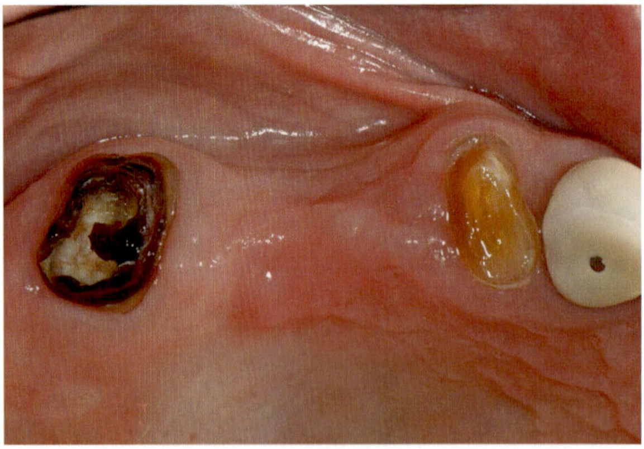

Fig. 1.14 Decay on posterior abutment is obvious likely because the posterior abutment became decemented, causing fracture of anterior abutment

missing teeth. Treatment planning is now quite different from the period prior to the widespread use of dental implants. There is quite a thirst for dentists to gain more knowledge about dental implants; the best venue for further enlightenment about dental implants would be with advanced programs within educational institutions that are accredited by the Commission on Dental Accreditation (CODA). Dental

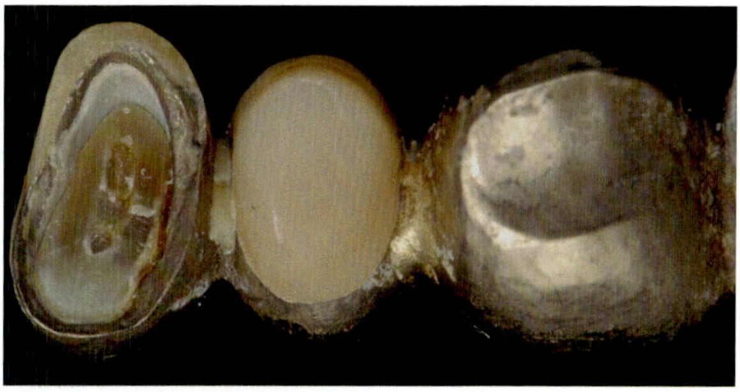

Fig. 1.15 Image of anterior abutment showing fractured anterior abutment; note that the cement is intact

organizations that tailor presentations for their members, continuing education venues and the like unfortunately are largely driven by dental implant manufacturers.

Compared to the other methods of replacing teeth, many more publications and studies have been presented and many more innovations have been made to simplify treatment modalities and improve the outcomes for patients.

Advantages of implants include:

1. Preservation of tooth structure
2. Preservation of bone surrounding integrated implants
3. Provision of support for restorations
4. No decay as there is no calcified tissue

1.5 Preservation of Tooth Structure

As described above, with fixed partial dentures (FPDs), significant amounts of tooth structure are removed to prepare abutment teeth (Figs. 1.10, 1.11 and 1.12). Restoration of missing teeth with dental implants will spare the removal of tooth structure of adjacent teeth. Removal of tooth structure weakens the abutment teeth further when longer span FPD abutments are prepared as the abutments need to accommodate the paths of insertion of the fixed partial denture abutments. Thus, more tooth structure needs to be removed; the added removal of tooth structure together with other factors has been reported to lead to about 6% of abutment teeth to require endodontic therapy [32–34].

Naert et al. reported a cumulative success rate of 96.5% over an 11-year period, and there are numerous other studies alluding to the longevity of single-unit implant restorations [35–38]. Single tooth implant survival has been demonstrated to be the most predictable method of tooth replacement. There have also been no reports of loss of adjacent teeth when single tooth implant restorations have been undertaken; this is vastly different compared to treatment rendered with an FPD.

Any procedure that reduces tooth structure weakens a tooth and shortens the lifespan of the tooth; this is a critical factor when making treatment decisions [26–29]. Using implants to replace missing teeth will preserve tooth structure unlike abutments that support FPDs. Implant-supported restorations in lieu of FPDs have

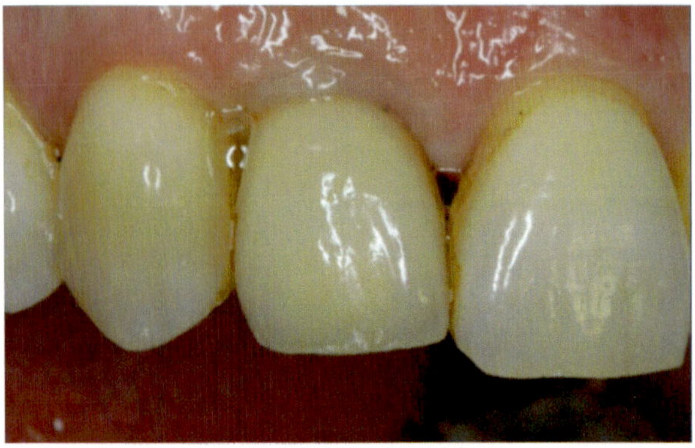

Fig. 1.16 Image of right lateral maxillary incisor restored with implant leaving both adjacent teeth unrestored

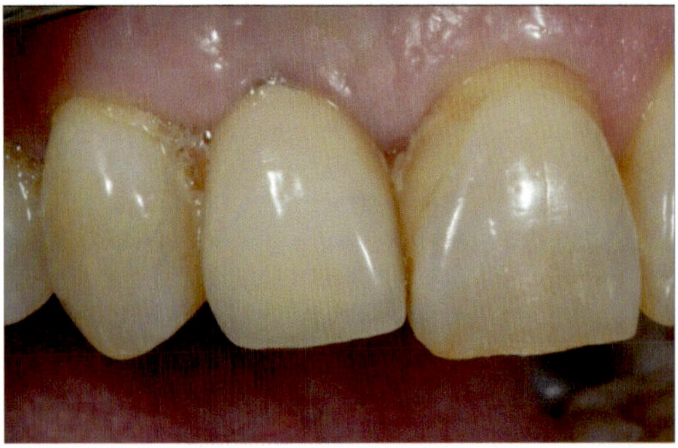

Fig. 1.17 Image of same tooth with some change in the mucosal margin of implant-supported restoration; adjacent teeth have discoloured over 28 years

been shown to have a good long-term success rate. Most importantly, the use of implants does not compromise the adjacent teeth, and additionally the implant will provide support of the restoration independent of the adjacent teeth (Figs. 1.16, 1.17 and 1.18).

1.6 Preservation of Bone Surrounding Integrated Implants

There is a close relationship between the tooth and the alveolar process throughout life. Tensional forces from the periodontal ligament preserve bone, and pressure causes resorption [39]. Similarly, function of muscle insertions into the retro-molar pad where tensional forces maintain the bone demonstrates this phenomenon. Bone requires tensional stimulation to maintain its form and density. When a tooth is lost, the lack of tension from the periodontal ligament removes stimulation to the residual bone causing a decrease in trabeculae and bone density in the area together with loss of the volume of bone in both dimensions of height and width. In a classical longitudinal study of edentulous patients by Tallgren using a radiographic method that demonstrated continued bone loss (Figs. 1.5 and 1.6), a fourfold greater bone loss was demonstrated in the maxilla compared to the mandible [40, 41].

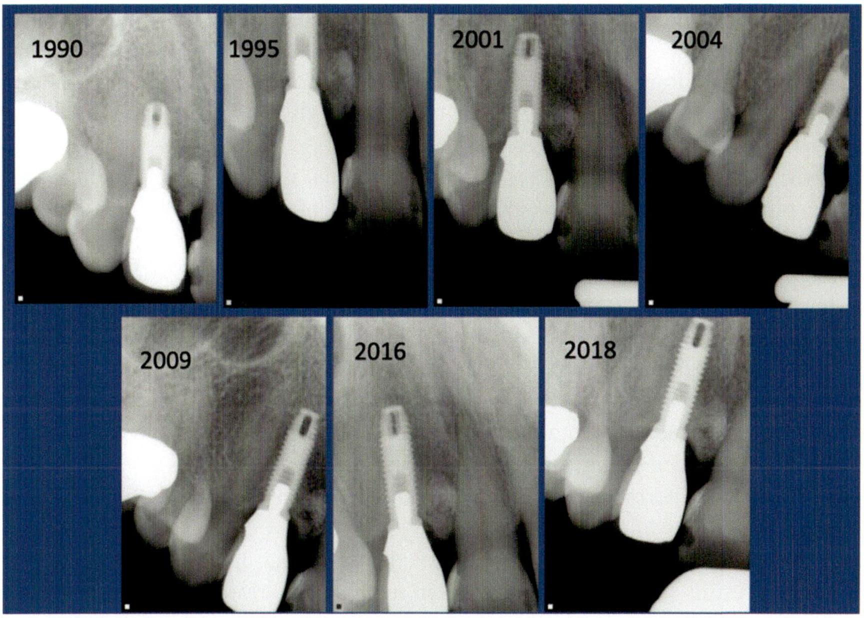

Fig. 1.18 Radiographs of implant-supported restoration in Figs. 1.16 and 1.17 demonstrating little bone loss around implant

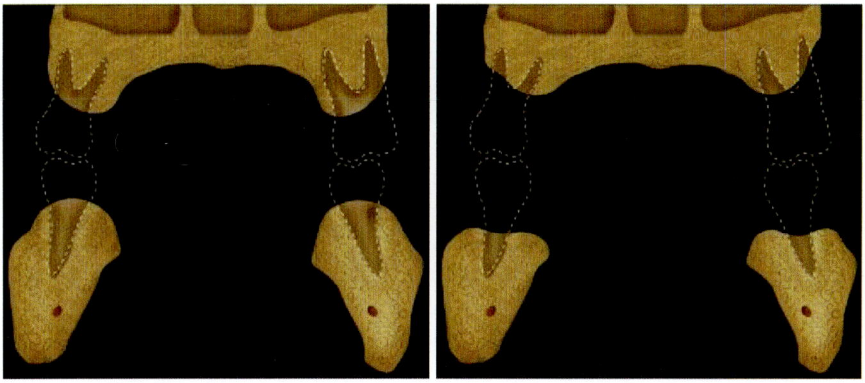

Figs. 1.19 and 1.20 Left diagram illustrating the direction of bone resorption when teeth are removed, right diagram illustrating longer term removal of teeth and a more severe change in the relationship of bone

In the edentulous patient, bone tends to resorb apically and medially in the maxilla and apically and laterally in the mandible. This often results in a jaw size discrepancy, which tends more toward a class III skeletal relationship. To respect this natural disproportion, teeth must be aligned differently with the maxillary molars being more facially positioned and the mandibular molars being more lingually positioned (Figs. 1.19 and 1.20). The literature concludes that periodontal attachment that provides a tensional force is required to maintain bone, and with loss of teeth, bone is no longer stimulated. In contradistinction, when using dentures that will cause pressure to supporting areas, these areas will resorb more quickly when pressure to the supporting mucosa is applied.

Over time with continuous resorption of the bone, it can be severe enough that sufficient bone may not be available for placement of implants. Most patients are unaware of the consequences of bone loss when teeth are removed; in addition, when they utilize removable prostheses that are supported by mucosa, the reduction of bone volume is exacerbated. Patients should be made aware and informed of the preventive nature of dental implants to bone loss. Dental implant-supported restorations will facilitate restoration of function and aesthetics and maintain the hard and soft tissues [42, 43].

With missing teeth or teeth to be extracted, the compromised state can affect a patient's overall well-being and quality of life. Restoring a patient's stomatognathic system to a more normal function may enhance their masticatory performance and improve the quality of their lives [44].

Transitioning a patient from a complete denture to an implant-supported fixed prosthesis results in a dramatic increase in maximal bite force. Complete denture patients are unable to exert equivalent forces due to pain when soft tissue is compressed between the denture base and underlying bone [45]. The patient with an implant-supported fixed prosthesis can exert an almost similar force to that of a patient with fixed restorations on teeth. The improved stability and retention of an implant-supported prosthesis are a vast improvement on soft tissue-supported dentures [46].

With patients who are missing posterior teeth and present with one or more signs of lack of posterior support, signs may include but are not limited to wear, splaying and fremitus of the anterior teeth. Traditionally, these restorative problems were addressed by splinting the anterior teeth and provision of a tooth- and mucosa-supported Kennedy class 1, removable partial denture. The function of the partial denture was to provide increased chewing surface and re-establish posterior support. Monteith reported that there is a marked difference in the viscoelastic response to loading of teeth and mucosa. The marked disparity between the 500 micron resilience of the residual ridge tissues and the 20 microns of teeth brings to light the questionable nature of providing posterior support with removable partial dentures [47]. Tooth- and mucosa-supported partial dentures cannot re-establish posterior support in the long term due to the resilient and like effect of the mucosa [48]. One additional advantage of implant-supported restorations is retrievability. Implant-supported restorations should be screw retained rather than cemented. Screw retention and its benefits will be described in more detail in a separate chapter (Chap. 3).

1.7 Resistance to Disease

The most common causes of tooth loss are caries and periodontal disease; when either of the disease processes causes teeth to be lost, implant-supported restorations are often the best choice to replace the lost tooth when necessary. There is however a differing consideration of treatment planning implants in the two main categories of tooth loss.

1.7.1 Tooth Loss Due to Decay

Four factors lead to tooth decay: bacteria, fermentable carbohydrates, susceptible tooth surfaces and time—ultimately, it is acid in contact with calcified tissues which causes the outcome that we know as tooth decay. Should a tooth be lost to severe decay and a replacement of the tooth with an implant-supported restoration, there will be no further calcified tissues to attack on the replaced tooth. Thus, implants and restorations will be the best replacement of a missing tooth or teeth for all the reasons discussed above.

In addition, when a risk-to-benefit analysis is used, clinicians should lean toward placing implants should multiple interventions such as endodontic treatment, crown lengthening, and post and core are needed to facilitate restoration; also as mentioned above, removal of tooth structure further weakens the tooth.

1.7.2 Tooth Loss Due to Periodontitis

The aetiology of periodontitis is generally caused by a susceptible host, one that has an exuberant response to insult such as bacteria; this strong inflammatory response can lead to attachment loss [49] (Chaps. 10 and 19).

With almost any population, there is a distribution of susceptibility to disease; for periodontitis, there is also a "bell-shaped curve" of a population. There will be those who are resistant and those who are susceptible to periodontitis. Those susceptible to periodontitis have their condition exacerbated by poor home care, smoking, diabetes, immune deficiencies and many other factors. These exacerbating factors will shift a subject toward suffering a more severe periodontitis.

Here is where decision-making plays a role with respect to using dental implants; with tooth loss due to caries, the substrate for decay is removed and dental implants are predictably integrated to bone and have a survival rate in the long term above 90% [50–52]. For teeth loss due to periodontitis, the host is still susceptible to peri-implant inflammation, and this population of patients are on the more vulnerable side of the "bell-shaped curve". It is well documented that these patients are similarly susceptible to peri-implant bone loss (peri-implantitis). It has also been reported that peri-implantitis causes more rapid bone loss than bone loss around teeth with periodontitis [53–55].

There is not a definitive protocol for treating progressing peri-implant bone loss; some have described resection of bone to facilitate cleanability of the peri-implant area to be effective in preventing the progress of peri-implant bone loss; the consequence of resection is exposure of the implant components that are severely disfiguring in visible areas. Treatment of teeth with attachment loss is much more predictable, and exposure of the root is much less disfiguring than exposure of implant components. When considering the risk-to-benefit analysis, more effort should be spent on treating periodontitis and preventing further attachment loss (Chaps. 10 and 19).

Examples of situations when implants are indicated for use are when patients with periodontitis are in functional discomfort, when periodontal lesions are exuding purulence and suffer recalcitrant periodontitis, when teeth exhibit class III mobility and can be depressed, when teeth have shifted significantly and when patients want to improve their aesthetics. Patients should be informed of how their susceptibility to periodontitis will also have susceptibility to peri-implantitis; consequently, their levels of home care and professional care need to increase. Peri-implantitis seems to progress more quickly than periodontitis due to a lack of attachment; implant is ankylosed to bone with no attachment apparatus as teeth have. Implants can be successfully delivered to patients with a history of peri-implantitis, but meticulous hygiene will be required for long-term success [56].

1.8 Summary

In the long past, loss of teeth, eventual edentulism and wearing of complete or partial dentures have been part of the expected course of ageing of the general population. Although patients may adapt well to both a complete and partial denture, the decrease in masticatory function in comparison to a patient with a natural dentition has been well documented. Use of a removable prosthesis results in progressive bone resorption in the denture bearing areas where bone resorption is accelerated. This bone loss leads to less support and stability for removable prostheses and in addition may reduce the opportunity for placement of implants.

When fixed restorations supported by teeth are provided, the abutments are compromised with tooth structure being removed to accommodate full coverage restorations, and a high percentage of them require endodontic treatment when pulps are compromised. Studies have demonstrated that decay and fracture of endodontically treated teeth are primary causes of failure for fixed partial dentures. Further, failures occur more rapidly with longer span fixed partial dentures.

Implant-supported restorations help to return patients to good oral function in a predictable manner; adjacent teeth are not compromised as the implant-supported restorations do not depend on adjacent teeth for support. Teeth that are not restored are teeth that will have the best longevity and that factor alone should help to maintain oral health. Implant-supported restorations indicated and delivered with proper diagnosis and treatment planning allow clinicians to deliver the most long-lasting support for prostheses. The implant body has been scrupulously studied and has been reported as the most durable prosthesis that health care can provide. We are not only able to provide support for restorations but also allowed with proper planning to provide functional and aesthetic restorations that are supported by the implants; these restorations are easily repaired or replaced when needed; newer materials are methods that will grant our profession the tools to achieve the goal of returning the patient to oral health, function and aesthetics predictably. The chapters in this book will describe treatment choices and procedures in further detail. Implant-supported prostheses offer a more predictable solution than traditional removable restorations. The many advantages passed on to the patient by use of implant-supported restorations allow a patient to function with confidence and enjoy a better quality of life.

References

1. DeVan MM. The nature of the partial denture foundation: suggestions for its preservation. J Prosthet Dent. 1952;2(2):210–8.
2. Ramfjord SP. Periodontal aspects of restorative dentistry. J Oral Rehabil. 1974;1(2):107–26.
3. Waerhaug J, Philos D. Periodontology and partial prosthesis. Int Dent J. 1968;18(1):101–7.
4. Käyser AF. Limited treatment goals—shortened dental arches. Periodontology. 2000;1994(4):7–14.
5. Wolfart S, et al. The randomized shortened dental arch study: influence of two different treatments on interdental spacing over 5 years. Clin Oral Investig. 2016;21:1945. https://doi.org/10.1007/s00784-016-1981-2.
6. Witter DJ, de Haan AF, Käyser AF, Van Rossum GM. A 6-year follow-up study of oral function in shortened dental arches. Part II: Craniomandibular dysfunction and oral comfort. J Oral Rehabil. 1994;21:353–66.
7. Witter DJ, de Haan AF, Käyser AF, Rossum GMV. A 6-year follow-up study of oral function in shortened dental arches. Part I: Occlusal stability. J Oral Rehabil. 1994;21:113–25.
8. Witter DJ, van Palenstein Helderman WH, Creugers NH, Käyser AF. The shortened dental arch concept and its implications for oral health care. Community Dent Oral Epidemiol. 1999;27:249–58.
9. Haraldson T, et al. Bite force and oral function in complete denture wearers. J Oral Rehabil. 1979;6(1):41–8.
10. Conny DJ, Tedesco LA. The gagging problem in prosthodontic treatment. Part II: Patient management. J Prosthet Dent. 1983;49(6):757–61.
11. Turner M, et al. Hyposalivation, xerostomia and the complete denture: a systematic review. J Am Dent Assoc (1939). 2008;139(2):146–50.
12. Papadaki E, Anastassiadou V. Elderly complete denture wearers: a social approach to tooth loss. Gerodontology. 2012;29(2):e721–7.
13. Kelsey CC. Alveolar bone resorption under complete dentures. J Prosthet Dent. 1971;25(3):152–61.
14. Pham NQ, et al. Average rate of ridge resorption in denture treatment: a systematic review. J Prosthodont Res. 2021;65(4):429–37.
15. Carlsson GE, et al. Studies in partial dental prosthesis. IV. Final results of a 4-year longitudinal investigation of dentogingivally supported partial dentures. Acta Odontol Scand. 1965;23(5):443–72.
16. Zlatarić DK, et al. The effect of removable partial dentures on periodontal health of abutment and non-abutment teeth. J Periodontol. 2002;73(2):137–44.
17. Tebrock OC, et al. The effect of various clasping systems on the mobility of abutment teeth for distal-extension removable partial dentures. J Prosthet Dent. 1979;41(5):511–6.

18. Kapur KK, et al. A randomized clinical trial of two basic removable partial denture designs. Part I: Comparisons of 5-year success rates and periodontal health. J Prosthet Dent. 1994;72(3):268–82.
19. Kapur KK, et al. A randomized clinical trial of two basic removable partial denture designs. Part II: Comparisons of masticatory scores. J Prosthet Dent. 1997;78(1):15–21. https://doi.org/10.1016/s0022-3913(97)70082-9.
20. Witter DJ, et al. The shortened dental arch concept and its implications for oral health care. Community Dent Oral Epidemiol. 1999;27(4):249–58.
21. Olley RC, Renton T, Frost PM. Observational study investigating tooth extraction and the shortened dental arch approach. J Oral Rehabil. 2017;44:610–6.
22. Armellini DB, Heydecke G, Witter DJ, Creugers NHJ. Effect of removable partial dentures on oral health-related quality of life in subjects with shortened dental arches: a 2-center cross-sectional study. Int J Prosthodont. 2008;21:524–30.
23. Armellini DB, et al. Effect of removable partial dentures on oral health-related quality of life in subjects with shortened dental arches: a 2-center cross-sectional study. Int J Prosthodont. 2008;21(6):524–30.
24. Thoma DS, Sailer I, Ioannidis A, Zwahlen M, Makarov N, Pjetursson BE. A systematic review of the survival and complication rates of resin-bonded fixed dental prostheses after a mean observation period of at least 5 years. Clin Oral Implants Res. 2017;28(11):1421–32.
25. Tanoue N, et al. Longevity of resin-bonded fixed partial dentures made of metal alloys: a review of the literature. J Prosthodont Res. 2021;65(3):267–72.
26. Edelhoff D, Sorensen JA. Tooth structure removal associated with various preparation designs for anterior teeth. J Prosthet Dent. 2002;87(5):503–9. https://doi.org/10.1067/mpr.2002.124094.
27. Edelhoff D, Sorensen JA. Tooth structure removal associated with various preparation designs for posterior teeth. Int J Periodontics Restor Dent. 2002;22(3):241–9.
28. Al-Fouzan A, Tashkandi E. Volumetric measurements of removed tooth structure associated with various preparation designs. Int J Prosthodont. 2013;26:545–8.
29. Reeh ES, et al. Reduction in tooth stiffness as a result of endodontic and restorative procedures. J Endod. 1989;15(11):512–6.
30. Creugers NHJ, Käyser AF, Hof MA. A meta-analysis of durability data on conventional fixed bridges. Community Dent Oral. 1994;22:448–52.
31. Glantz P-OJ, et al. Quality of fixed prosthodontics after 22 years. Acta Odontol Scand. 2002;60(4):213–8.
32. Lockard MW. A retrospective study of pulpal response in vital adult teeth prepared for complete coverage restorations at ultrahigh speed using only air coolant. J Prosthet Dent. 2002;88(5):473–8. https://doi.org/10.1067/mpr.2002.129380.
33. Mjör IA, Odont D. Pulp-dentin biology in restorative dentistry. Part 2: initial reactions to preparation of teeth for restorative procedures. Quintessence Int. 2001;32(7):537–51.
34. Murray PE, et al. Preserving the vital pulp in operative dentistry: 2. Guidelines for successful restoration of unexposed dentinal lesions. Dent Update. 2002;29(3):127–34.
35. Naert I, et al. Biologic outcome of single-implant restorations as tooth replacements: a long-term follow-up study. Clin Implant Dent Relat Res. 2000;2(4):209–18.
36. Schmitt A, Zarb GA. The longitudinal clinical effectiveness of osseointegrated dental implants for single-tooth replacement. Int J Prosthodont. 1993;6(2):197–202.
37. Haas R, et al. A long-term follow-up of 76 Bränemark single-tooth implants. Clin Oral Implants Res. 2002;13(1):38–43.
38. Henry PJ, et al. Osseointegrated implants for single-tooth replacement: a prospective 5-year multicenter study. Int J Oral Maxillofac Implants. 1996;11(4):450–5.
39. Van der Weijden F, Dell'Acqua F, Slot DE. Alveolar bone dimensional changes of post-extraction sockets in humans: a systematic review. J Clin Periodontol. 2009;36(12):1048–58.
40. Tallgren A, Lang BR, Walker GF, Ash MM Jr. Roentgen cephalometric analysis of ridge resorption and changes in jaw and occlusal relationships in immediate complete denture wearers. J Oral Rehabil. 1980;7(1):77–94.

41. Tallgren A. The reduction in face height of edentulous and partially edentulous subjects during long-term denture wear. A longitudinal roentgenographic cephalometric study. Acta Odontol Scand. 1966;24(2):195–239.
42. Carr AB, Laney WR. Maximum occlusal force levels in patients with osseointegrated oral implant prostheses and patients with complete dentures. Int J Oral Maxillofac Implants. 1987;2(2):101–8.
43. Rissin L, House JE, Manly RS, Kapur KK. Clinical comparison of masticatory performance and electromyographic activity of patients with complete dentures, overdentures, and natural teeth. J Prosthet Dent. 1978;39(5):508–11.
44. van de Rijt LJM, Stoop CC, Weijenberg RAF, de Vries R, Feast AR, Sampson EL, Lobbezoo F. The influence of oral health factors on the quality of life in older people: a systematic review. Gerontologist. 2020;60(5):e378–94.
45. Haraldson T, Karlsson U, Carlsson GE. Bite force and oral function in complete denture wearers. J Oral Rehabil. 1979;6(1):41–8.
46. Haraldson T, Carlsson GE. Bite force and oral function in patients with osseointegrated oral implants. Scand J Dent Res. 1977;85(3):200–8.
47. Monteith BD. Management of loading forces on mandibular distal-extension prostheses. Part I: Evaluation of concepts for design. J Prosthet Dent. 1984;52(5):673–81.
48. Tauchi Y, Yang TC, Maeda Y. Distribution of forces in distal-extension removable partial dentures with and without retromolar pad coverage: a pilot in vivo study. Int J Prosthodont. 2015;28(4):386–8. https://doi.org/10.11607/ijp.4239. PMID: 26218022.
49. Kwon T, Lamster IB, Levin L. Current concepts in the management of periodontitis. Int Dent J. 2021;71(6):462–76.
50. Jemt T. Implant survival in the posterior partially edentulous arch-30 years of experience. Part IV: A retro-prospective multivariable regression analysis on implant failures related to arch and implant surface. Int J Prosthodont. 2019;32(2):143–52.
51. Balshi TJ, et al. A long-term retrospective analysis of survival rates of implants in the mandible. Int J Oral Maxillofac Implants. 2015;30(6):1348–54. https://doi.org/10.11607/jomi.3910.
52. Jemt T, Johansson J. Implant treatment in the edentulous maxillae: a 15 year follow-up study on 76 consecutive patients provided with fixed prostheses. Clin Implant Dent Relat Res. 2006;8(2):61–9.
53. Roos-Jansåker AM, Lindahl C, Renvert H, Renvert S. Nine- to fourteen-year follow-up of implant treatment. Part I: implant loss and associations to various factors. J Clin Periodontol. 2006;33(4):283–9.
54. Roos-Jansåker AM, Renvert H, Lindahl C, Renvert S. Nine- to fourteen-year follow-up of implant treatment. Part III: factors associated with peri-implant lesions. J Clin Periodontol. 2006;33(4):296–301.
55. Heitz-Mayfield LJ, Lang NP. Comparative biology of chronic and aggressive periodontitis vs. peri-implantitis. Periodontology 2000. 2010;53:167–81.
56. Karoussis IK, Müller S, Salvi GE, Heitz-Mayfield LJ, Brägger U, Lang NP. Association between periodontal and peri-implant conditions: a 10-year prospective study. Clin Oral Implants Res. 2004;15(1):1–7.

2 Clinical Biomechanics for Implant Prosthodontics

Saj Jivraj and Winston Chee

2.1 Literature Review

A key determinant in prosthetic and biological complications of dental implants is the way mechanical stresses are transferred to the existing prosthesis and to the surrounding bone. The primary functional design objective is to manage the loads and to optimize the implant-supported prosthesis in function. Excessive loads on an osseointegrated implants may result in screw loosening and mobility of the prosthesis. If unnoticed, this may contribute to the fracture of implant prosthetic components, and in some instances the implant body.

The study of implant biomechanics is not an exact science. Numerous models have been created to predict loads and outcomes. These include but are not limited to the following:

(a) Mathematical models—which are theoretical.
(b) Finite element models—these models do have some limitations when it comes to living organic tissue. Assumptions about the physical properties of bone must be made, along with assumptions on the amount of bone-to-implant contact. This is impossible to model as every person has different bone densities and bone-to-implant contact with dental implants. Extrapolation from such literature is questionable.
(c) Strain gauge analyses.

Transferring these models to a biological setting is not exact but may serve as a starting point for further investigation.

S. Jivraj (✉)
Private Practice, Anacapa Dental Art Institute, Oxnard, CA, USA

W. Chee
Advanced Prosthodontics, Herman Ostrow School of Dentistry, University of Southern California, Los Angeles, CA, USA

W. Chee, S. Jivraj (eds.), *Treatment Planning In Implant Dentistry*, BDJ Clinician's Guides, https://doi.org/10.1007/978-3-031-68726-6_2

Due to the difficulty in scientific investigation, there is limited evidence to support a direct cause-effect relationship between adverse biomechanical design and biological complications with dental implants.

In treatment planning, a profound understanding of implant biomechanics is required that will impact the clinical outcome of a restoration.

The following subjects will be addressed, and clinical implications discussed.

1. **Differences between teeth and dental implants**
2. **Implant moment arms/forces on implants**
3. **Implant body design and connection**
4. **Screw mechanics**
5. **Axial vs. tilted implants**
6. **Cantilevers and anteroposterior spread**
7. **Crown/implant ratio**
8. **Misfit**
9. **Number of implants**
10. **Splinting vs. non-splinting**
11. **Material selection**
12. **Recommendations in treatment planning**

2.2 Differences Between Teeth and Dental Implants (Fig. 2.1)

Dental implants typically assume a high survival rate and have been a superior treatment option in the replacement of missing or hopeless teeth. If the biomechanics of the implant/prosthodontic complex is not understood, several complications can likely occur which may jeopardize longevity.

There are anatomical differences between teeth and dental implants which influence diagnosis, treatment planning and delivery of restorations [1–5].

The differences between teeth and implants include but are not limited to:

(a) Periodontal sulcus vs. peri-implant sulcus
(b) Periodontal attachment vs. peri-implant attachment
(c) Proprioception vs. osseoperception
(d) Healing response of tissue
(e) Tooth root vs. implant body

The specific difference that is pertinent to implant biomechanics is the attachment mechanism and how the complex responds to load. A periodontal ligament transfers loads to the bone through micromovement. The presence of mobility allows dissipation of loads. The pain reflex during overloading of teeth limits the loading capacity and provides a protective mechanism that guards against overload and possible breakdown. Tooth overload may result in wear, fracture and drifting. This varies from individual to individual.

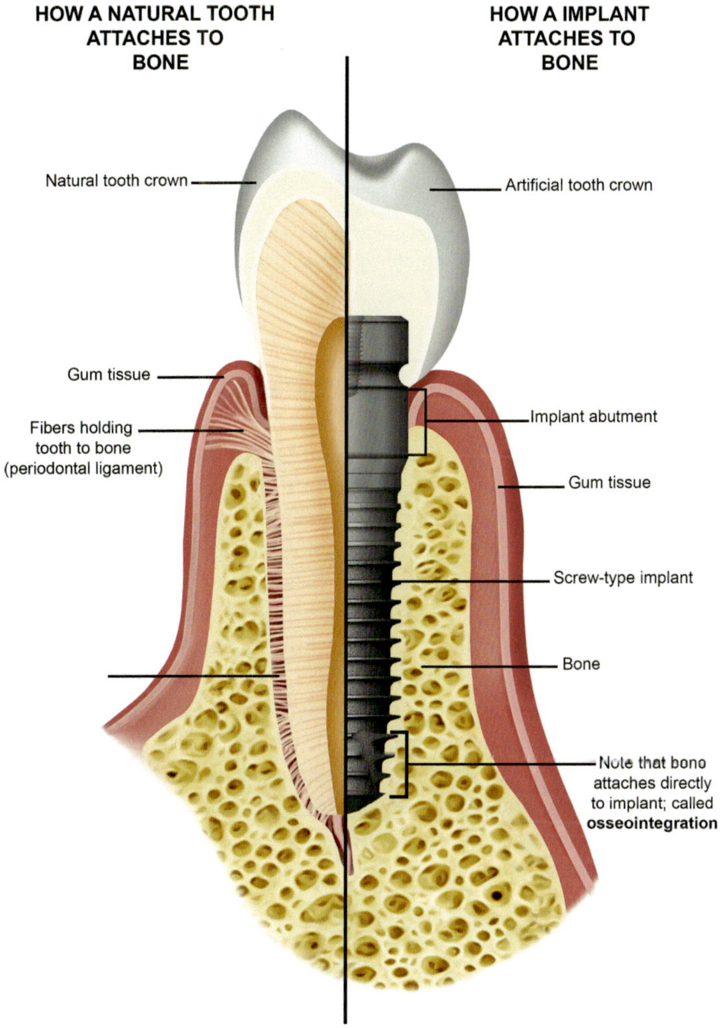

Fig. 2.1 Diagram illustrating differences between a tooth and an implant

With dental implants, there is a rigid almost ankylotic connection. Occlusal loads are transferred directly to the bone. The flexibility within the components of an implant/prosthodontic complex may dampen some of these loads. Due to the rigid connection, dental implants are more likely to have mechanical complications such as prosthetic screw loosening, screw fracture, fracture of components, fracture of the restoration and in extreme situations fracture of the implant body itself [6].

Biomechanical differences between implants and teeth [7]

Teeth	Implants
Has a periodontal ligament attachment	Ankylotic connection to bone
Flexible connection	Stiff connection
Stress distributed to surrounding bone	Stress distributed to crestal bone
Proprioception in the region of 20 microns	Osseoperception in the region of 48–64 microns
Apical intrusion 28 microns	Apical movement 10 microns
Lateral movement 50–108 microns	Negligible lateral movement

2.3 Implant Moment Arms and Forces on Implants

The magnitude of forces applied to an implant is based on the anatomical region, age, gender and state of the dentition. Misch, in 1980, described that the magnitude of bite force is greater in the molar region (200 lb.), decreases in the canine area (100 lb.) and is the least in the anterior incisor region (25–35 lb.). Occlusal forces can increase up to 1000 lb. in the presence of parafunctional habits such as bruxism, clenching and tongue thrusting [8]. These parafunctional habits increase the duration of bite forces that exceed the endurance limit of the implant components and can lead to screw loosening or fatigue failure.

The clinician should be aware that six moments (rotations) may develop around three clinical coordinate axes (occluso-apical, labiolingual and mesiodistal axes). Such loads may induce micro-rotations and stress at the crest of the ridge. These loads become more complex in nature depending on the opposing occlusion and whether the implant restorations are splinted (Fig. 2.2). Three clinical moment arms bear significance in implant dentistry:

(a) Occlusal height
(b) Cantilever length
(c) Occlusal width

There is minimal scientific evidence to support a direct cause-effect relationship between the above factors and complications in implant/prosthodontics. Concepts have been developed through a combination of dogma, expert opinion, in vitro studies, animal studies and extrapolation of concepts used for natural teeth. The astute clinician should exercise biomechanical caution when designing restorations on implants.

Author recommendations would be to analyse the following factors and ask the following questions:

1. Is it a high- or a low-function patient?
2. What is the nature of the opposing dentition? Natural, denture or implant supported?

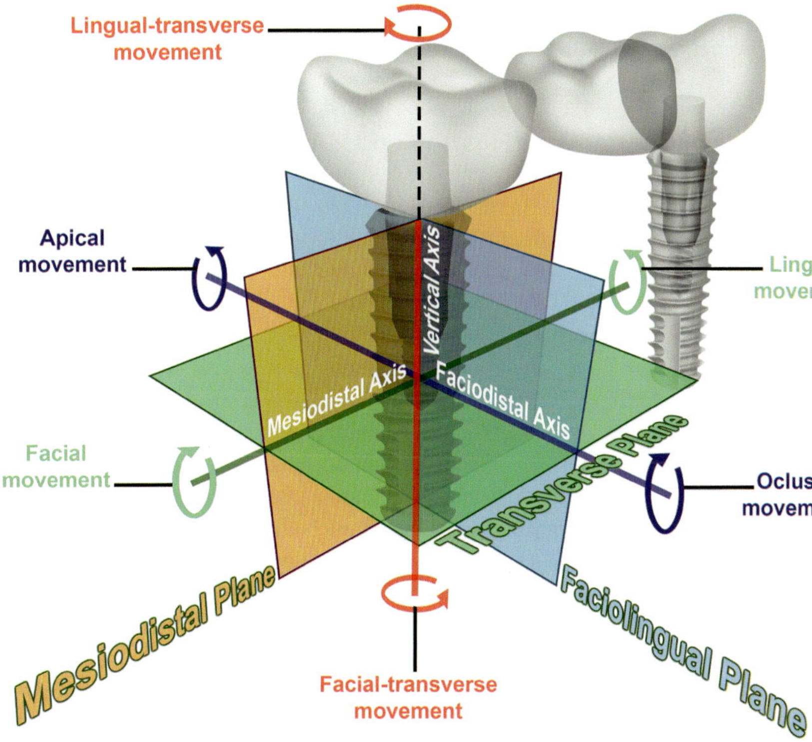

Fig. 2.2 Moment arms around implants

3. How many teeth does the patient have, and do they provide support for the occlusion?
4. Where in the mouth is the tooth located? Greater forces are exerted on posterior teeth.

2.4 Implant Body Design

An understanding of implant body design is critical in choosing an implant system. Dental implants are available in different materials, body shapes, diameters, lengths, platforms, surface properties and coatings. In particular, the area of implant surface modifications and coatings has been subjected to aggressive marketing aimed at establishing the superiority of a given surface over the others. The choice of system should not be based upon a manufacturer's advertising, or anecdotal presentations of individual cases by a clinician, but on sound clinical judgment available from the existing clinical and laboratory data.

This section will be divided into

(A) Type of connection—external vs. internal

(B) Platform switching—flat vs. conical interface
(C) Hex geometry and platform diameter

2.4.1 Type of Connection (Figs. 2.3 and 2.4)

One of the features that have been the subject of debate amongst the systems is the design of the connection that allows the prosthetic superstructures to be attached to the implants.

2.4.1.1 External Connections

The Branemark system was characterized by an external hexagon, which was developed to facilitate implant insertion. This external hexagon configuration has served well over the years, and it has been incorporated in several competing systems. However, it has some drawbacks due to its limited height and, therefore, limited effectiveness when subjected to off-axis loads. It has been postulated that, under high occlusal loads, the external hexagon might allow for micromovements of the abutment, thus causing instability of the joint, which may result in abutment screw loosening or even fatigue fracture. Eccentric lateral forces can cause more separation displacement at the implant/abutment junction than do forces down the long axis of the implant and not forces down the long axis when centric forces are applied. This is in reference to a single standing implant. When implants are splinted, forces applied will more often be directed axially to the splinted implants and reduce the forces on the retaining screws.

2.4.1.2 Internal Connections

It has been shown that internal implant/abutment connections demonstrate higher resistance to bending and improved force distribution over external configurations because of their ability to dissipate lateral loads deeply within the implant and to resist joint opening due to the deep and rigid connection which creates a unified

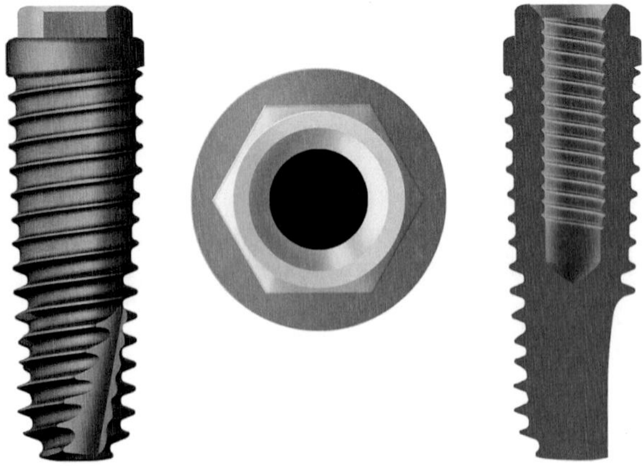

Fig. 2.3 External connection

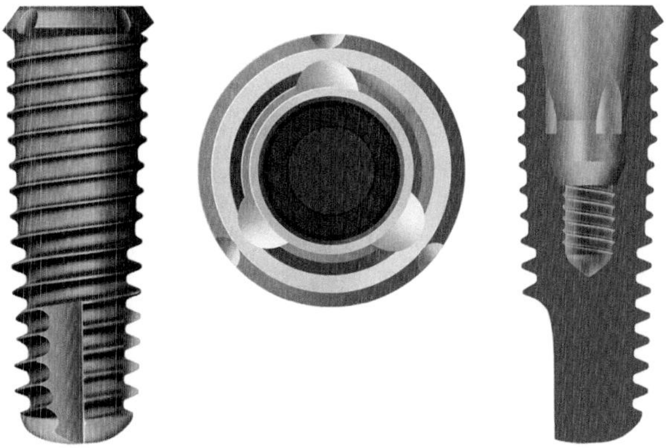

Fig. 2.4 Internal connection

body, thus displaying a more favourable load distribution in the connection area [8]. The incorporation of a conical abutment design optimized the ability of an implant-to-abutment joint to resist bending force. The internal conical implant/abutment joint has shown fatigue resistance superior to the hex-mediated butt joint. The stress dispersion over the joint interface may be the reason for the high resistance to repeated lateral loading. The reader should be aware that this advantage is applicable in single-unit restorations and does not apply to multiple splinted units with an internal connection. In multiple splinted units, engagement to the internal walls of the implant is absent.

2.4.1.3 Comparison Between External and Internal Connections

Accuracy of Impressions

A systematic review by Gracis et al. [9] compared internal and external connections in the area of accuracy of implant-level impressions and the incidence of technical complications. The results were inconclusive as no study directly compared impressions with internal vs. external hex connections. It should be noted that impression making of multiple implants with an internal connection differs in many aspects from that of implants with an external connection. Some internal connection configurations have an intimate fit with the respective impression copings, which may make withdrawal of the impression more difficult and, therefore, may generate a higher degree of distortion. Furthermore, external connection implants can accommodate a larger degree of divergence than internal connection systems due to the insertion of the impression copings into the internal connection implants.

Incidence of Screw Loosening

Screw loosening usually has a causative factor. The most common causes include but are not limited to:

(a) Excessive occlusal load
(b) Misfit

(c) Inadequate calibrated torque

Anecdotally, clinicians and companies have reported that dental implants with internal connections have a lower incidence of screw loosening than dental implants with external connections. In reference to the literature, screw loosening was by far the mechanical complication that occurred more frequently with single-implant restorations. This applied to both external and internal connections. The incidence, however, was statistically significantly lower for the internal connection than it was for the external connection. Some of these studies may be questioned in that standardized protocols were not applied for the tightening of the screws at predetermined torque levels. In the studies where standardize protocols were applied, the material of the screws (titanium) did not allow reaching clinically recommended preloads. One of the major advancements for the stability of the abutment-fixture joint has been the change of the screw's material and surface treatment to allow a sensible increase in preload, along with the recommendation to always tighten the screw with torque controller that applies a calibrated force. A retrospective study by experienced operators evaluated both internal and external connections over a period of 5 years. There was no difference in negative events, restoration fracture and screw loosening between internal and external implant connections [10–16].

Fracture Strength

Manufacturers have also reported anecdotally that implant systems with an internal connection have a higher resistance to fracture than systems with an external connection.

Multiple studies were conducted that yielded the following outcomes [17–23]:

1. The incidence fracture of metal-based and zirconia-based abutments does not seem to be influenced by the type of connection
2. The incidence of abutment screw fracture does not seem to be influenced by the connection
3. Loosening of the abutment screw was the most common complication. The type of connection does seem to have an influence on screw loosening. More screws were loosened in external connections. With that said, proper preload may decrease such loosening.

Conclusion

In summary, it seems that a steep and long internal connection-type joint does result in a stiffer and unyielding joint system compared to a flat-top external connection-type joint in a single-unit restoration. The clinician should also be aware that when implant restorations are splinted and screw is retained, the benefits of the internal connection are not realized. In this instance, the merit of utilizing an external connection for practicality and long-term patient maintenance should be considered.

2.4.2 Platform Switching

Platform switching is defined as a protocol that includes smaller diameter restorative components that have been placed onto larger diameter implant-restorative platforms—the outer edge of the implant/abutment interface is horizontally repositioned inwardly and away from the outer edge of the implant platform.

Multiple theories have been proposed:

(a) **The biomechanical theory**: Connecting the implant to a smaller diameter abutment may limit bone resorption by shifting the stress concentration zone away from the crestal bone implant interface and directing the forces of occlusal loading along the axis of the implant.
(b) **The biologic width theory**: Shifting the implant/abutment connection may medialize the location of the biologic width and minimize the marginal bone resorption. Placing the implant/abutment junction (IAJ) at or below the crestal bone level may cause vertical bone resorption to re-establish the biologic width.
(c) **The inflammation at IAJ theory**: This theory postulates that bone resorption is caused by an inflammatory infiltrate at the IAJ. The presence of peri-implant microbiota was suggested to influence the crestal bone resorption by maintaining the inflammatory cell infiltrate at the IAJ. The physical repositioning of the IAJ away from the outer external edge of the implant and neighbouring bone may limit bone resorption by shifting the leakage away from the adjacent crestal bone.

The reader should be aware that the points outlined above are theories. It is not scientifically known if crestal bone loss is caused by microleakage or stress concentration. On occasion, submucosal contours necessitate the implant to be placed deeper, which may be a benefit for aesthetics and contours but a detriment to biology.

Overloading has been proposed as a primary factor behind dental implant failure. The peak bone stresses normally appear in the marginal bone. The so-called platform-switching concept was introduced in an attempt to reduce this marginal bone loss. Multiple studies using finite element analysis have been used to compare both platform switching in external and internal connections. Maeda et al. (2007) used a finite element model in an external hex connection and suggested that platform switching has the biomechanical advantage of shifting the stress concentration away from the bone/implant interface [18].

Hansson also used a finite element model and compared a conical connection with a flat-top connection. The study found that the conical connection showed a decrease in the peak bone/implant shear stress compared to the flat-top interface. They concluded that the implant with the conical interface can theoretically resist a larger axial load than the implant with the flat-top interface [19].

Finite element analysis (FEA) has severe limitations when it comes to modelling living, organic tissue. Assumptions about the physical properties of bone must be made, along with assumptions on the amount of bone-to-implant contact. This is impossible to model as every person has different bone densities and bone-to-implant contact with dental implants. Furthermore, Maeda's study assumed that the abutment and the abutment screw were one piece, which is not the case. This severely limits the validity of the result. Manufacturers often cite FEA studies and "coronal stress" to justify the design of their particular implant system. The reader is advised to use caution when using FEA studies to make clinical judgements.

The clinician must evaluate the literature carefully and must not succumb to manufacturer bias and manufacturer-supported literature. As much as is known about osteointegration, there is still a lot that is unknown. Bone loss around implants does not have an exact aetiology. Authors continue to speculate the causes of bone loss, and manufacturers propose changes in implant design based on speculation since there is no true data to support their changes in implant design.

One specific study by Jacobs et al. [20] prospectively looked at marginal bone loss around and implant survival in internal (Astratech) and external (Branemark) implants in a randomized split-mouth design over a 20-year period. After 20 years of follow-up, marginal bone loss and implant survival between the two groups were insignificant. This study further questions the value of finite element models and puts into perspective clinical reality when making extrapolations from such studies.

2.4.3 Hex Geometry and Platform Diameter

Screws are an integral part of vitality of all implant-retained crown systems. One of the most common complications following successful implant therapy has been screw loosening. Not only is a minimum torque critical, but also excessive torque may exceed the yield strength of the screw, resulting in permanent deformation, loss of mechanical properties and ultimately screw fracture.

Complications such as chronic screw loosening and fracture, in addition to prosthesis and implant fracture, have been reported. Most fractures in prosthetic structures are the result of fatigue failure. Wider diameter implants have been proposed as a solution to stress reduction in both bone and the overlying prosthetic superstructures.

Multiple authors have studied the impact of cyclic loading with different load positions and periods on abutment rotational displacement [21–30].

The reported outcomes were the following:

(a) The rotational displacement of the external hexagon joint was more significant under eccentric lateral loading when compared to centric loading and more significant with longer periods of eccentric loading.
(b) It was postulated that in eccentric loading, the abutment twists within or over the play at the implant/abutment interface.
(c) Increasing the vertical height, increasing the degree of fit tolerance or eliminating the implant external hexagon did not significantly affect the reverse torque values of the abutment screws after fatigue testing.

Authors have also looked at platform diameter and how it affects mechanical strength of the abutment/implant interface [26, 27].

The reported outcomes were as follows:

(a) 5 mm diameter implant was found stronger in both static and fatigue conditions in comparison to the 4 mm.
(b) It was concluded that wide-diameter implants could be used to reduce the likelihood of long-term component fracture.

2.4.3.1 Conclusion

In summary, it seems that wider diameter implants are mechanically more advantageous. The decision on the use of wider diameter implants must be balanced with the available bone to place the said implant. Rotational displacement may affect preload in retaining screws, and it seems that longer term eccentric loading can produce more rotational displacement. Hex geometry has been shown to not affect reverse torque values, and it seems that the role of hex geometry in the stability of the screw joint is minimal. More details regarding stability of screw joints will be presented in the discussion on screw mechanics.

2.5 Screw Mechanics (Fig. 2.5)

It is important to understand the mechanics of preload and the factors that affect it. A screw is tightened by applying torque that develops a force within the screw called the preload. The torque wrench magnifies this force as does the screw thread as an inclined plane. As a screw is tightened, it elongates, producing tension. Elastic recovery of the screw pulls the two parts together, creating a clamping force. The preload in the screw, from elongation and elastic recovery, is equal in magnitude to the clamping force. The screw should not be stretched beyond its elastic limit. Excessive forces may stretch the screw beyond its elastic limit. If this occurs, the screw will lose its elasticity leading to complications of screw loosening and screw fracture.

Opposing the clamping force is a joint-separating force, which attempts to separate the screw joint. Screw loosening occurs when the joint-separating forces acting on the screw joint are greater than the clamping forces holding the screw unit together. Excessive forces cause slippage between threads of the screw resulting in a loss of preload; minimizing separating forces and maximizing clamping forces will act to prevent screw loosening.

Multiple forces act to separate the screw joint; these include but are not limited to:

1. Off-axis occlusal contacts
2. Lateral excursive contacts
3. Interproximal contacts between natural teeth and implant restorations
4. Protrusive contacts
5. Parafunctional force

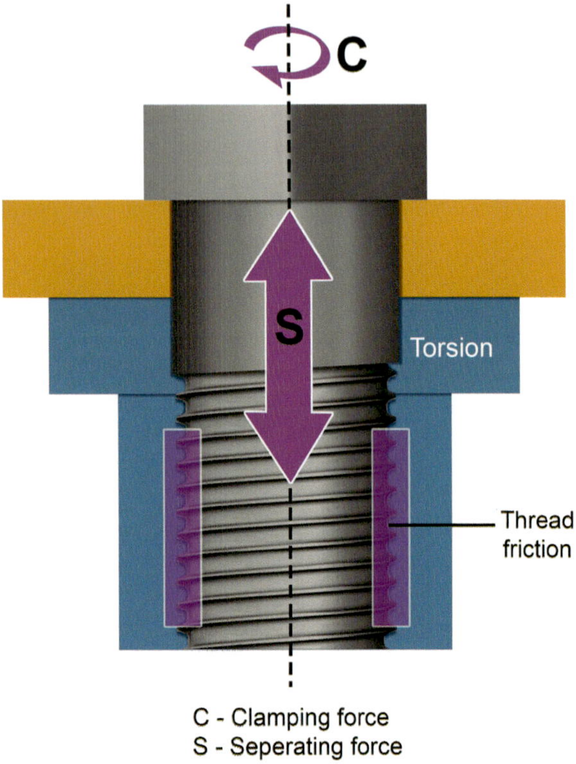

Fig. 2.5 Diagram illustrating preload, clamping force and joint-separating forces

6. Non-passive frameworks that attach to the implants

All these factors may exceed the load beyond the preload that is established, which causes the components to separate [31, 32].

The external load rapidly reduces the preload when the elastic limits of the screw are exceeded, resulting in vibration and micromovement that lead to screw loosening. The clinician must recognize the possible forces that will be acting on the screw joint, so that screw loosening and other possible complications can be minimized or avoided.

One of the simplest methods to avoid screw loosening is to make sure that the screw is tightened according to the manufacturer's recommendations.

Preload can be influenced by the following factors:

- Friction/lubricant
- Applied torque
- Screw alloy
- Screw head design
- Abutment alloy
- Abutment surfaces
- Ageing and fatigue

2.5.1 Influencing Factors

2.5.1.1 Friction

Implant prosthetic screw design has changed over the years. Earlier designs included gold screws. These screws provided more elasticity and less friction. Most of the applied load was spent on the elongation of the screw, which resulted in a higher preload. Today, prosthetic screws are gold or Teflon coated. The purpose of the coating is to reduce the friction to the screws.

Friction is a function of the surface texture of the screw threads, under the head of the screw, and abutment/implant interface. When the screw is tightened, the shank of the screw stretches and develops a clamping force. Friction is important in preventing loosening of the screw and loss of the clamping force.

To prevent bending of the joint, the screw must be sufficiently strong. Screw strength is a function of design and material of the screw. The material from which the screw is made should have a wide elastic range (to maintain the clamping force) and a high yield strength.

2.5.1.2 Applied Torque

Theoretically, the maximal preload is developed just before the screw's proportional limit. To increase preload and minimize the risk of screw fracture during use, optimal preload is calculated by multiplying the usable screw strength (75% of proof-load stress) by the tensile stress area of the screw's threaded section. Simply put, the optimal torque can be calculated by tightening a screw until it fails; 75% of this value is the optimal torque to place on the screw [33–35].

2.5.1.3 Screw Alloy and Material Properties

Given that the screw is the component that holds the abutment and fixture together, it stands to reason that its mechanical properties such as alloy type and surface characteristics will affect the ability of the screw to do its job.

Multiple authors [36–41] have studied materials and coatings on screws and have come to the following conclusions:

(a) Gold screws have higher preloads than titanium.
(b) Gold is softer than titanium, and long term, this may result in deformation of threads and loss of preload.
(c) Gold screws show a loss of preload initially but stay consistent thereafter.
(d) Although gold deforms, they are preferred to titanium due to the potential of galling in the latter.
(e) Titanium screws may cause damage to the internal threads of the implant.
(f) Gold screws may be indicated to achieve superior longevity of the screw joint and prosthetic restoration due to the greater preload achieved.
(g) Higher preloads are generated using the gold-coated screw. It is more likely that this type of screw will maintain a secure joint when tightened for the second or third time.

(h) Abutment screws with enhanced surfaces helped reduce the coefficient of friction and helped produce increased preload values than conventional screws.

In summary, while gold alloy screws have been shown to allow for higher preloads, the material choice for the retaining screw is usually determined by what the manufacturer provides. There is evidence for the lubrication of mating surfaces via surface modifications of screws to achieve higher preload values. There is insufficient evidence for the tightening of retaining screws beyond the manufacturer's recommended torque values.

2.5.1.4 Abutment Surfaces (Settling) (Fig. 2.6)

The settling effect (embedment relaxation) plays a critical role in screw stability. It is the result of no surface being completely smooth. No matter how carefully machined an implant surface is, it is slightly rough when viewed microscopically. Because of this microroughness, no two surfaces are completely in contact with one another. Settling occurs as the rough spots flatten under load, since they are the only contacting surfaces when the initial tightening torque is applied. When the screw interface is subjected to external loads, micromovement occurs between the surfaces. Wear of the contact areas brings the two surfaces closer together. It has been reported that 2–10% of the initial preload is lost as a result of settling.

As a result, the torque necessary to remove a screw is less than the torque initially used to place the screw. To reduce the settling effect, screws should be retightened 10 min after the initial torque application.

Early detection of prosthetic retaining and/or abutment screw loosening requires only a simple retightening to the recommended torque value; however, if screw

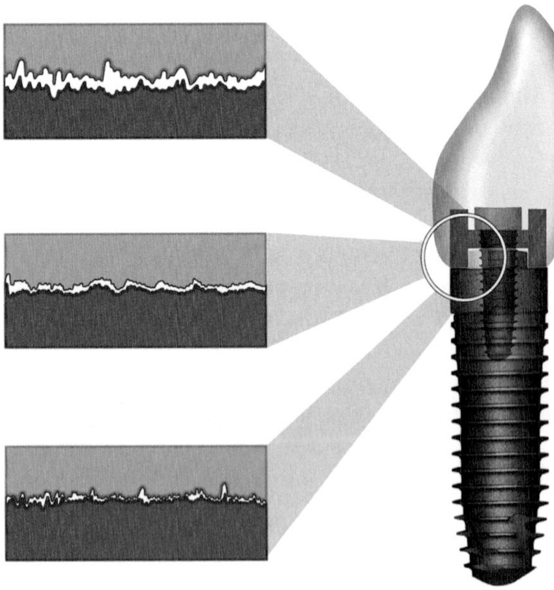

Fig. 2.6 Close-up of abutment and implant surface showing roughness

loosening goes undetected, it will lead to a more complicated, time-consuming, and expensive repair:

- To reduce the settling effect, implant screws should be retightened 10 min after the initial torque application.
- Short-term relaxation, sometimes called embedment relaxation or settling of prosthetic retaining screws, is the initial preload loss (about 10%) after the first tightening of the screw [42].

2.5.1.5 Ageing and Fatigue of Screws

Once preload has been established and the restoration delivered, the screw/preload is still influenced by several clinical and non-clinical factors.

The screw may be affected by:

- Adhesive wear and thermal changes
- Magnitude of occlusal forces
- Cantilever length
- Occlusal scheme
- Chewing patterns
- Short/long-term relaxations

Authors [43–46] have investigated the ageing of screws in full-arch restorations and when screws warrant replacement and have come to the following conclusions:

(A) Retorque retaining screws after the first 6 months of service and then retorque retaining screws annually. It was also recommended that the middle screws be rotated with the posterior screws each year at the same time that the clinician performs the retorquing.

(B) As a result of galling, the intended preload values of prosthetic retaining screws may decrease with increased in-service time.

(C) It is recommended not to interchange implant components between implant systems.

(D) Each implant screw joint "adapts" to its environment based on its design and material properties. Each joint develops unique characteristics and becomes work hardened, with an intimate adaptation of each of its components. Therefore, in the circumstance of a stable joint, the screw should not be replaced.

(E) It was shown that insufficient torque will lead to poor fatigue performance of dental implant/abutment assemblies, and abutment screws should be tightened to the torque recommended by the manufacturer.

(F) It is suggested that the use of a shorter abutment screw may be more beneficial than complete removal of a fractured screw if removing a fractured screw can potentially cause damage to surrounding tissues or to the implant itself.

In summary, preload does decrease with increasing in-service time. The establishment of an adequate preload and its maintenance over the service life of the restoration are important for long-term success of implant restorations.

2.5.2 Strategies to Minimize Screw Loosening

1. It has been suggested that placement of the implants must be ideally parallel to occlusal forces when unsplinted. The incidence of screw loosening is minimized by splinting multiple implants.
2. The associated prosthesis must be designed to direct occlusal forces through the long axis of the implant, when unsplinted.
3. Screw loosening can be limited by minimizing cantilever length, eliminating posterior working and balancing contacts, centralizing contacts and sharing anterior guidance with the natural dentition. Also, anti-rotational features must be engaged, and passively fitting frameworks for multiple units are essential.
4. Optimum preload maximizes the fatigue life of the retaining screw as the load is transferred from the abutment to the implant surface with minimal effect to the screw.

The clinician should not focus only on eliminating loose screws without eliminating the cause of screw loosening. Loose screws should be seen as a clinical symptom that may indicate that the forces are not appropriately balanced on an implant restoration. Fit and occlusion should always be checked first, before reassembling an implant restoration.

Clinicians often ask the following questions:

1. How do clinicians know if a screw is completely secured?
2. Can we increase the torque above the manufacturer's recommendations to increase the preload?
3. Can clinicians produce the recommended torque with handheld drivers?
4. How often should we replace a screw in a full-arch restoration?

Several authors [42–48] have addressed these questions, and the following conclusions are pertinent:

1. Spring torque drivers are the most consistent torque delivery devices.
2. Titanium screws produced a higher degree of reproducibility.
3. Gaps at the interface can be recognized by altered screw turn limits (underturn or overturn).
4. The screw position can be an indicator of fit in dental implant prostheses if the end point of screw rotation is adequately indexed by the manufacturer, specific to each assembly and screw.
5. What was found that the induced stresses to the screws when tightened to the recommended torques were 57.5% and 56% of the yield strengths for gold and

titanium alloys, respectively. It is suggested that tightening of screws beyond recommended levels may be possible without producing plastic deformation. However, the reader is cautioned on doing so routinely since studies only have predicted data and each manufacturer has specific materials and recommendations for torque values.

6. The data indicate that there is wide variation in the ability of clinicians to perceive adequate torquing forces applied to implant components and that calibrated torquing devices are mandatory if proper torquing procedures are to be accomplished.
7. The American College of Prosthodontists in a position paper recommended removal of a full-arch restoration on risk assessment. The clinician must evaluate the tissue, hygiene, and radiographs. The restoration should only be removed if there is a significant reason to do so.

In summary, establishing an adequate preload in the retaining screw is important for joint stability. There seems to be some room to exceed manufacturer's recommended torque values to increase preload in the screw, but there is no conclusive evidence on how much higher we can go in increasing the torque. The reader is advised to exercise caution and good judgement. The use of a calibrated torquing device to deliver the proper preload is an important step in ensuring success.

2.6 Axial vs. Tilted Implants

The introduction of a tilted implant protocol in full-arch fixed rehabilitation utilizing immediate loading put into question the need for universal axial implant placement. Since that time, these two implant-positioning regimens have been compared throughout the literature [49–52]. However, it is clear that in many instances, tilting of posterior implants in full-arch rehabilitations provides significant benefits [51].

Benefits of Tilted Posterior Implants (Fig. 2.7)

1. Implants are placed into denser and better quality bone.
2. Longer posterior implants can be utilized through tilting.
3. Marginal bone levels are maintained around tilted implants.
4. Similar success and survival rates when compared to axial implants.

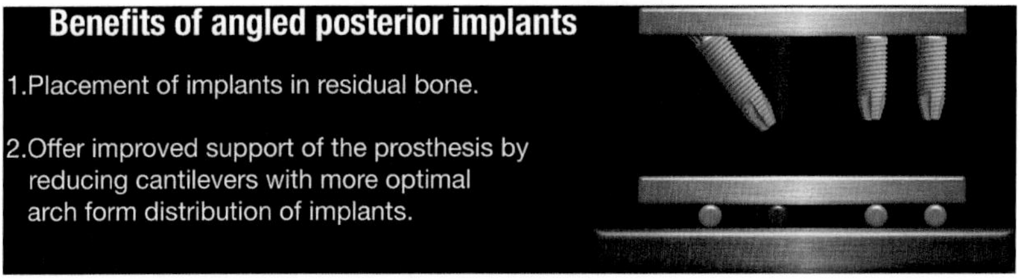

Fig. 2.7 Benefits of tilted implants

5. Vital anatomical structures are avoided by tilting posterior implants.
6. Tilting posterior implants minimizes the need for grafting procedures.

However, concerns about the consistency and clinical results using tilted implants continue to be present in the industry. Namely, three general areas of concern are prevalent:

1. Titled implants exhibit more bone loss.
2. There is increased stress concentration around tilted implants.
3. Restorations with tilted implants experience greater prosthetic complications.

It has now been thoroughly established that the use of tilted implants in an immediate loading protocol does not induce more bone loss compared to the use of an axially placed implant [49–52]. Many studies have indicated that the inclination of implants in a splinted structure aids in decreasing the stress in the arch [49–52]. There is no evidence to demonstrate a higher prosthetic complication rate in restorations that encompass tilted implants [52].

The reasons why splinted restorations utilizing a tilted implant protocol perform so well include the following:

1. Rigidity of the prosthesis counteracts the relatively small bending moments applied to the tilted implants.
2. Enough micro-motion for function not enough to prohibit osseointegration.
3. Off-axis loading is stabilized by cross-arch stability.

Tilting of implants does not seem to present any increased biological risk or technical risk when splinted. The benefits of the use of tilted implants to avoid anatomical structures and improve AP spread should be balanced with the considerations for rotational misfit, restorative space and material choice if the tilted implants have to be restored at the abutment level.

2.7 Cantilever and Anteroposterior Spread

Cantilevers in completely edentulous patients treated with implant-supported restorations have been used since the evolution of osseointegration. They have been associated with a high degree of success [53, 54].

AP spread was defined as the distance between a line connecting the distal of the most distal implants of a full-arch implant-supported prosthesis and a line through the centre of the most anterior implant [55, 56]. The evidence shows that the relationship between AP spread and cantilever length is not linear and is dependent on many variables (Figs. 2.8 and 2.9).

Variables to compute cantilever length include but are not limited to:

1. Maxilla vs. mandible

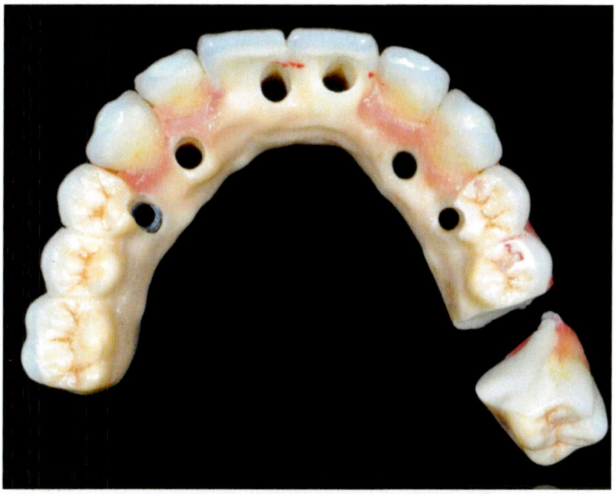

Fig. 2.8 Excessive cantilever in zirconia

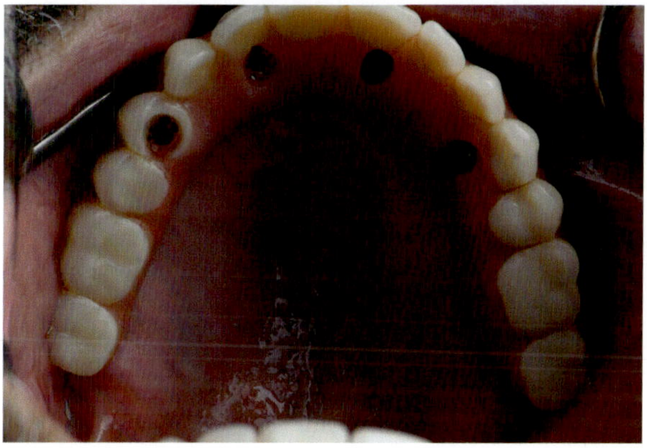

Fig. 2.9 Excessive cantilever in an acrylic titanium prosthesis intra-orally

2. Number and distribution of implants
3. Prosthetic materials
4. Framework design

Due to the number of variables, AP spread is only one of many factors that should be considered when computing cantilever length.

Cantilever length can be thought of in two ways: (1) the length of the suprastructure projecting distally or mesially from an implant and (2) the length of the suprastructure projecting buccally from an implant. It allows the clinician to provide additional teeth in areas where placement of an implant is not feasible. It has become quite commonplace in full-arch implant-supported restorations. Due to resorption, clinicians must consider mesial, distal and buccal cantilevers.

Cantilevers can broaden treatment options, simplify prosthetics rehabilitation and reduce the number of surgical procedures and associated costs.

Literature [55] on the mechanics of the cantilever and which materials are best suited for a cantilevered prosthesis is sparse.

The literature groups the information into three types of research methods:

1. Mathematical models—theoretical
2. 3D finite element analyses—questionable extrapolation to a clinical environment
3. Strain gauge analyses

All the above types of study have inherent problems since we are extrapolating mechanical formulae to a biological situation. What makes this problem difficult to solve is the fact that each implant is connected to both the bone and the prosthesis; computing the loads (and stresses and strains) in each part of the structure is a problem that is not solvable by statics alone, but also requires data on the material properties of the implants, bone and prosthesis as well as their stress–strain behaviours. Prosthesis rigidity, bone implant stiffness and deformation of the mandible also come into consideration.

More recent attempts to quantify cantilever length challenge the traditional empirical AP spread concept and propose a prosthesis-implant arch area ratio (Fig. 2.10). This concept allows a more systematic indexing of different full-arch implant clinical scenarios and allows for greater specificity and consistency [56].

The prosthesis-implant arch area ratio measures the area at the exits of the screw channel; this does not take into consideration the actual exit of the implant at bone level, which is a much more realistic indicator of the actual distribution of the implants.

An alternative proposal by the authors is to look at the arch area ratio at the implant level. This is the region where the implant exits the bone. Often, proposals have been made that tilting implants improve the anteroposterior spread, and this justifies a longer cantilever because of improved biomechanical stress distribution at implant level. Clinicians appear to be tilting implants even when there is an abundance of bone to accommodate a vertically placed implant. The tilt necessitates a pre-angled multiunit abutment. When the abutment is placed from a prosthetic perspective, the screw access channels appear to be in the correct position. This provides a stable restoration with limited screw loosening due to the splinting.

Fig. 2.10 (**a**) Prosthesis implant area-arch ratio. An alternative to calculate cantilever length. (**b**) Implant arch ratio with reduced AP spread and area. (**c**) Implant arch ratio with increase in AP spread and area. (**d**) Tilted implants do not improve stress distribution at implant level. (**e**) Preoperative panoramic radiograph showing excessive cantilever on the patient's left. (**f**) Fracture of implants illustrating force is transmitting at bone level. (**g**) Poor anteroposterior spread with excessive cantilever. One would expect the prosthetic screws to loosen. This scenario illustrated that forces are at bone level. (**h**) Implants removed and additional tissue-level implants placed. (**i**) Five implants with improved anteroposterior spread and reduced cantilever on the patient's left side. (**j**) Definitive restorations with night guard. (**k**) Panoramic radiograph. Short implant placed on right side due to proximity of inferior alveolar nerve

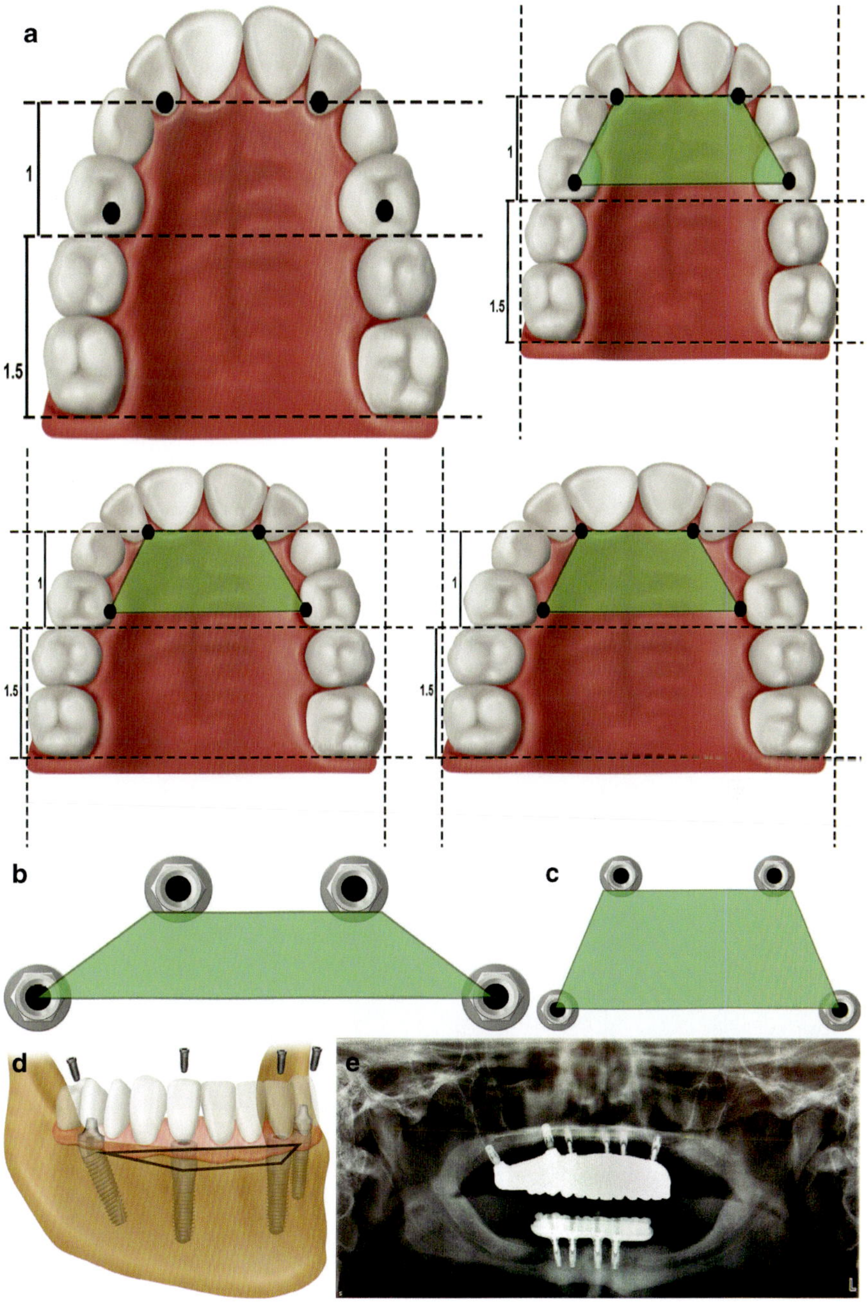
a
1
1.5
1
1.5
1
1.5
1
1.5
b
c
d
e
L

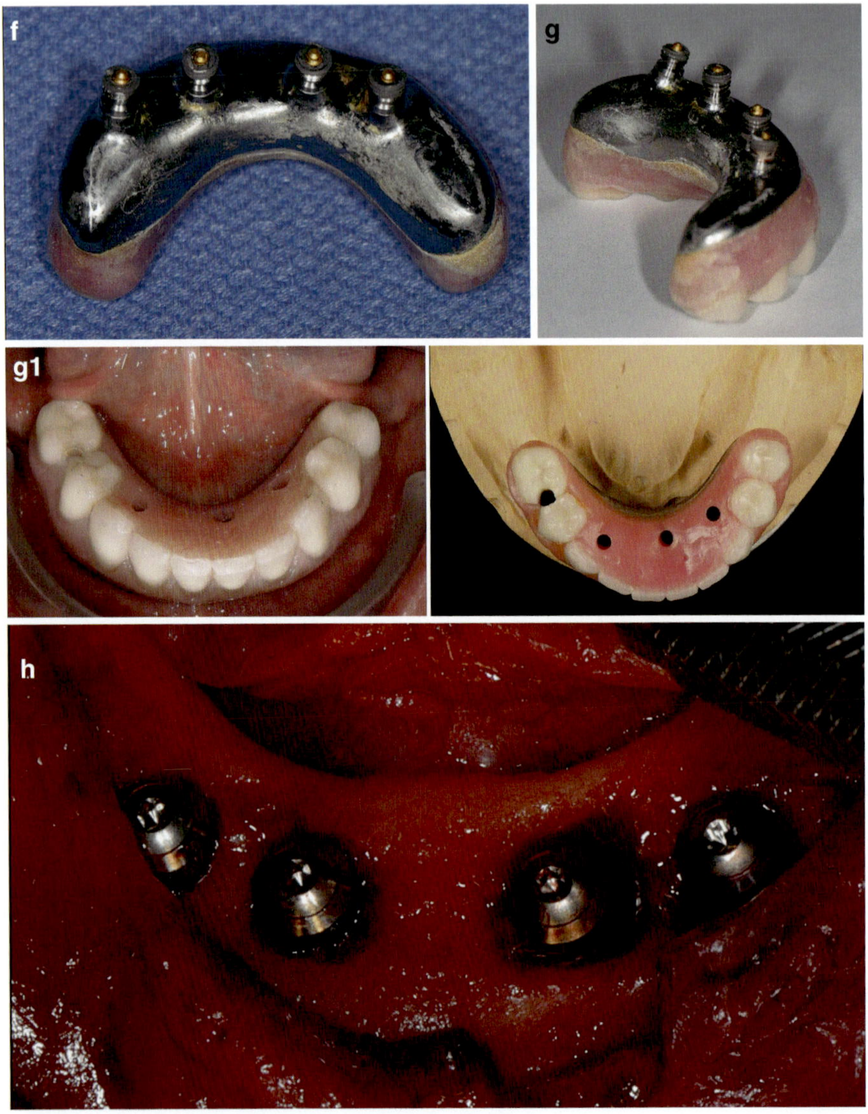

Fig. 2.10 (continued)

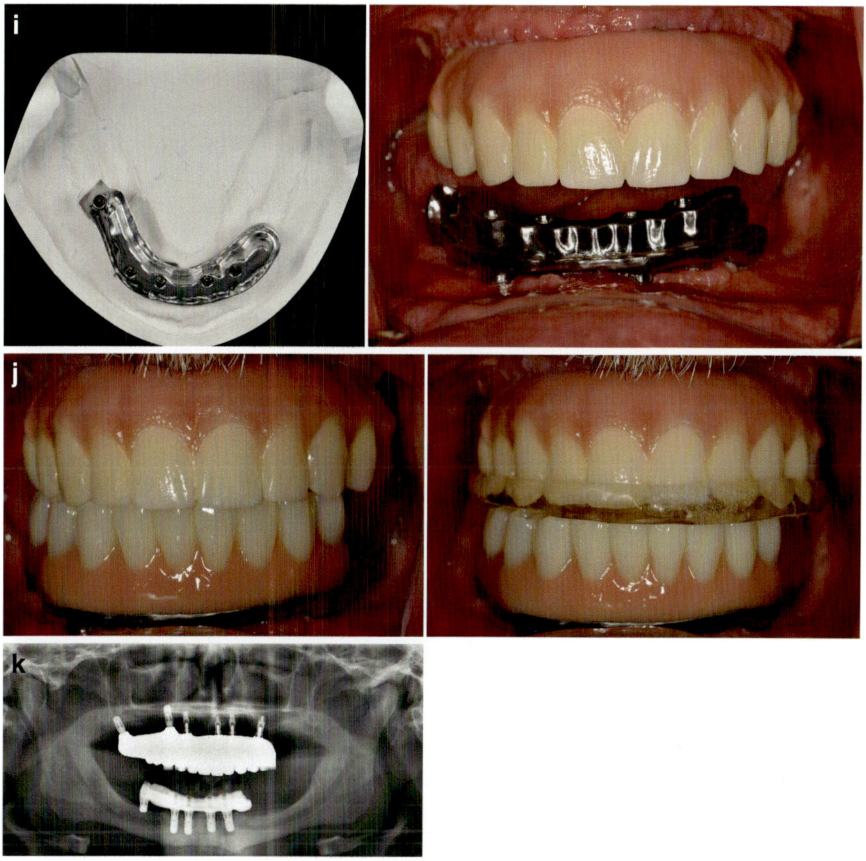

Fig. 2.10 (continued)

A consideration should be to measure the area at the exit of the bone level; this gives a true indication of the support provided by the implants. Tilting implants does not decrease stress at the bone level. The implant arch area at bone level should be a consideration. The larger the implant arch area, the better the biomechanical stress distribution of the implants. This is a biomechanical thought, and further study is required (Fig. 2.10a–k).

Biomechanically, cantilevers result in force magnification on the implant, and most clinicians would agree that the length of the cantilever should be as minimal as possible and occlusal contacts are minimized.

The literature [57–63] supports the following recommendations on cantilever length. The reader should keep in mind that these recommendations are not scientifically based due to reasons outlined above:

(a) Empirically, the cantilever length should be 1.5 times the AP spread in the mandible when five implants have been used with a maximum cantilever length of 10–12 mm. The clinician must attempt to maximize the AP spread.

(b) In full-arch scenarios, the opposing occlusion must be considered. It is known that implant vs. implant occlusion can generate higher forces. The clinician must consider the size, number, thread design and distribution of implants to distribute the occlusal forces.
(c) Implant distribution must be maximized to decrease the load per implant.
(d) Cross-arch splinting is beneficial.
(e) Use of rigid material for the framework.
(f) Studies on cantilevers in the maxilla are sparse.
(g) Cantilever length recommendations for more contemporary materials are lacking.
(h) Cantilevers with less than or equal to 15 mm had a better prosthesis survival rate.
(i) Anteroposterior spread of the implants is more important than the number of implants in determining cantilever length.
(j) Providing an excessive length of cantilever may result in prosthetic screw loosening.
(k) Excessive cantilever lengths are associated with more prosthetic problems.
(l) AP spread can be affected by the number and length of implants supporting the prosthesis, presence of cross-arch stabilization and masticatory forces generated by the patient (such as parafunctional forces); there is no consensus as to the optimal cantilever length as the function of implant length.
(m) When the number of implants was increased for the same AP spread, the length of the cantilever could also be increased.
(n) The law of beams indicates that if a cantilever is extended, the length of a beam, similar to its height, will flex to the cube power.
(o) Increase in height and thickness of the framework in the region of the cantilever provides more resistance to deformation.

2.8 Crown/Implant Ratio

In patients who have undergone severe resorption, there is obviously a limited amount of bone to place the implants and an obvious bulk of prosthetic structure and on occasion causing a tremendous prosthesis-to-implant ratio. Multiple systematic reviews on short implants have shown high survival rates. The advantage of short implants is reduced surgical procedures for the patient. A greater crown/implant ratio has been considered to be detrimental by some authors (Figs. 2.11a, b and 2.12a, b).

The theory is that in these patients with unfavourable crown/implant ratio, the prosthesis acts as a lever that causes a bending moment and transmits stress to the peri-implant crestal bone causing resorption.

The crown-to-implant ratio (CIR) was always seen as a key factor for success. While in natural teeth the optimal ratio is 1 (crown) to 2 (root), such ratios are

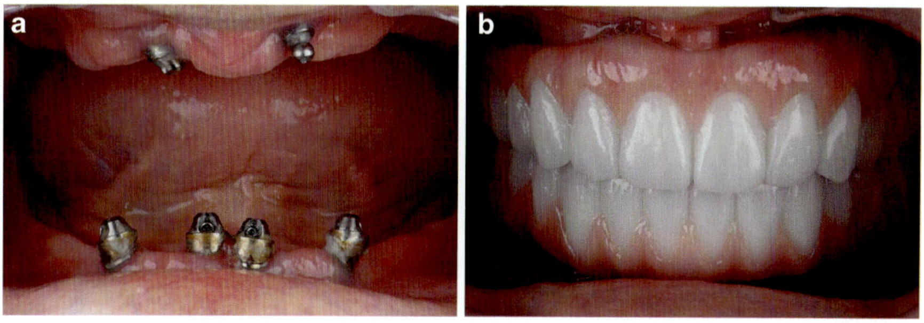

Fig. 2.11 (**a**) Failing full-mouth implant rehabilitation. Patient has lost a lot of bone. (**b**) Look at pink replacement. Restorations are splinted on zygomatic implants

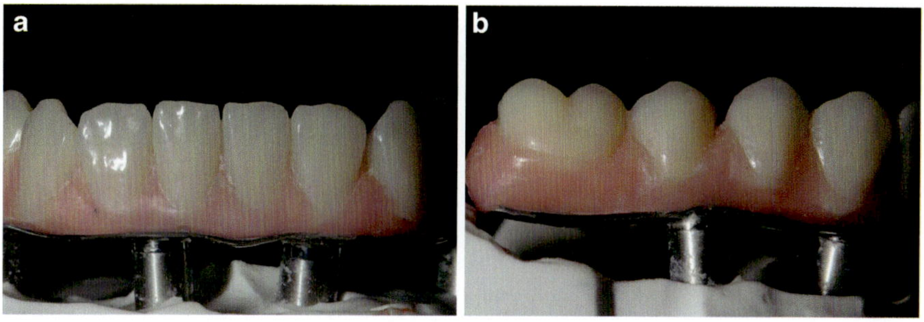

Fig. 2.12 (**a**) Lack of restorative space for an acrylic titanium prosthesis. (**b**) Lack of restorative space and excessive cantilever

almost never found in implant-supported restorations due to the frequently encountered ridge atrophy. A 1:1 CIR was considered favourable, and a ratio of 2:1 was considered as the limit of acceptance. This was due to the increase in alveolar ridge stress caused by the increase of momentum. Recent studies seem to only partially agree with this theory. A 5-year longitudinal cohort study published in 2019 [64] states that higher CIR values do not necessarily induce peri-implant bone loss and that using short implants may always be considered as an option in reduced bone heights. Other studies also state that increasing the CIR does not have a significant effect on marginal bone loss [65].

Recent systematic reviews that investigated the influence of crown/implant ratio on the success rate and marginal bone loss of dental implants showed that the higher the crown/implant ratio, the less the peri-implant marginal bone loss. Multiple studies have shown that crown/implant ratio is not a factor that causes bone loss, provided that there is a good fit of the prosthesis to the implants and cross-arch stabilization is maintained. The crown/implant ratio is theoretical and is dictated by aesthetics and the level of the occlusal plane. An increase in crown/implant ratio may result in increased prosthetic complications. Short implants may be considered as an alternative to standard implants due to their simplicity and lower cost. Their use may avoid unnecessary surgical procedures such as sinus lifts and nerve repositioning. Another advantage of short implants is that they can shorten the treatment time [66].

2.9 Misfit

Passive fit has been defined as the "adaptation of one component to another in a manner that does not impart strain". Achieving passive fit is desirable in implant prosthodontics.

Currently available clinical strategies to evaluate passivity include the following:

(a) Planning of visual examination
(b) Use of a disclosing medium
(c) Tactile feedback from palpation
(d) Tactile feedback from a one-screw test
(e) Tactile feedback from a screw clamping force
(f) Radiographs

None of the above methods have any scientific validation and are empirical. None of the above methods are reproducible or measurable. Evaluation of passive fit has no defined objective criteria. Passive fit is more difficult to discern in an implant with an internal connection than an external one.

The non-passive misfit of the prosthesis on implants is thought to cause technical and biological problems that result in marginal bone loss. The scientific evidence has shown no adverse effects on bone surrounding implants due to the misfit of prosthetic components. Non-passive fit does not appear to be a major risk factor to the health of the osseointegrated interface. Misfit of the prosthesis may have an impact on the prosthetic screws. If their preload is exceeded and the screw is stretched beyond its elastic limit, consequences may include screw loosening or screw fracture.

Some degree of misfit is present amongst all prosthetic components. The threshold for failure is unknown, having established that there exists a biological tolerance for prosthesis having misfit. Misfit does not seem to affect long-term survival or success of the implant prosthesis; the question remains on the technical complications that could arise from a prosthesis with misfit. Researchers have reported varying levels of prosthetic screw instability, and this may present as a prosthetic complication [67, 68].

2.10 Number of Implants

Rangert (1997) [30] described the differences between treatment planning for implants in a partially edentulous situation compared with a completely edentulous situation. In a partially edentulous situation, there is loss of cross-arch stabilization seen when restoring a fully edentulous arch with implants. The differences in mobility between teeth and implants in the same quadrant tend to force the implants to carry a major share of load. He described the different factors in treatment planning for implants and categorized them into geometric load factors, occlusal load factors, bone/implant support capacity and technological risk factors.

Positioning of the implants is also a key consideration. The load on an individual implant could vary based on the number of implants, their positioning and prosthetic design.

When deciding the optimal number of implants in a full- or partial-arch rehabilitation, we must give the term optimal a broader definition. The clinician should consider not just the number of implants, but where in the jaw they are placed and the quality of bone in which they are placed. The magnitude of stresses that develop in the bone, the implant and the prosthesis and the relationship of the stresses and strains to thresholds for damage to the bone and prosthetic components should also be given consideration. The treatment plan must be developed biomechanically. Thought must also be given to the material used in the reconstruction. Too many implants or implants placed too close together may compromise the material properties of the overlying restoration.

In a full-arch scenario, attempting to predict forces on four, five or six implants based on current literature becomes impossible. What makes this problem difficult to solve is the fact that each implant is connected to both the bone and the prosthesis; computing the loads (and stresses and strains) in each part of the structure is a problem that is not solvable by statistics alone, but also requires data on the material properties of the implants, bone and prosthesis as well as their stress-strain behaviours. Prosthesis rigidity, bone implant stiffness and deformation of the mandible also come into consideration. The use of fewer implants to rehabilitate an edentulous patient has been established. It should not be used as a panacea for all full-arch implant reconstructions.

It is the author's opinion that more than four implants are required when:

1. There is an abundance of bone and biomechanically cantilevers can be avoided.
2. The patient presents with a dentition that exhibits signs and symptoms of excessive force.
3. The patient has uncontrolled metabolic disease which compromises healing.
4. There is poor-quality bone.

The advantages and considerations of placing more implants and preserving bone include the following:

1. There is the ability to segment the prosthesis, and complication management becomes easier for the clinician.
2. If in the future an implant were to fail, there are enough implants where the patient may not have to undergo surgery again.
3. The thought process that making an impression on four implants is easier than making an impression on five or six does not hold merit. Today, with

advancements in digital technologies, analogue impression making may soon become obsolete at multi-unit abutment level.

4. When placing implants, the clinician must begin with the end in mind visualizing the definitive restoration. Zirconia requires specific connector dimensions and requires appropriate distance between implants. Zirconia also requires specific thickness for biomechanical integrity. The implants together with the multi-unit abutments must be positioned three dimensionally to allow for this.
5. Maintenance of bone in between the implants can be obtained by banking roots.
6. If a catastrophic failure were to occur and all the implants were lost, then the clinician still has the opportunity to retreat the patient.

Treatment planning should be based on a thorough diagnosis to culminate in an appropriate treatment plan for the patients presenting clinical situation.

2.11 Splinting vs. Non-splinting

The concept of splinting implants to decrease force magnification does not hold scientific merit. The decision to splint is primarily a clinical one which has advantages and disadvantages. On delivery of a 3/4-unit splinted implant restoration, the advantage for the clinician is that there are fewer proximal contacts to adjust. The disadvantage for the clinician is when complications such as porcelain fracture occur. The entire prosthesis must be removed and sent to the laboratory for porcelain addition (Fig. 2.13).

The disadvantage of splinting from a patient perspective is that maintaining hygiene becomes more difficult.

Indications for splinting may include the following:

1. Splinting has obvious biomechanical advantages when distal or mesial cantilevers are necessary. (It is the author's preference in partial-arch restorations to cantilever mesially and to place additional implants when distal cantilevers are required.)

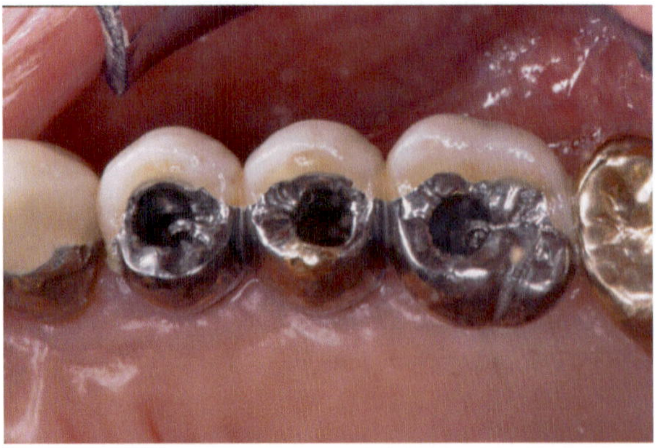

Fig. 2.13 Splinted implant restorations

2. Full-arch implant-supported restorations are done when additional teeth are required through distal cantilever and the patient's anatomy precludes the placement of additional implants. The clinician can take advantage of cross-arch stabilization.

Splinting of implants to natural teeth should be avoided due to the biomechanical differences in each structure. A separate chapter will discuss treatment planning thought process if connection to natural teeth is required. (Please refer Chap. 4.)

2.12 Material Selection

The most commonly used materials in implant dentistry are the following:

(a) Acrylic resin
(b) Composite resin
(c) Metal alloys (high noble, noble, base metal, milled titanium, milled co-chrome (cobalt-chromium)
(d) Feldspathic ceramics
(e) Monolithic materials (zirconia, lithium disilicate)

There is no scientific evidence for the breakdown of the osseointegration interface due to difference in occlusal material. There also appears to be no difference in the strain transmitted to the bone by different occlusal materials. This could be explained by the inherent flexibility in the restoration complex [69, 70].

The most commonly seen complication in implant restorations is fracture of the occlusal material [71].

Acrylic resin was most used as a restorative material for fixed implant-supported restorations primarily due to its cost. Clinicians also thought that acrylic resin may have a dampening effect reducing the force transmitted to the bone. There is no evidence to support this. Consequences with acrylic resin included wear and fracture of the teeth. As a result, clinicians explored the use of metal alloys overlaid with feldspathic porcelain in aesthetically conscious patients. Unfortunately, ceramic fractures were reported to be as high as 20.3%. Reasons for ceramic fracture included occlusal overload, lack of proprioception and in some instances inadequate design of the metal substructure supporting the ceramic (Figs. 2.14a–c and 2.15a, b) [72].

All ceramic materials have gained popularity in implant prosthodontics primarily due to improved aesthetics and reduced cost. Materials such as zirconia and lithium disilicate, both in monolithic and bi-layered forms, have been used extensively, and short- to medium-term results have been promising [73, 74].

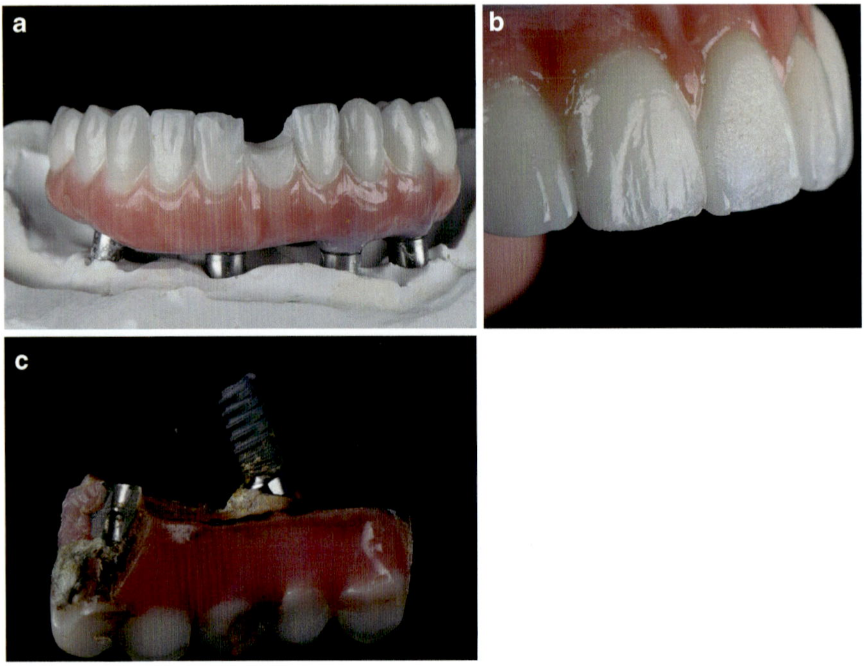

Fig. 2.14 (**a**) Monolithic zirconia fracture. (**b**) Layered ceramic chipping off a zirconia framework. (**c**) Fracture of framework and implant

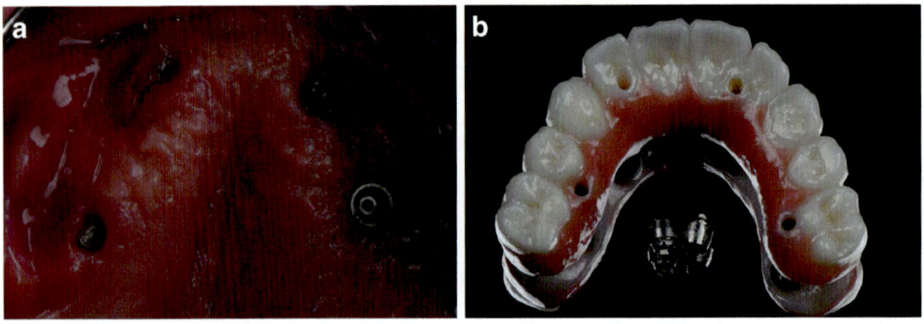

Fig. 2.15 (**a**) Screw and abutment fractures in a full-arch implant restoration. (**b**) Fracture of abutment and fracture of ceramics

2.13 Recommendations in Treatment Planning

Loads applied to teeth and implants during physiologic oral functions such as chewing, clenching, swallowing or grinding may vary because the anchorage of natural and artificial abutments in the jaw is not of the same type and quality.

Micromovement of the periodontal ligament allows the distribution of force along the surfaces of a natural tooth root around the centre of rotation in the apical third, but an osseointegrated implant has no equivalent micromovement and so forces are concentrated at the crest of the ridge.

A thorough evaluation of the patient and consideration of load control should be undertaken prior to embarking upon extensive therapy. Biomechanics is a part of implant treatment planning and ultimately will culminate in longevity of the restoration.

The clinician must give consideration to the following factors:

1. Number of implants—This will depend on the quality of bone, anticipated force on the prosthesis and an evaluation of the patient's medical history to identify additional risk factors.
2. Position of the implants—This will be dictated by bone quantity and quality and prosthetic design. Biomechanically reducing cantilever will be advantageous, as will splinting to minimize screw loosening.
3. Geometry of the prosthesis—Minimize anterior and posterior cantilever. Sufficient implants should be placed for equitable load distribution.
4. Lateral occlusal force components—Minimize lateral loads on unsplinted implant restorations. Flatter rather than steeper cusps with a narrower occlusal table should be designed on posterior teeth.
5. Parafunctional habits—Over-engineer in patients with parafunctional habits and provide a night-time appliance.
6. Occlusal relationships—A true cusp-to-fossa relationship should be created in centric occlusion, with no contact in working- or balancing-side relationships where possible. Torque should be reduced on the implant by decreasing the inclination of the occlusal impact area and allowing a cusp-to-fossa relationship. Consideration should be given to providing a crossbite in posterior regions if this results in occlusal forces being more in line with the implant.
7. Occlusal table—Narrowing of the occlusal surface could diminish implant loads considerably.
8. A cantilevered pontic extended from a free-standing implant-supported prosthesis should never exceed that which can be supported by the implants alone.
9. Mesial cantilevers are preferred to distal cantilevers.
10. A cantilever length of less than 15 mm results in less prosthetic complications.
11. Attachment of splinted natural teeth to an implant-supported cantilever increases the load on the implants rather than supporting them. The reader is advised to proceed with caution when connecting dental implants to teeth. Connecting implants to teeth is considered a last-resort option, and the authors advise against it (see Chap. 4 on implant-related tooth migration).
12. Vertical level of the implant location is dictated by anatomy and is not something that is avoidable. A good interface fit is required to reduce stress to the retaining screw.

Implants do not behave like natural teeth. Many of the theories that are applied to the natural teeth cannot be scientifically applied to dental implants. The astute practitioner must have a sound understanding on clinical implant biomechanics and maintain a simple approach to implant prosthodontics. Success is achieved with an adequate diagnosis and meticulous execution of the treatment plan.

Acknowledgments Figure 2.10e–k were provided by Dr. Chang-kai Chen.

References

1. Dhir S, Mahesh L, Kurtzman GM, Vandana KL. Peri-implant and periodontal tissues: a review of differences and similarities. Compend Contin Educ Dent. 2013;34(7):e69–75.
2. Cochran DL, Hermann JS, Schenk RK, Higginbottom FL, Buser D. Biologic width around titanium implants. A histometric analysis of the implanto-gingival junction around unloaded and loaded nonsubmerged implants in the canine mandible. J Periodontol. 1997;68(2):186–98.
3. Passanezi E, Sant'Ana AC, Damante CA. Occlusal trauma and mucositis or peri-implantitis? J Am Dent Assoc. 2017;148(2):106–12. https://doi.org/10.1016/j.adaj.2016.09.009.
4. Stimmelmayr M, Groesser J, Beuer F, et al. Accuracy and mechanical performance of passivated and conventional fabricated 3-unit fixed dental prosthesis on multi-unit abutments. J Prosthodont Res. 2017;61:403. https://doi.org/10.1016/j.jpor.2016.12.011.
5. Han A, Tsoi J, Rodrigues FP, Leprince JG, Palin WM. Bacterial adhesion mechanisms on dental implant surfaces and the influencing factors. Int J Adhes Adhes. 2016;69:58.
6. Higaki N, Goto T, Ishida Y, Watanabe M, Tomotake Y, Ichikawa T. Do sensation differences exist between dental implants and natural teeth? A meta-analysis. Clin Oral Implants Res. 2014;25(11):1307–10.
7. Prakash P, Narayanan A. Biomechanics in dental implants. IP Ann Prosthodont Restor Dentistry. 2021;7(3):131–6.
8. Misch CE, Strong T, Bidez MW. A scientific rationale for dental implant design. In: Misch C, editor. Contemporary implant dentistry. 3rd ed. St. Louis: Mosby; 1999. p. 200–29.
9. Gracis S, Michalakis K, Vigolo P, Vult von Steyern P, Zwahlen M, Sailer I. Internal vs. external connections for abutments/reconstructions: a systematic review. Clin Oral Implants Res. 2012;23(Suppl 6):202–16.
10. Cho SC, Small PN, Elian N, Tarnow D. Screw loosening for standard and wide diameter implants in partially edentulous cases: 3- to 7-year longitudinal data. Implant Dent. 2004;13(3):245–50.
11. Jemt T. Single implants in the anterior maxilla after 15 years of follow-up: comparison with central implants in the edentulous maxilla. Int J Prosthodont. 2008;21(5):400–8.
12. Theoharidou A, Petridis HP, Tzannas K, Garefis P. Abutment screw loosening in single-implant restorations: a systematic review. Int J Oral Maxillofac Implants. 2008;23(4):681–90.
13. Steinebrunner L, Wolfart S, Ludwig K, Kern M. Implant-abutment interface design affects fatigue and fracture strength of implants. Clin Oral Implants Res. 2008;19(12):1276–84.
14. Khraisat A, Stegaroiu R, Nomura S, Miyakawa O. Fatigue resistance of two implant/abutment joint designs. J Prosthet Dent. 2002;88(6):604–10.
15. Basten CH, Nicholls JI, Daly CH, Taggart R. Load fatigue performance of two implant-abutment combinations. Int J Oral Maxillofac Implants. 1996;11(4):522–8.
16. Merz BR, Hunenbart S, Belser UC. Mechanics of the implant-abutment connection: an 8° taper compared to a butt joint connection. Int J Oral Maxillofac Implants. 2000;15(4):519–26.
17. Norton MR. In vitro evaluation of the strength of the conical implant-to-abutment joint in two commercially available implant systems. J Prosthet Dent. 2000;83(5):567–71.
18. Maeda Y, Miura J, Taki I, Sogo M. Biomechanical analysis on platform switching: is there any biomechanical rationale? Clin Oral Implants Res. 2007;18(5):581–4.
19. Hansson S. Implant-abutment interface: biomechanical study of flat top versus conical. Clin Implant Dent Relat Res. 2000;2(1):33–41.
20. Jacobs R, Gu Y, Quirynen M, et al. In J Oral Implantol. 2021;14(4):421–30.

21. Khraisat A, Baqain ZH, Smadi L, Nomura S, Miyakawa O, Elnasser Z. Abutment rotational displacement of external hexagon implant system under lateral cyclic loading. Clin Implant Dent Relat Res. 2006;8(2):96–9.
22. Khraisat A, Hashimoto A, Nomura S, Miyakawa O. Effect of lateral cyclic loading on abutment screw loosening of an external hexagon implant system. J Prosthet Dent. 2004;91(4):326–34.
23. Cibirka RM, Nelson SK, Lang BR, Rueggeberg FA. Examination of the implant-abutment interface after fatigue testing. J Prosthet Dent. 2001;85(3):268–75.
24. Boggan RS, Strong JT, Misch CE, Bidez MW. Influence of hex geometry and prosthetic table width on static and fatigue strength of dental implants. J Prosthet Dent. 1999;82(4):436–40.
25. Weinberg LA. The biomechanics of force distribution in implant-supported prostheses. Int J Oral Maxillofac Implants. 1993;8(1):19–31.
26. Morneburg TR, Pröschel PA. In vivo forces on implants influenced by occlusal scheme and food consistency. Int J Prosthodont. 2003;16(5):481–6.
27. McGlumphy EA, Campagni WV, Peterson LJ. A comparison of the stress transfer characteristics of a dental implant with a rigid or a resilient internal element. J Prosthet Dent. 1989;62(5):586–93.
28. Chee W, Jivraj S. Connecting implants to teeth. Br Dent J. 2006;201(10):629–32.
29. Brunski JB, Hipp JA. In vivo forces on endosteal implants: a measurement system and biomechanical considerations. J Prosthet Dent. 1984;51(1):82–90.
30. Richter EJ. In vivo vertical forces on implants. Int J Oral Maxillofac Implants. 1995;10(1):99–108.
31. Rangert BR, Sullivan RM, Jemt TM. Load factor control for implants in the posterior partially edentulous segment. Int J Oral Maxillofac Implants. 1997;12(3):360–70.
32. Winkler S, Ring K, Ring JD, Boberick KG. Implant screw mechanics and the settling effect: overview. J Oral Implantol. 2003;29(5):242–5.
33. Sakaguchi RL, Borgersen SE. Nonlinear contact analysis of preload in dental implant screws. Int J Oral Maxillofac Implants. 1995;10(3):295–302.
34. Jörnéus L, Jemt T, Carlsson L. Loads and designs of screw joints for single crowns supported by osseointegrated implants. Int J Oral Maxillofac Implants. 1992;7(3):353–9.
35. Cantwell A, Hobkirk JA. Preload loss in gold prosthesis-retaining screws as a function of time. Int J Oral Maxillofac Implants. 2004;19(1):124–32.
36. Farina AP, Spazzin AO, Consani RL, Mesquita MF. Screw joint stability after the application of retorque in implant-supported dentures under simulated masticatory conditions. J Prosthet Dent. 2014;111(6):499–504.
37. Bakaeen LG, Winkler S, Neff PA. The effect of implant diameter, restoration design, and occlusal table variations on screw loosening of posterior single-tooth implant restorations. J Oral Implantol. 2001;27(2):63–72.
38. Siamos G, Winkler S, Boberick KG. Relationship between implant preload and screw loosening on implant-supported prostheses. J Oral Implantol. 2002;28(2):67–73.
39. Doolabh R, Dullabh HD, Sykes LM. A comparison of preload values in gold and titanium dental implant retaining screws. SADJ. 2014;69(7):316–20.
40. Stüker RA, Teixeira ER, Beck JC, da Costa NP. Preload and torque removal evaluation of three different abutment screws for single standing implant restorations. J Appl Oral Sci. 2008;16(1):55–8.
41. Byrne D, Jacobs S, O'Connell B, Houston F, Claffey N. Preloads generated with repeated tightening in three types of screws used in dental implant assemblies. J Prosthodont. 2006;15(3):164–71.
42. Martin WC, Woody RD, Miller BH, Miller AW. Implant abutment screw rotations and preloads for four different screw materials and surfaces. J Prosthet Dent. 2001;86(1):24.
43. Al Jabbari YS, Fournelle R, Ziebert G, Toth J, Iacopino AM. Mechanical behavior and failure analysis of prosthetic retaining screws after long-term use in vivo. Part 3: Preload and tensile fracture load testing. J Prosthodont. 2008;17(3):192–200.

44. Al Jabbari YS, Fournelle R, Ziebert G, Toth J, Iacopino AM. Mechanical behavior and failure analysis of prosthetic retaining screws after long-term use in vivo. Part 4: failure analysis of 10 fractured retaining screws retrieved from three patients. J Prosthodont. 2008;17(3):201–10.
45. Yousef H, Luke A, Ricci J, Weiner S. Analysis of changes in implant screws subject to occlusal loading: a preliminary analysis. Implant Dent. 2005;14(4):378–82.
46. Xia D, Lin H, Yuan S, Bai W, Zheng G. Dynamic fatigue performance of implant-abutment assemblies with different tightening torque values. Biomed Mater Eng. 2014;24(6):2143–9.
47. Al Jabbari YS, Fournelle R, Ziebert G, Toth J, Iacopino AM. Mechanical behavior and failure analysis of prosthetic retaining screws after long-term use in vivo. Part 1: Characterization of adhesive wear and structure of retaining screws. J Prosthodont. 2008;17(3):168–80.
48. Al Jabbari Y, Fournelle R, Ziebert G, Toth J, Iacopino A. Mechanical behavior and failure analysis of prosthetic retaining screws after long-term use in vivo. Part 2: Metallurgical and microhardness analysis. J Prosthodont. 2008;17(3):181–91.
49. Yeo IS, Lee JH, Kang TJ, Kim SK, Heo SJ, Koak JY, et al. The effect of abutment screw length on screw loosening in dental implants with external abutment connections after thermocycling. Int J Oral Maxillofac Implants. 2014;29(1):59–62.
50. Barbier L, Schepers E. Adaptive bone remodeling around oral implants under axial and nonaxial loading conditions in the dog mandible. Int J Oral Maxillofac Implants. 1997;12(2):215–23.
51. Celletti R, Pameijer CH, Bracchetti G, Donath K, Persichetti G, Visani I. Histologic evaluation of osseointegrated implants restored in nonaxial functional occlusion with preangled abutments. Int J Periodont Restor Dent. 1995;15(6):562–73.
52. Koutouzis T, Wennström JL. Bone level changes at axial- and non-axial-positioned implants supporting fixed partial dentures. A 5-year retrospective longitudinal study. Clin Oral Implants Res. 2007;18(5):585–90.
53. Krekmanov L, Kahn M, Rangert B, Lindström H. Tilting of posterior mandibular and maxillary implants for improved prosthesis support. Int J Oral Maxillofac Implants. 2000;15(3):405–14.
54. Branemark PI. Osseointegration and its experimental background. J Prosthet Dent. 1983;50(3):399–410.
55. Rodriguez AM, Aquilino SA, Lund PS. Cantilever and implant biomechanics: a review of the literature, part 2. J Prosthodont. 1994;3(2):114–8.
56. Kim KY. Prosthesis implant arch ratio. A new geometric paradigm, replacing the current AP spread of a cantilever in full arch implant prosthesis. A proof of concept experiment. J Prosthodont. 2022;32(3):227–33.
57. English CE. Critical A-P spread. Implant Soc. 1990;1(1):2–3.
58. Rangert B, Jemt T, Jörneus L. Forces and moments on Branemark implants. Int J Oral Maxillofac Implants. 1989;4(3):241–7.
59. Brosky ME, Korioth TW, Hodges J. The anterior cantilever in the implant-supported screw-retained mandibular prosthesis. J Prosthet Dent. 2003;89(3):244–9.
60. McAlarney ME, Stavropoulos DN. Determination of cantilever length-anterior-posterior spread ratio assuming failure criteria to be the compromise of the prosthesis retaining screw-prosthesis joint. Int J Oral Maxillofac Implants. 1996;11(3):331–9.
61. Romeo E, Lops D, Margutti E, Ghisolfi M, Chiapasco M, Vogel G. Implant-supported fixed cantilever prostheses in partially edentulous arches. A 7-year prospective study. Clin Oral Implants Res. 2003;14(3):303–11.
62. Hälg GA, Schmid J, Hämmerle CH. Bone level changes at implants supporting crowns or fixed partial dentures with or without cantilevers. Clin Oral Implants Res. 2008;19(10):983–90.
63. Aglietta M, Siciliano VI, Zwahlen M, Brägger U, Pjetursson BE, Lang NP, et al. A systematic review of the survival and complication rates of implant supported fixed dental prostheses with cantilever extensions after an observation period of at least 5 years. Clin Oral Implants Res. 2009;20(5):441–51.
64. Greenstein G, Cavallaro J Jr. Cantilevers extending from unilateral implant-supported fixed prostheses: a review of the literature and presentation of practical guidelines. J Am Dent Assoc. 2010;141(10):1221–30.

65. Ravidà A, Barootchi S, Alkanderi A, Tavelli L, Suárez-López Del Amo F. The effect of crown-to-implant ratio on the clinical outcomes of dental implants: a systematic review. Int J Oral Maxillofac Implants. 2019;34:1121–31. https://doi.org/10.11607/jomi.7355.
66. Meijer HJA, Boven C, Delli K, Raghoebar GM. Is there an effect of crown-to-implant ratio on implant treatment outcomes? A systematic review. Clin Oral Implants Res. 2018;29(Suppl 18):243–52.
67. Lee SA, Lee CT, Fu MM, et al. Systematic review and metal analysis of randomized controlled trials for the management of limited vertical height in the posterior region: short implants 5–8 mm. vs long implants >8 mm in vertically augmented sites. Int J Oral Maxillofac Implants. 2014;29(5):1085–97.
68. Carr AB, Gerrard DA, Larsen PE. The response of bone in primates around unloaded dental implants supporting prosthesis with different levels of fit. J Prosthet Dent. 1996;76(5):500–9.
69. Jemt T, Book K. Prosthesis misfit and marginal bone loss in edentulous implant patients. Int J Oral Maxillofac Implants. 1996;11(5):620–5.
70. Menini M, Conserva E, Tealdo T, Bevilacqua M, Pera F, Signori A, Pera P. Shock absorption capacity of restorative materials for dental implant prostheses: an in vitro study. Int J Prosthodont. 2013;26(6):549–56.
71. Stegaroiu R, Khraisat A, Nomura S, et al. Influence of superstructure material on strain around an implant under two loading conditions: a technical investigation. Int J Oral Maxillofac Implants. 2014;19(5):735–42.
72. Goodacrfe CJ, Bernal G, Rungcharassaeng K, et al. Clinical complications with implants and implant prosthesis. J Prosthet Dent. 2003;90(2):121–32.
73. Wittneben JG, Buser D, Salvi GE. Complications and failure rates with implant supported fixed dental prosthesis and single crowns: a 10 year retrospective study. Clin Implant Dent Relat Res. 2014;16(3):356–64.
74. Morton D, Gallucci G, Lin WS, Pjetursson B, Polido W, Roehling S, Sailer I, Aghaloo T, Albera H, Bohner L, Braut V, Buser D, Chen S, Dawson A, Eckert S, Gahlert M, Hamilton A, Jaffin R, Jarry C, Karayazgan B, Laine J, Martin W, Rahman L, Schlegel A, Shiota M, Stilwell C, Vorster C, Zembic A, Zhou W. Group 2 ITI consensus report: prosthodontics and implant dentistry. Clin Oral Implants Res. 2018;29(Suppl 16):215–23.

Screw-Retained vs. Cement-Retained Implant-Supported Restorations

3

Winston Chee and Saj Jivraj

3.1 Cement Residue with Cemented Implant-Supported Restorations

In 1982, osseointegrated implants were introduced to North America in a conference titled "Osseointegration in Clinical Dentistry". Dr. P. I. Brånemark collected clinical outcomes for 20 years prior to presenting this information. In those times, restorations presented were screw retained. After the introduction to osseointegration at this conference, most clinicians who were exposed to the use of dental implants to replace missing teeth provided mostly screw-retained restorations. In the 1980s, almost all dental schools did not have any types of implants, let alone osseointegrated cylindrical implants, as part of their curriculum. To make implant-supported restorations more similar to how tooth-supported restorations were fabricated, implant manufacturers encouraged cementation as the mode of attaching restorations to implants using cementable abutments. Clinicians who were conversant with conventional fixed prostheses on teeth then developed preferences to provide cement-retained restorations on implants. Up to the present time, manufacturers supply abutments that do not conform to the mucosal margins of the restoration as they are fabricated without variation of the cement margins. Later, clinicians fabricated customized abutments to have the cement margins follow the mucosal contours for aesthetics and easier removal of cement excess. Those who had preferences to deliver screw-retained restorations, when presented with implant trajectories that were not ideal in aesthetic zones, were forced to use cementable abutments. Figure 3.1 illustrates the Sharpey's fibres that attach bone and gingiva to the root

W. Chee (✉)
Advanced Prosthodontics, Herman Ostrow School of Dentistry, University of Southern California, Los Angeles, CA, USA

S. Jivraj
Private Practice, Anacapa Dental Art Institute, Oxnard, CA, USA

W. Chee, S. Jivraj (eds.), *Treatment Planning In Implant Dentistry*, BDJ Clinician's Guides, https://doi.org/10.1007/978-3-031-68726-6_3

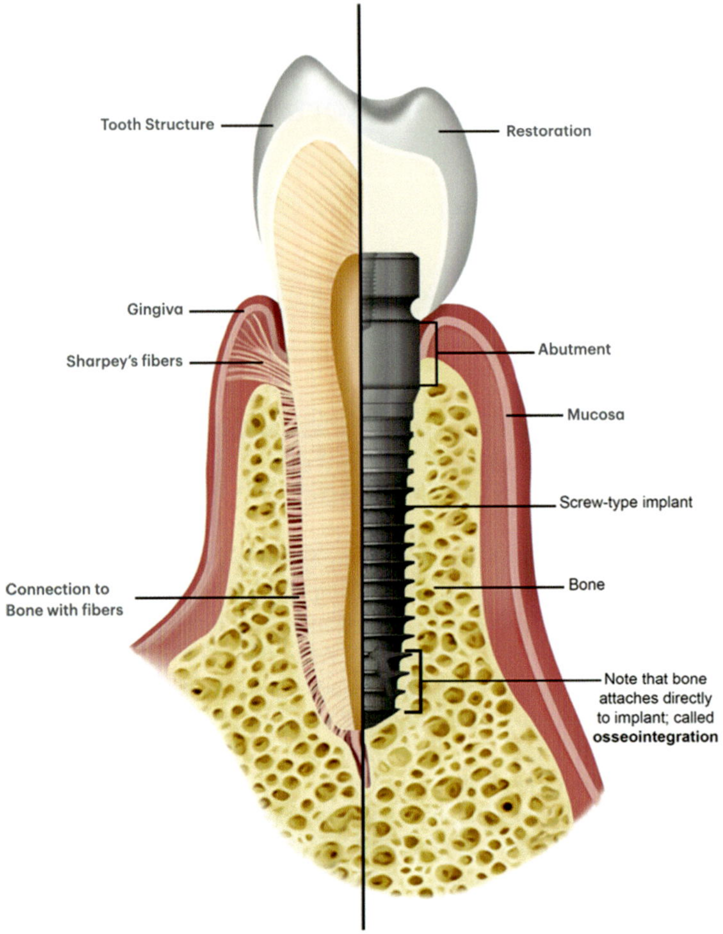

Fig. 3.1 Diagram of tooth and implant attachment to bone and soft tissue with different mechanisms. On the tooth side, bone and soft tissue are connected with Sharpey's fibres. On the implant side, the implant is connected directly to the bone and the soft tissues are connected only with hemidesmosomes

cementum, and with implants, there is only direct attachment of the implant to bone and only hemidesmosomal attachment between mucosa and the implant.

At minimum, when cemented restorations are used, the abutment should be formed to support the peri-implant mucosa and have the cement margin follow the mucosal contour to facilitate removal of cement.

When cementing implant-supported restorations, a critical issue is that cement residue is often found; this occurs because there is no barrier unlike teeth which have Sharpey's fibres that insert from alveolar bone to tooth roots. This prevents the cement from flowing apically when restorations are seated as crown preparations on teeth. With implant-supported cemented restorations, at best, a long junctional epithelial attachment to the abutment can be formed.

When crowns are cemented onto cementable implant abutments, the cement can flow and have proximity to the bone or come in direct contact with the peri-implant bone [1] (Fig. 3.1).

When seating the crown, the abutment serves as a plunger causing the cement to be extruded and forced apically toward the bone. It has been demonstrated in an in vitro study that cement could not be entirely removed when experienced clinicians were asked to remove cement around implant-supported restorations in a typodont with artificial soft tissue surrounding the cement margin [2]. Clinically, Wilson with the use of a dental endoscope found that peri-implant disease was related to cement remnants at up to 81% of patients when symptoms of peri-implant disease were manifest; this author reported that when cement was removed, signs of peri-implant disease were resolved 74% of the time, indicating that implant disease is caused by cement remnants when restorations are cemented onto implants. It has also been noted that peri-implant disease can manifest many years after cemented implant restorations are delivered [3] (Figs. 3.2 and 3.3).

In addition, further studies by other authors have revealed that a high percentage of cemented restorations exhibited cement residues in their respective clinical cohorts. In addition to these findings, others have evaluated the bacterial biofilms found in the cement that was removed and indicated that more aggressive biofilms were found when using resin cements compared to non-resin cements. Many of the implant companies have promoted the use of resin cements as being highly retentive for restorations; using resin-based cements is a disadvantage for the patients and clinicians because the use of resin cements which are radiolucent causes difficulty in removing excess cement and then detecting cement remnants that remain [4–7]. Cement remnants are recognized as a risk factor in peri-implant bone loss in publications; these remnants are considered an etiological factor in peri-implantitis-affected implants [8–10] (Figs. 3.3 and 3.4).

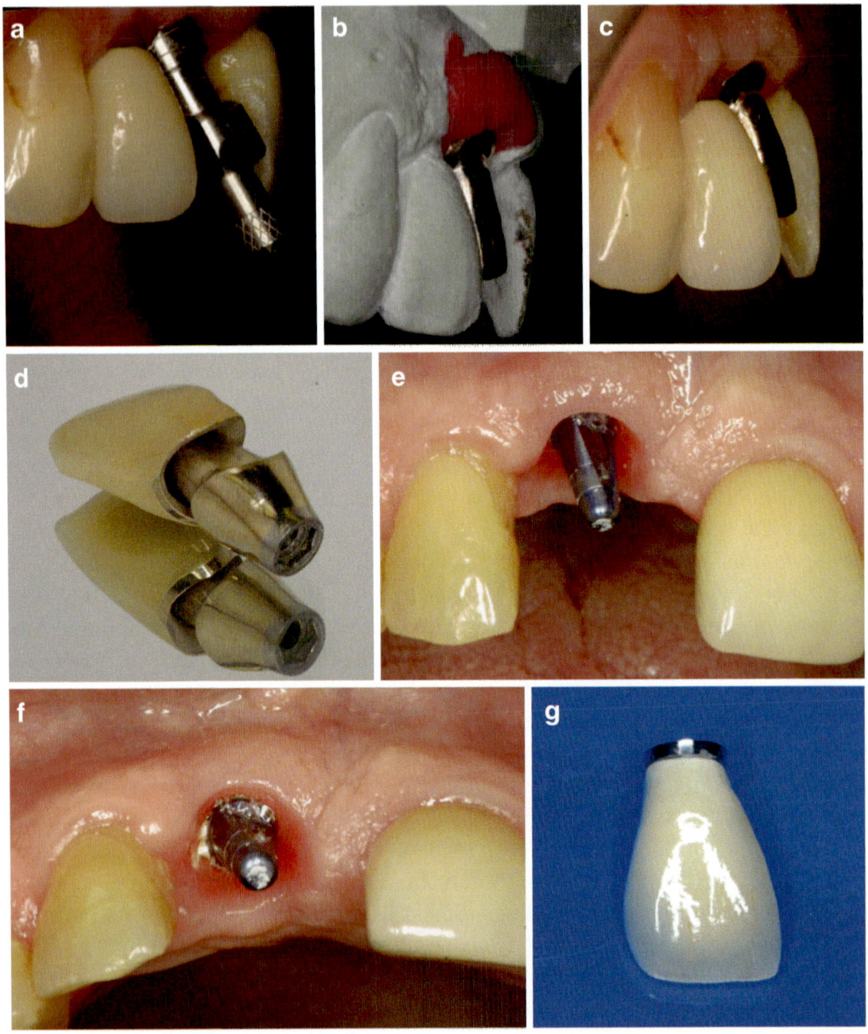

Fig. 3.2 (**a**) Impression coping demonstrating that the implant trajectory is exiting facially on implant-supported restoration. (**b**) Image of custom abutment on cast to receive restoration to be cemented. (**c**) Image of abutment intra-orally; the custom cemented abutments are fabricated to follow the mucosal margins to minimize cement entrapment when restorations are delivered. (**d**) Image of restoration to be delivered with customized abutment that follows the mucosal and the contours that support the soft tissues from the margin to the implant platform. (**e**) An example of a company-manufactured cement abutment that does not present with any mucosal margin to reduce cement entrapment and develop submucosal contours. (**f**) Occlusal view shows the deep margin and cement remnants when restorations are removed; in addition, submucosal contours are supported by the restoration that will be cemented. (**g**) Example of restoration to be cemented with no relationship to the mucosal margin

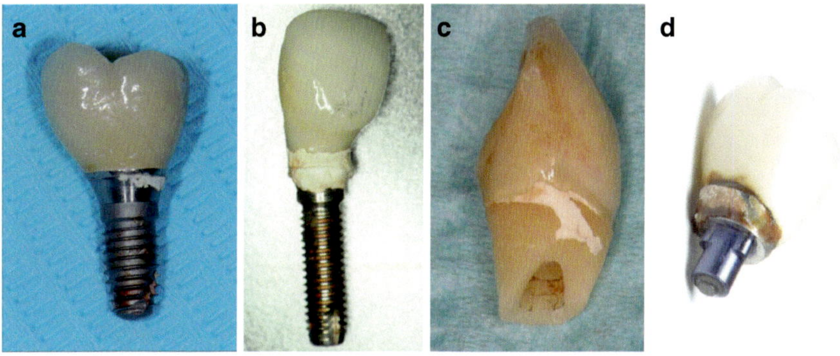

Fig. 3.3 (**a**) Cement retention on implant that failed; note that the cement margin is not conforming with mucosal margin. (**b**) A more severe accumulation of cement when the implant is explanted. (**c**) Cement retention seen when a ceramic abutment that has been in place for several years; the cement is unnoticed till the abutment is fractured. (**d**) Resin cement retention noted when the abutment screw fractures and abutment and restoration are displaced—resin cements are radiolucent and are not detected with radiographs

At times when cementation of restorations is required, for example with one-piece implants (implants that are fabricated with implant body and abutments in one piece) and two-piece implants with only available components for cemented restorations, Additionally when required to repair or refabricate cemented restorations where unknown implant types cannot be identified. Many methods of minimizing cement retention are from minimally coating restorations with cement to venting restorations. One method that is simple and has been shown to reduce cement extrusion at seating is by seating the restoration on an impression putty jig. The putty will form the cementation jig that will receive the restorations; the restorations can be filled with cement and seated on the jig to extrude the excess cement. Removal of the restorations will leave an even and minimal coating of the cement; seating of the restoration will minimize the excess cement extruded on cementation [11] (Fig. 3.5).

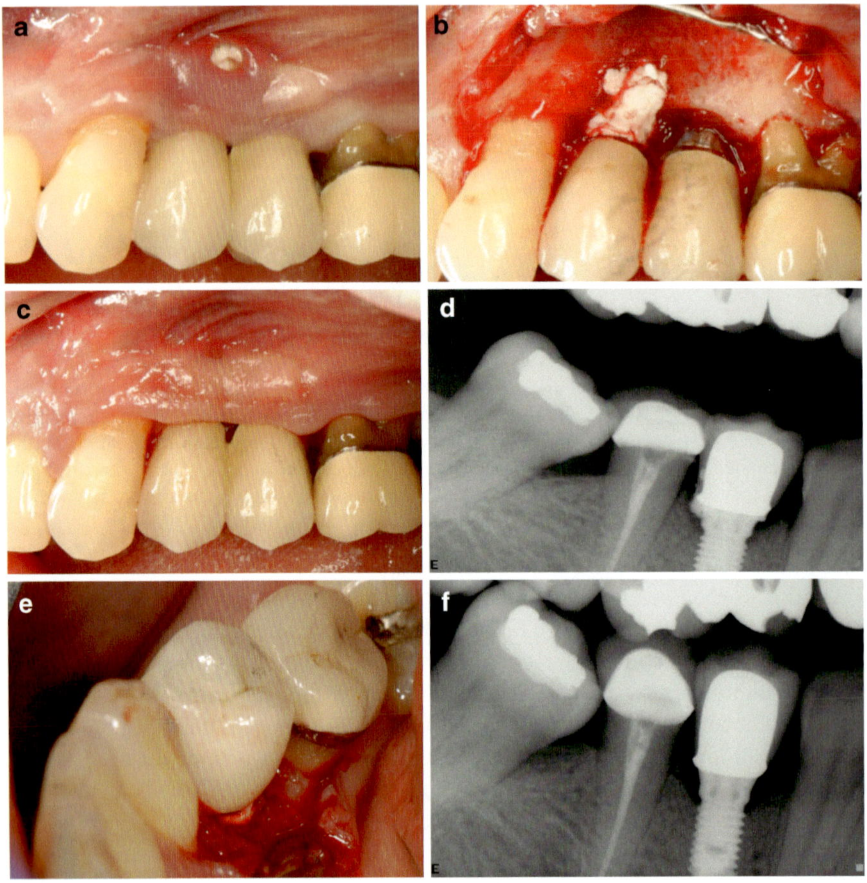

Fig. 3.4 (**a**) Cement extrusion is visible 5 mm apical to the mucosal margin of maxillary left first premolar. (**b**) Cement retention is evident when flap is retracted. (**c**) The cement is removed, but there is significant loss of soft tissue due to the cement extrusion. (**d**) Radiograph shows cement extruded in the mesial and distal sides of the cemented restoration on mandibular right first premolar. (**e**) An open flap exposes cement retention in the lingual area of the restoration. (**f**) Radiograph shows that cement is removed entirely from the margins of the cemented restoration

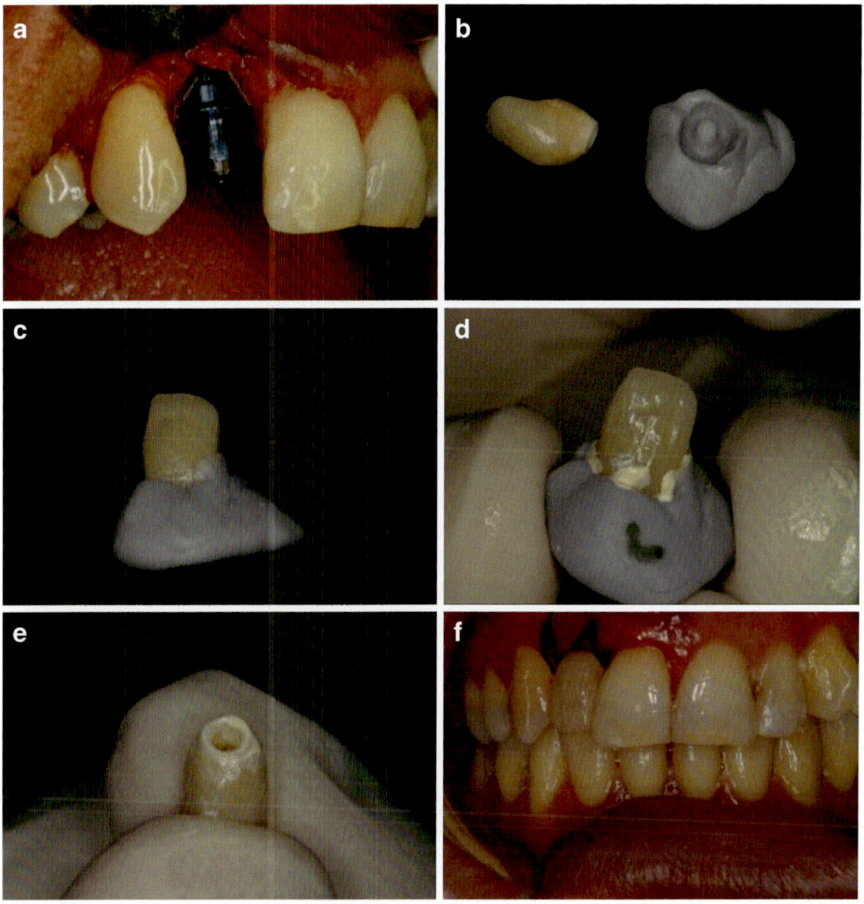

Fig. 3.5 (**a**) Implant placed to be immediately loaded. (**b**) The provisional restoration is filled with silicone putty to impress the internal and external of the provisional restoration to form the cementation jig. (**c**) The putty jig fills the cavity on the restoration and the peripheral surface of the restoration. (**d**) Excess cement that is extruded by the cementation jig is visible. (**e**) The provisional restoration is removed from the jig; the excess cement will be removed from the external surface of the restoration. (**f**) The restoration is seated onto the abutment with minimal cement extrusion

3.2 Retrievability

Removing implant-supported restorations that are cement retained is a subject that has received much attention with respect to preferences of cemented or screw-retained restorations. In the 1990s, many who were considered experts expressed that implant-supported restorations should be treated similarly to restorations cemented onto teeth, i.e. clinicians did not hesitate to destroy otherwise intact restorations to address the underlying problems of screw loosening or other maintenance.

Authors of this book have kept to delivering screw-retained restorations from the beginning of delivering implant-supported restorations from the start of exposure to osseointegration. Since implants are unlike teeth and with some care in planning of implant placement, restorations can be made to be retrievable; as clinicians, we should plan for this possibility.

An aspect of cementation of restorations on implants is the difficulty of removing the restorations when required; the most common cause to remove the restoration is when screw loosening occurs. A main reason for occurrence of screw loosening is the issue of settling; implant components are machine milled, and this process leaves some fretting (machining marks) during the process [11, 12].

Settling is a term used by machinists; when the abutment and implant are connected, the two fitting surfaces rub against each other with forces when occluding and chewing; this fretting of machined surfaces smoothens. This then brings the two components toward each other causing the elongation of the screw to be reduced; this reduces the preload (elongation of screw that develops clamping forces) of the screw leading to screw loosening. Some of the settling can be overcome with a 10-min wait after torquing the screw and then re-torquing. With a cemented restoration, the abutment is attached, and the restoration is cemented; there is no opportunity to re-torque the screw; this may increase the rate of screw loosening. With screw-retained restorations, restorations are delivered with suggested torque forces and then re-torqued after a few weeks of usage before sealing the screw access channel (Fig. 3.6).

When there are episodes of screw loosening or other causes, removal of the cemented restorations can be difficult and unpredictable. In order to be able to remove the restoration when it is cemented, it can be attempted to remove them with

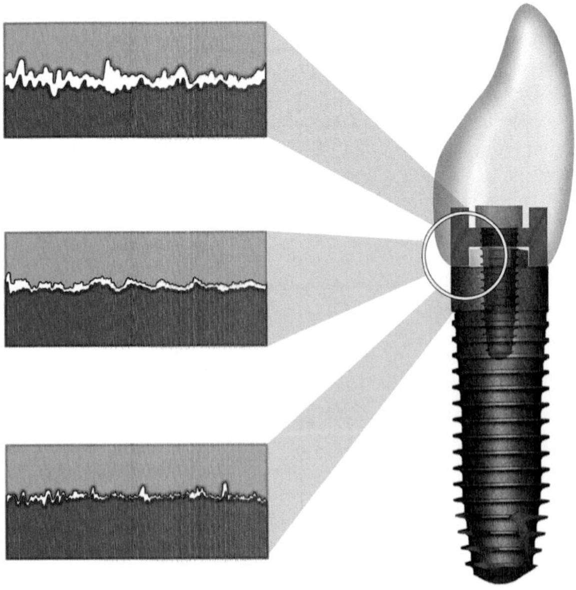

Fig. 3.6 Settling effects are seen as the abutment and the platform surface of the implant reduce the fretting over time causing the fit surfaces to become closer and reduce the screw elongation and reduce the preload that clamps the components together

hemostats or back-action devices. With back-action devices, there may be a better opportunity to remove splinted units as the connector areas can be engaged; single units are most difficult to remove when no purchase on the restoration is available. When restorations cannot be retrieved intact, the only option is to cut the restoration off in a similar fashion, as crowns are removed from teeth when required, or to access the retaining screw by cutting into the restoration by estimating the trajectory of the implant to access the abutment screw. The cemented restoration can be removed from the abutment extra-orally. Both methods usually render the restoration unserviceable and require that the restorations be remade (Fig. 3.7).

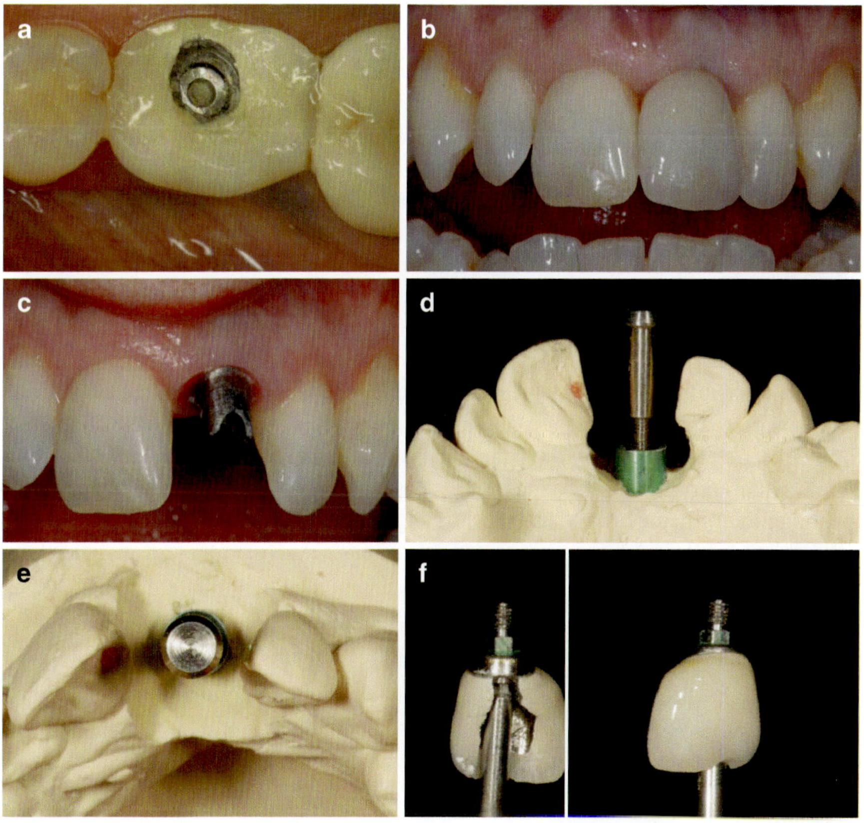

Fig. 3.7 (**a**) Cemented restoration with retentive screw loosened; the screw can be accessed by attempting to find the projection of the screw with radiographs, the screw can be exposed and the screw can be replaced if the existing restoration permits. (**b**) Image of maxillary left central incisor restoration that is cemented with retaining screw loosened. (**c**) Crown is removed after removing the restoration by accessing the screw. (**d**) One advantage of tracing the screw trajectory is having the master cast which was used to fabricate the abutment and restoration. (**e**) The trajectory of the implant can clearly be seen with the help of a long screw, with cemented restorations giving the casts to the patient or storing the casts being helpful when access to the screw is expedited. (**f**) Two views of the restoration and abutment will demonstrate the damage to the cemented restoration; the restoration is separated from the abutment extra-orally

Other methods of more predictably removing cemented restorations have been presented; one way offered to eliminate the use of cement was to use a set screw which would engage the abutment with threads within the restoration and then engage the set screw against the abutment for retention (Fig. 3.8). This illustration shows that the restoration is being delivered with engagement of the abutment with a set screw; however, it demonstrates that the set screw causes a tipping of the restoration when the screw is tightened against the abutment and the fit of the margin between the abutment and restoration is not ideal. This is due to some spacing between the restoration and the abutment.

A different use of set screw can be used to displace the restoration that has been cemented to the abutment. In this design, the set screw is placed in a position to displace the restoration from the abutment by tightening the set screw against the abutment causing the restoration to lift away from the abutment and cause the cement seal to break [13]. Figure 3.9 illustrates how a cemented restoration on an implant that is axially inclined facially is incorporating a set screw within the restoration. The abutment is designed to receive the restoration with the set screw that will be able to predictably remove the restoration when required.

Another method of removing a cemented restoration is to incorporate a slot in the lingual area of the restoration that will allow an instrument to be placed in the slot to allow the restoration to be separated from the abutment with leverage or torquing with an instrument when inserted [14] (Fig. 3.10).

When having to remove cemented restorations from abutments when a clinician is not responsible for delivering the restoration, the difficulty is increased significantly as there is no information about the cement used, the taper of the abutment, the height of the abutment, the trajectory of the implant and many other factors. Screw retention will simplify maintenance of implant-supported restorations with the major factor being able to use the suitable driver. One novel technique of identifying the suitable driver for screw-retained restorations from an unknown previous

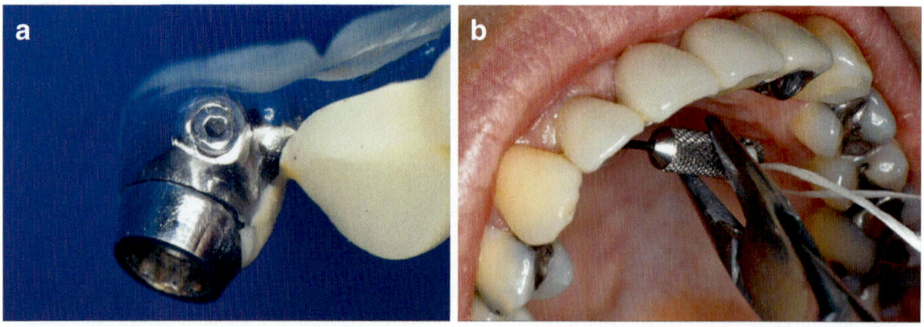

Fig. 3.8 (**a**) The set screw engaged often causes the restoration to lift from the abutment; the abutment and the restoration almost never fit perfectly. (**b**) The set screw is engaged palatally to retain the restoration to avoid cementation and can facilitate removal of the restoration by disengaging the set screw

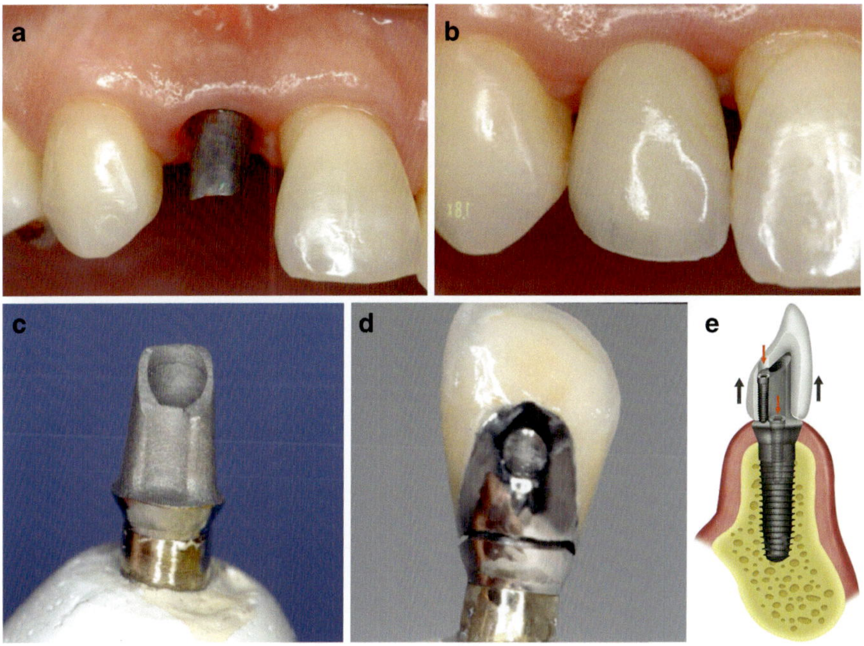

Fig. 3.9 (**a**) Cement abutment is in place to receive a restoration. (**b**) Image of restoration seated. (**c**) Image showing lingual screw slot that will receive the screw channel with the set screw housed in the restoration. (**d**) Image of the restoration on the abutment in (**c**); the restoration is displaced when the set screw is engaged; this is how the restoration that is cemented can be removed without damaging the restoration. (**e**) Diagram illustrates the vectors that will displace the restoration

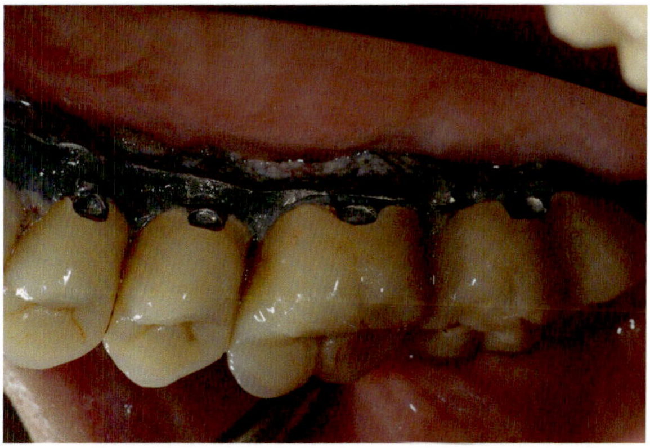

Fig. 3.10 Palatal image of feature to remove cemented restorations to abutment

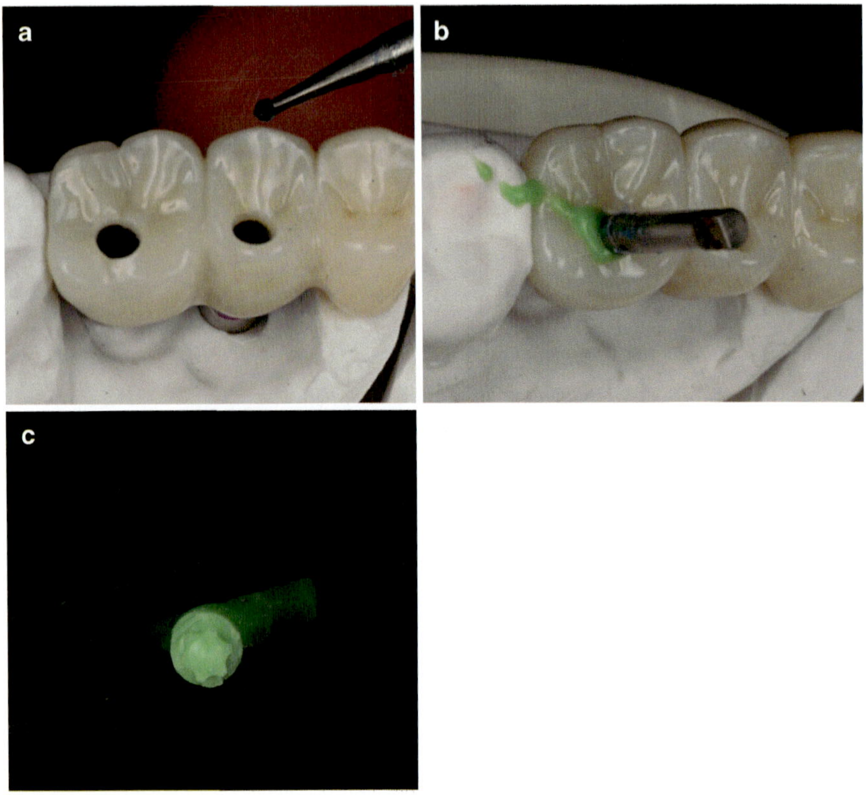

Fig. 3.11 (**a**) Image of restoration and burr as a demonstration extra-orally; the burr is coated with impression adhesive. (**b**) Light-bodied polyvinyl siloxane impression material is injected into the screw access followed by the burr. (**c**) The burr is removed after setting of the impression material, and the screw head is clearly visible to determine the correct driver to use. (Fig. 3.11a–c courtesy of Dr. Webster Felix)

provider is to use some impression material with a support that will be able to loosely traverse the screw channel to register the pattern of the screw head [15] (Fig. 3.11). This will help to identify a driver that will fit the retaining screw. If the cement abutment screw is not visible, this method can also be used.

It should also be considered that high-strength ceramics that are currently used to fabricate both abutments and cemented restorations are likely to fracture when removal of cemented units is attempted. With screw-retained ceramic restorations or abutments, the restorations can easily be removed.

3.3 Rotational Misfit of Cement Abutments

3.3.1 Screw-Retained Restorations

For most implant systems, implants and abutments are connected with a relocation feature; an example will be an implant with a hexagon which will engage with an abutment to position it in a specific trajectory. The two components will be connected with a drop screw; the abutment will need to be fully seated to the implant without binding of two parts. The implants and abutments need to be machined to have some tolerance in order to allow the components to seat without interference and allow the drop screw to avoid binding to attain the required preload. This required tolerance will allow anywhere from one to three degrees of freedom [16] (Fig. 3.12).

When multiple restorations are screw retained, non-engaging components (by passing the relocation features) are used to connect the restorations to the implants. When metal ceramic units are used, they can be evaluated for fit in the framework phase and be confirmed for fit with radiographs at the interface of the restoration and implant. Another method to evaluate a passive fit is using the "torque turn analysis"; once frameworks are seated with screws engaging, the screws are then torqued to the manufacturer's requirements; if the framework is deemed passive, the screws should not be rotated by more than a half turn of the screw [17]. After ceramics for metal ceramic restorations or for zirconia-based restorations are delivered, screws are torqued to the manufacturer's specifications and patients will be asked to return in 2 weeks or more. Patients with screw retained restorations are assessed and then re-torqued to the prior torque values. If there is no more than a quarter turn of any of the screws, the screw access will be closed with Teflon tape and a composite resin filling. Ideally, a mechanical torque wrench should be used; the most consistent is

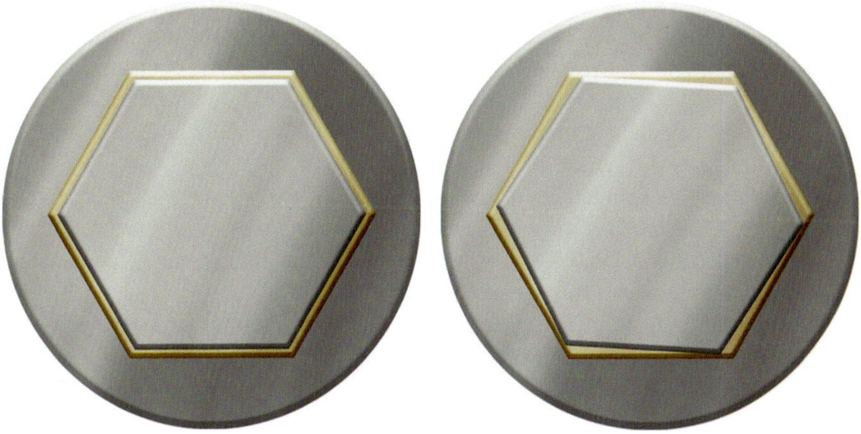

Fig. 3.12 (**a**) Diagram of freedom of rotation with milled components with a relocation feature; components are machined to prevent any binding when connected

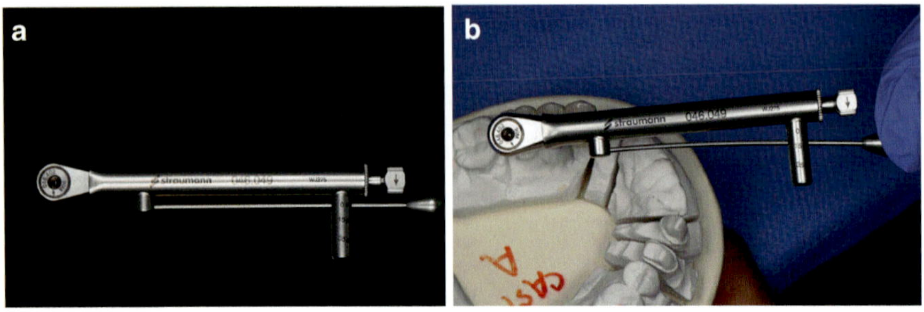

Fig. 3.13 (**a**) Image of a beam torque wrench. (**b**) Flexible bar will consistently provide torque to the screw. (Fig. 3.13a, b courtesy of Dr. Webster Felix)

the beam or spring type. This type of wrench has a rigid bar and a flexible metal bar; this flexible bar will indicate torque forces on the rigid part of the wrench [18] (Fig. 3.13).

3.4 Cement-Retained Restorations

There is always some tolerance that manifests rotational play between the location features of the implant and abutment; this feature allows cement abutments to be placed in specific positions. The cement abutments are required to be placed repeatedly in the same position as the angulations and marginal configurations of the abutments to receive the restorations to be placed. The fit of the restoration to the abutment may be adequate when single-unit restorations are fabricated; however, when multiple splinted restorations are supported by more than one implant, it would be difficult to have the cemented restoration seat perfectly on the abutments. This is because the rotational positions of the abutments can be in dissimilar positions from the cast where the restoration is fabricated to the patient. Several phases where the rotational play can occur include the following: (1) rotational play of the impression coping on the implant, (2) rotational play of the impression coping with the analogue and (3) rotational play of the restoration abutment or Ti base. After these phases, the cement abutments may be in dissimilar positions when compared to the master casts and intra-orally.

For multiple-unit splinted cemented restorations, the rotational misfits can cause margins of the cemented restorations to be opened when restorations are delivered. In addition, the misfit can also affect the occlusal and interproximal contacts to adjacent teeth to require adjustments (Fig. 3.14).

This is well documented by Semper et al. [19] where it is demonstrated that when there is a rotational misfit of the abutment that is angulated, there is a significant opening of the margin between the restoration and the abutment (Fig. 3.14).

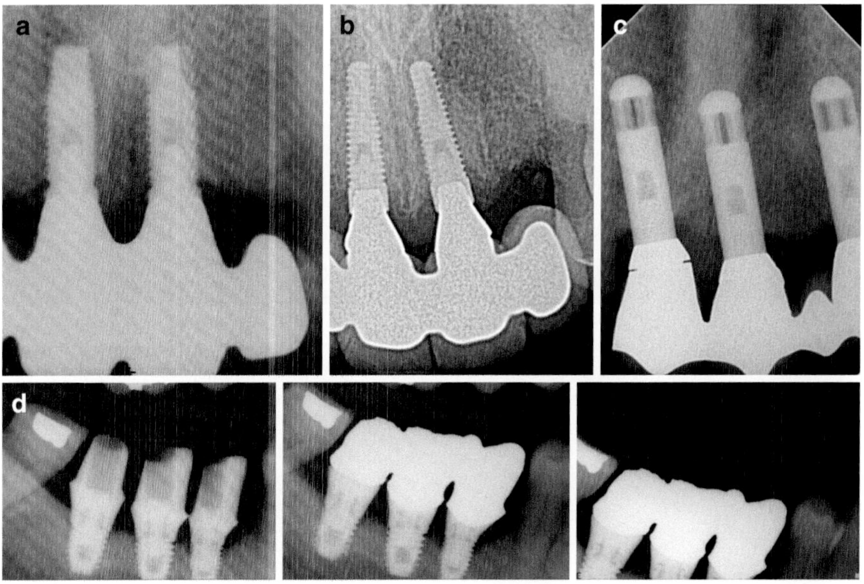

Fig. 3.14 (**a**) Radiograph of splinted screw-retained restoration; the restorations are seated on the implants. (**b**) Radiograph of splinted restorations seated on two cementable abutments; it can be seen on the radiograph that the restorations are not fully seated to the abutments. (**c**) Radiograph showing open margins with splinted units on abutments. (**d**) Radiographs show splinted restorations open in the most distal of the three implants in the middle image and then cut and reassembled to fit on all three abutments

3.4.1 Aesthetics

Currently, objections to screw-retaining restorations to implants due to aesthetics are mostly unfounded; there are few situations where screw retention is not possible due to implant positions. Components are available today where the screw channel for screw-retained restorations can be shifted away from areas that will compromise aesthetics. Additionally, these components can shift the screw access to areas where restorative materials are of adequate dimensions in order to reduce mechanical fracture of the restorations.

Obviously in some situations, having a screw access in a visible area is unacceptable. When screw access to the implants is in aesthetic areas, cemented restorations can be considered to improve aesthetics but have drawbacks that are discussed early in this chapter. Similar to the use of abutments for cementation, intermediary pre-angled abutments will also require that implants are placed more apically to accommodate the added space required by the abutment. Figures 3.15 and 3.16 show the added dimensions of the two types of intermediary abutments at the facial portion of the abutment as it emerges from the implant platform (Figs. 3.15 and 3.16).

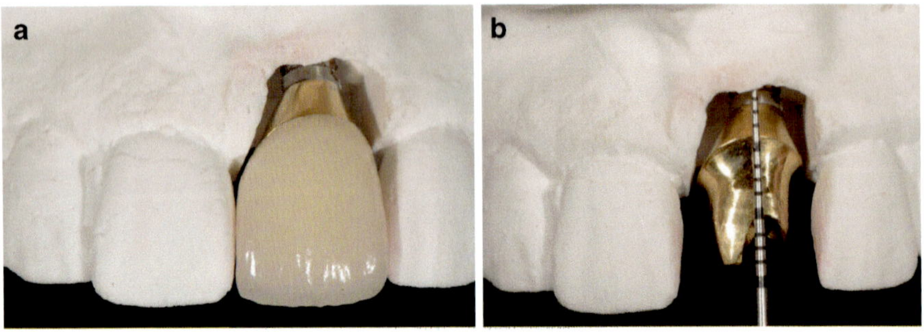

Fig. 3.15 (**a**) Image of cemented restoration on custom abutment. (**b**) Image of abutment showing the thickness of the abutment as it redirects the cement abutment palatally; this sometimes can expose some metallic components if the implant is not placed more apically

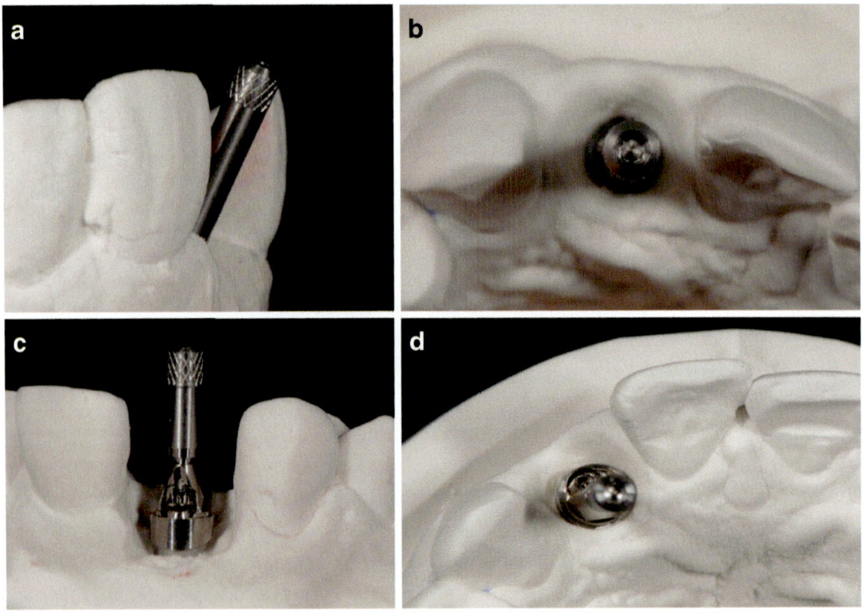

Fig. 3.16 (**a**) Image of implant trajectory illustrated with a long screw; the trajectory is toward the incisal edge. (**b**) Occlusal image of the long screw and incisal trajectory. (**c**) Image of the pre-angled screw-retained abutment; the thickness of the buccal area is required to compensate for the angle change. (**d**) Occlusal image of the abutment trajectory to receive the restoration is shifted to the palatal area

An example of implant that has been placed and integrated with the trajectory that points toward the buccal surface exiting at the facial cusp is shown in Fig. 3.17c, which illustrates the trajectory with provisional cylinder attached; there are several methods to deliver a restoration to have acceptable aesthetics. Images in Fig. 3.17e demonstrate the use of a pre-angled abutment that can provide an altered screw channel to retain a restoration using a secondary screw to engage the abutment. One disadvantage of using a pre-angled abutment is the thickness of the component on the facial side of the abutment. A display of an angulated abutment can be compensated for by having the implant placed more apically (Fig. 3.17d).

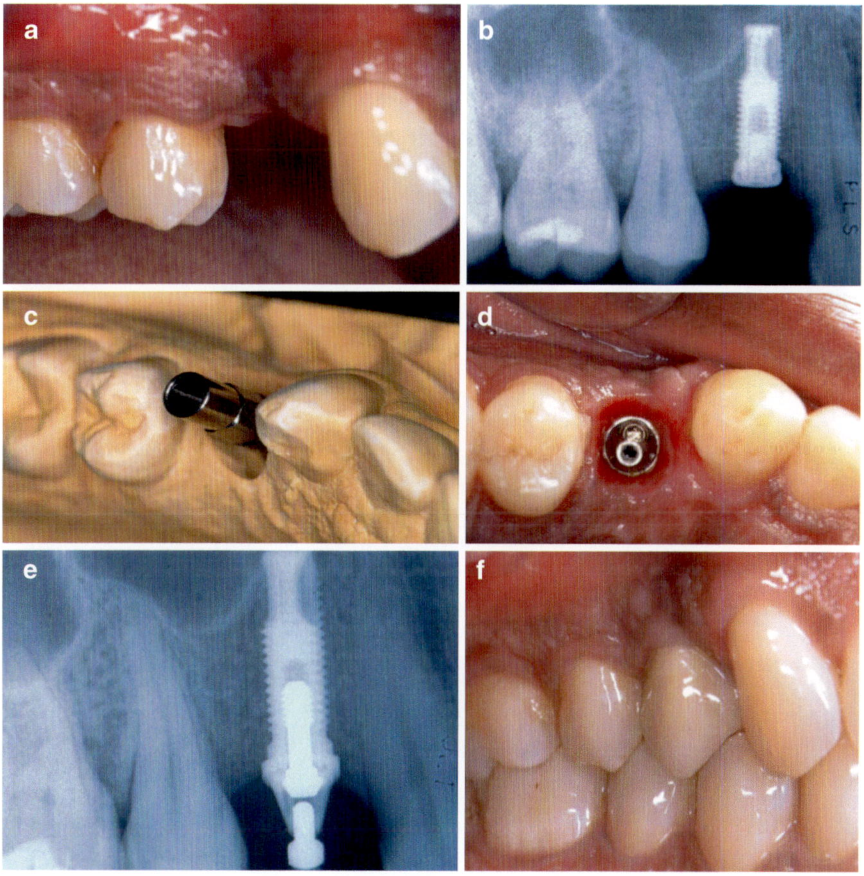

Fig. 3.17 (**a**) Lateral view of missing tooth prior to implant placement. (**b**) Radiograph of implant placed; the depth of the implant platform will accommodate pre-angled abutment; the implant was placed into host bone to avoid grafting. (**c**) A provisional abutment shows a buccal trajectory for a screw channel exiting too facial. (**d**) A pre-angled abutment to receive a screw-retained restoration is placed; the primary screw that retains the abutment to the implant is visible, and the secondary screw threads will accept the screw retaining the definitive restoration. (**e**) Radiograph with a provisional restoration in place shows the primary screw retaining the abutment and the secondary screw retaining the provisional restoration. (**f**) Lateral view of the definitive restoration in occlusion

There is another component that has been introduced that will eliminate the intermediary abutment; Fig. 3.18 illustrates how this component functions. This component (Dynamic Abutment Solutions, Lleida, Spain) can be used without involving digital dentistry. The screw channel can be shifted and then wax added and cast as in metal ceramic restorations [20].

Figures 3.18 and 3.19 illustrate the change in trajectory of the screw channel with the wax-up that will eventually lead to a screw-retained restoration. Note the minimal display of metal on the facial area of the abutment (Fig. 3.19a).

With the onset of digital dentistry, Ti bases that will accommodate shifting screw channels can be designed on various available software to accommodate positions of screw channels; the next examples of restorations will illustrate the versatility of these types of components that will replace cementation of implant-supported restorations.

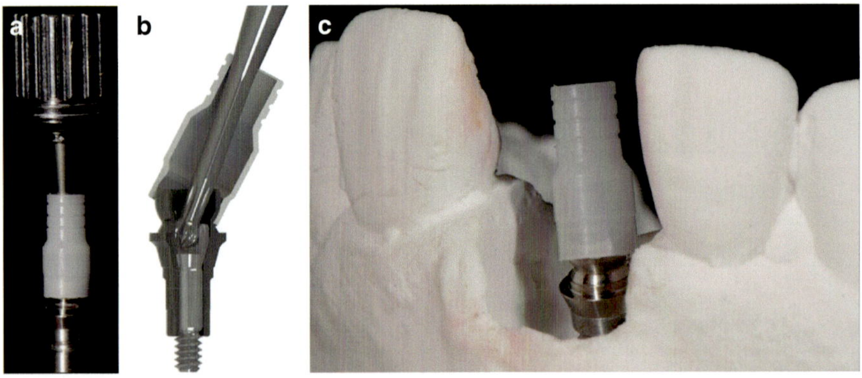

Fig. 3.18 (**a**) Image of abutment in axial direction. (**b**) Image of abutment with screw channel that can be shifted in any direction to receive the screwdriver. (**c**) Abutment on cast to demonstrate shifting of screw channel palatally

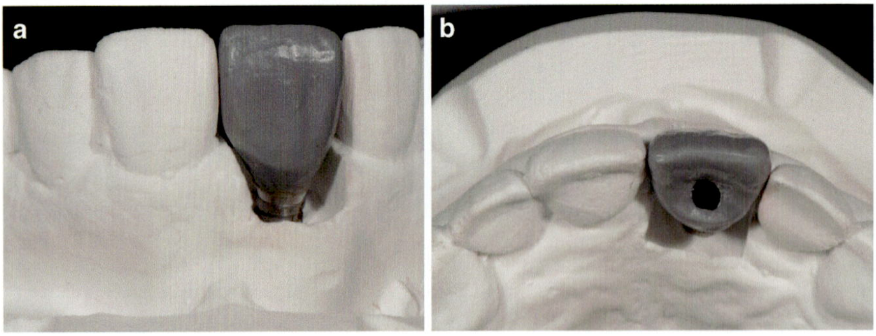

Fig. 3.19 (**a**) Waxed-up central incisor on Fig. 3.17c to show the submucosal contours and a minimum display of implant components and only one screw to retain the restoration (courtesy of Dr. Jack Goldberg for 19a, b). (**b**) Incisal view of wax-up showing the screw channel being shifted palatally

Figure 3.20a illustrates a patient presented with implants placed poorly; the screw accesses of the provisional restorations that were delivered had screw channels exiting the maxillary right central incisor in the incisal area and the maxillary left central incisor in the mid-facial area (Fig. 3.20b, c). The screw access openings needed to be sealed with polymethylmethacrylate to provide acceptable aesthetics for the patient (Fig. 3.20d).

The abutment that facilitated alteration of the trajectory of the screw channel was used (Fig. 3.21b) (Dynamic Abutment Solutions, Lleida, Spain). The zirconia restoration was milled with the screw channels incorporated and then cemented onto the abutment with screw channel shifted palatally. The images illustrate the screwdriver engaging the screws from the palatal screw channels. Figure 3.21b–d shows the definitive restorations with no screw access in the facial areas.

It should be noted that the screws which are torqued with a driver that is inserted at an angle to the implant have been tested in vitro with simulated cyclic loading. In

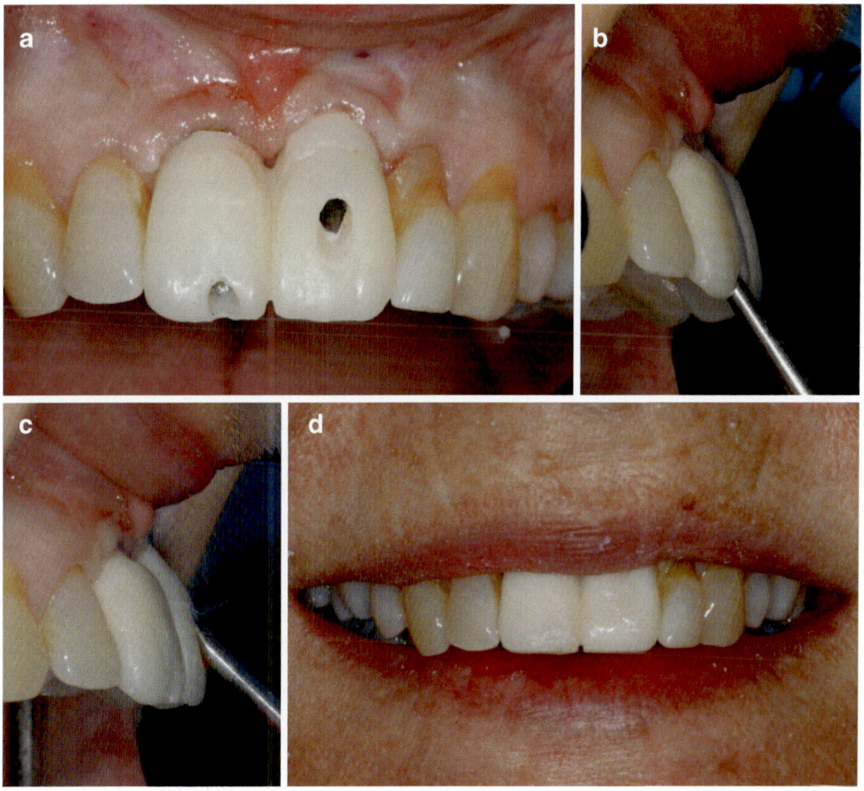

Fig. 3.20 (**a**) Facial view of provisional restorations with trajectories of implants projected facially. (**b**) Lateral view of maxillary right central incisor illustrates screw channel on the incisal area of tooth. (**c**) Lateral view of maxillary left central incisor illustrates the exit of screw channel on mid-facial area of tooth. (**d**) Sealed provisional restoration screw access with polymethylmcthacrylate

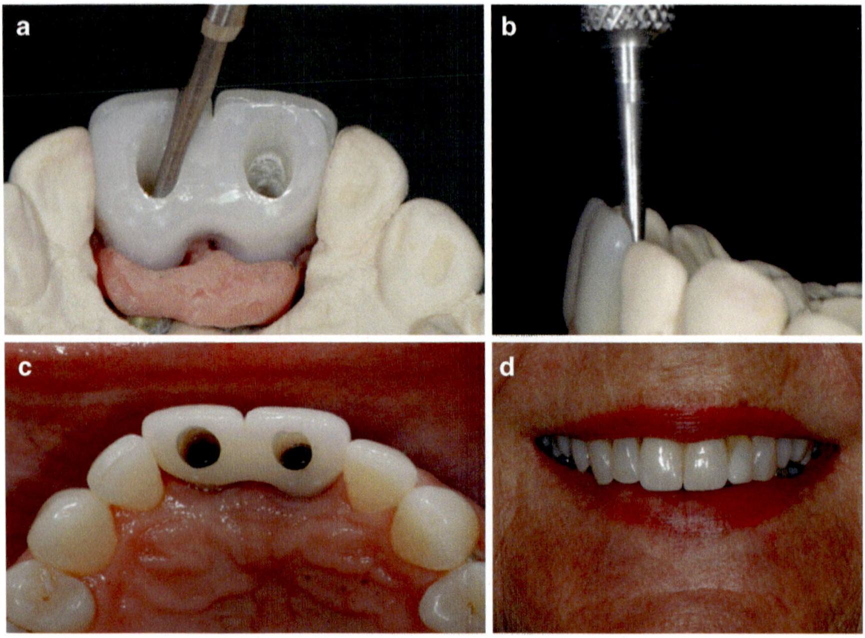

Fig. 3.21 (**a**) Image of definitive restorations with screw channels shifted apically for both incisors. (**b**) Image of screwdriver engaging screw from the palatal aspect of definitive restoration. (**c**) Image of definitive restorations from occlusal view intra-orally. (**d**) Image of central restorations from anterior

an article where external hexagon implants were used, the simulated restorations were connected in various degrees of angulation that span from 0° to 28° of deviation. The angled screws were torqued to 25 Ncm and the 0° control group torqued to 32 Ncm. Screw removal torque was recorded then using a mastication simulator for 1,200,000 cycles to mimic 5 years of mastication. At the end of the cycles, the screw removal torques were measured again. After re-torquing the screws, the samples were loaded to failure. The removal torque values of the various angulated screws were comparable to the control screws at 0°, and with load to failure, five screws fractured and the remaining samples fractured in the body of the implant. This in vivo study informs that the angled screw channels allow clinicians to provide adequate retaining forces by the screws that are angulated [21]. In other studies, similar outcomes have been presented [22].

Another example of having the advantage of being able to provide screw-retained restorations as compared to cemented restorations is presented. When screw channels can be altered to accommodate implant trajectories that are limited by the existing bony anatomy, the advantage of screw-retaining restorations is beneficial. Figure 3.22a illustrates a provisional restoration with screw accesses facially presented. This patient had a history of severe periodontal disease resulting in extraction of all of the remaining teeth due to poor response from periodontal therapy. Due to the significant attachment loss of the teeth removed, severe resorption of the ridges took place. Because of the advantage of shifting the screw channel, bone grafting procedures were avoided and the implants were able to be placed into host bone. Figure 3.22b shows the Ti base that is used, Fig. 3.22c shows the abutments attached to implant analogues on the cast and Fig. 3.22d shows the screw channels that would accommodate the shift in screw access palatally on the designing software (Exocad GmbH).

Figure 3.23 indicating maxillary arch shows screenshots of designing where the trajectories of the implants and screw channels shifted can be evaluated. Milled provisional restorations are shown with the screw channels transported to the palatal and occlusal aspects or the restoration.

Figure 3.24 indicating mandibular arch illustrates the path of the screw channels that are designed and the milled provisional restorations with the facial perspective (Fig. 3.24d) and screw channels in the lingual and occlusal areas of the restoration (Fig. 3.24e).

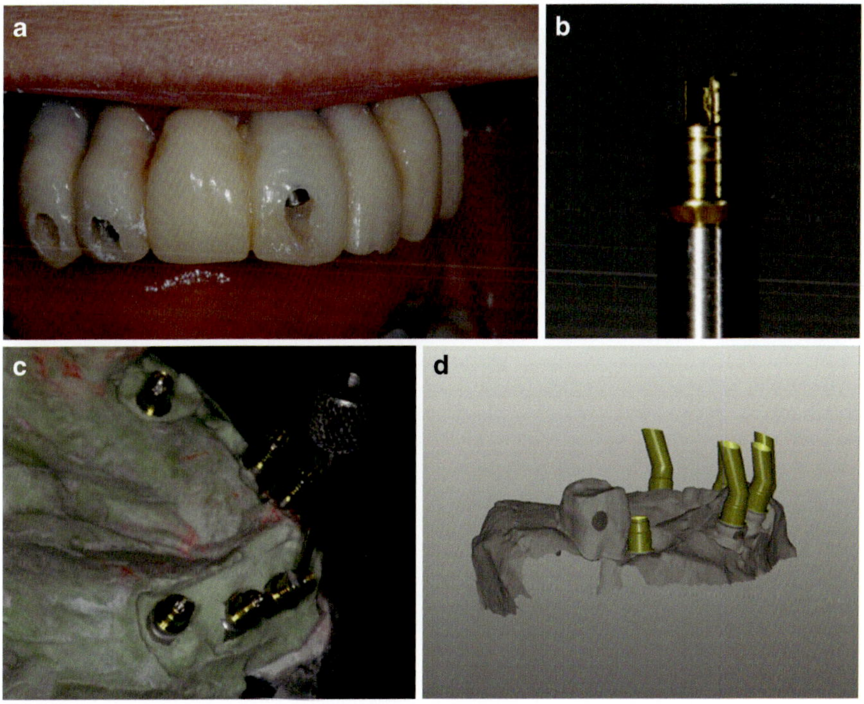

Fig. 3.22 (**a**) Intra-oral image of screw channels due to facially directed implants. (**b**) Image of Ti base to accommodate screw approaching from palatal direction. (**c**) Ti bases are attached to implant analogues and direction of screwdriver approaching palatally. (**d**) Screenshot of screw channels that are designed to show altered screw channels

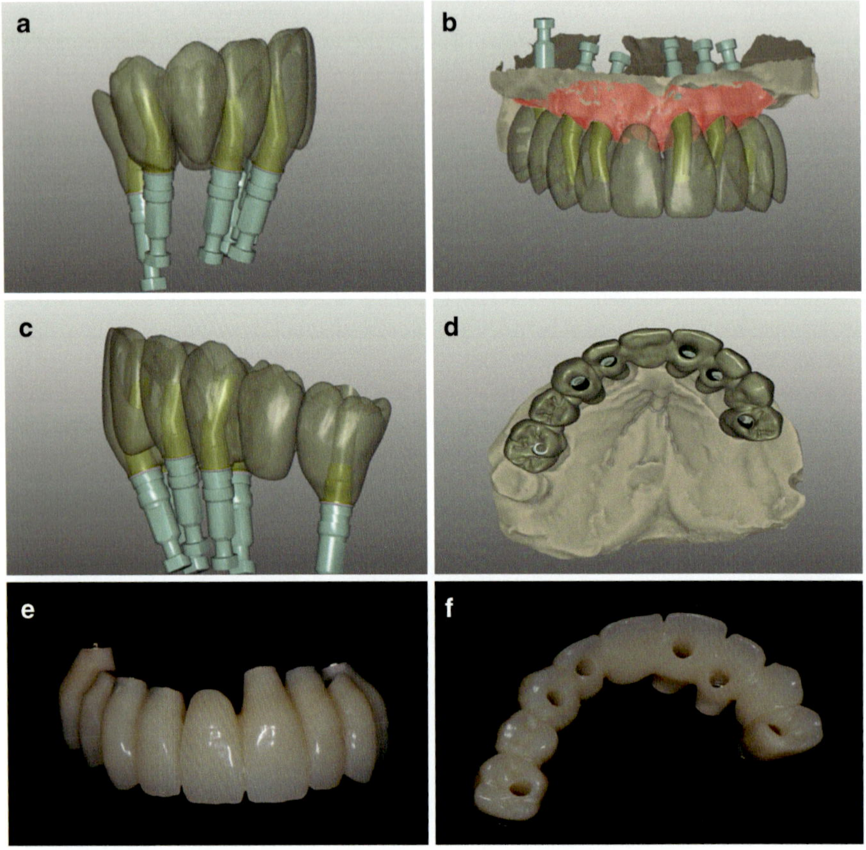

Fig. 3.23 (**a**) Screenshot showing the trajectory of screw channels with restorations adjusted to be translucent. (**b**) Screenshot from facial perspective with soft tissue. (**c**) Screenshot from lateral view showing screw channels shifted. (**d**) Occlusal image of transported screw channels. (**e**) Milled provisional restorations with Ti bases luted—note the minimal display of metallic components. (**f**) Occlusal aspect of provisional restorations milled after designing in Fig. 3.21d

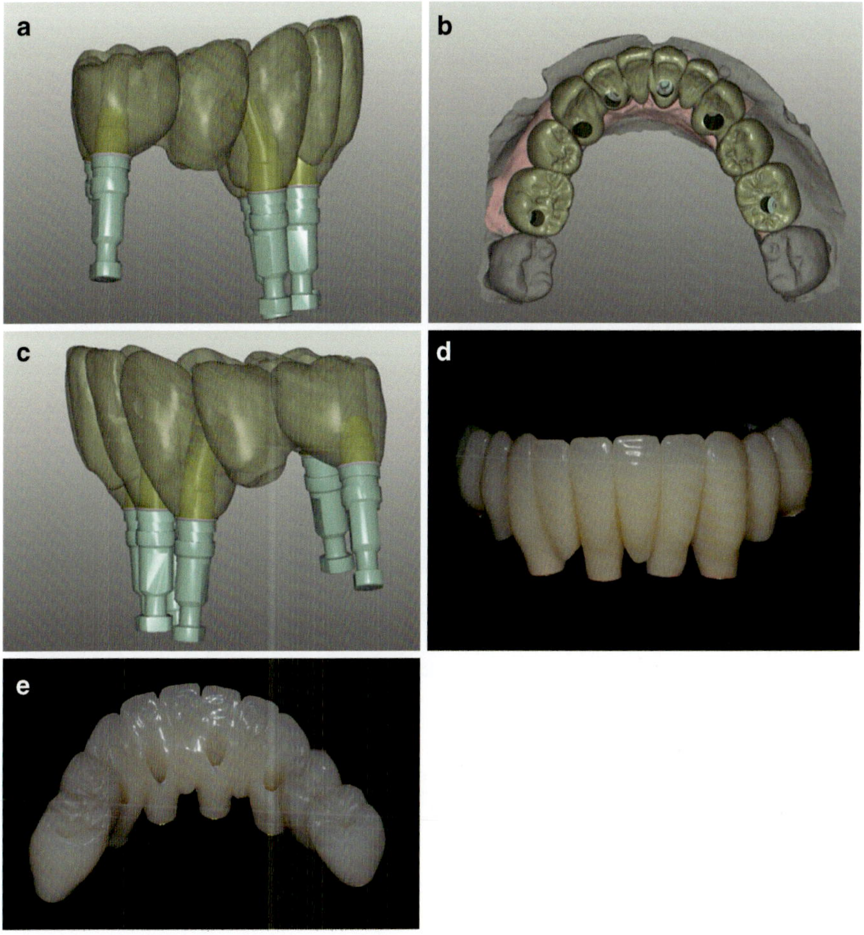

Fig. 3.24 (**a**) Screenshot showing the trajectory of screw channels with restorations adjusted to be translucent. (**b**) Screenshot from occlusal aspect showing altered screw channels. (**c**) Screenshot from lateral view showing screw channels planned. (**d**) Anterior view of milled provisional restorations. (**e**) Occlusal view of milled provisional restoration with Ti bases luted to the milled provisional restoration

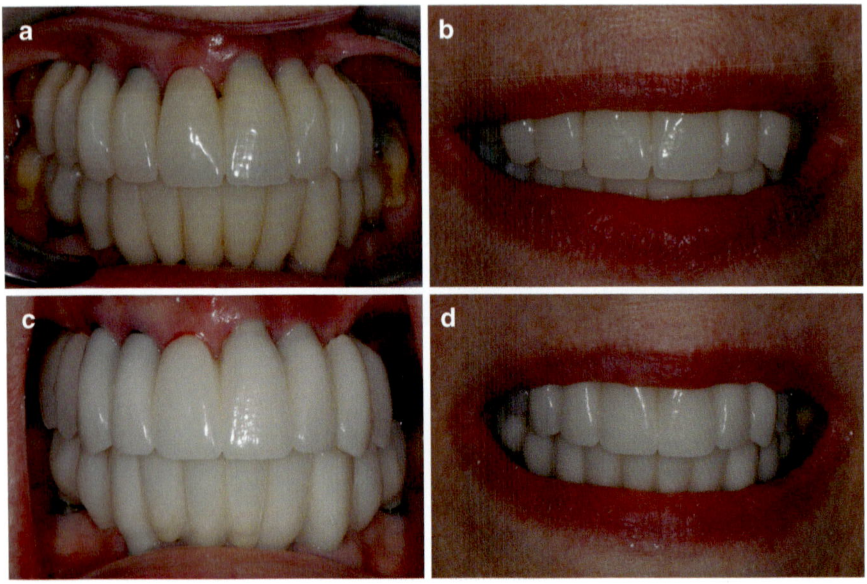

Fig. 3.25 (**a**) Intra-oral view from the anterior aspect of milled provisional restorations. (**b**) Extra-oral view from the anterior aspect of milled provisional restorations. (**c**) Intra-oral view from the anterior aspect of definitive restorations in zirconia. (**d**) Extra-oral view from the anterior aspect of definitive restorations

These provisional restorations also perform as prototypes of the restorations; if needed, changes can be made for aesthetics or soft tissue relationships to the restoration. The prototypes can be scanned, and the modifications can be incorporated in the definitive restorations. Figure 3.25 illustrates the provisional restorations and definitive restorations.

3.5 Summary

The benefits of screw-retained implant-supported restorations outweigh the benefits of cementing restorations onto implants. Cement retention, rotational misfits and needing to have implants placed deeper to facilitate cement abutments are shortcomings of cemented restorations.

With the newer materials and components that will allow minimal display of metal when the Ti base is cemented into zirconia restorations as seen in Fig. 3.19, there is almost no need to cement restorations on cement abutments that are attached to implants. In addition, with the newer components described earlier, the implants can be placed into host bone to avoid bone grafting, and with the screw channels being able to have screw channels altered up to 30° from the implant axis, the screw channels can be placed in areas that will not compromise aesthetics.

References

1. Linkevicius T, Vindasiute E, Puisys A, Peciuliene V. The influence of margin location on the amount of undetected cement excess after delivery of cement-retained implant restorations. Clin Oral Implants Res. 2011;22(12):1379–84.
2. Agar JR, Cameron SM, Hughbanks JC, Parker MH. Cement removal from restorations luted to titanium abutments with simulated subgingival margins. J Prosthet Dent. 1997;78(1):43–7. https://doi.org/10.1016/s0022-3913(97)70086-6.
3. Wilson TG Jr. The positive relationship between excess cement and peri-implant disease: a prospective clinical endoscopic study. J Periodontol. 2009;80(9):1388–92. https://doi.org/10.1902/jop.2009.090115.
4. Linkevicius T, Puisys A, Vindasiute E, Linkeviciene L, Apse P. Does residual cement around implant-supported restorations cause peri-implant disease? A retrospective case analysis. Clin Oral Implants Res. 2013;24(11):1179–84.
5. Quaranta A, Lim ZW, Tang J, Perrotti V, Leichter J. The impact of residual subgingival cement on biological complications around dental implants: a systematic review. Implant Dent. 2017;26(3):465–74.
6. Korsch M, Walther W. Peri-implantitis associated with type of cement: a retrospective analysis of different types of cement and their clinical correlation to the peri-implant tissue. Clin Implant Dent Relat Res. 2015;17(Suppl 2):e434–43.
7. Staubli N, Walter C, Schmidt JC, Weiger R, Zitzmann NU. Excess cement and the risk of peri-implant disease—a systematic review. Clin Oral Implants Res. 2017;28(10):1278–90.
8. Wilson TG Jr, Valderrama P, Burbano M, Blansett J, Levine R, Kessler H, Rodrigues DC. Foreign bodies associated with peri-implantitis human biopsies. J Periodontol. 2015;86(1):9–15.
9. Burbano M, Wilson TG Jr, Valderrama P, Blansett J, Wadhwani CP, Choudhary PK, Rodriguez LC, Rodrigues DC. Characterization of cement particles found in peri-implantitis-affected human biopsy specimens. Int J Oral Maxillofac Implants. 2015;30(5):1168–73.
10. Karl M, Irastorza-Landa A. In vitro characterization of original and nonoriginal implant abutments. Int J Oral Maxillofac Implants. 2018;33(6):1229–39. https://doi.org/10.11607/jomi.6921.
11. Chee WW, Duncan J, Afshar M, Moshaverinia A. Evaluation of the amount of excess cement around the margins of cement-retained dental implant restorations: the effect of the cement application method. J Prosthet Dent. 2013;109(4):216–21.
12. Winkler S, Ring K, Ring JD, Boberick KG. Implant screw mechanics and the settling effect: overview. J Oral Implantol. 2003;29(5):242–5. https://doi.org/10.1563/1548-1336(2003)029<0242:ISMATS>2.3.CO;2.
13. Chee WW, Torbati A, Albouy JP. Retrievable cemented implant restorations. J Prosthodont. 1998;7(2):120–5.
14. Okamoto M, Minagi S. Technique for removing a cemented superstructure from an implant abutment. J Prosthet Dent. 2002;87(2):241–2.
15. Real-Voltas F, Figueras-Alvarez O, Barrocal-Rodriguez S. Straight forward tip for identifying the type of screwdriver needed for screw-retained implant-supported prostheses. J Prosthet Dent. 2022;128(3):539–40.
16. Binon PP. The effect of implant/abutment hexagonal misfit on screw joint stability. Int J Prosthodont. 1996;9(2):149–60.
17. Wicks RA, deRijk WG, Windeler AS. An evaluation of fit in osseointegrated implant components using torque/turn analysis. J Prosthodont. 1994;3(4):206–12.
18. Britton-Vidal E, Baker P, Mettenburg D, Pannu DS, Looney SW, Londono J, Rueggeberg FA. Accuracy and precision of as-received implant torque wrenches. J Prosthet Dent. 2014;112(4):811–6.
19. Semper W, Kraft S, Mehrhof J, Nelson K. Impact of abutment rotation and angulation on marginal fit: theoretical considerations. Int J Oral Maxillofac Implants. 2010;25(4):752–8.

20. Berroeta E, Zabalegui I, Donovan T, Chee W. Dynamic abutment: a method of redirecting screw access for implant-supported restorations: technical details and a clinical report. J Prosthet Dent. 2015;113(6):516–9. https://doi.org/10.1016/j.prosdent.2014.11.009. Epub 2015 Mar 18.
21. Goldberg J, Lee T, Phark JH, Chee W. Removal torque and force to failure of non-axially tightened implant abutment screws. J Prosthet Dent. 2019;121(2):322–6.
22. Mulla SH, Seghi RR, Johnston WM, Yilmaz B. Effect of cyclic loading on reverse torque values of angled screw channel systems. J Prosthet Dent. 2022;128(3):458–66. https://doi.org/10.1016/j.prosdent.2020.12.020. Epub 2021 Feb 19

Implant-Related Tooth Intrusion and Migration

4

Winston Chee and Saj Jivraj

4.1 A Review of the Literature

Studies have been equivocal about the efficacy of this connection of teeth to implants; some studies indicate when there are non-rigid connections and rigid connection of implants to teeth that this is an acceptable procedure. When non-rigid connections are utilized, there are fewer complications when rigid connections are used [1–8]. More recent studies indicate that restorations with tooth and implant support are not as successful as earlier authors have opined [9–14]. In these articles, more complications have been reported like screw loosening, screw fracture, crestal bone loss on implants, unscheduled appointments and variability of the tooth mobility due to periodontal inflammation or attachment loss that reduces any support that is provided by teeth to the prostheses.

One manufacturer's approach to the problem had been the inclusion of an "intramobile element" into the implant. This resilient component was to provide flexibility to the implant to compensate for the mobility of the tooth. When this system was evaluated for that feature in an in vitro study, it was demonstrated that the "intramobile element" did not contribute to the flexibility of the system; furthermore, bending forces were transmitted to the retaining screw of the implant [15–17].

When teeth are connected to implants, two methods are proposed: one is when non-rigid connections are used with attachments (Fig. 4.1), and the other is a rigid connection when a cemented restoration is cemented on the implant cement abutment and the tooth (Fig. 4.2).

W. Chee (✉)
Advanced Prosthodontics, Herman Ostrow School of Dentistry, University of Southern California, Los Angeles, CA, USA

S. Jivraj
Private Practice, Anacapa Dental Art Institute, Oxnard, CA, USA

W. Chee, S. Jivraj (eds.), *Treatment Planning In Implant Dentistry*, BDJ Clinician's Guides, https://doi.org/10.1007/978-3-031-68726-6_4

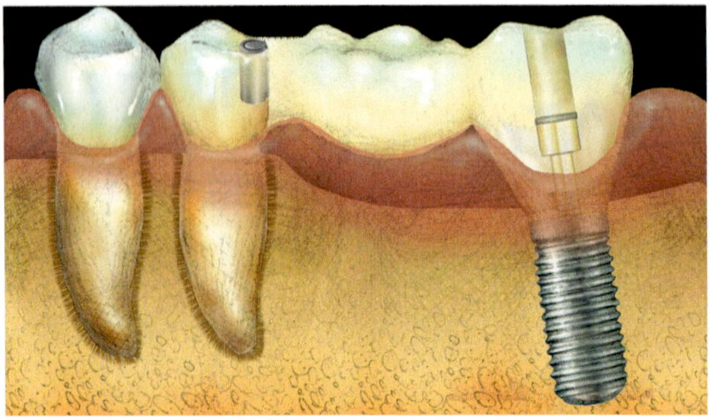

Fig. 4.1 Diagram of tooth connected to implant with pontic attached to the implant-supported restoration with the key attached and the restoration on the tooth with the keyway as part of the crown

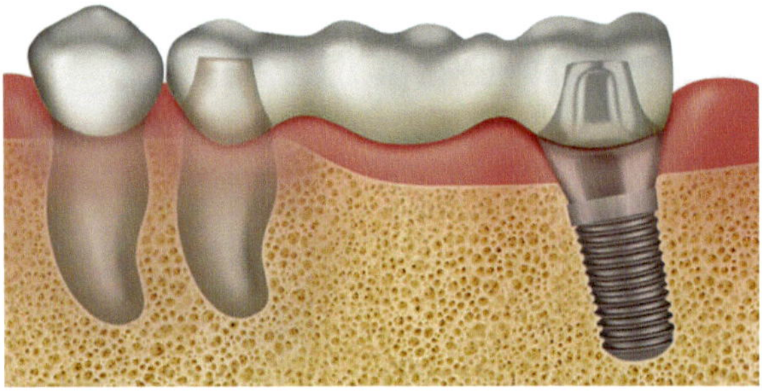

Fig. 4.2 Diagram of a rigidly connected fixed partial denture cemented to abutments that are on implant and the tooth

4.2 Intrusion of Teeth Connected to Dental Implants

Authors have discussed using a non-rigid connecting system to allow teeth to move independently of the implant while still being connected; key and keyway (matrix and patrix) types of connections have often been used. When non-rigid connectors are used, tooth intrusion has been observed frequently [5, 14]. The keyway is housed on the tooth, and the key is attached to the implant or pontic that is attached to the implant. Possible causes of this intrusion have been assigned to friction between the key and keyway of the attachment where occlusal forces depress the tooth. Friction between the non-rigid components prevents rebound of the tooth; this causes eventual intrusion of teeth (Figs. 4.1, 4.3 and 4.4). Similarly, micro-jamming of food particles at the bottom of the matrix is said to cause a similar intrusion as impaction of particles will prevent the tooth from rebounding to its original position. In addition, clinicians should take into account the physiologic mobility of the tooth and the level of the attachment and understand that the mobility of the tooth can be altered depending on any inflammation or attachment loss that can occur. It has also been postulated that flexion of the mandible could generate forces which cause intrusion of teeth connected to implants; however, intrusion has been documented in the maxillary and well as mandibular arches [13].

Other clinicians who have used rigid connections have had a lower frequency of intrusion but greater marginal bone loss. A high success rate of the connection has been seen with fewer unscheduled visits but greater marginal bone loss [7, 18].

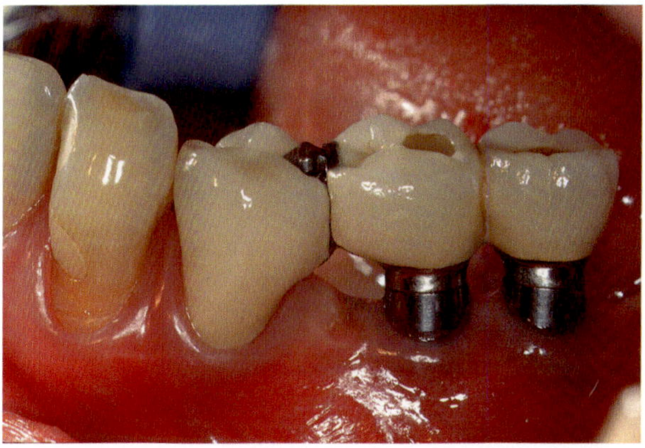

Fig. 4.3 Intra-oral image of a tooth that is intruded while connected to two implant-supported restorations

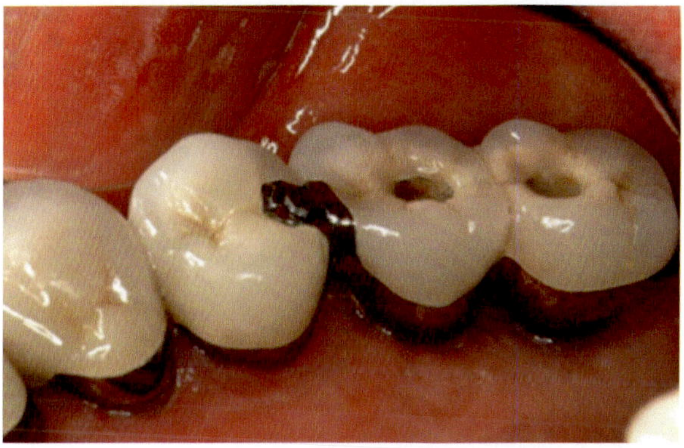

Fig. 4.4 A similar example of a tooth being intruded when connected to implant-supported restorations

When comparing the two types of connections, non-rigid connections have a higher intrusion risk, more prosthetic complications and more unscheduled visits to rectify complications that occur.

The most significant complication is the intrusion of the tooth when connection of tooth and implant takes place. But the phenomenon of intrusion when no forces have been applied to the intruded tooth in question is a mystery. Telescopic crowns on remaining teeth that are between implants have been used to incorporate the teeth into implant-supported restorations. It has been reported that intrusion of these teeth can occur in these situations even though there are no direct forces to the teeth when occluding [14]. An example of no direct forces to the tooth is presented in Fig. 4.5a–e; in these images, a patient who had several remaining teeth support a full-arch prosthesis in transition to a full-arch implant-supported restoration. After the implants were integrated, the treatment plan was to extract the remaining teeth. The patient refused to extract them and asked for them to be maintained. Copings were made over the remaining teeth and telescopic crowns that were rigidly splinted to implant-supported restorations; no occlusal forces were directed to the remaining teeth. After about 4 months, it was found clinically and radiographically that the teeth under the crowns intruded significantly. We informed the patient that the

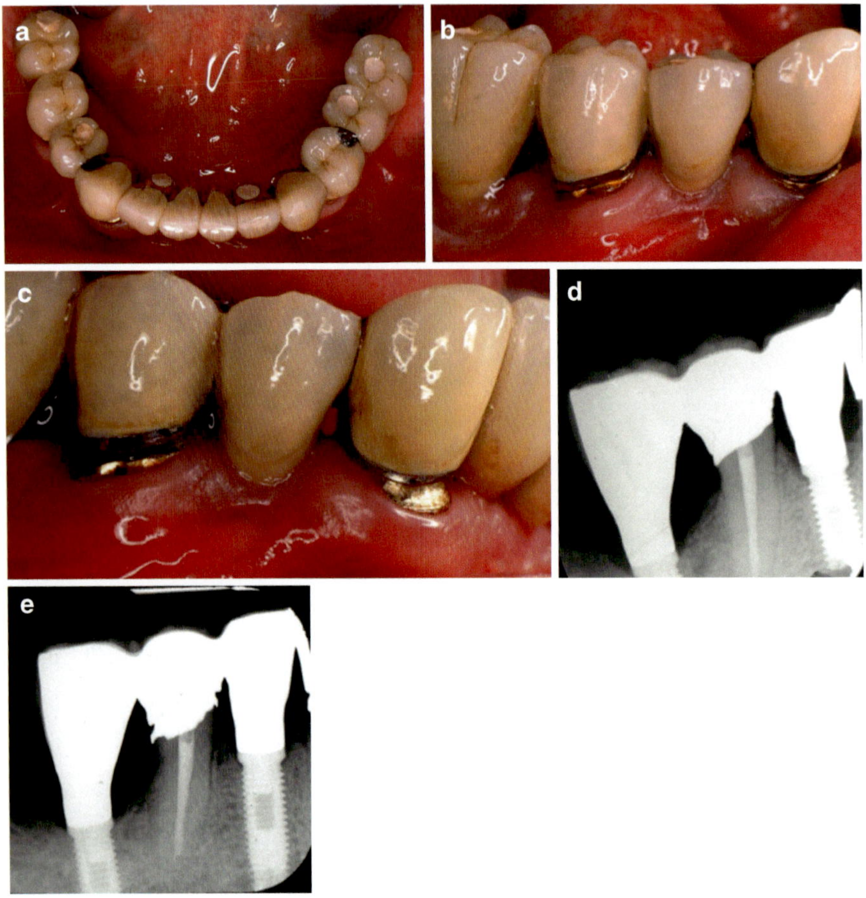

Fig. 4.5 (**a**) Intra-oral image from occlusal perspective on the mandibular right quadrant; the implant restorations #30 (mandibular right first molar) and #28 (mandibular right first premolar) are implant-supported restorations that are connected to the pontic that is telescoped over #29 (mandibular right second premolar). (Images 5a–e courtesy of Dr. George Cho). (**b**) Intra-oral image from buccal view shows #29 "pontic" with a metal margin seated well on the gold coping that was fabricated over #29. (**c**) Intra-oral image from buccal view shows that #29 tooth with coping has intruded. (**d**) Radiograph at the time of delivery of the definitive restoration shows telescopic pontic well seated to #29 coping. (**e**) Radiograph at 4 months post-delivery clearly shows the separation of #29 with coping that has intruded

intruded teeth did not support the restoration, and the patient agreed to have the teeth removed after which the telescopic crowns were filled with composite resin to eliminate the cavity of the telescopic crown and to make contact with the ridge as a pontic.

Two theories have been presented to describe this phenomenon. One proposes that the periodontal ligament atrophies due to disuse or lack of stimulation. There are so far no publications that can document the disuse atrophy of periodontal ligament when attached to implants [18–20]. Another proposed course describes the transfer of shock waves to the natural tooth, which forces the tooth into the socket [21]. This latter cause of intrusion is also not proven clinically or with any in vivo data.

Rigid connection of teeth to implants is not rational due to the adverse effects to the implants in the long term; non-rigid connection has the potential of intrusion of teeth [14, 22–24]. A review of the literature will reveal that there are many authors who advocate this tooth-implant connection despite this mismatch of mobility. This connection is used to potentially gain support from the tooth, to help to stabilize the tooth or to have the tooth reduce forces of rotation to the implant restoration-retaining screw [25].

Clinicians who advocate connecting teeth to implants rigidly accept the differential mobility of the implant and natural tooth. They deem that there is sufficient flexibility in the implant stack to allow sharing of the load. For this to occur, the implant components and their retaining screws must exhibit some degree of flexibility; the periodontal support of the natural tooth must be adequate and constant; in addition, the amplitude of movement of the prostheses must be minimal. This amplitude of movement will also affect the magnitude of the force to the screw joint that retains the restoration to the implant; this must be below the threshold of the preload of the retaining screw to prevent screw loosening. Constant bending of the screw will likely lead to metal fatigue and failure of the implant components [16, 26].

Others believe that a non-rigid connection placed between the pontic and the tooth will alleviate the biomechanical mismatch of mobility between the implant and tooth; different methods of this connection have been described. However, when this type of connection occurs, the phenomenon of intrusion of the tooth has been reported [3, 27, 28].

One rational method has been reported that can potentially allow sharing of load between tooth and implant and eliminate the problem of intrusion of teeth [29, 30]. This technique has been modified and will be described in the following patient presentation.

A patient with a history of periodontal disease had implants placed and restored in the mandibular left posterior sextant; the two implant-supported restorations were placed to restore #19 (mandibular left first molar) and #20 (mandibular left second premolar). After 10 years, the patient presented with significant bone loss around the implant #20 with purulence and bone loss peri-implant when examined. The treatment plan was to remove #20; it was not feasible to place an implant at the site after healing. Due to the occluso-gingival dimensions of #19, a cantilever of #20 as a pontic would not be a good indication (Fig. 4.6).

It was determined that a fixed partial denture would constitute #19 as an implant-supported restoration, #20 as a pontic and #21 as an abutment tooth. A non-rigid connection in the form of a deep removable partial denture (RPD)-type spoon-shaped rest was fabricated on the distal side of the pontic (Fig. 4.6); the pontic was rigidly connected to the tooth-supported crown (Fig. 4.7). A corresponding rest seat was prepared on the implant restoration #19 (Figs. 4.8 and 4.10). To allow retrieval

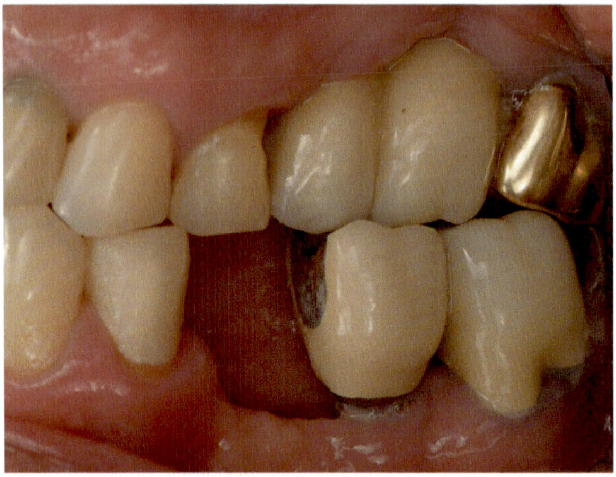

Fig. 4.6 Intra-oral image from the buccal view illustrating the bone loss in the area of #20 (mandibular left second premolar) to preclude a replacement of an implant, and a rest seat can be seen on #19 (mandibular left first molar). (Figs. 4.6, 4.8–4.11 courtesy of Dr. Joon Park)

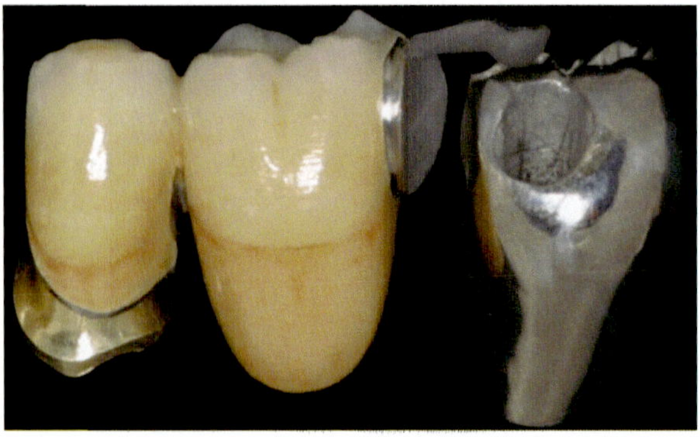

Fig. 4.7 Image of components from another patient's treatment illustrating parts of the restoration that connects implant to tooth; from the left, a gold coping to be cemented to the tooth, the crown attached to the pontic rigidly and the rest fabricated as part of the pontic; on the right is the implant-supported restoration with a rest seat to support the pontic. (Courtesy of Dr. Nikitas Mordohai)

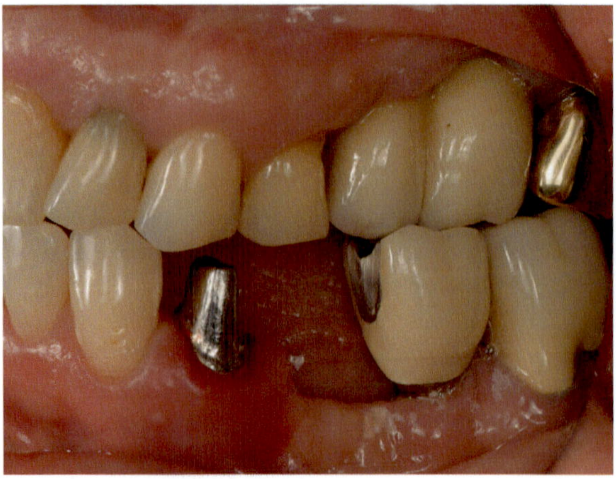

Fig. 4.8 Buccal view of the coping cemented on #21(mandibular left first premolar) and implant-supported restoration #19 with rest seat

of the implant restorations, a telescopic crown was cemented onto tooth #20 and the superstructures #20 and 21(crown and pontic) were cemented with a soft cement over the telescopic coping (Figs. 4.9, 4.10 and 4.11). This allowed removal of the superstructure from the tooth and removal of the implant-supported restoration if required. Mechanically, this system allowed loading of the implant and tooth when loads were applied to the pontic and free movement of the tooth when occlusal forces were applied to the implant alone; minimal movement due to direct integration with bone would manifest, when occlusal forces were directed to the tooth, and the tooth would be able to intrude and then rebound (Fig. 4.12a–c). No intrusion of the teeth or adverse effects to the abutments have been noted in restorations with this design.

With this restoration, the design addresses the problem of overloading the implant as the abutment on this fixed partial denture. When forces are directed to the

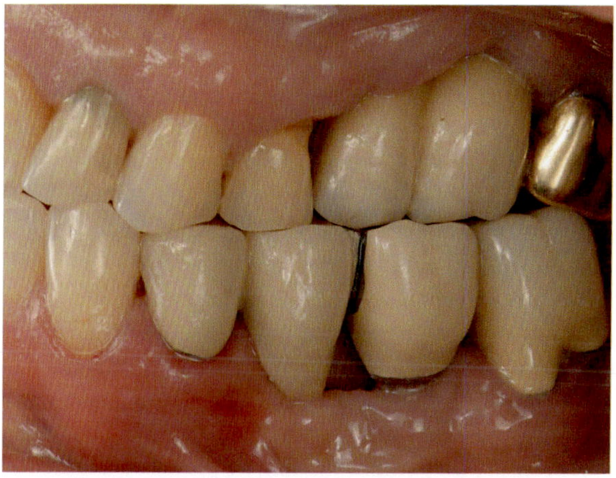

Fig. 4.9 Buccal view of the crown onto the coping of #21 with pontic connected to the crown and the rest seated onto the rest seat on #19

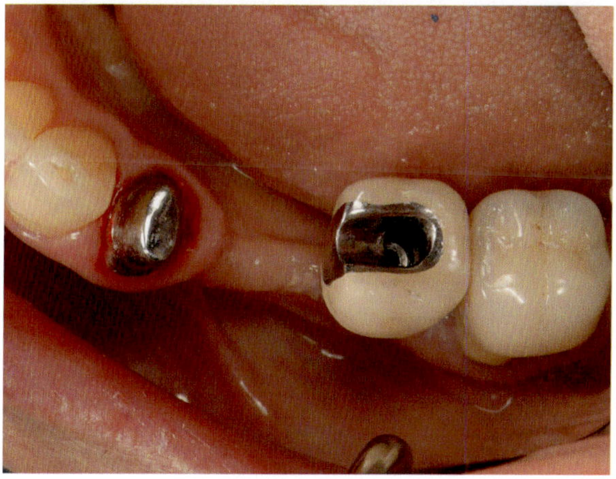

Fig. 4.10 Occlusal image of the coping cemented to #20 with rest seat on #19

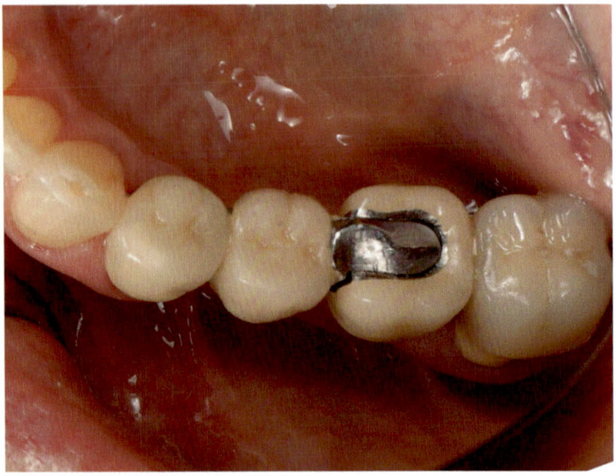

Fig. 4.11 Occlusal view of pontic connected to the crown that is supported by #21 tooth and the rest seated on the rest seat of #19 implant-supported restoration

tooth abutment, the rest seat on the implant will share the load as the tooth intrudes and the forces to the implant are directed axially. The axial direction of the forces to the retaining screws does not cause bending forces that may cause screw loosening, work hardening or fracture. When forces are directed to the pontic, both abutments can share the load as the rest can allow free movement of the pontic and tooth abutment—the rest seat will direct forces to the implant axially. When forces are directed to the implant abutment, it will accept loading axially (Fig. 4.12a–c).

Figure 4.1 diagrammatically illustrates how most clinicians connect implants to teeth; in this system, if we assume that the pontic is attached to the implant-supported restoration, when the pontic is loaded, almost no load sharing is possible with the tooth due to the rigidity of the implant connected to bone. There may be only a slight movement of the implant, and if the forces on the cantilevered pontic overcome the preload of the screw that retains the restoration to the implant, the screw can bend to allow minor loading of the tooth. Figure 4.2 illustrates rigid connection of a tooth and implant abutments in another configuration; in this situation, there is less incidence of intrusion of the tooth when connected to an implant; however, bending forces are directed to the implant and implant components due to the increased "cantilever effect" of the pontic and the cemented crown that is rigidly connected.

Another observation informs that the intrusion of teeth when connected to an implant can be reversed if the tooth and implant are disconnected; this has been reported in the literature [24]. As an example, Fig. 4.13 illustrates an implant that is poorly placed too palatally and coronally. This image was obtained when the implant-supported restoration was removed. The patient presented with a tooth #9 (maxillary left central incisor) that appeared to be significantly shorter than tooth #8 (maxillary right central incisor) (Fig. 4.14).

Fortunately, the implant-supported restoration was screw retained and could be removed easily. The contours of the implant-supported restoration showed the severe ridge lap of the restoration and demonstrated an anterior cantilever (Fig. 4.15).

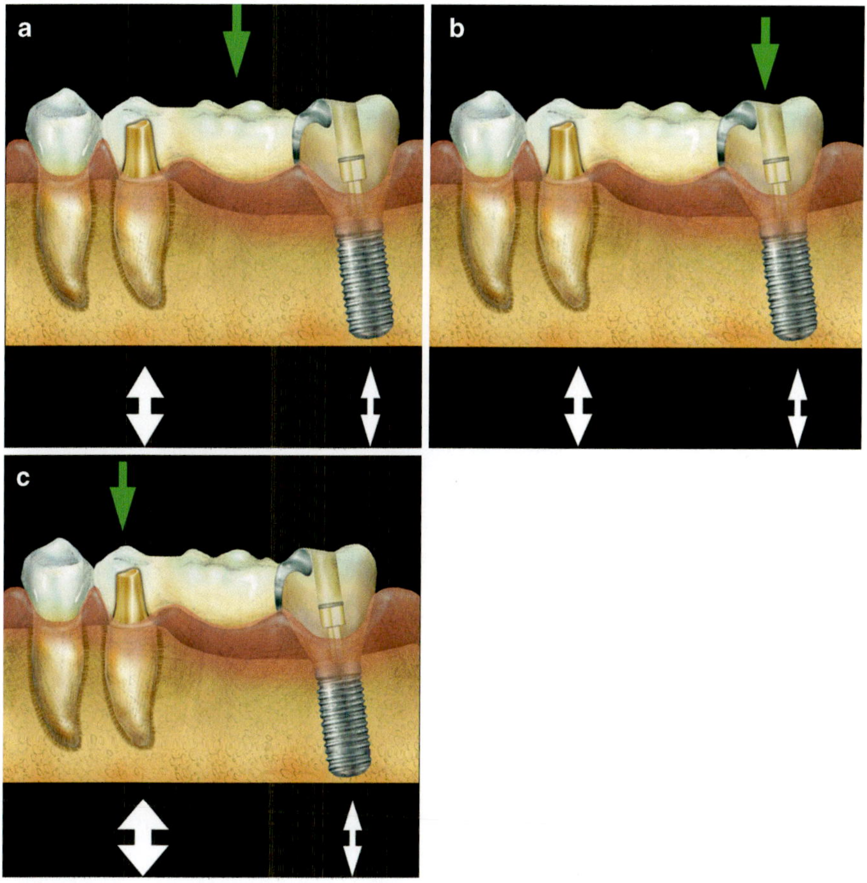

Fig. 4.12 (**a**) Diagram of occlusal forces applied to the pontic will allow sharing of forces to both tooth and implant—the tooth attached to the pontic will be able to move freely with more intrusion and will freely rebound when forces recede the implant can receive some forces that will be directed axially with no cantilever forces applied to the retaining screw or the implant. (**b**) Diagram of occlusal forces applied to implant-supported restoration; minimal forces would be applied to the tooth as the rest would allow minimal free movement. (**c**) Diagram of occlusal forces applied to the tooth will cause the tooth to take most of the load with some distributed to the pontic and implant again due to the design of the restoration; the tooth can move freely and rebound to the tooth's position prior to loading

The implant-supported restoration had a key that was incorporated into the restoration and inserted into the keyway that in turn was incorporated into the crown "supported" by the adjacent tooth #9. It was suggested by the prior provider that the tooth would provide support to the implant-supported restoration due to the malposition of the implant. With the intrusion of the tooth-supported restoration connected with the slot attachment, it is clear that teeth connected to implants do not provide support (Fig. 4.16). The reasons for the intrusion of the tooth are not known, as

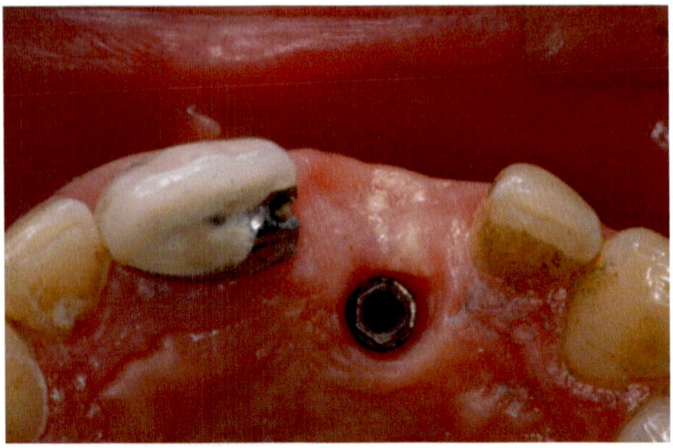

Fig. 4.13 Occlusal view of poorly placed implant in position #8 (maxillary right central incisor) that was placed too far palatal and too coronal; the adjacent tooth #9 (maxillary left central incisor) has a crown placed and has incorporated a keyway

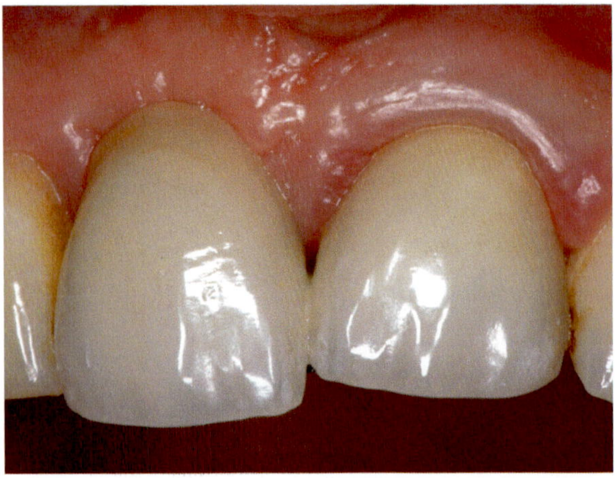

Fig. 4.14 Buccal view of #9 intruded by approximately 2 mm

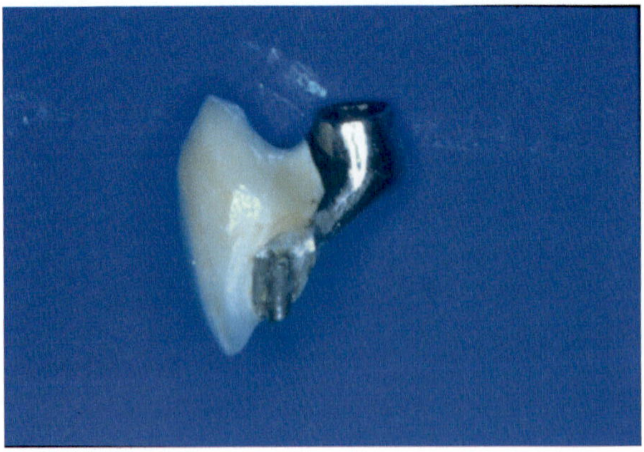

Fig. 4.15 Image of the implant-supported restoration was removed, and a key was seen on the mesial side and was inserted into the keyway of the crown on #9

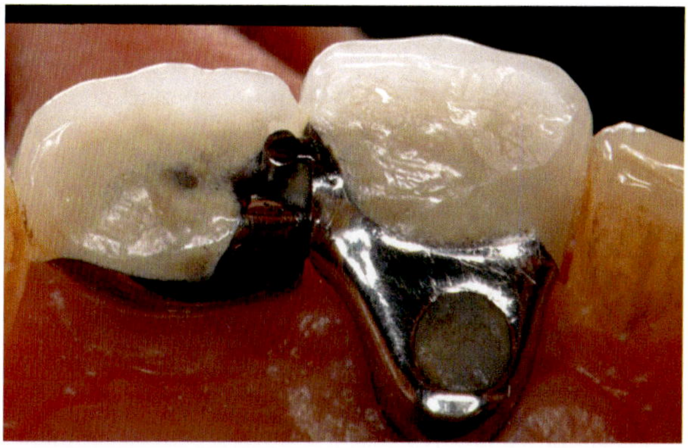

Fig. 4.16 A close-up image of #8 in position to illustrate the depth that #9 intruded

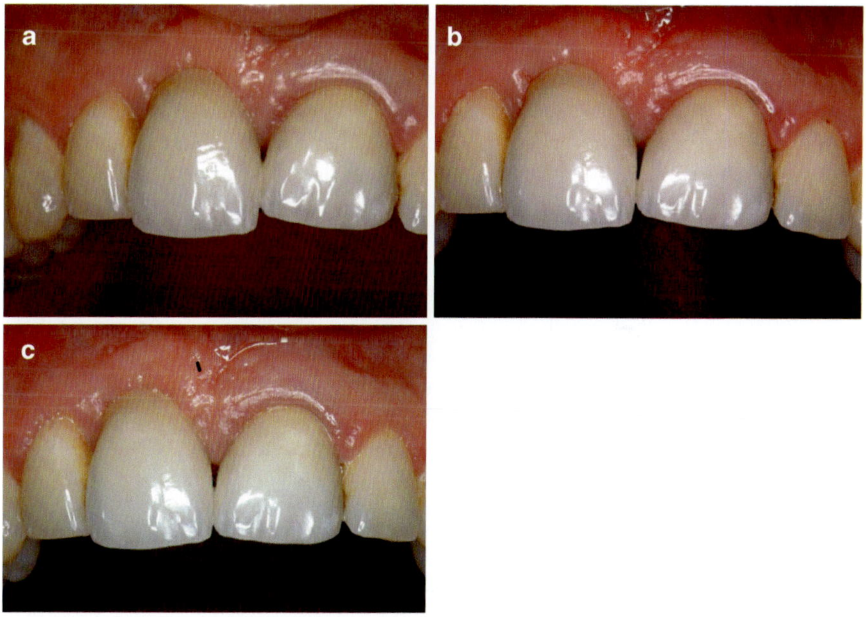

Fig. 4.17 (**a**–**c**) This collage of three images taken about 6 weeks apart; #9 rebounded to a position closer to #8

discussed earlier in the chapter; however, it was decided to disconnect the tooth-supported restoration from the implant-supported restoration. The key on the restoration was removed, and the keyway was filled with composite resin. Figure 4.17a–c demonstrates that over a period of 4 1/2 months, the teeth that have intruded can rebound; in this situation, the mandibular incisors that opposed the intruded tooth had to be re-contoured to accommodate the rebound eruption of the intruded tooth. The patient declined any further removal of tooth structure from the mandibular opposing incisors that might allow further eruption of the tooth and accepted the position of the tooth-supported restoration as in Fig. 4.17c.

Another example of teeth intruding though not connected to implants does occur; a patient was restored with a tooth that was restored in between two implant-supported restorations. After a 6-month period, the patient complained about having difficulty flossing between the tooth and implant both mesially and distally; after intra-oral inspection, it was discovered that the tooth between the implants intruded significantly (Fig. 4.18a). The proximal contacts were lightened to allow floss to pass freely, and this allowed the tooth to rebound (Fig. 4.18b, c). The intrusion could be caused by friction between proximal contacts that prevented the tooth from rebounding after increments to intrusion that took place during mastication [22].

Implant-supported restorations can be considered the most ideal replacement of a missing tooth; with some skills and experience, the restorations will present with both aesthetics and function. Intrusion of teeth connected to implants has been discussed earlier in this chapter. When patients have arches that have some missing teeth that are restored with implant-supported restorations, teeth adjacent to the fixed restorations often migrate mesially or distally. Publications have informed that up to 40% of adjacent teeth to implant-supported restorations cause proximal contacts to open, with more frequency of proximal contacts opening teeth migrating mesially. When teeth lie mesial to multiple splinted implants, the frequency of proximal contact opening is more. It has also been reported that proximal contact opening can occur within 3 months post-delivery of definitive restorations. Factors that

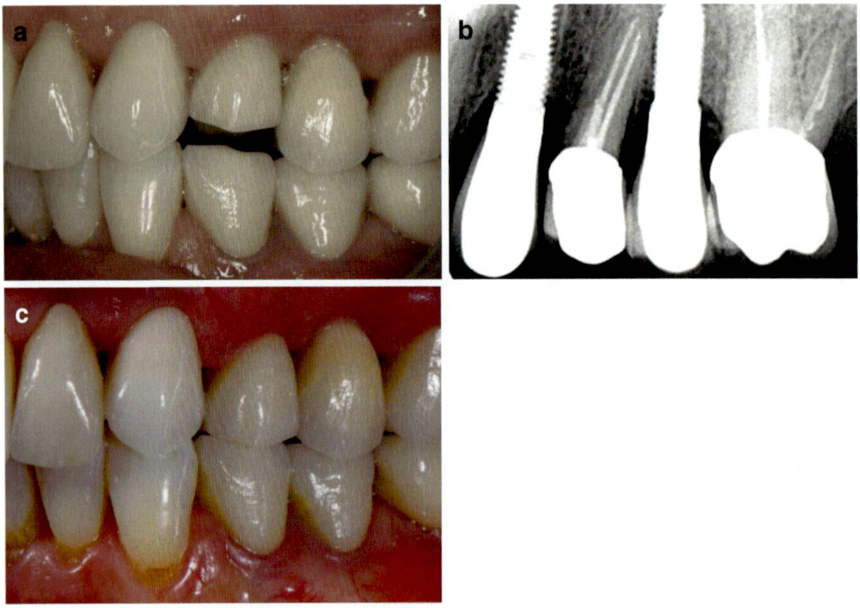

Fig. 4.18 (**a**) Buccal image of tooth that is intruded in between two implant-supported restorations. (Fig. 4.18a–c courtesy of Dr. Eva Beroetta). (**b**) Radiograph of tooth intruded between two implant-supported restorations. (**c**) The tooth rebounded after adjusting interproximal contacts to allow floss to pass freely

affect the magnitude of proximal contact opening are time of delivery of the prostheses and age of the patient [31, 32].

When patients have been re-called after delivery of the restoration, clinicians have often noticed the opening of proximal contacts. At other times, patients have complained of the issues of loose flossing, food packing and pain with trauma to the soft tissues in the interproximal areas between teeth and implants. Development of a notable diastema in areas where aesthetics is critical is an added problem [33, 34].

Publications of long-term follow-ups and systematic reviews demonstrate the high level of occurrences of open proximal contacts between implant-supported restorations and teeth; at present, there are no clear causes that can affect the migration of teeth. In situations of trauma to interproximal soft tissues or difficulty to remove entrapment of food, interventions to re-establish proximal contacts can be provided [35–37].

A patient presented with a concern about food impaction between a single molar implant-supported restoration #19 (mandibular left first molar) and #20 (mandibular left second premolar). The implant-supported restoration was fabricated of cast gold, and the adjacent tooth was restored with a small CL I amalgam restoration (Fig. 4.19). Fortunately, the implant-supported restoration was screw retained and could easily be removed; two choices were available: one was to add composite to the proximal surface of the tooth, and the other was to add composite to the mesial proximal surface of the implant-supported restoration. It was decided to prepare a cavity in the gold restoration to be retentive and accept addition of composite; this would allow the addition of the proximal contact to be extra-orally prepared, adjusted and polished with ease; it would also allow addition to more material should the proximal contact reopen in the future (Fig. 4.20). The added composite was adjusted to close the proximal contact, and the restoration was polished and replaced (Figs. 4.21 and 4.22).

When there are proximal contacts that are opened, screw-retained implant-supported restorations can easily be removed and contacts can be closed depending on the material that is used to fabricate the restoration. As presented above, the restoration can have added material to close the proximal contact by providing a

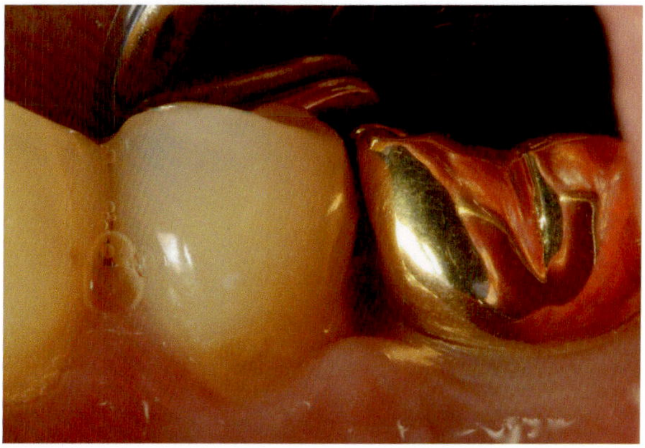

Fig. 4.19 Buccal view of the premolar migrating mesially to develop an open proximal contact

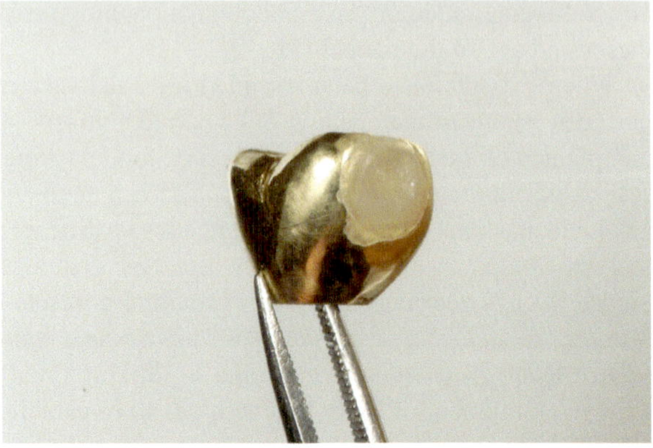

Fig. 4.20 Mesial contact of the implant-supported restoration re-contoured with composite resin to close the proximal contact

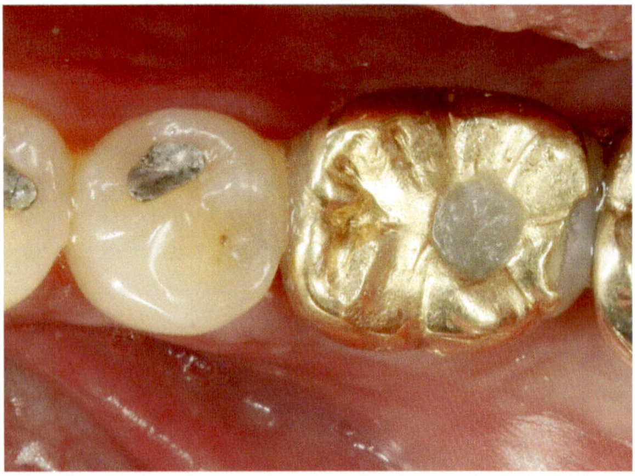

Fig. 4.21 Occlusal view of #19 implant-supported restoration that is seated with composite closing of the proximal contact with #20

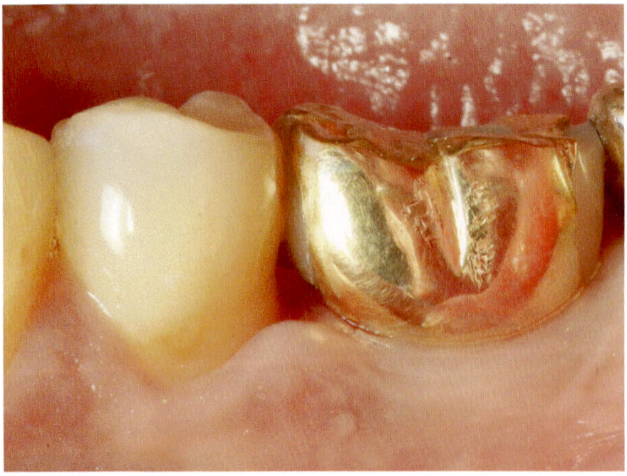

Fig. 4.22 Buccal view of #19 implant-supported restoration that is seated with composite closing of the proximal contact with #20

retentive cavity to retain the composite resin. If the material was fabricated with feldspathic porcelain bonded to metal or lithium disilicate, using hydrofluoric acid to etch the proximal surface would reliably add composite resin to the proximal surface to close the contact. Should the restoration be fabricated with zirconia, a protocol of mild air abrasion with silane can predictably bond composite to close the proximal contact; also occlusal forces are not severe to displace these additions [38–40].

If the adjacent teeth have proximal tooth structure facing the open proximal contact, adding composite to close the proximal contact would also be feasible. Should the adjacent tooth to the proximal site be restored with a full-coverage restoration, then bonding to the implant-supported restoration would be required to regain proximal contact.

The above methods depend on screw-retained restorations to re-establish the proximal contacts; with cement-retained restorations, there may be difficulty removing the restoration, and the restoration may have to be destroyed and replaced to close the proximal contact. It would be advisable to replace the restoration with a screw-retained restoration as the proximal contacts may require closure in time (refer to Chap. 3).

4.3 Summary

A review of the literature and discussion of the effects of connecting teeth to implants with different modalities have been presented. There is no doubt that the free-standing implant-supported restorations where teeth are not connected to implants are the preferred method of restoring missing teeth. In a situation when teeth do need to be connected to implants, a method of implementing the connection of teeth to implants has been described. It has also been shown that intruded teeth can rebound when disconnected. Opening of proximal contacts between implant-supported restorations and teeth is commonplace with more frequent contacts when teeth migrate mesially than distally. The only remedy for these open contacts is to be able to remove implant-supported restorations and then adding material to the tooth or the restoration in order to close the proximal contacts. Having screw-retained restorations would close proximal contacts with less difficulty if cemented restorations were delivered.

References

1. Kay H. Free standing vs. implant - tooth - interconnected restorations: understanding the prosthodontic perspective. Int J Perio Rest Dent. 1993;13:47–68.
2. Astrand J, Astrand P, Ahlen K, Borg K, Olsson M. Implants in partially edentulous patients. A longitudinal study of bridges supported by both implants and natural teeth. Clin Oral Impl Res. 1992;3:49–56.
3. Ericsson I, Lekholm U, Branemark PI, Lindhe J. A clinical evaluation of fixed-bridge restorations supported by the combination of teeth and osseointegrated titanium implants. J Clin Periodontol. 1986;13:307–12.

4. Olsson M, Gunne J, Astrand P, Borg K. Bridges supported by free-standing implants versus bridges supported by tooth and implant. A five-year prospective study. Clin Oral Implants Res. 1995;6(2):114–21.
5. Nickenig HJ, Schäfer C, Spiekermann H. Survival and complication rates of combined tooth-implant-supported fixed partial dentures. Clin Oral Implants Res. 2006;17(5):506–11.
6. Naert IE, Duyck JA, Hosny MM, Quirynen M, van Steenberghe D. Freestanding and tooth-implant connected prostheses in the treatment of partially edentulous patients Part II: an up to 15-years radiographic evaluation. Clin Oral Implants Res. 2001;12(3):245–51.
7. Naert IE, Duyck JA, Hosny MM, Van Steenberghe D. Freestanding and tooth-implant connected prostheses in the treatment of partially edentulous patients. Part I: an up to 15-years clinical evaluation. Clin Oral Implants Res. 2001;12(3):237–44.
8. Hoffmann O, Zafiropoulos GG. Tooth-implant connection: a review. J Oral Implantol. 2012;38(2):194–200.
9. Nickenig HJ, Spiekermann H, Wichmann M, Andreas SK, Eitner S. Survival and complication rates of combined tooth-implant-supported fixed and removable partial dentures. Int J Prosthodont. 2008;21(2):131–7.
10. Lang NP, Pjetursson BE, Tan K, Brägger U, Egger M, Zwahlen M. A systematic review of the survival and complication rates of fixed partial dentures (FPDs) after an observation period of at least 5 years. II. Combined tooth--implant-supported FPDs. Clin Oral Implants Res. 2004;15(6):643–53.
11. Ting M, Faulkner RJ, Donatelli DP, Suzuki JB. Tooth-to-implant-supported fixed partial denture: a comprehensive overview of systematic reviews. Implant Dent. 2019;28(5):490–9.
12. La Monaca G, Pranno N, Annibali S, Massimo C, Polimeni A, Patini R, Paola CM. Survival and complication rates of tooth-implant versus freestanding implant supporting fixed partial prosthesis: a systematic review and meta-analysis. J Prosthodont Res. 2021;65(1):1–10.
13. Block MS, Lirette D, Gardiner D, Li L, Finger IM, Hochstedler J, Evans G, Kent JN, Misiek DJ, Mendez AJ, Guerra L, Larsen H, Wood W, Worthington P. Prospective evaluation of implants connected to teeth. Int J Oral Maxillofac Implants. 2002;17(4):473–87.
14. Cho GC, Chee WW. Apparent intrusion of natural teeth under an implant-supported prosthesis: a clinical report. J Prosthet Dent. 1992;68(1):3–5.
15. Babbush CA, Kirsch A, Mentag HB. Intramobile Cylinder (IMZ) two stage osteointegrated implant system with the intra mobile element (IME): part 1. Its rationale and procedure for use. Int J Oral Maxillofac Implants. 1987;2:203–16.
16. McGlumphy EA, Mendel DA, Holloway JA. Implant screw mechanics. Dent Clin North Am. 1998;42(1):71–89.
17. Pesun IJ. Intrusion of teeth in the combination implant-to-natural-tooth fixed partial denture: a review of the theories. J Prosthodont. 1997;6(4):268–77.
18. Pesun IJ, Steflik DE, Parr GR, Hanes PJ. Histologic evaluation of the periodontium of abutment teeth in combination implant/tooth fixed partial denture. Int J Oral Maxillofac Implants. 1999;14(3):342–50.
19. Cohn SA. Disuse atrophy of the periodontium in mice. Arch Oral Biol. 1965;10:909–19.
20. Cohn SA. Disuse atrophy of the periodontium mice following partial loss of function. Arch Oral Biol. 1966;11:95–105.
21. Sheets CG, Earthman JC. Tooth intrusion in implant-assisted prostheses. J Prosthet Dent. 1997;77(1):39–45.
22. Wang T-M, Lee M-S, Kok S-H, Lin L-D. Intrusion and reversal of a free-standing natural tooth bounded by two implant-supported prostheses: a clinical report. J Prosthet Dent. 2004;92:418–22.
23. Garcia LT, Oesterle LJ. Naturel tooth intrusion phenomenon with implants: a survey. Int J Oral Maxillofac Implants. 1998;13:227–31.
24. Chee WW, Cho GC. A rationale for not connecting implants to natural teeth. J Prosthodont. 1997;6(1):7–10.
25. Velásquez-Plata D, Lutonsky J, Oshida Y, Jones R. A close-up look at an implant fracture: a case report. Int J Periodontics Restorative Dent. 2002;22(5):483–91.

26. Rangert B, Gunne J, Glantz P-O, Svensson A. Vertical load distribution on a three unit prosthesis supported by a natural tooth and a single Branemark implant an in vivo study. Clin Oral Impl Res. 1995;6:40–6.
27. Lundgren D, Laurell L. Biomechanical aspects of fixed bridgework supported by natural teeth and endosseous implants. Periodontology. 2000;1994(4):23–40.
28. Rangert B, Gunne J, Sullivan DY. Mechanical aspects of a Branemark implant connected to a natural tooth: an in vitro study. Int J Oral Maxillofac Implants. 1991;6:177–85.
29. Cohen SR, Orenstein JH. The use of attachments in combination implant and natural-tooth fixed partial dentures: a technical report. Int J Oral Maxillofac Implants. 1994;9(2):230–4.
30. Chee WW, Mordohai N. Tooth-to-implant connection: a systematic review of the literature and a case report utilizing a new connection design. Clin Implant Dent Relat Res. 2010;12(2):122–33.
31. Liang CH, Nien CY, Chen YL, Hsu KW. The prevalence and associated factors of proximal contact loss between implant restoration and adjacent tooth after function: A retrospective study. Clin Implant Dent Relat Res. 2020 Jun;22(3):351–8.
32. Koori H, Morimoto K, Tsukiyama Y, Koyano K. Statistical analysis of the diachronic loss of interproximal contact between fixed implant prostheses and adjacent teeth. Int J Prosthodont. 2010;23(6):535–40.
33. Varthis S, Randi A, Tarnow DP. Prevalence of interproximal open contacts between single-implant restorations and adjacent teeth. Int J Oral Maxillofac Implants. 2016;31(5):1089–92.
34. Manicone PF, De Angelis P, Rella E, Papetti L, D'Addona A. Proximal Contact Loss in Implant-Supported Restorations: A Systematic Review and Meta-Analysis of Prevalence. J Prosthodont. 2022 Mar;31(3.):201-209(30% open contacts, can damage inter prox tissues)
35. Bompolaki D, Edmondson SA, Katancik JA. Interproximal contact loss between implant-supported restorations and adjacent natural teeth: A retrospective cross-sectional study of 83 restorations with an up to 10-year follow-up. J Prosthet Dent. 2022;127(3):418–24. (35% open contacts, no inflammation peri implant
36. Goldstein G, Goodacre C, Brown MS, Tarnow DP. Proposal regarding potential causes related to certain complications with dental implants and adjacent natural teeth: Physics applied to prosthodontics. J Prosthodont. 2024; Epub ahead of print
37. Sfondouris T, Prestipino V. Chairside management of an open proximal contact on an implant-supported ceramic crown using direct composite resin. J Prosthet Dent. 2019;122(1):1–4.
38. Kern M, Swift EJ Jr. Bonding to zirconia. J Esthet Restor Dent. 2011;23(2):71–2.
39. Kern M, Passia N, Sasse M, Yazigi C. Ten-year outcome of zirconia ceramic cantilever resin-bonded fixed dental prostheses and the influence of the reasons for missing incisors. J Dent. 2017;65:51–5.
40. Al-Akhali M, Al-Dobaei E, Wille S, Mourshed B, Kern M. Influence of elapsed time between airborne-particle abrasion and bonding to zirconia bond strength. Dent Mater. 2021 Mar;37(3):516–22.

Impression Techniques for Implant Dentistry

5

Winston Chee and Saj Jivraj

5.1 The Conventional Method of Using Impression Materials

The object of making an impression in implant dentistry is to accurately relate an analogue of the implant or implant abutment to the other structures of the dental arch. This is affected by use of an impression coping, which is attached to the implant or implant abutment. This impression coping is then incorporated in an impression, and then in turn an analogue of the implant or abutment is connected to the impression coping. After the impression is poured, the analogues are then spatially related to the oral structures. In addition, the analogues are oriented with their relocation features that will be able to locate angled abutments when required. With implant impression copings, the coping is usually attached to the implant or abutment with screws. The impression material used is usually an elastomeric impression material; the most widely used and shown to be the most appropriate due to its characteristics is polyvinyl siloxane (PVS) impression material [1, 2].

The impression coping takes two general forms. One is the transfer impression coping, which is retained in the mouth, when the set impression is removed. The other type, known as the pickup impression coping, is incorporated in the set impression and removed from the mouth together. For both types of impression coping, a radiograph should be taken to confirm seating when the impression coping implant interface is submucosal.

Characteristics of the transfer-type impression coping are that it remains in the mouth on removal of the set impression, the coping is then removed from the patient and then the implant analogue is connected to the transfer impression coping. This

W. Chee (✉)
Advanced Prosthodontics, Herman Ostrow School of Dentistry, University of Southern California, Los Angeles, CA, USA

S. Jivraj
Private Practice, Anacapa Dental Art Institute, Oxnard, CA, USA

W. Chee, S. Jivraj (eds.), *Treatment Planning In Implant Dentistry*, BDJ Clinician's Guides, https://doi.org/10.1007/978-3-031-68726-6_5

assembly is then replaced in the indentations recorded in the set impression. Custom trays are not required when transfer impression copings are used (Figs. 5.1, 5.2 and 5.3).

With the pickup impression copings, a custom tray is fabricated to expose the impression coping screws; after the impression material is set, the impression copings are unscrewed and removed together with the set impression. The analogues are then attached to the impression copings that are embedded in the impression when removed from the mouth (Figs. 5.4, 5.5 and 5.6).

It has been documented that the pickup-type impression coping is more accurate than transfer copings, as errors occur on removal and replacement of the transfer-type impression copings, especially in the coronal-apical direction [3–5].

However, there are indications to use the transfer-type impression coping; for example, when there is limited mouth opening, there may not be sufficient space for access to the screws that need to be tightened and released with pickup-type impression copings. Patients with an exaggerated gag reflex would indicate the usage of transfer impression copings in anticipation to a patient requiring the impression tray to be removed due to a gag reflex or to facilitate a more comfortable experience with transfer-type impression copings as the impression can be removed more quickly than with the use of pickup impression copings.

The fidelity of the impression with respect to dimensional stability is critical; small discrepancies can lead to difficulty when the restoration is fabricated and delivered. Figure 5.7 illustrates a situation where a transfer-type impression coping was used, demonstrating that a slight error resulted in poor seating of the restoration due to interference with the proximal contacts. The impression was repeated with a pickup impression coping; the accuracy allowed a better fit of the proximal contacts and allowed a more efficient delivery of the completed restoration with minimal adjustments. These errors are more obvious when compared to conventional tooth-supported fixed prosthodontics compared to dental implants, due to the precise

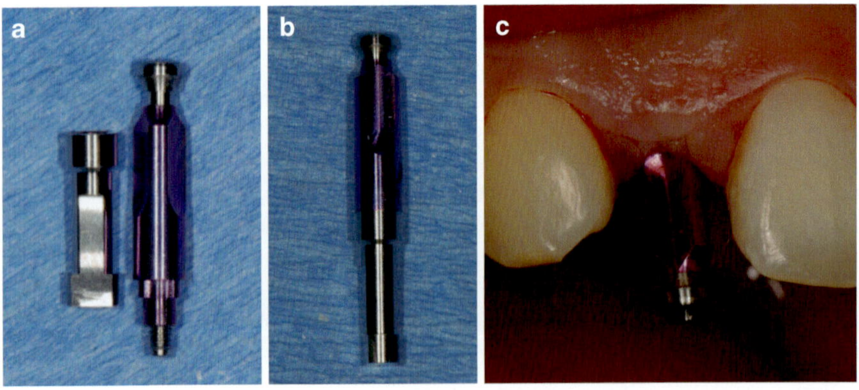

Fig. 5.1 (**a**) Transfer impression coping and implant analogue disassembled. (**b**) Transfer impression coping assembled. (**c**) Transfer impression coping attached to implant intra-orally

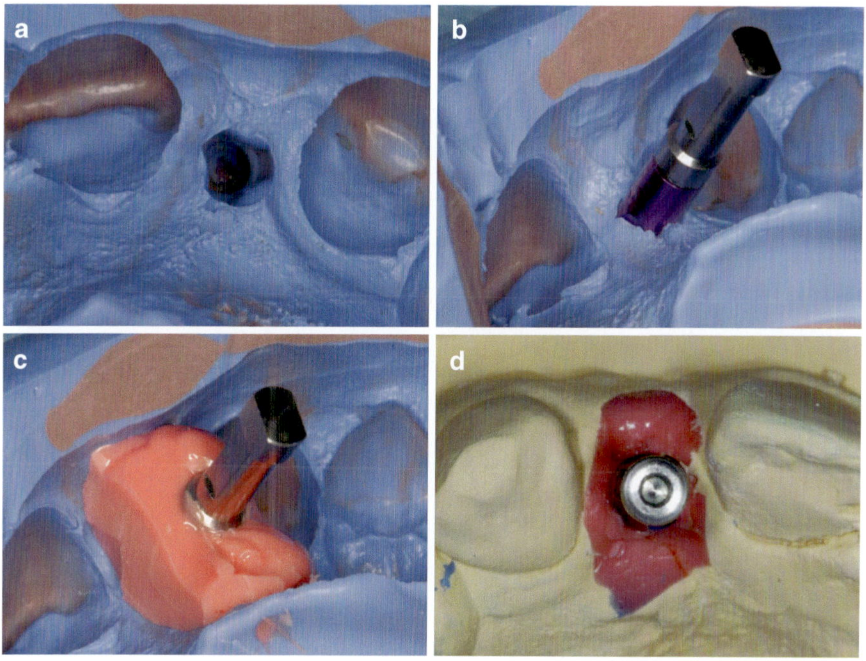

Fig. 5.2 (**a**) After removal of the impression, a clear imprint of the transfer impression coping is recorded. (**b**) The transfer impression coping attached to the implant analogue is wetted and then placed into the imprint recorded in the impression material. (**c**) Prior to pouring the impression, a soft tissue cast is formed around the analogue to facilitate soft tissue contours being formed. (**d**) A set cast with the impression coping in place

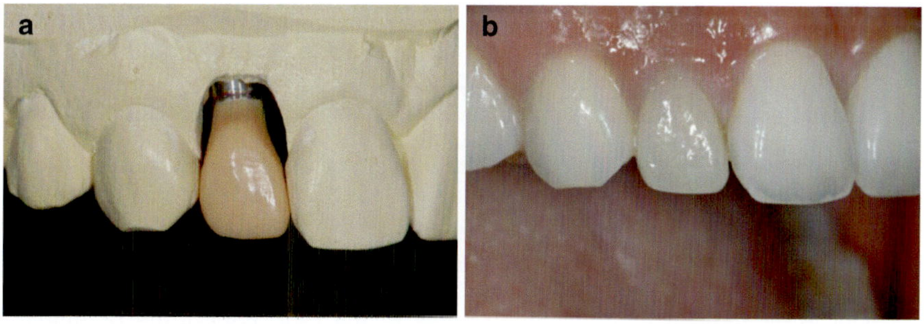

Fig. 5.3 (**a**) A wax-up of the restoration after removal of the soft tissue cast allows forming the submucosal contours. (**b**) Provisional restoration is fabricated from the wax-up with the contours supporting the soft tissue profile for an ideal aesthetic outcome. (Courtesy of Dr. George Cho Figs. 5.1–5.3)

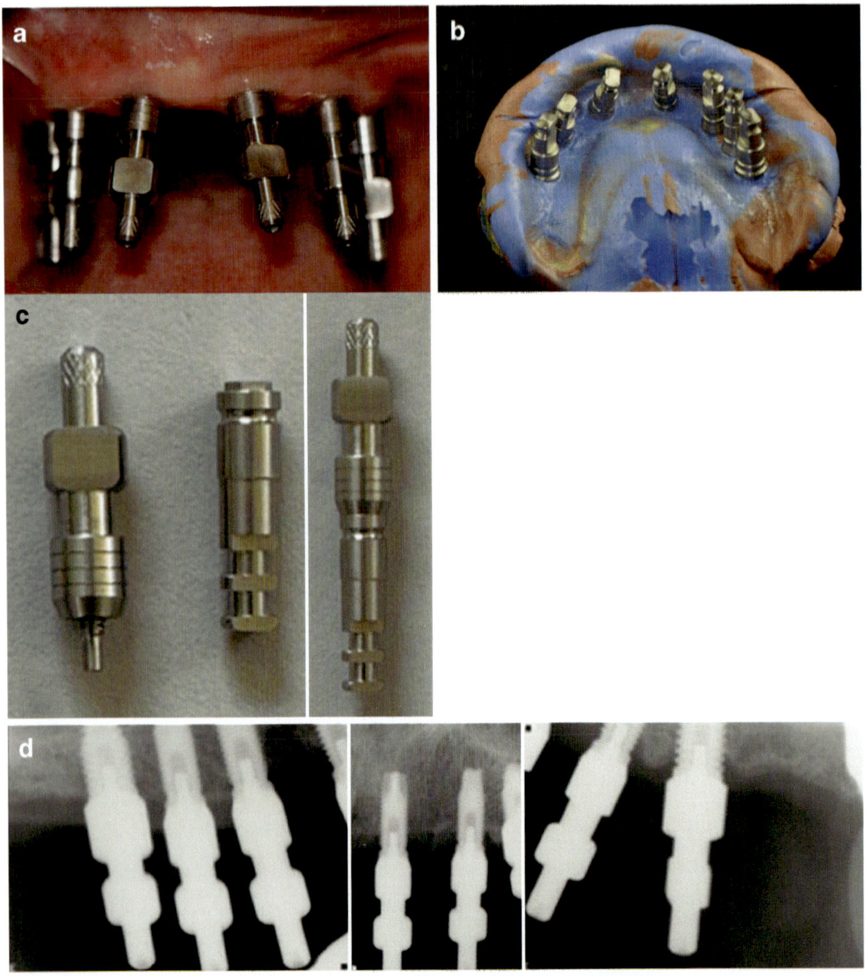

Fig. 5.4 (**a**) Intra-oral image of pickup impression copings attached to implants. (**b**) Implant analogues attached to the impression copings that are embedded into the impression material. (**c**) Images of the pickup impression copings disassembled and assembled. (**d**) Radiographs to confirm seating of the impression copings to the implants

machine fit of implant components and due to the rigid connection of implant to bone.

When impressions are required for multi-implant restorations such as full-arch restorations, the precision of the impression is even more critical. This is because cast frameworks or milled zirconia restorations will be constructed from the master cast; misfit in the frameworks or milled zirconia restorations can lead to stress applied to the implants and restoration when passivity of the screw-retained restoration is not achieved.

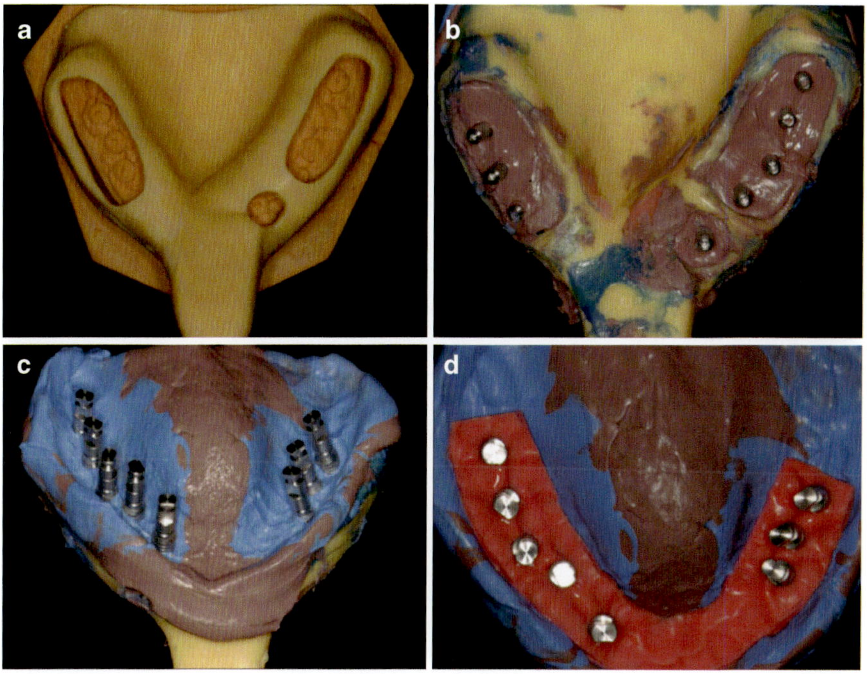

Fig. 5.5 (**a**) Custom tray fabricated to allow retention screw of the pickup impression copings to be released in order to remove the impression copings together with the custom tray. (**b**) The set impression material with the screws exposed to facilitate removal of the impression copings. (**c**) Implant analogues are attached to the pickup impression copings. (**d**) Soft tissue cast is placed around the implant analogues to allow submucosal contours to be developed

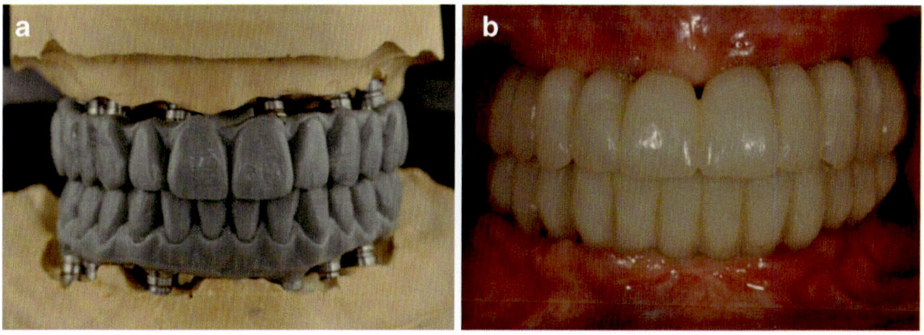

Fig. 5.6 (**a**) Casts from the impression are shown with the soft tissue cast removed in order to develop the submucosal contours of the restoration. (**b**) Intra-oral view of the provisional restorations fabricated from the impressions made

Though pickup-type impression copings have been documented to be more precise than transfer impression copings, many articles have been written with in vitro studies that have been carried out to evaluate methods to improve the fidelity of

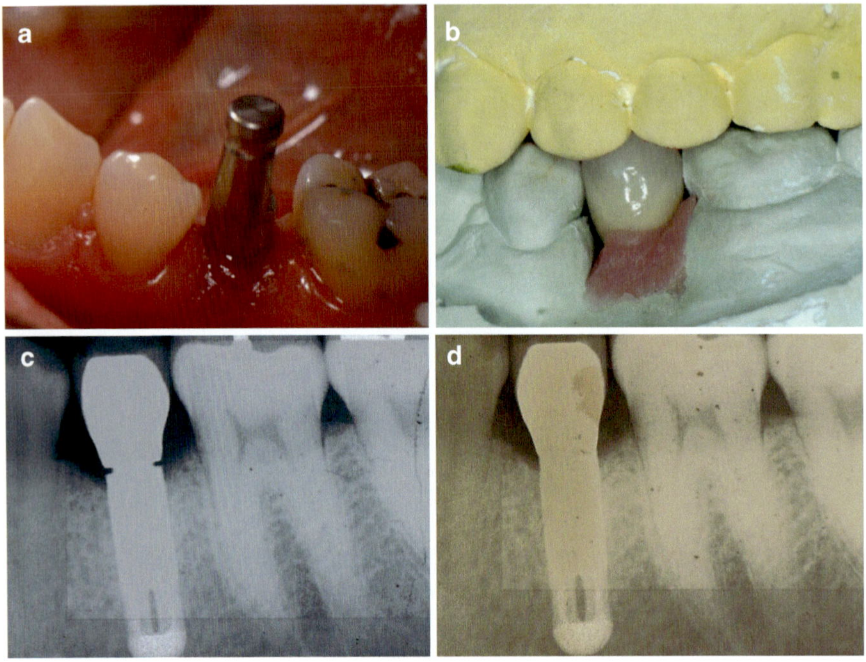

Fig. 5.7 (**a**) Intra-oral placement of transfer impression coping. (**b**) Restoration fabricated from cast poured from impression using transfer impression coping. (**c**) Radiograph of restoration not seating due to malposition of implant analogue. (**d**) Radiograph of restoration seated after remaking impression with pickup impression coping

impressions with the use of pickup-type impression copings alone. Some advocate connecting the impression copings together intra-orally prior to impression making with acrylic resin. There are studies that are equivocal; some indicate that impression copings that are splinted with acrylic are more precise, and others indicate that non-splinted impression copings are equally precise [6–8]. Others advocate the use of impression plaster to connect the impression copings [9]. Manufacturers have developed impression copings with "metal wings" that can be connected with acrylic resin to reduce the bulk of shrinking acrylic to further improve dimensional stability of the impression in order to obtain a cast that has high fidelity to the implant positions [10]. Yet others have advocated corrected impression techniques where impression copings are connected then with only one impression coping related to the cast; the other analogues are retrofitted to the cast to compensate for distortions of the impression material, and the distortions of the setting die master cast material. Other authors have demonstrated that none of the above procedures are likely to improve the fidelity of the impression over the use of a rigid custom tray and pickup-type impression copings with an elastomeric impression material [6–8].

Another consideration is that impressions made of implants with internal connections might cause difficulty in removal of diverging implants when pickup impression copings are splinted. When the pickup impression copings are used in significantly diverging internal connection implants, it has been reported that impressions can be less accurate [11]. In this situation with diverging implants with internal connections, transfer impression copings might be indicated.

Based on the above, the authors' suggestion is to use a custom tray which is rigid with openings to allow access to the retaining screws of pickup impression copings and use of a polyvinyl siloxane impression material. With the use of this technique, a cast is poured with implant analogues in place.

This method of making impressions of multiple implants is favourable; however, other methods as discussed might be used due to limitations described above. The next step to test the fidelity of the cast obtained by any of the above methods is best verified with a "verification jig". This is a wafer of mounting plaster that has minimal setting expansion; the wafer is connected to temporary cylinders that will be fabricated on the cast obtained (Fig. 5.8). It will be 4–5 mm thick and attached to metal provisional restoration abutments; this verification jig will be transferred to the implants intra-orally, placed on the implants and then torqued to the recommended torque forces to seat the jig; if the cast is accurate, the verification jig will not fracture. Should it fracture, the impression will need to be retaken and the process repeated till a cast which is verified can be used to fabricate restorations.

Once verified, definitive restorations can be confidently used for fit, metal ceramic restoration frameworks can be sectioned and soldered to fit, and zirconia restorations would need to be used as the cast to cement the Ti bases to the zirconia restoration. When zirconia restorations are sintered to cause the allotropic change from monoclinic to tetragonal, though the shrinkage can occur and be compensated by algorithms, the errors occurred are compensated by cement space to accommodate the Ti bases. The verified cast will allow the Ti bases to both seat to the implant analogues and be cemented to the restoration; any discrepancy of the fit of the zirconia restoration can be compensated with the cement space programmed around the Ti bases to accommodate the zirconia restoration for an accurate and passive fit.

The above describes only making an impression that is poured to have a cast with implant analogues that have fidelity to the implants that are intra-oral. This only provides the technician with part of the information he or she needs to fabricate the restoration in the supramucosal area. Another information that the technician will require is the submucosal soft tissue contours that will mould and shape the peri-implant mucosa to provide the aesthetics. This information will be provided by recording the submucosal contours of the provisional restorations and presenting them on the working casts.

Manufacturer-supplied impression copings do not take into consideration soft tissue morphology formed by provisional restorations. Impressions using manufacturer-supplied impression copings merely relate the implant or implant abutment to oral structures.

Customized impression copings that can replicate the submucosal contours are formed by provisional restorations; using these customized impression copings, these submucosal contours can be provided to the technicians who will in turn fabricate the restorations that will replicate both sub- and supramucosal forms [12].

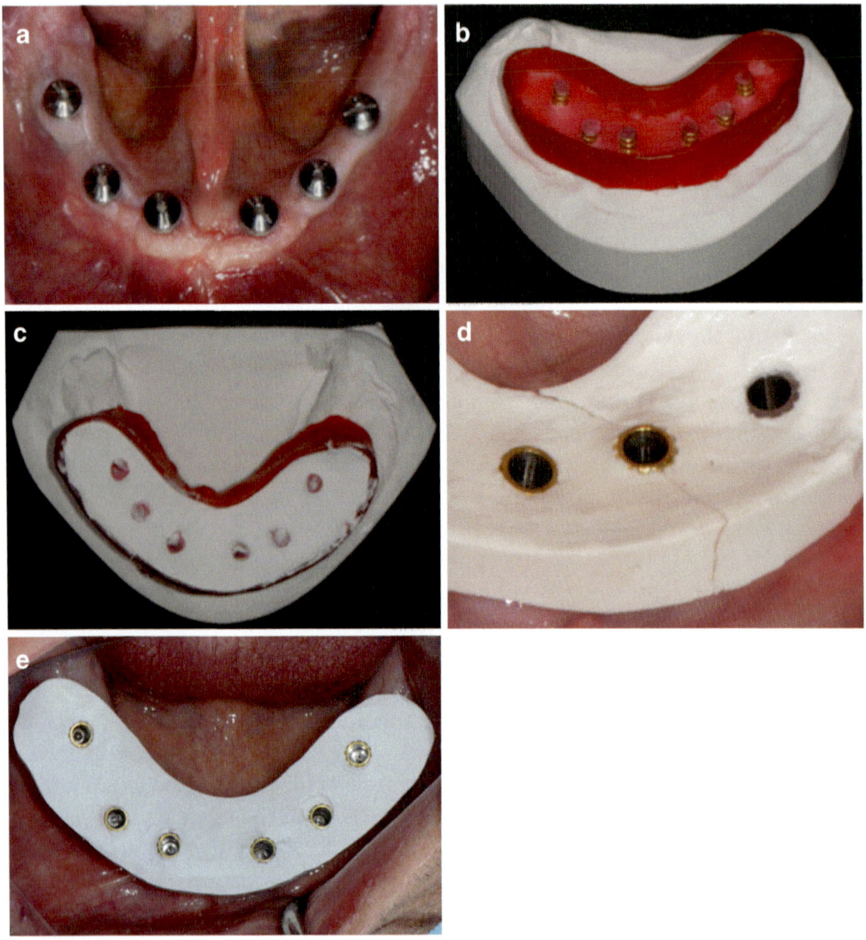

Fig. 5.8 (**a**) Intra-oral view of implants in mandibular arch. (**b**) Wax form to make wafer with abutments for provisional restorations. (**c**) Plaster is poured into the wax form. (**d**) Plaster verification jig is placed intra-orally, and screws are tightened to specifications; in the image, the jig is fractured, and the implant analogues on the cast are not accurately placed. (**e**) A new impression is made, and cast poured; the verification jig is seated and torqued to specifications leaving the jig intact; this demonstrates the fidelity of the cast

Submucosal contours will collapse rapidly when implant-supported restorations are removed; several authors have used a method of placing an impression coping on the implant immediately on removal of the implant-supported provisional restoration and then injecting a bis-acryl composite material into the sulcus around the impression coping in order to record the submucosal contour to be transferred to the cast. This procedure is not precise because of the rapid change in soft tissue contours after removal of the implant-supported restoration [13–15].

A more precise method is to replicate the submucosal contours by modifying an impression coping extra-orally. After a provisional restoration is delivered and the submucosal contours are established to satisfy aesthetics, the provisional restoration is removed and then attached to an implant analogue; this analogue is set into a gypsum base, and then the analogue and provisional restoration are embedded in silicone putty up to the level where the restoration exits the soft tissue. The provisional restoration is then removed, and the space surrounding the impression coping is filled with acrylic resin. This modified impression coping is then used as any other impression coping; this allows both the position of the implant and the submucosal contours to be captured in the impression. Figures 5.9 and 5.10 illustrate the steps toward fabricating a custom impression coping.

Another method of replicating submucosal contours when screw-retained provisional restorations are utilized is to use the provisional as a customized impression coping. The retaining screw of the provisional restoration is removed, and a long screw—usually the screw that retains a pickup impression coping—is used; an open tray is used to facilitate tightening and loosening of the screw; this assembly will be removed together with the impression, and the cast can be poured to record the submucosal contours. One drawback of this procedure is that the patient will be without the provisional restoration and will have to wait till the cast is set to have the restoration redelivered [16–19] (Fig. 5.11).

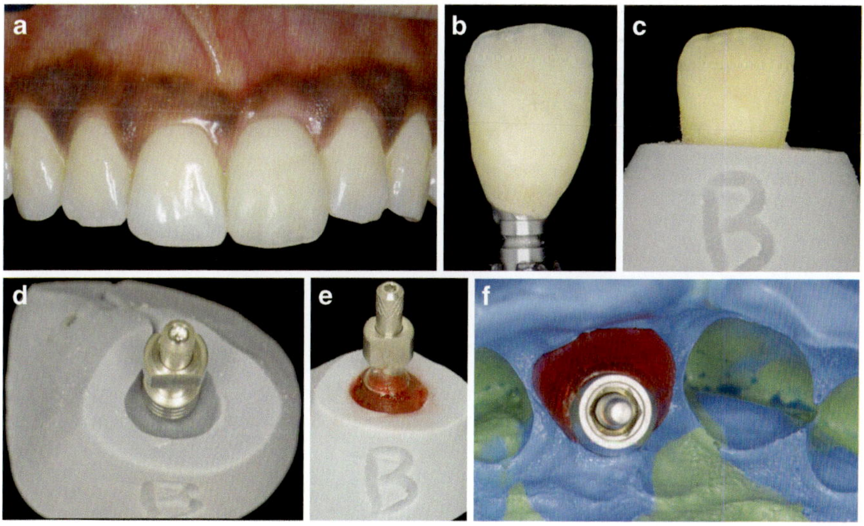

Fig. 5.9 (**a**) Intra-oral image of a provisional restoration on maxillary left central dental implant. (**b**) The provisional is removed and attached to an implant analogue. (**c**) The provisional is embedded into an additional silicone putty to replicate the submucosal contours of the restoration. (**d**) The provisional restoration is removed, and a pickup impression coping is placed onto the implant analogue. (**e**) Polymethylmethacrylate is placed around the implant and takes the form of the provisional restoration. (**f**) The customized impression is picked up in the impression to replicate the submucosal contours and the position of the implant

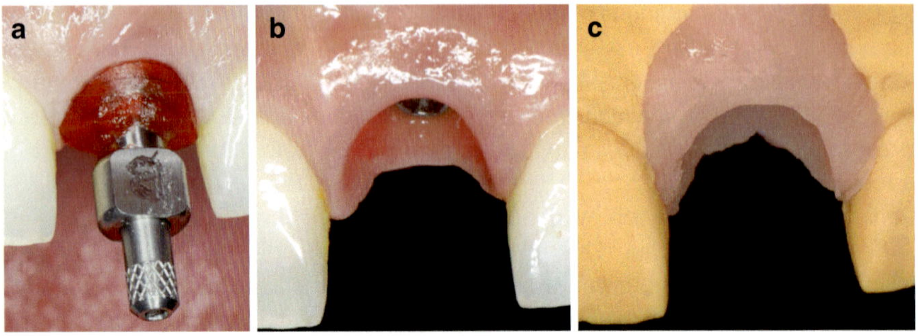

Fig. 5.10 (**a**) Intra-oral view of the customized impression coping in place. (**b**) Soft tissue morphology is supported by the provisional restoration. (**c**) The soft tissue cast is an exact replica of the soft tissue contours. (Figs. 5.9 and 5.10 Courtesy of Dr. Nikitas Mordahai)

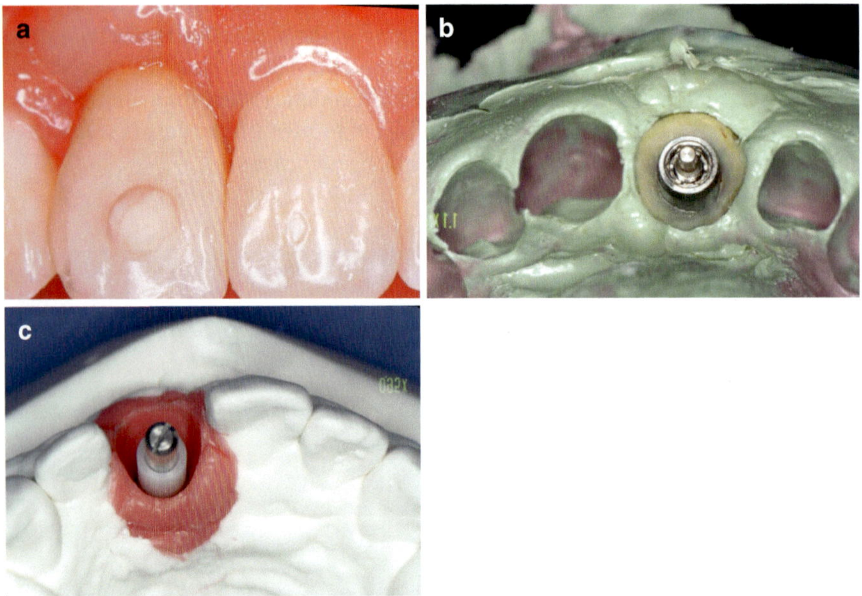

Fig. 5.11 (**a**) Implant-retained provisional in maxillary right central incisor with added feature to become a pickup impression coping. (**b**) Provisional restoration is picked up in impression. (**c**) Cast is poured showing the submucosal contours

With screw-retained restorations, the submucosal form of the soft tissue collapses almost immediately after removal of the provisional restoration. During the removal of restoration for any chairside purposes, for example, there is a need to repair the provisional or a need to scan the provisional to obtain a Standard Tessellation Language (STL) file. Using healing caps to keep the screw access patent is not sufficient to maintain the submucosal contours. A simple way to facilitate keeping the submucosal contours in place is to air-dry the peri-implant areas and then inject a light-bodied polyvinyl siloxane impression material in the submucosal areas related to the restoration immediately on removal of the provisional restoration. The set material is self-retained by the impression material engaging the screw channels or internal connection space of implants; the soft tissue template can be removed and replaced. In addition, the soft tissue template can be retained and used if the provisional restoration needs to be removed again on another clinical appointment. This is a useful and effective technique that saves chair time when placing and removing healing caps when removing restorations; healing caps need to be obtained specifically for the implant types, and impression material would compensate for the use of healing caps. When using a soft tissue template, maintaining the soft tissue contours is much more expedient. Replacing the provisional or definitive restoration without maintaining the soft tissue contours can be uncomfortable with collapse of the soft tissues; at times, local anaesthetic may have to be administered on replacement [20] (Fig. 5.12).

There are situations when there are difficulties in making impressions of teeth and implants simultaneously; implant impression copings can reduce access to prepared teeth when making impressions; it may be difficult to manage the cord packing for teeth and extruding impression material around the margins of the prepared teeth without the implant impression copings impeding access. The goal of the impression will be to have dimensional fidelity of the implants and fine detail reproduction of prepared teeth [21].

A preliminary impression is taken and poured to form a cast; separate impressions are made of the prepared teeth using custom trays that are made closely fitting with five layers of rubber sep with film thickness of 12–15 microns on the tooth preparations (George Taub Products and Fusion Co, Jersey City, NJ) and with retentive features to facilitate pickup by an over-impression tray that will also accommodate the pickup impression copings.

The individual impression trays (Fig. 5.13a) are coated with impression material adhesive. Retraction cords are used for tooth preparations that are deeper than 1 mm. With the use of this coping technique, avoiding use of retraction cords is also beneficial if patients are prone to bleeding. Each tray is loaded with a heavy-body PVS material, then removed and evaluated for completeness after setting and then perforated in the occlusal aspect with a #6 round burr (Fig. 5.13b, c). After confirming a good impression and venting, light-body PVS material is loaded in each tray and replaced on the preparations and left in place; implant impression copings are attached, and then the over-impression tray is loaded with impression material and seated over the impression copings and individual impression copings over tooth preparations; when set, the impression copings are released, and the impression is removed (Fig. 5.13d–f).

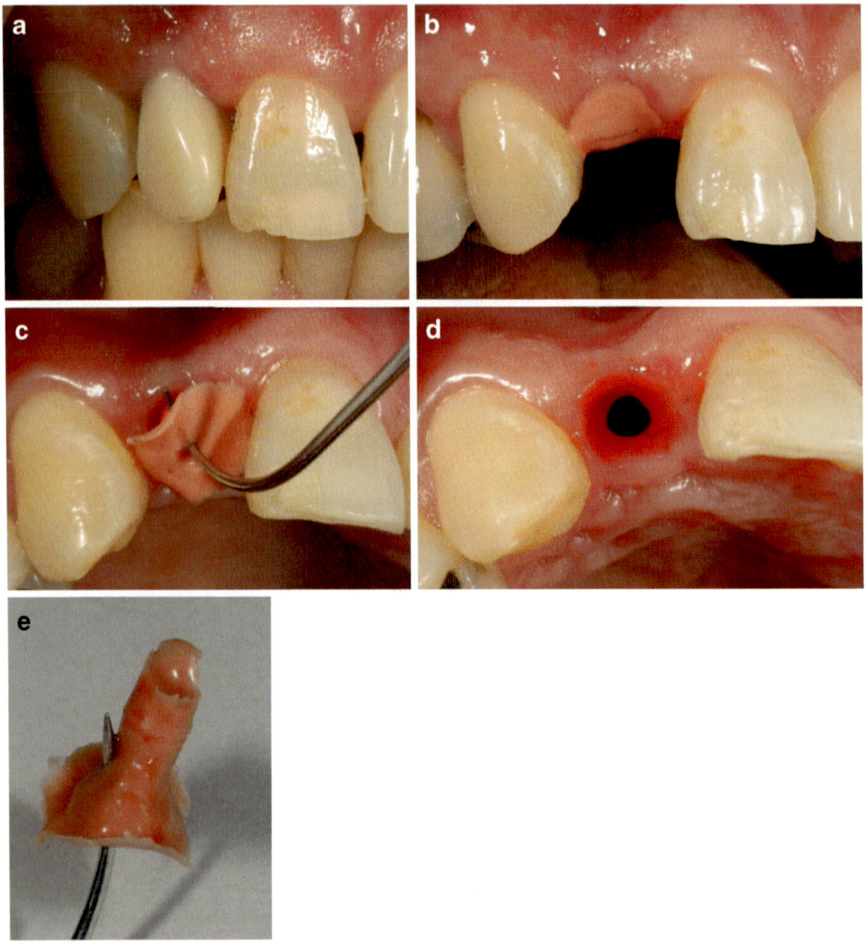

Fig. 5.12 (**a**) Intra-oral view of maxillary right lateral provisional restoration. (**b**) Polyvinyl siloxane impression material is expressed into the submucosal area. (**c**) The submucosal template is removed to replace the restoration. (**d**) The submucosal contours are maintained. (**e**) An image of the soft tissue template

5.2 Summary

A review of the literature concerning impression making in implant dentistry was presented along with suggestions for a predictable implant impression technique; when aesthetics is of concern, methods of transferring the soft tissue information formed by provisional restorations to the master cast were also described.

Use of digital methods of scanning dental implants and restorations will be described in more detail in Chap. 8.

However, it should be made clear that full digital workflows are not currently feasible in some situations. With a full digital workflow for implant-supported

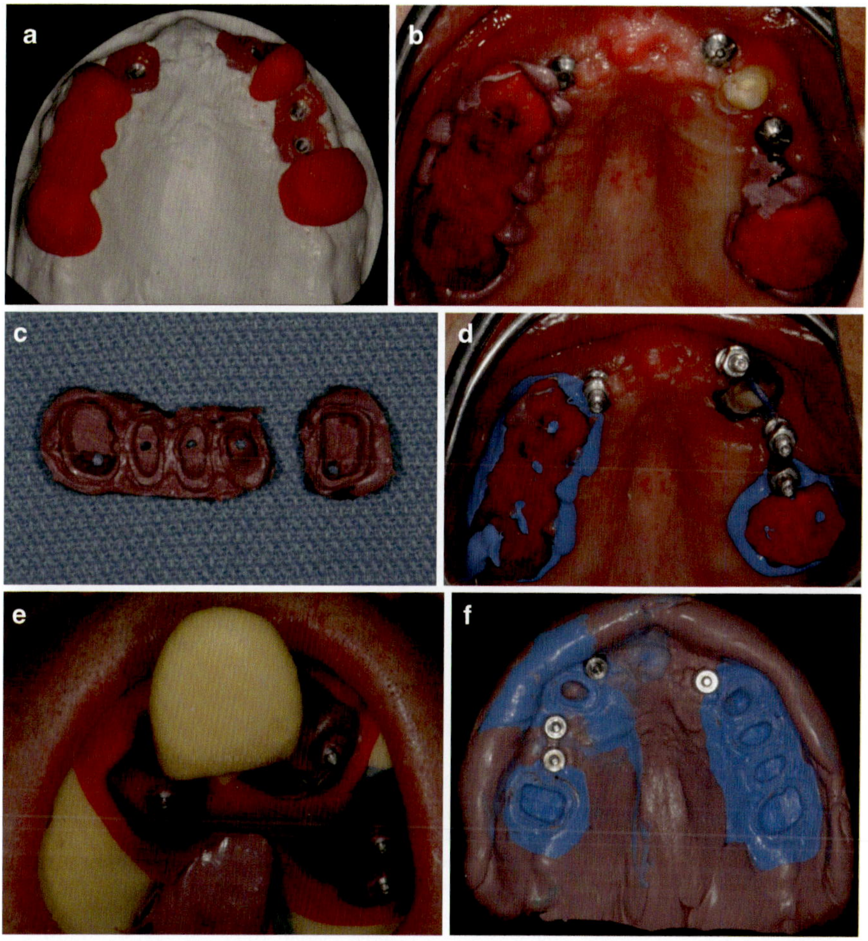

Fig. 5.13 (**a**) Copings for teeth prepared with a spacer of about 60–90 micron spacer. (**b**) Copings are loaded with heavy-bodied polyvinyl siloxane impression material and then placed onto the prepared teeth after drying. (**c**) The trays are removed, and the impression can be evaluated for completeness of impression, and then the impressions and copings are perforated. (**d**) The impression copings are placed on the trays that are filled with light-body polyvinyl siloxane impression material and replaced onto the respective tooth preparations again after drying. (**e**) An over tray is used to relate the implant positions and tooth preparations. (**f**) The completed impression after setting is removed; the clearly recorded impression for prepared teeth and the pickup impressions that are well related. (Fig. 5.13 courtesy of Dr. Derek Tan)

restorations, they are limited at present to accommodate implant-supported restorations that are fabricated with monolithic materials. If there are prepared teeth in the same arch or layered restorations, there is some difficulty using a full digital workflow. Laboratory technicians will have no guides to proximal contacts, submucosal contours and cementations of Ti bases with implant restorations. At present, a milled or printed cast to accurately receive an implant analogue secured into the cast in the correct position is not yet developed, including the locating feature such as a hexagonal feature to be oriented precisely. In addition, with layered restorations on teeth and implants, casts may have to be poured with conventional implant methods to allow mixes of crowns, veneers and implants to be fabricated simultaneously. In time, development of digital features will progress.

References

1. Wee AG. Comparison of impression materials for direct multi-implant impressions. J Prosthet Dent. 2000;83(3):323–31.
2. Chee WW, Donovan TE. Polyvinyl siloxane impression materials: a review of properties and techniques. J Prosthet Dent. 1992;68(5):728–32. https://doi.org/10.1016/0022-3913(92)90192-d.
3. Liou AD, Nicholls JI, Yuodelis RA, Brudvik JS. Accuracy of replacing three tapered transfer impression copings in two elastomeric impression materials. Int J Prosthodont. 1993;6(4):377–83.
4. Assif D, Fenton A, Zarb G, Schmitt A. Comparative accuracy of implant impression procedures. Int J Periodontics Restor Dent. 1992;12(2):112–21.
5. Barrett MG, de Rijk WG, Burgess JO. The accuracy of six impression techniques for osseointegrated implants. J Prosthodont. 1993;2(2):75–82. https://doi.org/10.1111/j.1532-849x.1993.tb00387.x.
6. Ma Y, Al-Radhi RYZ, Jiang L, Yu H. Does splinting the direct copings increase the impression accuracy of two-unit nonparallel implant restorations? A systematic review and meta-analysis. Int J Oral Maxillofac Implants. 2022;37(4):653–9.
7. Baig MR. Accuracy of impressions of multiple implants in the edentulous arch: a systematic review. Int J Oral Maxillofac Implants. 2014;29(4):869–80. https://doi.org/10.11607/jomi.3233.
8. Kim JH, Kim KR, Kim S. Critical appraisal of implant impression accuracies: a systematic review. J Prosthet Dent. 2015;114(2):185–92.e1. https://doi.org/10.1016/j.prosdent.2015.02.005. Epub 2015 Apr 30. PMID.
9. Assif D, Nissan J, Varsano I, Singer A. Accuracy of implant impression splinted techniques: effect of splinting material. Int J Oral Maxillofac Implants. 1999;14(6):885–8.
10. Carr AB, Master J. The accuracy of implant verification casts compared with casts produced from a rigid transfer coping technique. J Prosthodont. 1996;5(4):248–52. https://doi.org/10.1111/j.1532-849x.1996.tb00507.x.
11. Mpikos P, Kafantaris N, Tortopidis D, Galanis C, Kaisarlis G, Koidis P. The effect of impression technique and implant angulation on the impression accuracy of external- and internal-connection implants [Erratum in: Int J Oral Maxillofac Implants. 2013;28(1):43. Kafantaris, Nikolaos [added].]. Int J Oral Maxillofac Implants. 2012;27(6):1422–8.
12. Chee W, Jivraj S. Impression techniques for implant dentistry. Br Dent J. 2006;201(7):429–32.
13. Li J, Chen Z, Wang M, Wang HL, Yu H. Dynamic changes of peri-implant soft tissue after interim restoration removal during a digital intraoral scan. J Prosthet Dent. 2019;122(3):288–94. https://doi.org/10.1016/j.prosdent.2018.07.020. Epub 2019 Mar 15.
14. Polack MA. Simple method of fabricating an impression coping to reproduce peri-implant gingiva on the master cast. J Prosthet Dent. 2002;88(2):221–3. https://doi.org/10.1067/mpr.2002.127895.
15. Schoenbaum TR, Han TJ. Direct custom implant impression copings for the preservation of the pontic receptor site architecture. J Prosthet Dent. 2012;107(3):203–6.
16. Neale D, Chee WW. Development of implant soft tissue emergence profile: a technique. J Prosthet Dent. 1994;71(4):364–8.
17. Chee WW, Cho GC, Ha S. Replicating soft tissue contours on working casts for implant restorations. J Prosthodont. 1997;6(3):218–20.

18. Chee WW, Cho GC, Ikoma MM, Arcidiacono A. A technique to replicate soft tissues around fixed restoration pontics on working casts. J Prosthodont. 1999;8(1):44–6.
19. Tsai BY. A method for obtaining peri-implant soft-tissue contours by using screw-retained provisional restorations as impression copings: a clinical report. J Oral Implantol. 2011;37(5):605–9. https://doi.org/10.1563/AAID-JOI-D-10-00026.1. Epub 2010 Jun 16.
20. Pawlak A, Chee WW, Park CJ. Use of polyvinyl siloxane to maintain peri-implant submucosal contours on removal of screw-retained implant-supported restorations. J Prosthet Dent. 2023; https://doi.org/10.1016/j.prosdent.2023.03.027. Epub ahead of print.
21. Chee WW, Alexander ML. Impression technique for arches requiring both implant and natural tooth restorations. J Prosthodont. 1998;7(1):45–8.

The Decision to Restore a Tooth or Extract It and Replace It with a Single Implant

6

Geneviève Guertin

6.1 The Compromised Tooth with a Questionable to Poor Prognosis

In the medical field, once a diagnosis has been established, the prognosis of a disease is one of the criteria used to support a clinician's decision in treatment planning. In dentistry, prognosis corresponds to the expected success of therapy and maintenance of the tooth's condition over time. While there is no single universally accepted classification system for all the dental disciplines, prognosis typically can be categorized in different levels of possibility of an optimistic outcome (excellent, good, favourable prognosis) to a more pessimistic outcome (guarded, poor, hopeless prognosis).

Prognosis of a tooth is determined by the identification of the various risk factors associated with disease and whether these factors can be managed or controlled through therapy.

6.1.1 Prognostication

- A favourable prognosis (excellent–good–fair) indicates that treatment success is likely and that the tooth's condition should be maintained in good function and health over time
- A questionable prognosis indicates that treatment success is uncertain or less predictable and that the maintenance of the tooth's condition over time is uncertain due to risk factors that may or may not be controlled
- An unfavourable prognosis indicates that treatment success is unlikely and that the tooth's condition is expected to deteriorate over time despite the intervention
- A hopeless prognosis indicates that the tooth cannot be effectively treated or maintained, and extraction is the most appropriate course of action

G. Guertin (✉)
Private Practice, Centre Prosthodontique Mont-Royal, Montreal, QC, Canada

W. Chee, S. Jivraj (eds.), *Treatment Planning In Implant Dentistry*, BDJ Clinician's Guides, https://doi.org/10.1007/978-3-031-68726-6_6

The situations that are of interest in this chapter are those where success of treatment or maintainability in the long term is less predictable (questionable or poor prognosis). It is important to understand that while a less than good prognosis indicates a less favourable outcome, there is no exact way of forecasting accurately when treatment failure will occur or cause the tooth to require extraction [1–4].

6.1.2 Risk Factors

With proper patient interview and clinical examination, an experienced clinician will be able to identify the many risk factors that affect the onset and progression of a specific disease [5]. These factors include but are not limited to:

The patient's systemic condition	Genetics, medical conditions and use of medication, smoking, oral hygiene, oral pH, parafunction
The patient's hard tissue condition	Caries, tooth structure loss, type of restoration, missing teeth
The patient's periodontal condition	Attachment loss, single- or multi-rooted teeth, tooth position, furcation involvement, mobility, root anatomy, gingival thickness and presence of keratinized tissue
The patient's endodontic condition	Tooth vitality, root anatomy, root resorption, quality of endodontic treatment, access for treatment, remaining tooth structure
The patient's occlusal risk factors	Type of occlusion, arch form, occlusal plane, occlusal vertical dimension, posterior support

Other important risk factors that need to be identified are the factors that are associated with treatment success; these factors include, but are not limited to:

The operator	Use of appropriate therapeutic armamentarium Knowledge, experience
The patient's compliance	Home care Wear of occlusal appliance Dental maintenance appointments
The patient's psychosocial risk factors	Anxiety, expectations, motivation, ability to pay
The patient's aesthetic risk factors	Position of the teeth in relation to facial anatomy, lip mobility, gingival architecture, position of neighbouring teeth

Some examples of situations where the question of whether to treat a tooth or extract it and place an implant typically arises:

- The treatment required is considered straightforward; however, the prognosis remains questionable because of specific risk factors that cannot be eliminated (Fig. 6.1a–c).
- The treatment required is considered complex, and its success is dependent on technical aspects of treatment planning and execution, including the skill and experience of the dental professional; the prognosis remains questionable because of the uncertain outcome of the procedure (Fig. 6.2a, b).

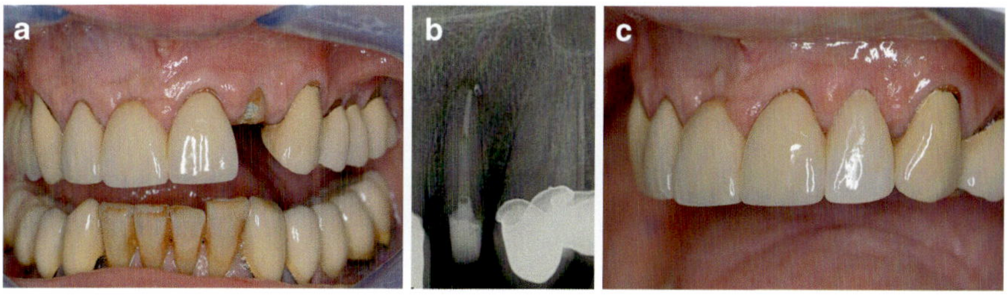

Fig. 6.1 (**a**) Restore or extract? This 79-year-old patient was referred for extraction of tooth 22 (FDI) (maxillary left lateral incisor #9) and implant placement. The tooth has little tooth structure remaining, an unfavourable prognosis. (**b**) When presented with treatment options, the patient decided to restore the tooth. Although the post and core offer adequate retention and stress distribution, little to no ferrule is present, making this tooth to be at high risk of fracture. (**c**) When compared to implant or fixed partial denture, this solution is time and cost efficient. Reducing mechanical risk factors such as reducing occlusal load and providing a night guard is imperative

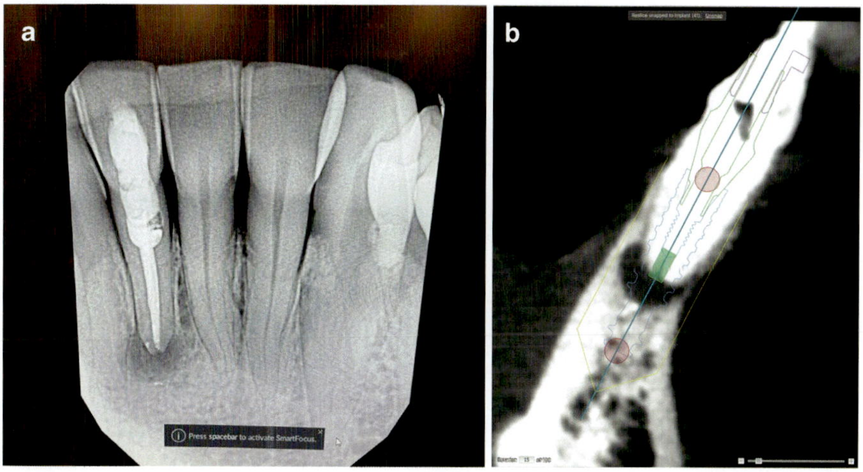

Fig. 6.2 (**a**) Restore or extract? This 50-year-old male was referred for extraction and implant placement of tooth 42 (FDI) (mandibular right lateral incisor #26). Although the tooth has an unfavourable prognosis, extraction and implant placement of this tooth are a complex treatment that offers an uncertain outcome. (**b**) Radiograph illustrates the apical lesion of (**a**) and the thin buccal and lingual bone. Extraction could result in an important bone defect that will be difficult to graft

- Many treatments are required putting to question the cost/benefit ratio. The prognosis remains questionable because of the interdependent prognosis of the multiple therapies (Fig. 6.3a, b).

6.1.3 Impact on the Global Treatment Plan

When deciding on the maintenance of a specific tooth with a less favourable prognosis, assessment of how the tooth's success or failure will impact a comprehensive treatment plan or how its deterioration could affect the oral condition is of capital

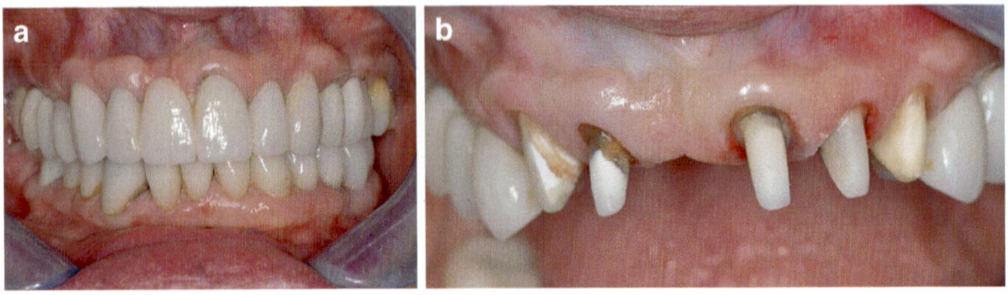

Fig. 6.3 (**a**) Restore or extract? This multi-unit anterior fixed partial denture (FPD) is defective and must be replaced. (**b**) Restore or extract? Upon removal of bridge, we notice that the most anterior abutments have weak tooth structure with little to no ferrule. Although individually these abutments are restorable, the restoration of the FPD will be as strong as the weakest link

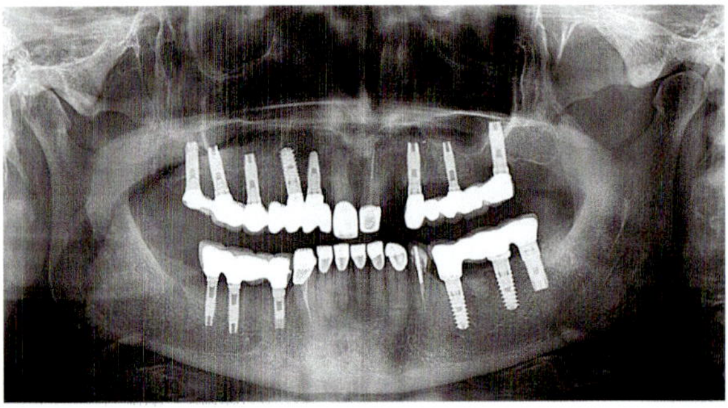

Fig. 6.4 Strategic extraction—removing the maxillary incisors would have made this treatment plan more predictable. Now that No. 22 (FDI) (maxillary left lateral incisor #10) is fractured, additional complex treatment is required

importance. This is where the decision of extraction can be recommended or postponed for strategic reasons [6–8].

Extraction of a tooth should be considered if:

- The complications of the questionable tooth will negatively impact the prognosis of the neighbouring teeth
- Maintaining the tooth may cause the situation to deteriorate to the point where other options are compromised
- The treatment plan will need major revision if this tooth fails (Fig. 6.4)
- The root's position is of strategic value and might better serve as an implant site in a global treatment plan when considering the whole oral environment (Fig. 6.5a, b)
- The tooth is in malposition and removing it will allow for a better treatment result and improved implant distribution (Fig. 6.6a–c)

Examples of situations where the preservation of a compromised tooth may be recommended are the following:

- To help support or retain a provisional transitioning restoration
- To maintain occlusal vertical dimension (Fig. 6.7)
- To postpone tooth extraction to a better timing according to patient age or life circumstances

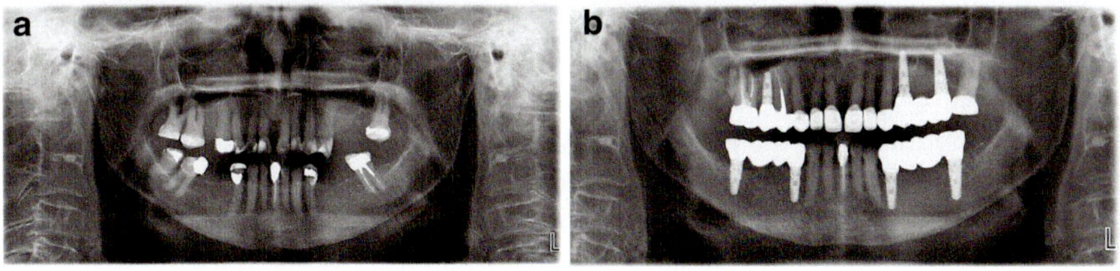

Fig. 6.5 (**a**) Strategic extraction—this patient has insufficient bone to place implants in the edentulous posterior segments. (**b**) Strategic extraction of some restorable teeth offers the possibility to place implants where bone remains, resulting in improved posterior support and a more predictable restoration

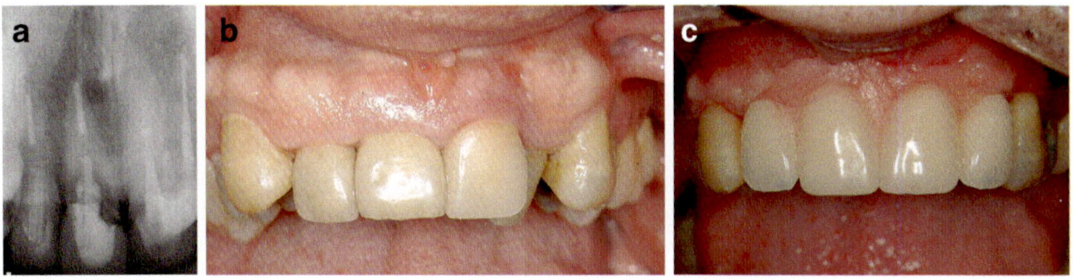

Fig. 6.6 (**a**) Strategic extraction—tooth 11 (FDI) (maxillary right central incisor #8) has a large carious lesion and is about to be extracted. Tooth 12 (FDI) (maxillary right lateral incisor #7) is heavily restored. (**b**) Teeth 12 (FDI) (#7) and 22 (FDI) (maxillary left lateral incisor #10) are not in an optimal aesthetic and functional position. (**c**) Strategic extraction of 21 (FDI) (maxillary left central incisor #9) and 22 (FDI) (#10) offers a better restorative position for the implants

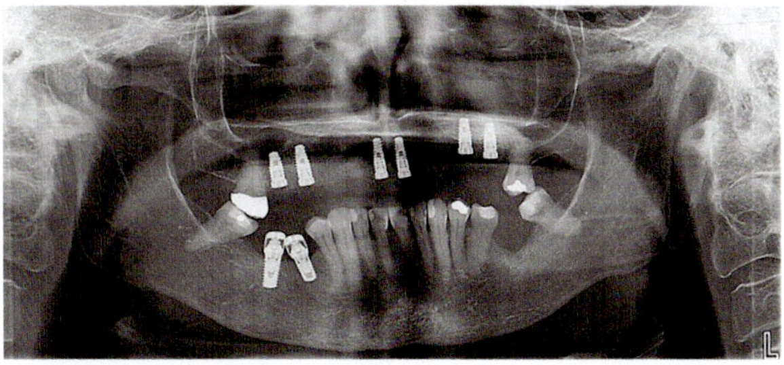

Fig. 6.7 Strategic maintenance of molars has helped this patient retain her partial denture and maintain OVD during the healing of both bone grafting and implants

- To maintain support and comfort of the edentulous extension of a removable partial denture

6.2 Restoring the Compromised Tooth

6.2.1 Tooth Structure Loss

The main cause of tooth structure loss in people of all ages worldwide is dental caries. The three main factors that increase the risk of developing caries, also known as the caries triangle, are the presence of bacteria, consumption of sugary foods and drinks and a susceptible tooth surface. Oral hygiene instructions in a motivated patient combined with changes in dietary habits will help control the two primary factors and usually succeed in resolving the problem of tooth decay.

Unfortunately, certain systemic conditions and medications can cause a periodic or persistent reduction in the patient's salivary flow, leading to a reduced capacity of the saliva to cleanse the oral cavity and buffer acids present in the mouth [9]. This pH imbalance will lead to chemical erosion of the tooth structure, leaving the tooth surface more susceptible to dental erosion and tooth decay (Fig. 6.8).

An acidic oral environment can also be related to a patient's diet [10] or an increased contact of the teeth with acids of intrinsic source. Erosive tooth structure lesions are a frequent occurrence in patients with gastro-oesophageal reflux disorder (GERD) or eating disorders such as bulimia nervosa where patients repeatedly have stomach acids in contact with their teeth (Fig. 6.9).

As tooth structure is progressively lost to dental decay, the remaining enamel and dentin are weakened and more prone to fracture under functional loading. Teeth with moderate to severe damage will often require cuspal coverage for better load distribution and protection from fracture. In situations where tooth structure remaining does not offer proper retention, some teeth will require root canal therapy for the added retention offered by an endodontic post or the pulp chamber itself (Table 6.1).

When preparing a tooth for a crown, it is general consensus that a 2 mm ferrule of coronal dentin above the margin of a crown preparation significantly increases the failure threshold of endodontically treated teeth. When restoring compromised teeth, an effort to obtain adequate tooth structure encirclement through crown lengthening or orthodontic extrusion should be attempted. When such a ferrule cannot be obtained, the tooth will have a significantly diminished capacity to withstand functional loading making its prognosis less favourable [9, 14–16].

In cases where the tooth is subject to an increased functional load, chances of fracture are amplified. Causes of an increase in functional loading can be related to an unfavourable occlusal scheme, occlusal interferences or lack of posterior support. Also, endodontically treated teeth that act as removable partial denture abutments have been shown to have a higher risk of failure when used as RPD abutments

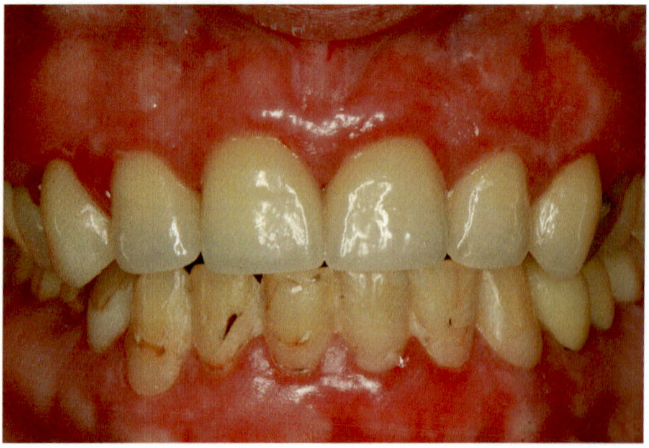

Fig. 6.8 Caries-susceptible patient—carious lesions on atypical tooth surfaces are often indicative of a high-caries-risk patient

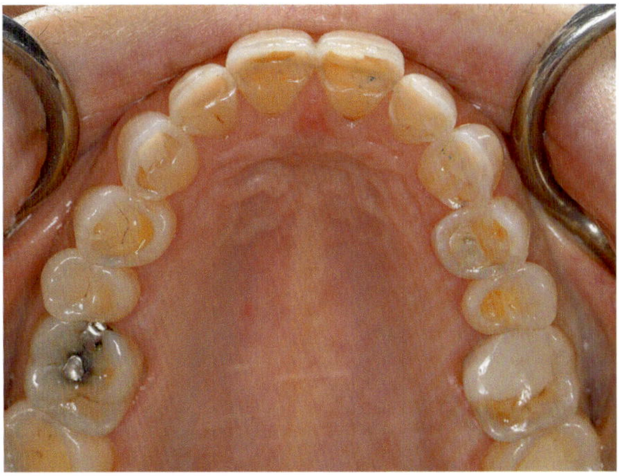

Fig. 6.9 Tooth structure loss caused by erosion of intrinsic source—in this case, a bulimic patient

Table 6.1 Systemic and local risk factors associated with xerostomia [10–13]

Medications that are associated with xerostomia	Anticholinergic agents Antidepressants and antipsychotic agents Diuretic agents, antihypertensive agents Sedative and anxiolytic agents Muscle relaxants, analgesic agents Antihistamine agents, bronchodilators Antiacne agents, appetite suppressants Anticonvulsants, antimigraine drugs
Systemic conditions associated with xerostomia	Primary and secondary Sjögren syndrome HIV, AIDS Graft vs. host disease Renal dialysis Anxiety, depression, stress Diabetes Anaemia, Parkinson's, Alzheimer's
Damage to salivary glands	Radiotherapy Chemotherapy

[17]. Efforts should be made to decrease the load on the compromised tooth by correcting the occlusion or providing posterior support (Fig. 6.10a, b).

Unfortunately, certain individuals present with bruxism that causes an increase in masticatory muscle activity of varied severity, leading to tooth fracture and wear (Fig. 6.11). It has been proposed that the aetiology of bruxism is multifactorial with risk factors related to genetics, stress and anxiety, and some exogenous factors (alcohol, medication, smoking). In sleep bruxism, central nervous system activation may be the primary factor involved [18, 19] (Table 6.2).

6.2.1.1 Recommendations

In cases of recurrent tooth decay where tooth structure loss is severe and caused by an oral condition that the patient is incapable of managing, implants may offer a more predictable treatment option as they show a high rate of survival in patients

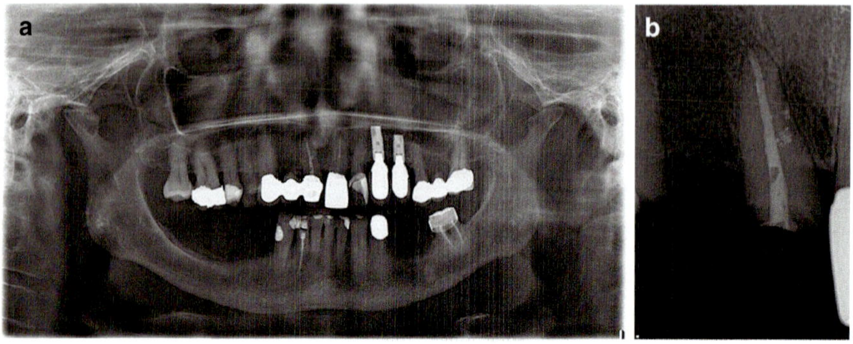

Fig. 6.10 (**a**) The lack of posterior support creates an increase in load on the anterior teeth. (**b**) Fracture of the fixed partial denture abutments is a consequence of lack of posterior support

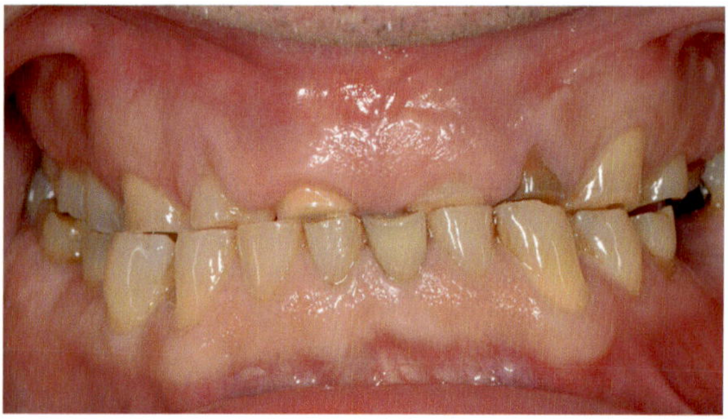

Fig. 6.11 Tooth structure loss caused by parafunctional activity

Table 6.2 Mechanical risk factors that may accelerate tooth fracture

Tooth structure loss (reduction in capacity to withstand functional load)	For example, less than a 2 mm ferrule of coronal dentin above the margin of a crown preparation
Increased functional load on tooth	For example, unfavourable occlusion, malocclusion, lack of posterior support Tooth will be abutment for RPD
Parafunction (pathological load)	Medications: Antidepressants, antipsychotics and stimulants Medical conditions: Bruxism Parkinson's disease, Tourette syndrome, stroke

with most common systemic conditions that would cause xerostomia or oral pH imbalance.

In cases where it is impossible to control the mechanical risk factors, extraction and implant placement will not necessarily offer an advantage over the natural compromised tooth. Higher rates of mechanical complications with implant restorations have been reported in patients with parafunctional activity. One must understand that the implant restoration complex presents no proprioception in these patients and is rigidly attached to bone offering a reduced capacity for shock absorption.

6.2.2 Endodontic Infections

An endodontic infection occurs when bacteria have infected the pulp. Causes of the endodontic infections are often related to deep carious lesions infecting the pulp or damage to the pulp following dental trauma or iatrogenic dental treatment.

Root canal therapy consists of removal of the pulp tissue, shaping and obturation of the root canal space. Often paired with the use of antibiotic therapy, this treatment will help resolve periapical infections.

Many local factors will influence the capacity of the restorative dentist to properly obturate the root canal and prevent future bacterial infiltration from occurring. These include number of roots, root anatomy and root canal access. Systematic reviews have shown that the success rate of initial endodontic therapy is high and will offer higher success rates in situations where there was absence of an apical periodontal lesion.

Other factors related to a tooth's dental history will influence the outcome of endodontic therapy [20–24] such as

- Presence of periapical lesions and extent of infection
- Previous endodontic treatment and their quality
- Presence of calcified canals or presence of root resorption

When a conventional root canal therapy has failed to resolve persistent infection or inflammation, surgical endodontic therapies may be required to better access the infected root tip, remove the inflamed or infected tissues (cysts or granulomas) and resect and seal the infected root tip (Fig. 6.12a, b) (Table 6.3).

6.2.2.1 Recommendations

When both conventional and surgical endodontic therapies have failed to resolve the infection and the tooth continues to show symptoms of discomfort, the decision to extract the problematic tooth may be recommended. Evaluation of the site to

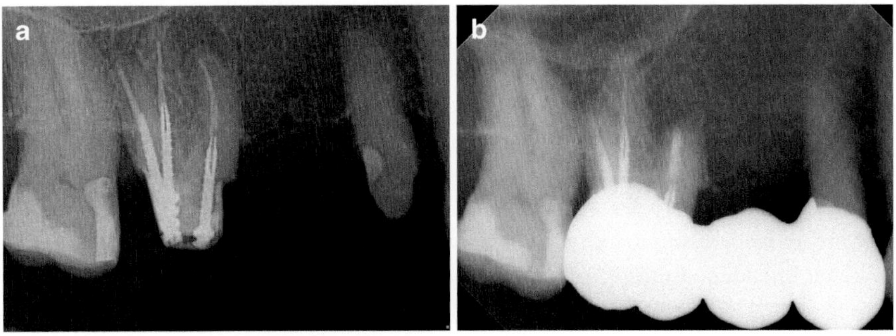

Fig. 6.12 (**a**) MB root with apical lesion; tooth has been restored with multiple posts, and retreatment is improbable. (**b**) Apical resection and retrograde filling offer a second chance at this tooth serving as an abutment for a fixed partial denture

Table 6.3 Endodontic risk factors [20]

Local factors	Number of roots, root anatomy and root canal access
Dental history	Presence/extent of periapical lesions or infections Presence of calcified canals Previous endodontic treatment and their quality History of trauma, presence of root resorption
Systemic health conditions	Conditions that compromise the ability to fight infections (uncontrolled diabetes, immunodeficiency, autoimmune disease)

determine if the conditions are conducive to a successful tooth replacement with dental implants is necessary prior to extraction.

6.2.3 Periodontal Disease

The primary cause of periodontal disease is bacterial plaque accumulation on the root surfaces. These bacteria produce enzymes and toxins that destroy periodontal tissue. In order to help control the progression of the disease and tooth loss, systematic reviews confirm that enforcement of consistent oral hygiene habits paired with professional cleaning and close monitoring of the periodontal condition is effective. Tooth-related factors such as tooth type, tooth location and presence of furcation involvement are identified as relevant risk factors towards an increased risk of tooth loss during periodontal maintenance [25, 26].

When periodontal attachment loss has progressed and the anatomy of the tooth or defect makes it difficult to provide adequate hygiene to the area, the outcome of therapy becomes less predictable. In these cases, surgical interventions may be required to either remove or regenerate bone and create a more favourable anatomy for easier hygiene.

Although any patient may develop periodontal attachment loss, certain individuals are more susceptible to this disease. Pooled estimates from prospective studies could identify that both smoking and diabetes are significant factors towards tooth loss during periodontal maintenance. In these higher risk patients and in certain forms of aggressive periodontitis that show a rapid rate of destruction, patients will require a shorter maintenance interval (Table 6.4).

6.2.3.1 Recommendation

When conventional therapy and surgical therapy have failed to create a healthy and stable periodontal attachment and tissues continue to show signs that the disease process is active (periodontal probing depths, bleeding on probing and increased mobility), the decision to extract a tooth with a questionable to poor prognosis may be recommended. Leaving the disease to progress could negatively impact the neighbouring teeth and the residual bone volume required for the future stabilization of a dental implant (Fig. 6.13a, b).

Table 6.4 Periodontal risk factors [25, 26]

Local tooth-related factors	Multi-rooted teeth Root anatomy Tooth position Bone loss, furcation involvement Occlusion, number of teeth remaining Parafunction, mobility
Patient social habits	Smoking Patient compliance
Periodontal host risk factors that reduce the patient's immune response	Genetic predispositions Medical conditions (diabetes or immune disorders)

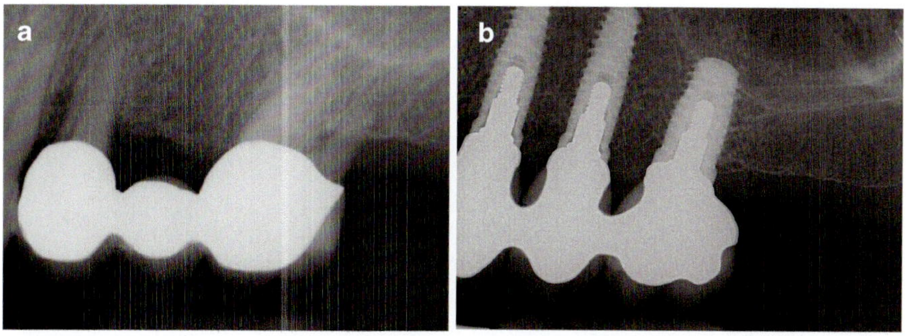

Fig. 6.13 (**a**) Periodontally involved teeth—bone loss and furcation involvement in posterior teeth on compliant patient—extraction is recommended while bone is still available for implant placement. (**b**) Implant replacements showing bone stability over time (over 10 years)

However, the same risk factors that contribute to periodontal disease, such as poor oral hygiene, smoking, diabetes and genetic predisposition, can also increase the risk of peri-implantitis.

6.2.4 Trauma

Traumatic injury to teeth is frequent and can occur at all ages in various contexts: falls, sports activities, bicycle accidents, car accidents or physical brawls. These traumatic accidents are more prevalent in the permanent dentition of boys and often involve the more prominent maxillary central and lateral incisor teeth [27] (Fig. 6.14a, b).

Damage caused by the trauma may be limited to the tooth's coronal structure but may also include damage to the root and pulpal tissues and in more severe cases damage to the periodontal tissues and surrounding bone when trauma causes tooth displacement or avulsion.

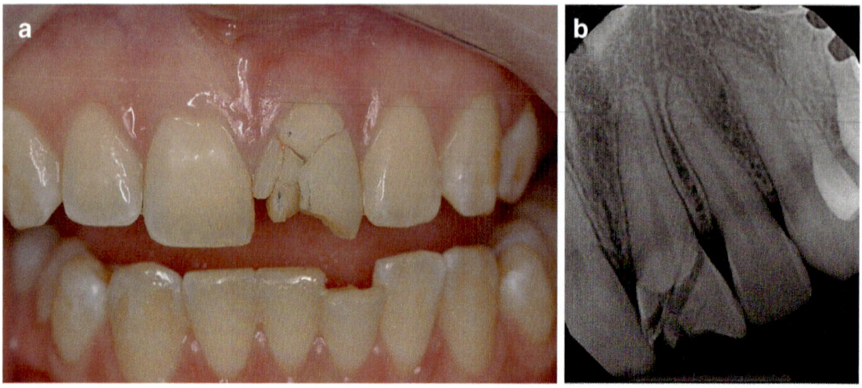

Fig. 6.14 (**a**) Trauma—catastrophic fracture of tooth 21 (maxillary left central incisor #9) requiring immediate extraction of the incisor. (**b**) Radiograph of fracture extending below bone level

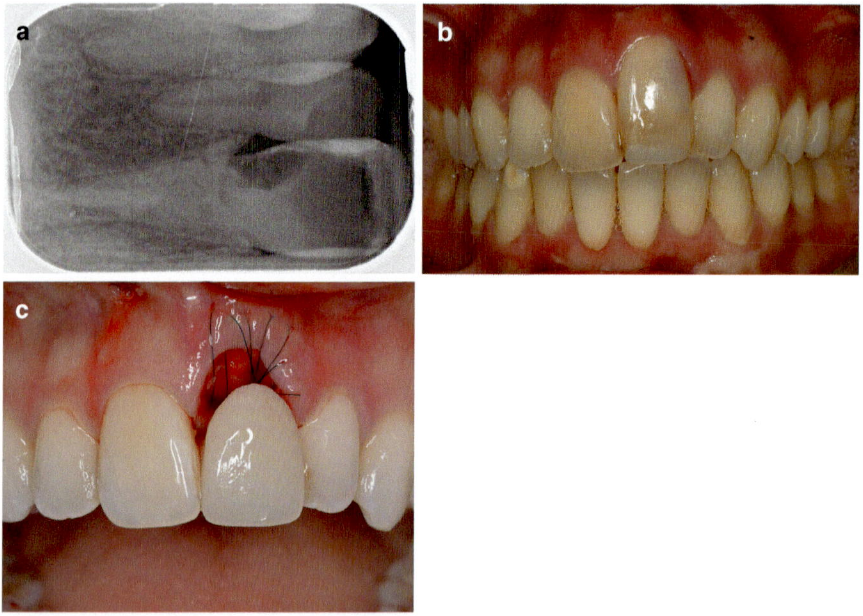

Fig. 6.15 (**a**) Traumatic injury has led to ankylosis and external root resorption of the central incisor. (**b**) Ankylosis of the tooth has hindered the skeletal growth pattern in the maxilla and will require bone augmentation. (**c**) Bone augmentation following tooth extraction to regain bone and soft tissue

In the short term, emergency restorative, endodontic and periodontal therapies may stabilize the situation and, in certain cases, show complete healing. However, traumatic injuries are often accompanied by complications of different types and severities that can occur several months or even years after the injury (Fig. 6.15a, (Table 6.5).

Table 6.5 Risk factors associated with traumatic tooth injuries [27]

Type/severity of injury	Hard tissue and pulp injury	Lateral luxation Intrusion/avulsion
Time delay prior to treatment and quality of treatment	Rapid replantation Proper endodontic therapy	Delayed replantation inappropriate handling of root
Treatment of complicated crown fractures	Pulpotomy	Pulp capping

Dental traumas have been shown to cause the body to initiate excessive inflammatory response that may result in root canal calcification, surface resorption or replacement resorption/ankylosis or internal root resorption. As a result of these mechanisms, tooth discoloration, alterations in dental alignment and occlusion, discomfort and recurrent infection may be observed (Fig. 6.15b, c).

6.2.4.1 Recommendations

When adequate restorative, periodontal and endodontic therapies have failed to provide the patient with a comfortable, functional and aesthetic tooth, extraction and placement of a dental implant are recommended as long-term survival of the tooth is doubtful. In the case of younger patients, as long as it does not cause complications for the future implant site, close monitoring of the traumatized tooth is recommended until patients have completed their skeletal growth and bone development.

6.3 Extraction and Implant Placement

When considering implant therapy, the tooth to be replaced must first be extracted and an implant fixture placed in the bone. The endosseous root form implant is the most common type of dental implant and has been used for over five decades now. This prosthetic device is intended to retain and support the dental restoration much like a natural dental root would. Once the implant is positioned, bone remodelling and soft tissue healing can begin, and osseointegration is the most likely outcome. Survival of dental implant restorations is high and well documented with reports of osseointegration in the high 90% [28–33].

Some systemic factors have been associated with higher rates of implant failure and complications, including impaired osseointegration, increased risk of infection and peri-implantitis. These risk factors include certain medical conditions and medications that affect bone healing and remodelling, diabetes, radiated bone in cancer patients, smoking and tobacco use and medications that affect the patient's immune response (Table 6.6).

6.3.1 Prosthetically Driven Implant Therapy

Although implant osseointegration and survival was considered the main objective when implant dentistry was at its early stages, it is considered an insufficient

Table 6.6 Risk factors that affect implant survival and success

Local factors	Complexity of extraction Presence or absence of bone lesion
	The patient's biotype Thickness of buccal bone Implant position
Systemic factors	Smoking and tobacco use Diabetes Radiated bone in cancer patients Medications that affect the patient's immune response Medications that affect bone healing and remodelling Medical conditions that affect bone healing

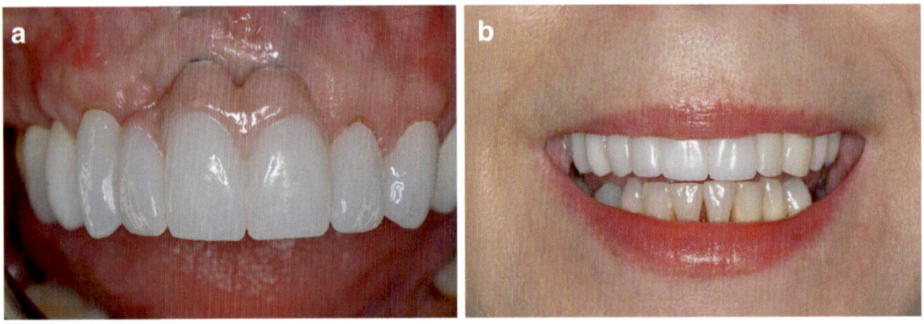

Fig. 6.16 (**a**) Implant placement—aesthetic failure in this anterior restoration. (**b**) Lower aesthetic risk: fortunately, the patient's lip line hides the aesthetic problem

criterion to determine success in the modern implant therapy era (Fig. 6.16a, b). Outcome measures are related to a multitude of factors that will affect patient satisfaction such as the implant's morbidity and cost of therapy, time of treatment, comfort when in function and aesthetic appearance, particularly in the aesthetic zone [34].

It has been demonstrated that the extraction of a tooth and its periodontal ligament will result in the breakdown of the bundle bone that contributes to the maintenance of the integrity and architecture of the surrounding bone tissue. As bone remodels, dimensional changes are to be expected, and these will affect the soft tissue contours leading to loss of papilla and often appearance of longer tooth proportions (Fig. 6.17).

The extent of these changes will depend on various local factors relative to the patient's biotype, thickness of buccal bone, presence or absence of bone lesion, complexity of extraction and capacity of bone to heal.

Ridge preservation techniques can be performed at the time of extraction to minimize bone resorption and maintain the dimensions of the alveolar ridge for future implant placement. This requires placement of a bone graft material in the socket and use of a membrane or barrier to maintain the graft in place [35–37].

When socket preservation is unlikely to provide sufficient bone quantity for implant placement or proper gingival contours, guided bone regeneration also known as bone augmentation has proven to help restore adequate bone volume for implant placement and help recreate aesthetically pleasing gingival contours (Fig. 6.15c).

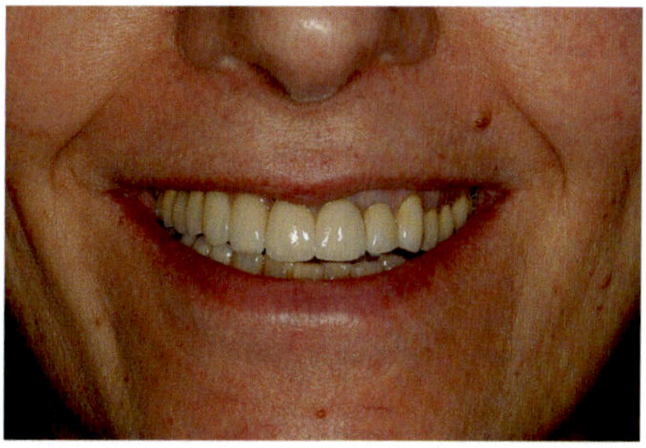

Fig. 6.17 Changes in bone after extraction: implant restorations look longer on this patient's right compared to left side

Table 6.7 Implant-associated procedures to maintain soft tissue contours and increase chances of implant success and longevity

Virtual treatment planning and guided implant placement	Virtual treatment planning software and use of surgical guides are highly recommended and will ensure precise prosthetically driven implant positioning
Reduction of bone collapse	Socket preservation
Bone volume augmentation	Guided bone regeneration Sinus lift procedures
Soft tissue augmentation	Free gingival graft Connective tissue graft
Immediate implant placement	Combination of tooth extraction, bone graft, socket barrier or seal

In the posterior maxilla, bone augmentation can be executed to gain bone volume vertically within the sinus. During a sinus lift procedure, the sinus's Schneiderian membrane is gently elevated, and bone graft material is placed into the space created between the sinus floor and the membrane [37].

Soft tissue augmentation is another type of surgery that can help modify peri-implant soft tissue phenotype to compensate and withstand the expected changes over time or treat peri-implant marginal mucosa defects. In areas where minimal bone loss can be of great consequence on the aesthetic outcome, the use of these additional surgical procedures is considered inevitable [38–40] (Table 6.7).

In specific situations where the patient's tissue contours are initially satisfactory, where the patient's biotype is thick, buccal bone is preserved and no acute infection is present, immediate implant placement has been identified as a way of maintaining soft tissue architecture. This procedure combines extraction, implant placement and bone grafting all at once with the placement of a personalized abutment or temporary crown to seal the socket from the oral environment. Studies provide promising short-term results in the aesthetic zone [41] (Fig. 6.18a–d).

Immediate implant placement significantly reduces the treatment time for patients. Although patient satisfaction with quick intervention may be increased, it is important that the use of the technique does not prevent the operator from placing the implant in the optimal three-dimensional position.

6.3.1.1 Recommendations

In order to be successful and obtain a restoration that will integrate harmoniously with the adjacent teeth and soft tissue, implant therapy will involve more than the

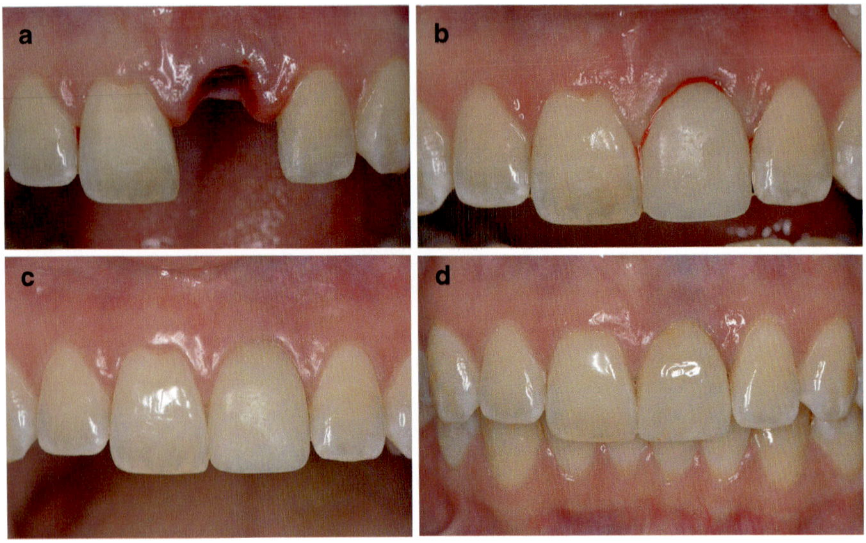

Fig. 6.18 (**a**) Immediate implant at the day of extraction. (**b**) Immediate loading of the implant with a temporary crown. (**c**) 5 weeks of healing. (**d**) Definitive restoration—1 year after definitive crown

act of extraction and implant placement. Initial analysis of CBCT scans and careful planning of the implant position with modern software (Fig. 6.19a, b) and the use of guided surgery will allow for placement of implants in a prosthetically appropriate position. Bone preservation, bone augmentation and soft tissue procedures may require additional time for healing and additional costs for therapy. However, they will increase the likelihood of treatment success.

6.3.2 Implant Complications [42–48]

When dental implants have fully osseointegrated and have re-established function and aesthetics, they can provide reliable long-term satisfaction for patients. However, much like a natural tooth, complications may arise in the medium to long term. These complications of various natures are usually foreseeable when risk factors have been previously identified. The main risk factors that affect implants are:

Risk factor type	Risk factors that may affect implants	Complications
The patient's systemic condition	Diabetes, smoking Hygiene	Implant loss Peri-implantitis
The patient's tooth structure condition	Highly restored teeth that may not withstand functional loading in the long term	Tooth fractures Mechanical complications, screw loosening, screw fractures

Risk factor type	Risk factors that may affect implants	Complications
The patient's periodontal condition	Bone support and crown height-space over 15 mm Biotype Hygiene	Mechanical complications Soft tissue inflammation Dehiscence, bleeding on probing Bone loss
The patient's endodontic condition	Persistent chronic infections that are in the vicinity of the implant	Implant loss Immediate implant placement should not be performed when acute infections are present
The patient's occlusal risk factors	Type of occlusion Occlusal vertical dimension Posterior support Missing teeth Parafunctional activity	Mechanical complications Acrylic or porcelain veneer fracture Screw loosening, screw fracture, fracture of abutment, decementation of crown from titanium base, fracture of implant
The patient's aesthetic risk factors	Lip mobility, tooth position, gingival biotype, inadequate bone support, inadequate amount of space for implant	Appearance of longer tooth, loss of papilla, disharmonious gingival architecture, tissue texture and colour changes, inadequate tooth proportions
The patient's psychological risk factors	Exacting patients High expectation Adaptive capacity	Dissatisfaction with restoration Dissatisfaction with phonetics

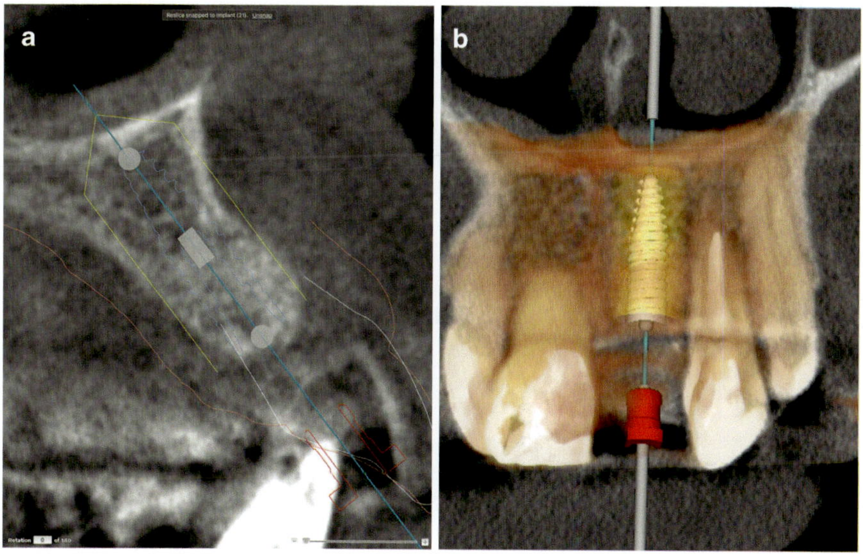

Fig. 6.19 (**a**) Modern implant planning: the software helps virtually position the implant in the optimal location. (**b**) Modern implant surgery: the software designs a surgical guide in order to precisely place the implant

6.4 Conclusion

When faced with the decision to restore or extract a tooth, the clinician's role is to determine if, within a comprehensive treatment plan, conventional dental therapy can provide adequate function and aesthetics for a sufficient amount of time that will be satisfactory to the patient. Having multiple treatment options is always an advantage. When choosing to maintain a tooth, a patient can also retain the possibility of placing implants in the future. Contrarily, when we choose to extract teeth before they have completed their useful life cycle in order to place implants, we reduce the patient's dental treatment options for the future.

Advantages of maintaining a natural tooth
The proprioceptive and viscoelastic properties of the periodontal ligament offer sensory function and shock absorption that help regulate bite force and offer the natural feeling of bite comfort that implants lack
The possibility of dynamic remodelling of the bone and periodontal ligament allows for tooth movement and offers the possibility of orthodontic tooth repositioning for optimal alignment and occlusion
Retaining a restorable tooth in the aesthetic zone may offer the advantages of a more predictable aesthetic outcome where the restoration of hard and soft tissue may be costly, challenging and time consuming with dental implants

In the proper circumstances, circumstances permitting, if no perilous biological risks are taken, retaining teeth allows for maintenance of the advantages offered by the periodontal ligament, and postponing extraction to a later date can be considered a reasonable objective. Communicating clearly with the patient regarding therapeutic modalities and their expected outcomes and the advantages and limitations of implant restorations is essential if the clinician wants to guide the patient in decision-making and achieve patient satisfaction.

Both teeth and implants have risk of complications. Identifying the risk factors specific to the patient will help the clinician determine which therapy may offer a more predictable outcome and guide the patient into making an informed decision.

Communicating the advantages and disadvantages of the dental implant to the patient will help manage expectations and increase chances of a successful therapy.

Advantages of implants
Titanium does not deteriorate when in a low-pH (acidic) environment
In normal functional conditions, implants have a good capacity to withstand functional loading

When placed in the proper position with adequate restoration, implants are easy to maintain and care for

When a tooth is not in the ideal position, implants may be positioned in a more ideal prosthetic location

Disadvantages of implants

Implant therapy may require more treatment time and added costs

Implant sites often require bone augmentation prior to implant placement

Soft tissue phenotype often must be modified to offer mucosal stability

The surgical interventions may have associated morbidity

Implants will act as an ankylotic tooth and will not be displaceable

Implants do not offer the same proprioception or shock absorption in function and may feel unnatural

Implant success depends on many variables that the operator must evaluate for each patient presentation and control the many factors regarding decision-making, treatment, delivery and maintenance; it may be challenging to obtain a satisfactory aesthetic result for a long term

References

1. McGuire MK. Prognosis versus actual outcome: a long-term survey of 100 treated periodontal patients under maintenance care. J Periodontol. 1991;62(1):51–8. https://doi.org/10.1902/jop.1991.62.1.51.
2. McGuire MK, Nunn ME. Prognosis versus actual outcome. II. The effectiveness of clinical parameters in developing an accurate prognosis. J Periodontol. 1996;67(7):658–65. https://doi.org/10.1902/jop.1996.67.7.658.
3. McGuire MK, Nunn ME. Prognosis versus actual outcome. III. The effectiveness of clinical parameters in accurately predicting tooth survival. J Periodontol. 1996;67(7):666–74. https://doi.org/10.1902/jop.1996.67.7.666.
4. McGuire MK, Nunn ME. Prognosis versus actual outcome. IV. The effectiveness of clinical parameters and IL-1 genotype in accurately predicting prognoses and tooth survival. J Periodontol. 1999;70(1):49–56. https://doi.org/10.1902/jop.1999.70.1.49.
5. Lee SJ, Chung D, Asano A, Sasaki D, Maeno M, Ishida Y, Kobayashi T, Kuwajima Y, Da Silva JD, Nagai S. Diagnosis of tooth prognosis using artificial intelligence. Diagnostics (Basel). 2022;12(6):1422. https://doi.org/10.3390/diagnostics12061422. PMID: 35741232; PMCID: PMC9221626.
6. Mordohai N, Reshad M, Jivraj SA. To extract or not to extract? Factors that affect individual tooth prognosis. J Calif Dent Assoc. 2005;33(4):319–28.
7. Kao RT. Strategic extraction: a paradigm shift that is changing our profession. J Periodontol. 2008;79(6):971–7. https://doi.org/10.1902/jop.2008.070551.
8. Kao RT, Lin GH, Kapila Y, Sadowsky S, Curtis DA. A commentary on strategic extraction. J Periodontol. 2022;93(1):11–9. https://doi.org/10.1002/JPER.20-0855. Epub 2021 Oct 26.
9. Magne P, Lazari PC, Carvalho MA, Johnson T, Del Bel Cury AA. Ferrule-effect dominates over use of a fiber post when restoring endodontically treated incisors: an in vitro study. Oper Dent. 2017;42(4):396–406. https://doi.org/10.2341/16-243-L. Epub 2017 Apr 12.
10. Carvalho TS, Schmid TM, Baumann T, Lussi A. Erosive effect of different dietary substances on deciduous and permanent teeth. Clin Oral Investig. 2017;21(5):1519–26. https://doi.org/10.1007/s00784-016-1915-z. Epub 2016 Jul 23.
11. Donovan T, Nguyen-Ngoc C, Abd Alraheam I, Irusa K. Contemporary diagnosis and management of dental erosion. J Esthet Restor Dent. 2021;33(1):78–87. https://doi.org/10.1111/jerd.12706. Epub 2021 Jan 6.
12. Guggenheimer J, Moore PA. Xerostomia: etiology, recognition and treatment. J Am Dent Assoc. 2003;134(1):61–9.; quiz 118–9. https://doi.org/10.14219/jada.archive.2003.0018.
13. Tanasiewicz M, Hildebrandt T, Obersztyn I. Xerostomia of various etiologies: a review of the literature. Adv Clin Exp Med. 2016;25(1):199–206. https://doi.org/10.17219/acem/29375.
14. Sorensen JA, Engelman MJ. Ferrule design and fracture resistance of endodontically treated teeth. J Prosthet Dent. 1990;63(5):529–36. https://doi.org/10.1016/0022-3913(90)90070-s.
15. Tan PL, Aquilino SA, Gratton DG, Stanford CM, Tan SC, Johnson WT, Dawson D. In vitro fracture resistance of endodontically treated central incisors with varying ferrule heights and configurations. J Prosthet Dent. 2005;93(4):331–6. https://doi.org/10.1016/j.prosdent.2005.01.013.
16. Sorensen JA, Martinoff JT. Endodontically treated teeth as abutments. J Prosthet Dent. 1985;53(5):631–6. https://doi.org/10.1016/0022-3913(85)90008-3.
17. Wegner PK, Freitag S, Kern M. Survival rate of endodontically treated teeth with posts after prosthetic restoration. J Endod. 2006;32(10):928–31. https://doi.org/10.1016/j.joen.2006.06.001. Epub 2006 Jul 26.
18. Melo G, Duarte J, Pauletto P, Porporatti AL, Stuginski-Barbosa J, Winocur E, Flores-Mir C, De Luca CG. Bruxism: an umbrella review of systematic reviews. J Oral Rehabil. 2019;46(7):666–90. https://doi.org/10.1111/joor.12801. Epub 2019 May 7.
19. Goldstein G, DeSantis L, Goodacre C. Bruxism: best evidence consensus statement. J Prosthodont. 2021;30(S1):91–101. https://doi.org/10.1111/jopr.13308.

20. Ferrari M, Pontoriero DIK, Ferrari Cagidiaco E, Carboncini F. Restorative difficulty evaluation system of endodontically treated teeth. J Esthet Restor Dent. 2022;34(1):65–80. https://doi.org/10.1111/jerd.12880. Epub 2022 Feb 8.
21. Baba NZ, Goodacre CJ, Kattadiyil MT. Tooth retention through root canal treatment or tooth extraction and implant placement: a prosthodontic perspective. Quintessence Int. 2014;45(5):405–16. https://doi.org/10.3290/j.qi.a31544.
22. Torabinejad M, Landaez M, Milan M, Sun CX, Henkin J, Al-Ardah A, Kattadiyil M, Bahjri K, Dehom S, Cortez E, White SN. Tooth retention through endodontic microsurgery or tooth replacement using single implants: a systematic review of treatment outcomes. J Endod. 2015;41(1):1–10. https://doi.org/10.1016/j.joen.2014.09.002. Epub 2014 Oct 11.
23. Torabinejad M, Anderson P, Bader J, Brown LJ, Chen LH, Goodacre CJ, Kattadiyil MT, Kutsenko D, Lozada J, Patel R, Petersen F, Puterman I, White SN. Outcomes of root canal treatment and restoration, implant-supported single crowns, fixed partial dentures, and extraction without replacement: a systematic review. J Prosthet Dent. 2007;98(4):285–311. https://doi.org/10.1016/S0022-3913(07)60102-4.
24. Parirokh M, Zarifian A, Ghoddusi J. Choice of treatment plan based on root canal therapy versus extraction and implant placement: a mini review. Iran Endod J. 2015;10(3):152–5. https://doi.org/10.7508/iej.2015.03.001. Epub 2015 Jul 1. PMID: 26213535; PMCID: PMC4509120.
25. Kwok V, Caton JG. Commentary: prognosis revisited: a system for assigning periodontal prognosis. J Periodontol. 2007;78(11):2063–71. https://doi.org/10.1902/jop.2007.070210.
26. Carvalho R, Botelho J, Machado V, Mascarenhas P, Alcoforado G, Mendes JJ, Chambrone L. Predictors of tooth loss during long-term periodontal maintenance: an updated systematic review. J Clin Periodontol. 2021;48(8):1019–36. https://doi.org/10.1111/jcpe.13488. Epub 2021 May 29.
27. Zaleckiene V, Peciuliene V, Brukiene V, Drukteinis S. Traumatic dental injuries: etiology, prevalence and possible outcomes. Stomatologija. 2014;16(1):7–14.
28. Levin L, Halperin-Sternfeld M. Tooth preservation or implant placement: a systematic review of long-term tooth and implant survival rates. J Am Dent Assoc. 2013;144(10):1119–33. https://doi.org/10.14219/jada.archive.2013.0030.
29. Chappuis V, Buser R, Brägger U, Bornstein MM, Salvi GE, Buser D. Long-term outcomes of dental implants with a titanium plasma-sprayed surface: a 20-year prospective case series study in partially edentulous patients. Clin Implant Dent Relat Res. 2013;15(6):780–90. https://doi.org/10.1111/cid.12056. Epub 2013 Mar 18.
30. Pjetursson BE, Asgeirsson AG, Zwahlen M, Sailer I. Improvements in implant dentistry over the last decade: comparison of survival and complication rates in older and newer publications. Int J Oral Maxillofac Implants. 2014;29(Suppl):308–24. https://doi.org/10.11607/jomi.2014suppl.g5.2.
31. Schimmel M, Srinivasan M, McKenna G, Müller F. Effect of advanced age and/or systemic medical conditions on dental implant survival: a systematic review and meta-analysis. Clin Oral Implants Res. 2018;29(Suppl 16):311–30. https://doi.org/10.1111/clr.13288.
32. French D, Ofec R, Levin L. Long term clinical performance of 10,871 dental implants with up to 22 years of follow-up: a cohort study in 4247 patients. Clin Implant Dent Relat Res. 2021;23(3):289–97. https://doi.org/10.1111/cid.12994. Epub 2021 Mar 25. PMID: 33768695; PMCID: PMC8359846.
33. Mozzati M, Gallesio G, Del Fabbro M. Long-term (9–12 years) outcomes of titanium implants with an oxidized surface: a retrospective investigation on 209 implants. J Oral Implantol. 2015;41(4):437–43. https://doi.org/10.1563/AAID-JOI-D-13-00211. Epub 2013 Oct 31.
34. Furhauser R, Florescu D, Benesch T, Haas R, Mailath G, Watzek G. Evaluation of soft tissue around single-tooth implant crowns: the pink esthetics core. Clin Oral Implants Res. 2005;16:639–44. https://doi.org/10.1111/j.1600-0501.2005.01193.x.
35. Barone A, Ricci M, Tonelli P, Santini S, Covani U. Tissue changes of extraction sockets in humans: a comparison of spontaneous healing vs. ridge preservation with secondary soft tissue healing. Clin Oral Implants Res. 2013;24(11):1231–7. https://doi.org/10.1111/j.1600-0501.2012.02535.x. Epub 2012 Jul 12.

36. Ten Heggeler JM, Slot DE, Van der Weijden GA. Effect of socket preservation therapies following tooth extraction in non-molar regions in humans: a systematic review. Clin Oral Implants Res. 2011;22(8):779–88. https://doi.org/10.1111/j.1600-0501.2010.02064.x. Epub 2010 Nov 22.
37. Esposito M, Grusovin MG, Rees J, Karasoulos D, Felice P, Alissa R, Worthington H, Coulthard P. Effectiveness of sinus lift procedures for dental implant rehabilitation: a Cochrane systematic review. Eur J Oral Implantol. 2010;3(1):7–26.
38. Tavelli L, Barootchi S, Avila-Ortiz G, Urban IA, Giannobile WV, Wang HL. Peri-implant soft tissue phenotype modification and its impact on peri-implant health: a systematic review and network meta-analysis. J Periodontol. 2021;92(1):21–44. https://doi.org/10.1002/JPER.19-0716. Epub 2020 Aug 9.
39. Zucchelli G, Tavelli L, McGuire MK, Rasperini G, Feinberg SE, Wang HL, Giannobile WV. Autogenous soft tissue grafting for periodontal and peri-implant plastic surgical reconstruction. J Periodontol. 2020;91(1):9–16. https://doi.org/10.1002/JPER.19-0350. Epub 2019 Oct 6.
40. Avila-Ortiz G, Couso-Queiruga E, Pirc M, Chambrone L, Thoma DS. Outcome measures and methods of assessment of soft-tissue augmentation interventions in the context of dental implant therapy: a systematic review of clinical studies published in the last 10 years. Clin Oral Implants Res. 2023;34(Suppl 25):84–96. https://doi.org/10.1111/clr.13927. Epub 2022 Jul 11.
41. Chen ST, Buser D. Esthetic outcomes following immediate and early implant placement in the anterior maxilla—a systematic review. Int J Oral Maxillofac Implants. 2014;29(Suppl):186–215. https://doi.org/10.11607/jomi.2014suppl.g3.3. PMID: 24660198.
42. Do TA, Le HS, Shen YW, Huang HL, Fuh LJ. Risk factors related to late failure of dental implant—a systematic review of recent studies. Int J Environ Res Public Health. 2020;17(11):3931. https://doi.org/10.3390/ijerph17113931. PMID: 32498256; PMCID: PMC7312800.
43. Atieh MA, Alsabeeha NH, Faggion CM Jr, Duncan WJ. The frequency of peri-implant diseases: a systematic review and meta-analysis. J Periodontol. 2013;84(11):1586–98. https://doi.org/10.1902/jop.2012.120592. Epub 2012 Dec 13.
44. Berglundh T, Armitage G, Araujo MG, Avila-Ortiz G, Blanco J, Camargo PM, Chen S, Cochran D, Derks J, Figuero E, Hämmerle CHF, Heitz-Mayfield LJA, Huynh-Ba G, Iacono V, Koo KT, Lambert F, McCauley L, Quirynen M, Renvert S, Salvi GE, Schwarz F, Tarnow D, Tomasi C, Wang HL, Zitzmann N. Peri-implant diseases and conditions: consensus report of workgroup 4 of the 2017 world workshop on the classification of periodontal and peri-implant diseases and conditions. J Clin Periodontol. 2018;45(Suppl 20):S286–91. https://doi.org/10.1111/jcpe.12957.
45. Schou S, Holmstrup P, Worthington HV, Esposito M. Outcome of implant therapy in patients with previous tooth loss due to periodontitis. Clin Oral Implants Res. 2006;17(Suppl 2):104–23. https://doi.org/10.1111/j.1600-0501.2006.01347.x.
46. Goodacre CJ, Bernal G, Rungcharassaeng K, Kan JY. Clinical complications with implants and implant prostheses. J Prosthet Dent. 2003;90(2):121–32. https://doi.org/10.1016/S0022-3913(03)00212-9.
47. Sailer I, Karasan D, Todorovic A, Ligoutsikou M, Pjetursson BE. Prosthetic failures in dental implant therapy. Periodontology 2000. 2022;88(1):130–44. https://doi.org/10.1111/prd.12416. PMID: 35103329; PMCID: PMC9305548.
48. Jung RE, Zembic A, Pjetursson BE, Zwahlen M, Thoma DS. Systematic review of the survival rate and the incidence of biological, technical, and aesthetic complications of single crowns on implants reported in longitudinal studies with a mean follow-up of 5 years. Clin Oral Implants Res. 2012;23(Suppl 6):2–21. https://doi.org/10.1111/j.1600-0501.2012.02547.x.

Occlusion for Implant Prosthodontics

7

Saj Jivraj and Winston Chee

Occlusion on implant-supported restorations is a subject that lacks substantial evidence. Most occlusal philosophies espouse to concepts that have been taken from the natural dentition.

Commonly held beliefs in regard to occlusion on natural teeth include the following:

1. Stable stops on all teeth when the condyles are seated in the most superior anterior position against the articular eminence
2. An anterior guidance that is in harmony with the border movements of the envelope of function
3. Disclusion of all posterior teeth on the balancing side
4. Disclusion of all posterior teeth in a protrusive movement

The above principles are based on biomechanics rather than sound scientific literature. Implant occlusion is similar in this regard. The practitioner must understand that with implant-supported restorations, the goal is to minimize stress in the system so that the implant/abutment junction stays tight, and the preload of the screw is not exceeded.

When deciding on occlusal schemes, the clinician must differentiate between two clinical scenarios:

1. Does the patient have existing natural teeth and how many? Do the existing natural teeth provide definitive support? How many implants have been placed?

S. Jivraj (✉)
Private Practice, Anacapa Dental Art Institute, Oxnard, CA, USA

W. Chee
Advanced Prosthodontics, Herman Ostrow School of Dentistry, University of Southern California, Los Angeles, CA, USA

W. Chee, S. Jivraj (eds.), *Treatment Planning In Implant Dentistry*, BDJ Clinician's Guides, https://doi.org/10.1007/978-3-031-68726-6_7

2. Is the restoration totally implant supported in which circumstance distribution of tooth contacts is based solely on biomechanics rather than adapting to a specific occlusal scheme?

In all aspects, teeth need to come together in an intercuspal position—using the condylar position as a reference.

The following concepts will be discussed in order to come to an understanding of the occlusal schemes recommended:

1. Differences between teeth and implants
2. Factors that can cause overload—bruxism, excessive contact, inadequate number of implants, large occlusal table, steep cuspal inclination, inadequate number of implants and overextended cantilevers
3. Factors that can reduce stress in the system—timing of occlusal contacts, surface area, axial vs. tilted implants, crown cusp angle, crown height, occlusal contact position, implant/abutment connection and implant tooth connection
4. Confirmative occlusion—being conforming to the existing occlusal contacts vs. reorganized occlusion where the clinician has control of the entire occlusal scheme
5. Type of support intended—implant supported or implant and mucosa supported
6. Recommendations for single teeth, FPD, overdentures, fixed full-arch implant-supported restorations

7.1 Differences Between a Tooth and a Dental Implant

To begin to understand the dynamics of implant occlusion, the clinician must have a clear understanding of the physiological and mechanical differences between a tooth and an implant (Fig. 7.1).

7.1.1 Presence of a Periodontal Ligament (PDL)

A natural tooth has a support design which reduces transfer of forces to the crestal bone. A tooth is suspended in the socket by a periodontal ligament, whereas the implant is in direct contact with the bone. The average value of displacement of tooth within a socket is 25 microns [1]. The range of displacement around an implant has been reported to be 3–5 microns [2].

When a load is applied to a tooth, it gets displaced in the socket 25 microns, whereas an implant is displaced much less. The periodontal ligament is also functionally oriented towards an axial load, which leads to physiological adjustment of stress along the vertical axis of the tooth [3].

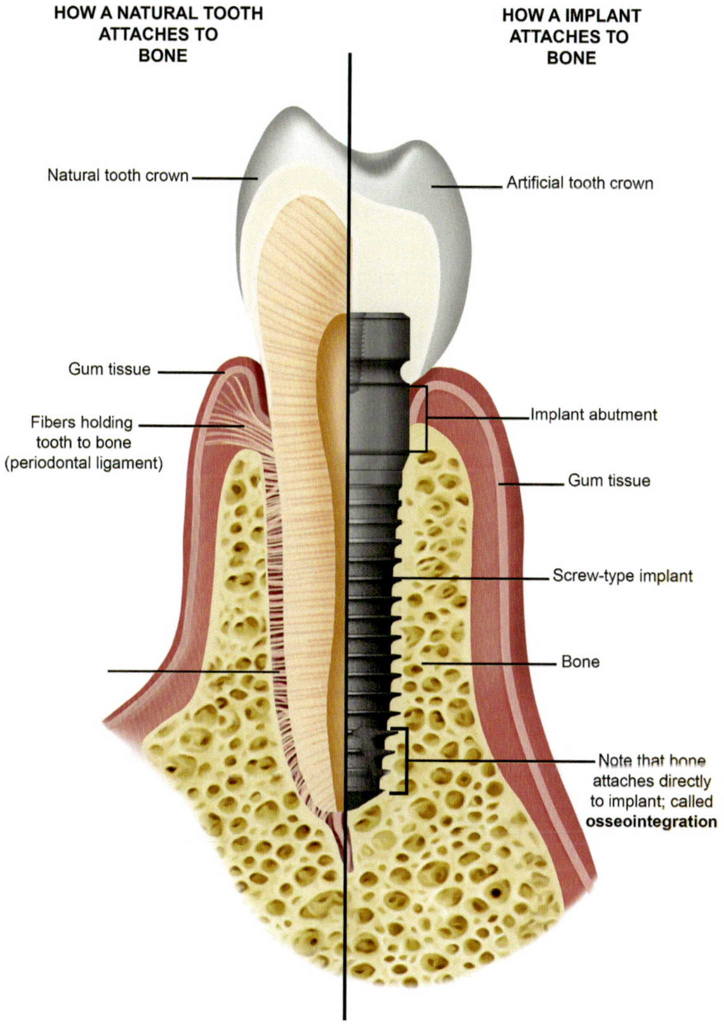

Fig. 7.1 Differences between a tooth and an implant

7.1.2 Tooth Mobility

The periodontal ligament provides the tooth with mobility, allowing it to move from high loads. Restorations on implants lack these benefits.

When the tooth is subject to lateral stresses, it rotates at the apical third of the root [4] and moves in a 56–108 micron range. The lateral force also immediately decreases from the bone crest and is transferred down the root [5]. There are no such instantaneous movements seen with the implant. It only displays secondary movements that are dependent on the viscoelasticity of bone and in the range of 10–50 microns.

This suggests that because of its mobility, the tooth moves far more than the implant when subjected to lateral stresses.

7.1.3 Proprioception

The presence of the PDL provides increased protection against occlusal overload by sending information to the central nervous system, which provides feedback to the elevator muscles that elicit a protective reflex to reduce occlusal forces.

In addition, the PDL offers additional protection by absorbing pressure when heavy occlusal forces are applied to the tooth. A natural tooth can be displaced 25–100 μm in the axial direction and 56–108 μm horizontally, compared to a dental implant, which can only be displaced 3–5 μm axially and 10–50 μm horizontally. The PDL also allows the tooth to adapt to excessive forces through intrusion or rotation and by distributing the load along the entire root surface. In contrast, because a dental implant is connected directly to the bone, it does not have the same adaptive capabilities.

7.1.4 Cross-Sectional Anatomy

The width of any implant replacing the tooth is much smaller than the natural teeth. The cross-sectional shape of the tooth is such that it resists the lateral loads very effectively. However, for the ease of surgical placement of the implant, they are round in cross section. They are thus less effective in resisting lateral bending forces in the crestal region.

The shape and size of the teeth are as per the functional requirements of the body.

The size of the implant is decided mostly by the amount of bone available to place implants rather than direction and magnitude of forces. The appropriate size of implant must be selected to have an abundance of bone around the implant and to support the type of tooth being replaced. The clinician must exercise caution in choosing a narrow-diameter implant for posterior teeth. In this circumstance, excessive forces will not lead to a loss of osseointegration but rather to a possible fracture of the implant.

7.1.5 Elastic Modulus (Stiffness of the Material)

The elastic modulus of tooth is closest to the bone compared to the available implant materials.

Titanium is at least five times stiffer than bone. The closer the value of elastic moduli of two dissimilar structures, the lesser the likelihood of relative motion at the bone–implant interface on application of loads.

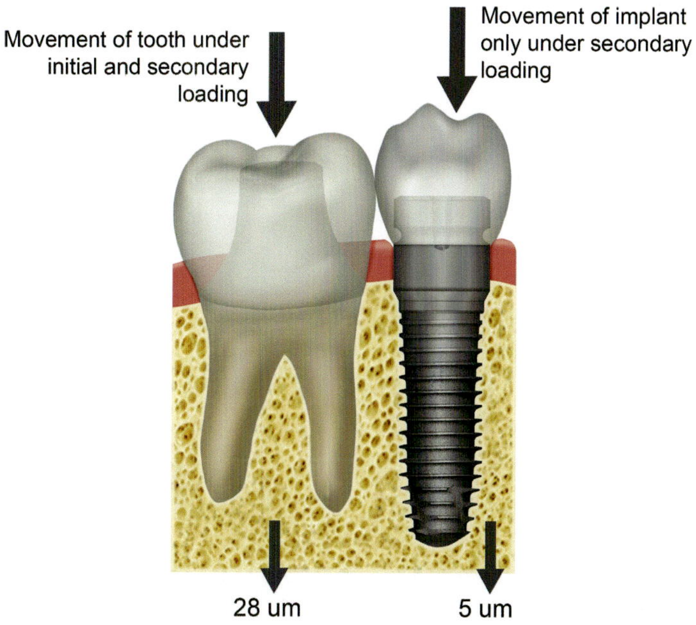

Fig. 7.2 Difference between tooth and an implant in terms of intrusion

Hence, under similar loading conditions, implants generate greater stresses and strain at the crest of bone than natural tooth due to severe difference in modulus of elasticity (stiffness) between titanium and bone (Fig. 7.2).

7.1.6 Signs of Occlusal Overload

Occlusal trauma is evident on natural teeth. It is seen in the form of enamel wear facets, stress lines, cervical abfractions, increase in periodontal membrane thickness, fremitus and tooth fracture, which may be associated with pain. These signs are absent in dental implants. Signs of overload may be prosthetic screw loosening, which results in a mobile prosthesis. This if undetected may result in prosthetic screw fracture. Additional sequelae may result in mechanical complications with the abutment, the titanium base or sometimes even the implant body (Table 7.1).

7.2 Factors That Can Cause Overload

(a) Parafunctional habits: Parafunctional habits are an important factor which may be responsible for occlusal overload. Treatment of patients who brux will require an in-depth education of the patient, risk management, clinical precautions and lifelong professional maintenance. Bruxism and clenching, and improper force distribution, are correlated with screw loosening, prosthesis

Table 7.1 Differences between a tooth and an implant [6]

	Natural tooth	Implant
Connection	Periodontal ligament	Functional ankylosis
Proprioception	Periodontal mechanoreceptors	Osseoperception
Tactile sensitivity	High	Low
Axial mobility	25–100 microns	3–5 microns
Movement patterns	Primary—non-linear and complex Secondary—linear and elastic	Primary—linear and elastic
Movement phases	Primary—immediate Secondary—gradual	Primary—gradual
Fulcrum to lateral force	Apical third of root	Crest of bone
Load-bearing characteristics	Shock absorbing/stress distribution	Stress concentration at crestal bone
Signs of overloading	PDL thickening, mobility, wear, fremitus, pain	Screw loosening, abutment screw, Ti base or implant fracture, prosthesis fracture

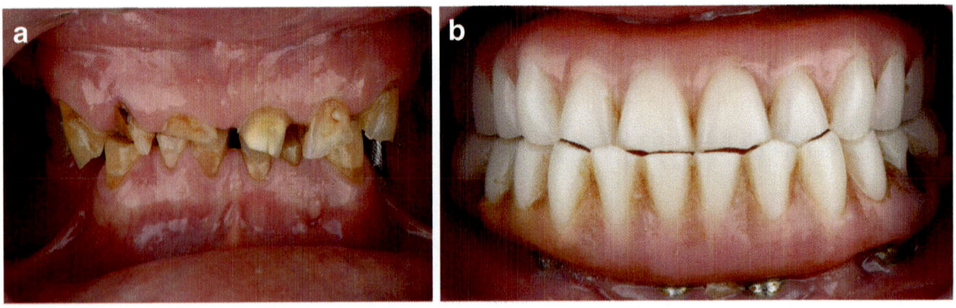

Fig. 7.3 (**a**) Picture of a high-function patient. (**b**) Picture of prosthesis in a high-function patient

mobility, prosthetic screw fracture and, in extreme situations, implant fracture [7] (Fig. 7.3a, b).

Management of dental occlusion in a bruxism patient may include some of the following measures:

1. Injection of botulinum toxin in their muscles of mastication.
2. Mutually protected occlusion with canine guidance for posterior disclusion. This is based purely on biomechanics with the thought that the teeth nearer the joint do not touch in lateral excursion. Forces on teeth towards the joint are much higher.
3. Avoidance of cantilevers.
4. Over-engineering the number of implants for increased force distribution.
5. Screw-retained prosthesis for retrievability and repairs.
6. Fabrication of a protective occlusal device.

(b) Cantilevers: This has been discussed at length in a previous chapter. Cantilevers serve to magnify loads. Cantilevers are useful in situations where anatomical constraints make it difficult to place the implant. Based on four RCTs with small sample sizes and long observation periods, no difference in marginal bone level between reconstruction with or without cantilevers was reported; however, more technical complications were frequently observed with cantilevers than without cantilevers (Fig. 7.4a–c). Therefore, prostheses with cantilevers should be checked not only for changes in the marginal bone level, but also for screw loosening or other changes in the occlusal contact and vertical dimension of the prosthesis [8–11].

Precautions to reduce overload in cantilevered prosthesis include the following:

1. Place cantilever in infra-occlusion.
2. Use low cusp angles and narrow occlusal tables.
3. Direct forces axially as much as possible.
4. Use a protective night-time device.

(c) Large occlusal table: The clinician when designing the restoration should understand that it may not be possible to give the patient similar contours which existed in the natural dentition. This often occurs in molars which are large mesiodistally and buccolingually. Contours should be designed with a slightly narrower occlusal table and shallower cuspal inclines to decrease loads on the

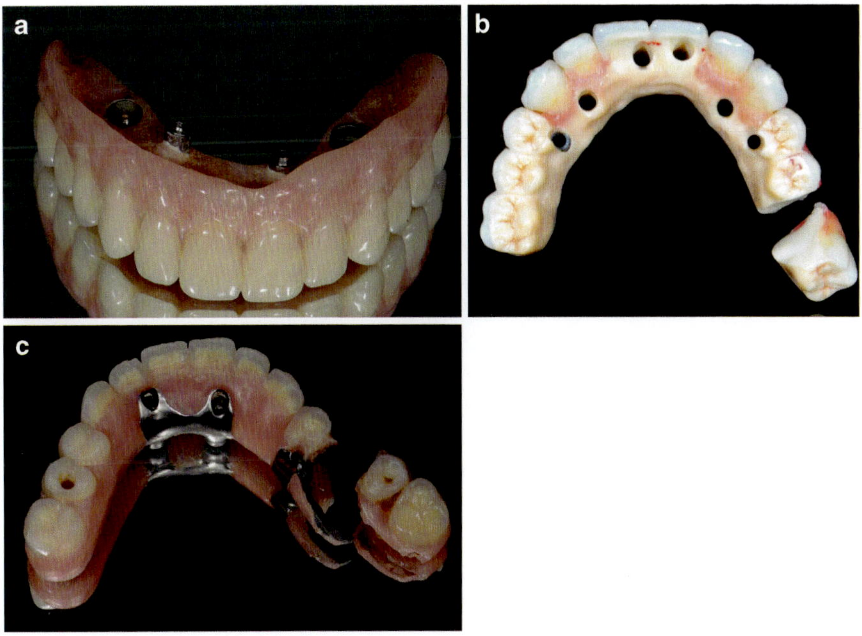

Fig. 7.4 (**a**) Excessive cantilever and incorrect support. This has been designed as an implant-supported restoration with unhygienic contours. (**b**) Excessive cantilever in zirconia. (**c**) Excessive cantilever and inadequate framework design

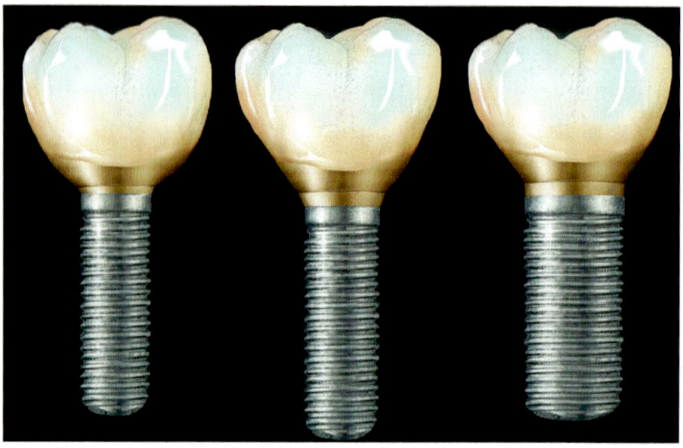

Fig. 7.5 For molars, it is preferable to have wider body implants if bone allows. This allows better stress distribution and development of an appropriate emergence profile

restoration. If the patient insists on a similar sized tooth, it should be given through either wider body implants or two implants to replace a molar (Fig. 7.4a–c).

(d) Inadequate number of implants: There is always going to be a debate over how many implants should be placed in an edentulous arch or partially edentulous arch. The answer to that question is "It depends". It depends on the patient's medical history, it depends on the quality of bone, it depends on the anticipated occlusal force on the restoration and it depends on the operator's skill. Where higher occlusal loads are anticipated, it is prudent to use additional implants so that the load distribution is divided amongst the fixtures (Fig. 7.5).

(e) Poor crown-to-implant ratio: In implant-borne restorations, crown-implant ratio is merely theoretical. The height of the crown is dictated by aesthetics and the distance of the occlusal plane from the head of the fixture. Multiple systematic reviews on short implants have shown high survival rates and marginal bone loss comparable to regular length implants. Once integrated, short implants appear to be just as efficacious as a long implant, and within the scope of dental occlusion, clinicians can ignore the concept of crown-to-implant ratio [12, 13].

(f) Excessive premature contacts: Contacts that divert the mandible from the normal path of closure, interfere with normal smooth gliding mandibular movements and/or deflect the position of the condyle, teeth or prosthesis are referred to as premature contacts. Premature contacts if excessive in nature may result in prosthetic complications such as screw, prosthesis mobility and prosthesis material fracture. The literature does not support a cause-effect relationship between premature contacts and marginal bone loss around implants (Figs. 7.6 and 7.7).

7.3 Factors That Can Decrease Stress in the System

(a) Premature contacts: During maximum intercuspation and centric occlusion, no occlusal contacts should be premature, especially in an implant-supported prosthesis.

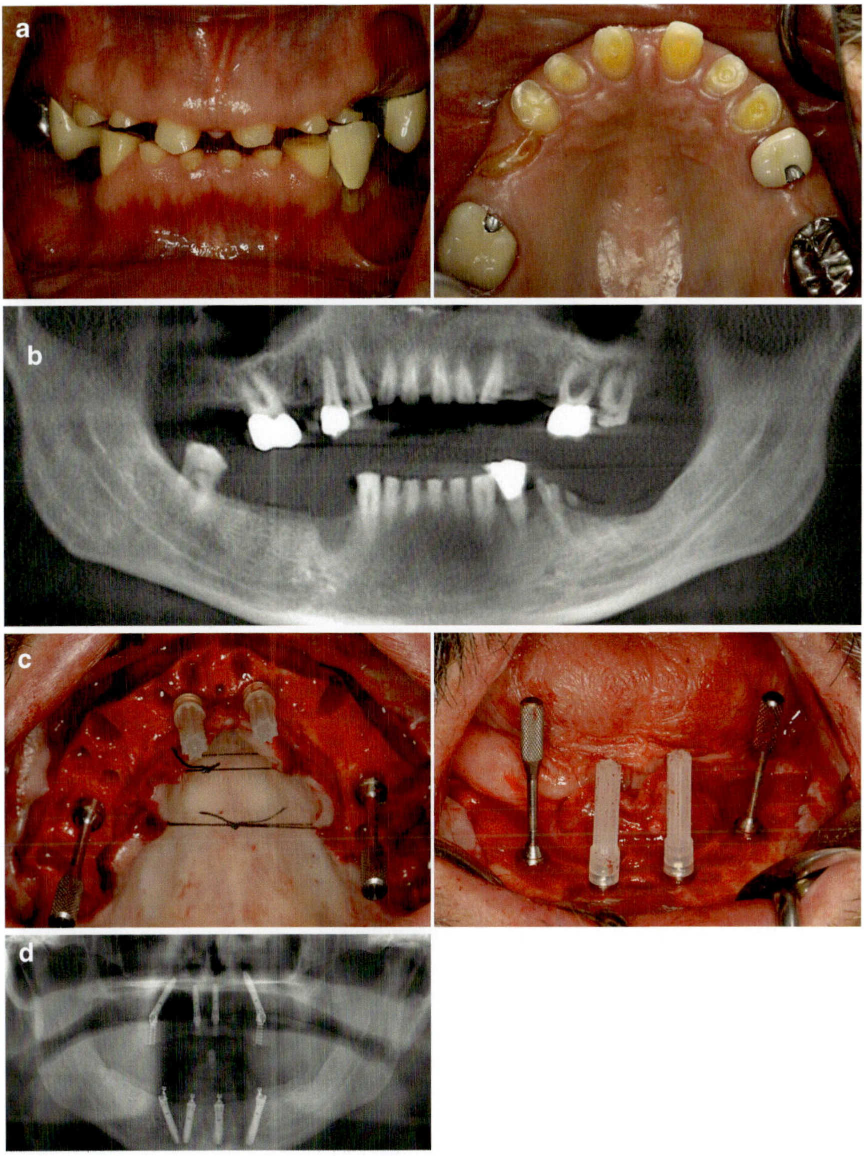

Fig. 7.6 (**a**) High-function patient with terminal dentition. (**b**) Panoramic radiograph shows abundance of bone. (**c**) Patient treated irrationally with the All on 4 ™ treatment concept. (**d**) In this scenario, it would have been preferable to place additional implants

(b) Timing of occlusal contacts: The initial occlusal contact should account for the difference in vertical movement between the tooth and the implant. If it does not, the implant will sustain greater loads than the adjacent teeth. When teeth are subjected to sudden occlusal load, the tooth movement ranges from 8 to 25

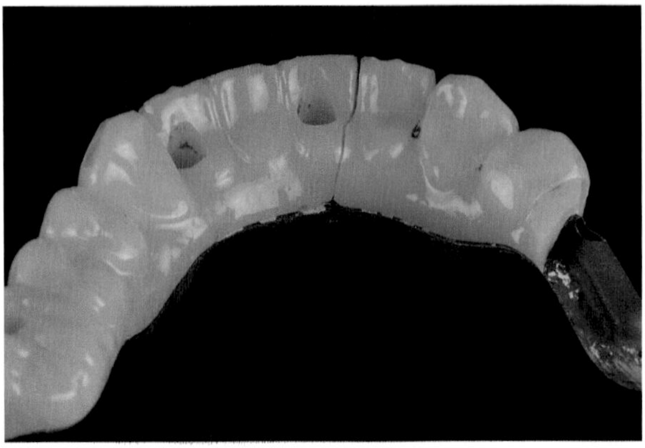

Fig. 7.7 Prosthesis fracture due to inadequate design and inadequate stress distribution

microns under 3–5 lbs. of load, depending on the anatomy and number of roots and also the time lapse since the last load application. Once the initial tooth movement occurs, the secondary tooth movement occurs in the surrounding bone. This is similar to bone–implant movement. The implant does not have any initial movement, and the 3–5 micron movement is due to bone resiliency. Hence, when teeth oppose each other, the combined intrusion may be 56 microns (28 + 28 microns). The teeth opposing an implant will have combined intrusion of 28 microns (28 + 0 microns). In case of implants opposing implant, the total combined intrusion may remain 0 microns compared with 56 microns in the rest of the arch. Teeth move immediately even with light loads, whereas implants move only under heavy occlusal loads. So even though the occlusion may be ideal, premature contacts on the implant may still occur because of the sudden initial movement of the teeth away from occlusal forces. The prosthesis should be checked with shim stock and thin articulating paper in light occlusion (less than 25 microns). If the implant prosthesis is between adjacent teeth, the prosthesis should barely contact. The adjacent teeth should exhibit greater occlusal contacts. In heavier occlusion, similar contacts should exist between the implant prosthesis and the adjacent teeth. There should be equitable load distribution. In a situation where the implants are in a distal extension and have been placed to restore posterior support, occlusal contacts should be distributed equitably between the teeth and implants in both light and heavy occlusion. This is based on biomechanics rather than science.

(c) Surface area and number of implants: Wider implants have a greater area of contact with the bone at the crest than narrower implants potentially reducing the mechanical stresses. The width of the occlusal table is directly related to the size of the implant (Fig. 7.5). Larger occlusal tables will transmit more loads to the bone, so narrowing the width of the table reduces the load. Stress and strain can also be reduced by using an increased number of implants in the area of concern and splinting the implants to increase the area of support (Figs. 7.6a–d and 7.7) [14].

(d) Crown cusp angle: Developing tooth morphology to induce axial loading is an important factor to consider when constructing an implant prosthesis. Weinberg [15] claimed that in the production of bending moment, cusp inclination is one of the most significant factors. The resultant bending moment can be decreased by reduction of cusp inclination with a lever-arm reduction and improvement of axial loading force. The occlusal contact over an implant crown should be ideally on a flat surface perpendicular to the implant body. This can be accomplished by widening the central fossa of the posterior teeth by 2–3 mm. The opposing cusp should be recontoured to occlude the central fossa directly over the implant body. The occlusal scheme and crown occlusal anatomy should be designed to direct axial loads to implant bodies.

(e) Implant crown contour: When contouring an implant crown, the position of the implant should be taken into consideration. When teeth are lost, the position of the ridge shifts both for the maxilla and the mandible. The maxillary ridge resorbs medially (towards the midline). Due to this, the implant may be placed palatally as compared to the mandibular teeth. In the mandibular arch, resorption in the lingual direction of the arch results in more lingual placement of the implants. The implant is narrower buccolingually as compared to the natural teeth. The centre of the implant most often is placed in the centre of the edentulous ridge, which is actually lingual to the rest of the teeth in the arch. Most often, the crown fabricated has cantilevered buccal cusps, which are formed to get the implant crown in alignment with the rest of the arch. This may place more load on the bone. In case of buccal bone resorption, palatal placement of the implant in posterior maxilla may be advocated. A significant buccal cantilever in a biomechanically poor environment (heavy bite, poor bone- and poor crown-implant ratio) can be created by normal contour on palatally placed implant. In this case, utilization of cross-bite occlusion can avoid the buccal cantilever and improve axial loading. The above can be avoided should the clinician choose to augment the ridge horizontally so that the implant can be placed in a similar position required for tooth morphology of the adjacent teeth (Fig. 7.8).

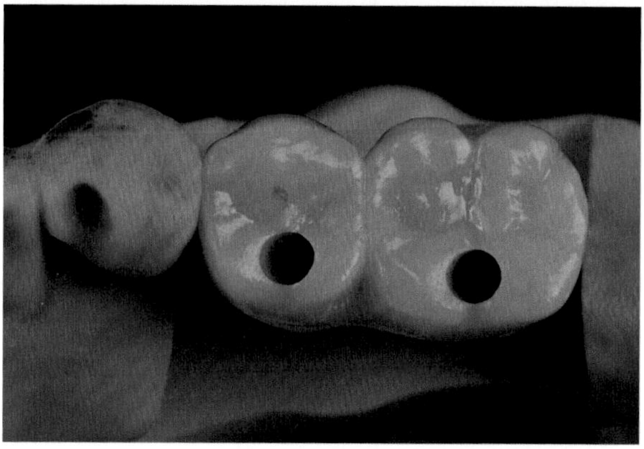

Fig. 7.8 Picture of molars with excessive buccal cantilever

(f) Occlusal contacts: The implant crown often exceeds the diameter of the implant. In both the maxilla and mandible, occlusal contacts are placed on either the palatal or the buccal cusps. This results in a cantilever. In posterior screw-retained restorations, often cantilever contacts are present. The primary occlusal contact should be within the diameter of the implant within the central fossa, and the secondary occlusal contact should remain with 1 mm of the periphery of the implant to decrease adverse loading.

7.4 Conformative or Reorganized Occlusion

Implant occlusion per se has limited scientific basis. Most philosophies have been adapted from the natural dentition. The design of the occlusal scheme depends on many factors. This to a large degree is based on clinical experience and clinical judgement.

The clinician must ask the following questions prior to implementing a specific occlusal philosophy/scheme:

1. How many natural teeth does the patient have?
2. What is the level of bony support around the existing dentition?
3. Does the patient have opposing sets of teeth to provide posterior support?
4. How many implants need to be restored?
5. Are the implant restorations going to be bounded by teeth?
6. Is the purpose of the implants to restore posterior support?
7. Are the restorations splinted or unsplinted?
8. Does the clinician have control of a few occlusal contacts or the entire occlusion?

Depending on the number of units being restored and the purpose of the units, the occlusion may be organized in such a way that it is:

(A) Conformative—conforming with the existing natural dentition.
(B) Reorganized—developing a complete occlusal scheme based on biomechanics.

Both occlusal schemes must ensure that the teeth come together simultaneously in the intercuspal position using the condyles as a reference.

7.5 Recommendations

The recommendations outlined below are based on biomechanics and not scientific evidence regarding occlusal schemes related to dental implants. Regular recall of the patient is required to verify the occlusal contacts and make adjustments as needed. Occlusal contacts are tested with articulating paper and shimstock. Shimstock is approximately 10 microns in thickness. In many articles, the phrase "shimstock should pull through" is used. The clinician should feel a slight resistance as the shimstock is pulled through. The shimstock should not tear or freely pull through. This is definitely a clinical judgement and requires practice to discern.

For the sake of minimizing repetition, in all situations where the patient has existing natural dentition, the occlusal contacts on the teeth should be verified prior to delivering the restoration.

Occlusal contacts are tested on the teeth anterior, posterior and on the contralateral side. All natural teeth should hold shimstock in the maximum intercuspal position with the patient closed with medium intensity. Following insertion of the implant restoration, these natural tooth contacts should still be the same. If the contacts on the implant restoration are heavy, thin-film articulating paper 27 microns in thickness should be introduced to mark the implant restorations. This should be adjusted until the natural tooth contact is conformative. A night-time protective appliance should also be delivered.

The following recommendations assume that the implants have been placed in an abundance of bone and sufficient implants have been placed after biomechanical risk assessment of the patient.

The opposing occlusion may also need to be adjusted. The recommendations assume opposing teeth in ideal positions:

1. Posterior single-tooth implant restorations bounded by teeth
2. Two posterior splinted implant restorations bounded by natural teeth
3. Kennedy class 1
4. Kennedy class 2
5. Implant in canine region
6. Occlusion when canine is missing
7. Full-arch immediate load
8. Full-arch opposing denture
9. Full-arch opposing teeth
10. Full-arch implants opposing full-arch implants
11. Overdentures implant retained and mucosa supported

7.5.1 Posterior Single-Tooth Implant Restorations Bounded by Teeth

Natural teeth—shimstock hold.

Implant restoration—shimstock drag.

When the patient moves into lateral excursion, there should be no contacts on the implant. Over time, the opposing tooth may overerupt bringing the implant restoration into contact. The astute practitioner should always look for excessive contacts at recall and adjust as necessary.

7.5.2 Kennedy Class 3—Two Posterior Splinted Implant Restoration Bounded by Natural Teeth

Natural teeth—shimstock hold.

Implant restorations—shimstock drag.

Splinting the implants distributes the loads over a wider area minimizing horizontal forces to the implant/abutment junction.

On lateral excursion, there should be no contacts on the implant restoration. The lateral excursion should be conformative with the patient's existing dentition.

7.5.3 Kennedy Class 1

Natural teeth—shimstock hold.

Implant restorations—shimstock hold.

Splinting the implants distributes the loads over a wider area minimizing horizontal forces to the implant/abutment junction.

The reason for shimstock hold is that in distal extension situation, implants are often placed to provide posterior support.

On lateral excursion, there should be no contacts on the implant restoration. The lateral excursion should be conformative with the patient's existing dentition.

7.5.4 Kennedy Class 2

Natural teeth—shimstock hold.

Implant restorations—shimstock hold.

Splinting the implants distributes the loads over a wider area minimizing horizontal forces to the implant/abutment junction.

The reason for shimstock hold is that in distal extension situation, implants are often placed to provide posterior support.

On lateral excursion, there should be no contacts on the implant restoration. The lateral excursion should be conformative with the patient's existing dentition.

7.5.5 Kennedy Class 4

Natural teeth—shimstock hold.

Implant restorations—shimstock drag.

Splinting the implants distributes the loads over a wider area minimizing horizontal forces to the implant/abutment junction.

On lateral excursions, the anterior implant restorations should guide the mandible in both lateral and protrusive excursions.

In the anterior maxilla, special attention must be given to vertical and horizontal overlap.

Attention must also be given to the amount of buccal cantilever. Often with significant bone resorption, implants are placed more apically and palatally, whilst the aesthetic requirements are more buccal. In such scenarios, the occlusion must be designed to be lighter on the implant-supported restorations.

7.5.6 Single Canine Implant Restoration

Natural teeth—shimstock hold.

Implant restoration—shimstock drag.

On lateral excursion, as much as possible guidance should be directed towards the premolars so as to avoid horizontal forces on the canine alone. Protrusive guidance is transferred to the central and lateral incisors. If the contour of the canine does not allow, then guidance should be distributed amongst multiple teeth.

In many situations, the overlap of the canine implant restoration is deep enough that transferring the guidance to the premolars is not possible. With deep overlap, there is a likelihood of horizontal forces impacting the screw joint resulting in screw loosening. In this scenario, the clinician is advised to utilize screw-retained restorations so complications can be managed more efficiently. A night-time appliance is also recommended. The patient must also be educated that loosening of the implant restoration may occur and if any mobility is experienced to call the office to re-torque the restoration.

7.5.7 Full-Arch Immediate Load

Agreement on the occlusal scheme to be utilized in the interim prosthesis has not been established in the literature. There is no evidence to show that one occlusal scheme is superior to another; one type of tooth form is more efficient than another or one type of occlusal scheme is preferred by patients.

Most occlusal schemes advise on avoiding non-axial loading on implants. If we evaluate the recommendations critically, we become aware that loading of implants almost never occurs along the long axis of the implant. Together with well-distributed splinted implants, function occurs on various areas of the prosthesis with the development of complex bending moments within the restorative implant components and within the surrounding bone.

Factors that affect distribution of occlusal forces include but are not limited to:

(a) Number of implants involved
(b) Biomechanical design of the implant
(c) Nature of the bolus of food
(d) Design and fit of the prosthesis
(e) Nature of the opposing occlusion
(f) Deformation of the bone and the prosthesis

Unfortunately, there are no randomized controlled clinical trials guiding the clinician to develop the occlusal scheme on the immediate load provisional prosthesis. Most occlusal schemes are based on biomechanics and distribution of the occlusal forces over areas which are most likely able to tolerate them.

Clinical guidelines for developing occlusion include but are not limited to:

(a) Good distribution of implants
(b) Minimum vertical overlap of anterior tooth restorations
(c) Bilateral simultaneous contact
(d) No interferences in lateral excursion
(e) Cross-arch stabilization with a passive screw-retained acrylic prosthesis which has sufficient rigidity to withstand occlusal forces without breaking
(f) No cantilevers
(g) Occlusal contacts from canine to canine only with shimstock drag on the posterior teeth. The rationale for this approach is centred around bone quality and occlusal forces. The posterior implants are in the weakest bone quality. The occlusal forces increase as we go further back in the mouth. The rationale is to protect the implants in the weakest quality bone being subjected to the highest occlusal forces. If this requires developing a ramp on the palatal aspect of the anterior teeth, this should be completed with cold-cured acrylic resin. If the patient has a severe class 2 incisor relationship, the above will not be possible in which case occlusal contacts are evenly distributed around the arch.

7.5.8 Full Arch Opposing a Denture

On light closure, there should be bilateral simultaneous contacts between opposing restorations. If the implant-supported restorations include cantilevers, there should be 100 micron clearance on the cantilever. Cantilevers serve as load magnification. On firm closure, all contacts should be maintained.

7.5.9 Full Arch Opposing Natural Dentition

On light closure, there should be simultaneous contacts between the natural teeth and the opposing restorations. Contact towards the incisors and canines should exhibit a shimstock drag. Patients with implant-supported restorations can exert significantly higher forces than those with a natural dentition. Often posterior teeth will wear, and heavy occlusal contacts will be directed towards the anterior teeth causing fracture of teeth or the restoration. The purpose of having lighter occlusion on anterior teeth is to delay this consequence.

In lateral excursion, the canine and incisors should disclude all posterior teeth in both lateral and protrusive excursions. The rationale for this is that forces are higher in the posterior part of the mouth and having horizontal forces on implant restorations on posterior teeth may result in fracture of the restoration and/or the prosthetic screw.

7.5.10 Full Arch Implant Rehabilitations

Patients with full implant-supported occlusion can exert much more force than those with a natural dentition. The arrangement of an occlusal scheme is based on biomechanics rather than scientific evidence.

The following guidelines can be provided:

1. Posterior cusps flattened to minimize bending and torsional forces.
2. Evaluation of the opposing occlusion: If the full-arch interim prosthesis opposes natural teeth, it may be feasible to adjust the natural teeth to minimize steep inclines and lateral forces.
3. Bilateral simultaneous contact.
4. Shallow protrusive disclusion.
5. Anterior group function.
6. Steep anterior disclusion is not recommended as this may create destructive deflective forces, which may result in prosthesis fracture.
7. Minimal contact on cantilevers: Cantilevers have been found to create greater risk in restoration fracture.

On a practical level, all posterior teeth should hold shimstock. Anterior teeth should drag shimstock.

On lateral excursion, the restoration should have canine guidance with progressive group function should the canines wear.

All the above design elements attempt to reduce stress within the overall system to ensure a biomechanically favourable restoration in the long term.

7.5.11 Implant- and Mucosa-Supported Overdentures

Occlusion may differ depending upon the opposing dentition and materials selected [16].

(a) Denture—conventionally, this should be treated as complete denture occlusion with bilateral simultaneous contact on both sides. The anterior teeth should drag shimstock. The rationale for this is that posterior teeth will wear resulting in heavier anterior occlusal contact. This may result in tooth fracture. The occlusal scheme is designed to delay this consequence. In lateral excursion, a balanced occlusion is considered favourable. This in realty is academic. When the patient inserts a bolus of food in the mouth, the benefits of bilateral balance are not realized. The academic rationale for a bilateral balance is that teeth come into contact many times a day when the patient swallows.

(b) Natural dentition—bilateral simultaneous contact on light closure. Anterior teeth should drag shimstock. The rationale is similar to the above scenario. In lateral excursions, limitations may exist based on the position of the opposing dentition. It is always recommended to get at least a unilateral progressive group function.
(c) Opposing implant-supported restorations—bilateral simultaneous contact on light closure. Anterior teeth should drag shimstock. The rationale is similar to the above scenario. In lateral excursion, canine guidance wears into progressive group function.

7.6 Conclusion

The limitation of these guidelines is the lack of long-term clinical data to provide strong evidence. The guidelines are largely based on the compilation of occlusal concepts from natural teeth, fixed and implant prosthodontics. By application of biomechanical principles such as reducing the cantilever length, passive fitting of prostheses, narrowing the buccolingual/mesiodistal dimensions of the prosthesis, reducing cusp inclination, eliminating excursive contacts and centring occlusal contacts, these complications can be reduced.

The differences between a natural tooth and an implant alter the way the occlusal forces impact the bone surrounding them. The lack of proprioception from dental implants allows higher forces to be exerted, which results in prosthetic complications.

To increase long-term prosthetic success, post-treatment considerations should include periodic recall exams, occlusal guard and patient education. During recall exams, centric and excursive contacts should be evaluated, along with structural and hygiene status of the prostheses. More frequent recall schedule is recommended for high-risk patients.

References

1. Sekine H, Komiyama Y, Hotta H, Yoshida K. Mobility characteristics and tactile sensitivity of osseointegrated fixture supporting systems. In: van Steenberghe D, editor. Tissue integration in oral and maxilla facial reconstruction. Amsterdam: Excerpta Medica; 1986. p. 326–32.
2. Schulte W. Implants and the periodontium. Int Dent J. 1995;45:16–26.
3. Llindhe J, Karring T. Anatomy of periodontium. In: Lindhe J, Karring T, Lang NP, editors. Clinics periodontology and implant dentistry. 3rd ed. Copenhagen: Munksgard; 1998. p. 45–9.
4. Parrtt GJ. Measurement of physiological mobility of individual teeth in axial direction. J Dent Res. 1960;39:608–18.
5. Hiliam DG. Stresses in the periodontal ligament. J Periodontal Res. 1973;8:51–6.
6. Siddhartha P, Deepesh S, Rohit M, Shivangi C. Occlusal principles and considerations for implants: an overview. J Acad Dent Educ. 2014;1(2):17–21.
7. Naert I, Quirynen M, van Steenberghe D, et al. A study of 589 consecutive implants supporting complete fixed prostheses. Part II: Prosthetic aspects. J Prosthet Dent. 1992;68:949–56.

8. Wenstrom J, Zurdo J, Karlsson S, Ekestubbe A, Gröndahl K, Lindhe J. Bone level change at implant-supported fixed partial dentures with and without cantilever extension after 5 years in function. J Clin Periodontol. 2004;31:1077–83.
9. Bragger U, Karoussis I, Persson R, Pjetursson B, Salvi G, Lang NP. Technical and biological complications/failures with single crowns and fixed partial dentures on implants: a 10-year prospective cohort study. Clin Oral Implant Res. 2005;16:326–34.
10. Kreissl ME, Gerds T, Muche R, Heydecke G, Strub JR. Technical complications of implant-supported fixed partial dentures in partially edentulous cases after an average observation period of 5 years. Clin Oral Implant Res. 2007;18:720–6.
11. Romeo E, Tomasi C, Finini I, Casentini P, Lops D. Implant-supported fixed cantilever prosthesis in partially edentulous jaws: a cohort prospective study. Clin Oral Implant Res. 2009;20:1278–85.
12. Lee SA, Lee CT, Fu MM, et al. Systematic review and meta-analysis of randomized controlled trials for the management of limited vertical height in the posterior region: short implants (5–8 mm) vs longer implants >8 mm in vertically augmented sites. Int J Oral Maxillofac Implants. 2014;29(5):1085–97.
13. Srinivasan M, Vazquez L, Rieder P, et al. Survival rate of short (6 mm) micro-rough surface implants. A review of literature and meta-analyses. COIR. 2014;25(5):539–45.
14. Rangert B, Krogh PH, Langer B, Van Roekel N. Bending overload and implant fracture: a retrospective clinical analysis. Int J Oral Maxillofac Implants. 1995;7:40–4.
15. Weinberg LA. Reduction of implant loading with therapeutic biomechanics. Implant Dent. 1998;7:277–85.
16. Taylor TD, Wiens J, Carr A. Evidence based considerations for removable prosthodontic and dental implant occlusion: a literature review. J Prosthet Dent. 2005;94(6):555–60.

Digital Workflows for Implants, from Single Tooth to Full Arch

8

Anas Aloum

8.1 Digital Tools

Digital tools have been introduced to the dental world for the last 30 years, and the trajectory of availability of the equipment and the usage have increased exponentially.

However, we have seen a major shift in contemporary practice in the last few years. Updated new printers, scanners, milling machines and face scanners are developed with more accuracy and are becoming more user friendly. Software are also improved and are showing better results that provide added value in daily dentistry.

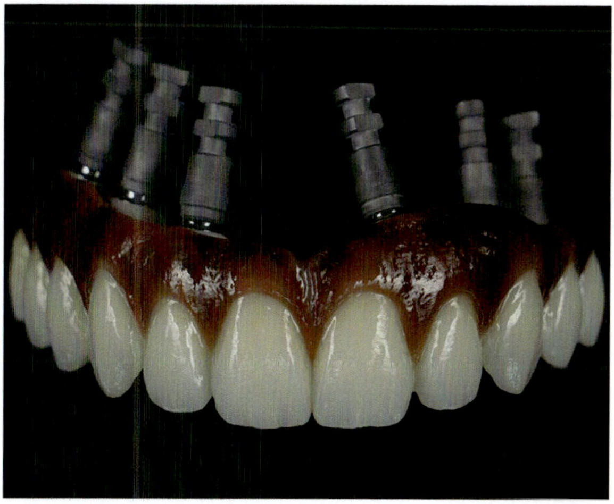

A. Aloum (✉)
Hikma Medical Center, Abu Dhabi, UAE

W. Chee, S. Jivraj (eds.), *Treatment Planning In Implant Dentistry*, BDJ Clinician's Guides, https://doi.org/10.1007/978-3-031-68726-6_8

Example of digital workflow: Full-arch zirconia monolithic structure with layered pink porcelain. The teeth are strained, glazed and polished. All are digitally designed and manufactured using natural tooth libraries.

For example, to add photos, image galleries, audio clips, videos, charts and customizable tooth shapes, Fig. 8.46, with a tap or click on one of the insert buttons in the toolbar or drag and drop of the objects onto the page, a clinician can layer objects, resize them and place the items anywhere appropriate on the screen.

Digital dentistry has allowed us as clinicians to visualize treatment plans instead of just imagining them. Case planning and case presentation to patients have become more objective and digital. Facially driven designs and planning the definitive prosthesis initially are what make digital dentistry appealing to many. Planning in 2D (2 dimensionally) and 3D (3 dimensionally) using numerous software is never easier today.

8.2 Introduction to Digital Dentistry

With contemporary dental care, digital dentistry requires the growing incorporation of computer-based or digital technologies and tools in place of classic traditional modalities. This evolution has not only revolutionized the way dentists diagnose, plan and provide treatments but also enhanced the precision and convenience; in addition, it can provide much better experiences to patients, as they are able to understand treatment plans and sequences of treatment and be able to visualize treatment outcomes. Due to the many innovations within digital dentistry, the realm of dental implants has been particularly noteworthy when using advancements in treatment planning and execution of treatments.

8.3 Dental Implant Digital Tools

1. Digital impressions: Having impression trays inserted with various impression materials can be uncomfortable for patients. With digital impression systems, like intra-oral scanners (IOSs) and photogrammetry, dentists can now take accurate digital images of the mouth, reducing patient discomfort and enhancing data accuracy.
2. 3D (3 dimensional) imaging and cone beam computed tomography (CBCT): CBCT offers a 3D view of the patient's jaws, allowing for precise implant planning and placement. This replaces traditional 2D (2 dimensional) radiographs, offering a more comprehensive view with less radiation exposure.
3. Computer-aided design/computer-aided manufacturing (CAD/CAM): This technology allows dentists to design custom crowns, fixed partial dentures and even some orthodontic devices within the premises of the practice facility, even allowing for same-day restorations.
4. Digital treatment planning: Software solutions now enable dentists to simulate the desired outcome in 2D and 3D, replacing traditional wax-ups with virtual ones and making treatment decisions that lead to truly prosthetically driven implant placement.

5. Therefore, implant therapy becomes more predictable and safer. Moreover, dentist-patient communication becomes more relevant and objective. Figures 8.1, 8.2, 8.3, 8.4, 8.5, 8.6, 8.7, 8.8, 8.9, 8.10, 8.11, 8.12, 8.13, 8.14, 8.15, 8.16, 8.17, 8.18, 8.19, 8.20, 8.21, 8.22 and 8.23 explain the usage of digital planning in single tooth implant surgical and restoration predictability.
6. Guided surgery templates: Using digital planning data, these templates are useful guides to facilitate the dentist for precise implant placement, reducing potential risks and achieving ideal implant positions.
7. Allowance of using monolithic materials: Using monolithic materials such as zirconia which is a material that is a ceramic that is biocompatible and has excellent properties to be utilized with implants as support. Zirconia is resistant to fracture and has overcome the many issues of using feldspathic porcelains and metal substructures. Improved aesthetics and milling or printing zirconia have made the process more predictable with less human interaction. Computers programmed by humans will direct the machines that form the restorations that are more durable and aesthetic (Fig. 8.132).

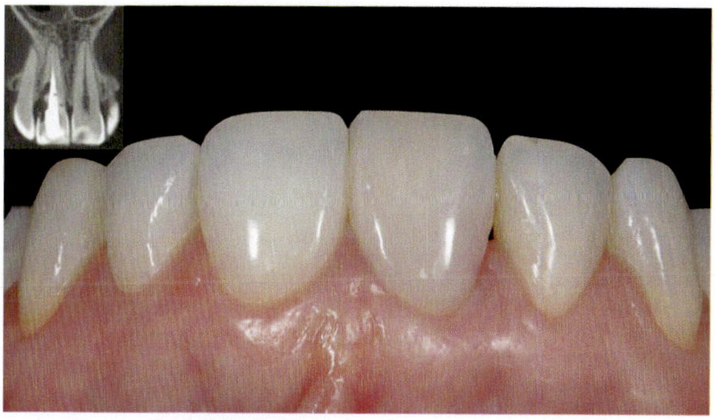

Fig. 8.1 This image illustrates a slightly discoloured maxillary right central incisor; the radiograph shows significant external root resorption

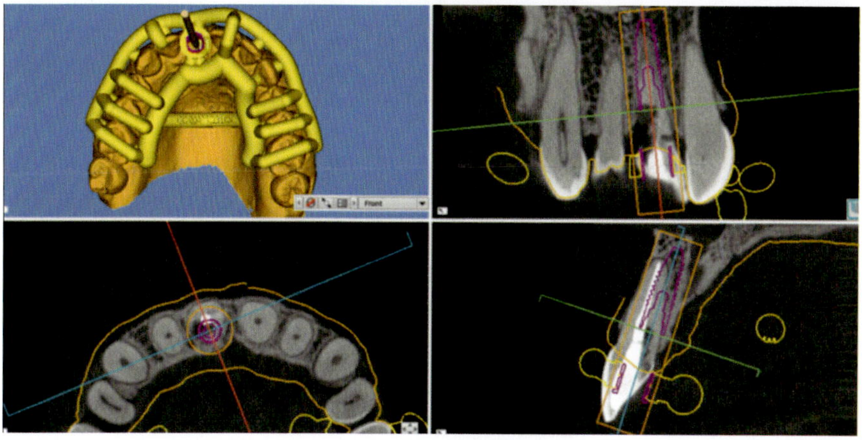

Fig. 8.2 The CBCT scan images clearly show the amount of resorption and also virtually placing the implant in the most ideal location to fabricate the surgical guide for precise placement

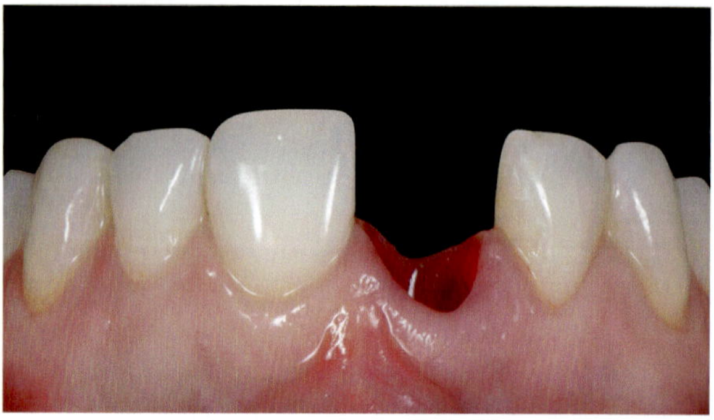

Fig. 8.3 The tooth is extracted without elevating a flap

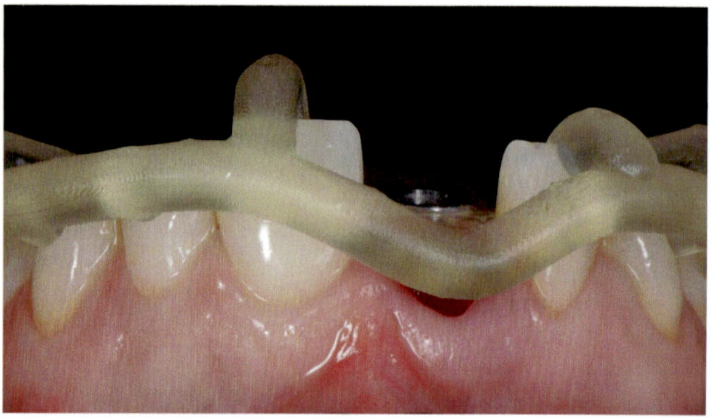

Fig. 8.4 Surgical guide placed

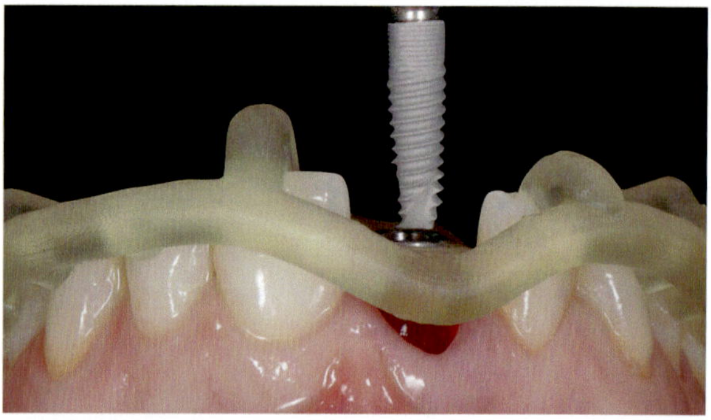

Fig. 8.5 Implant site is ready to receive the fixture

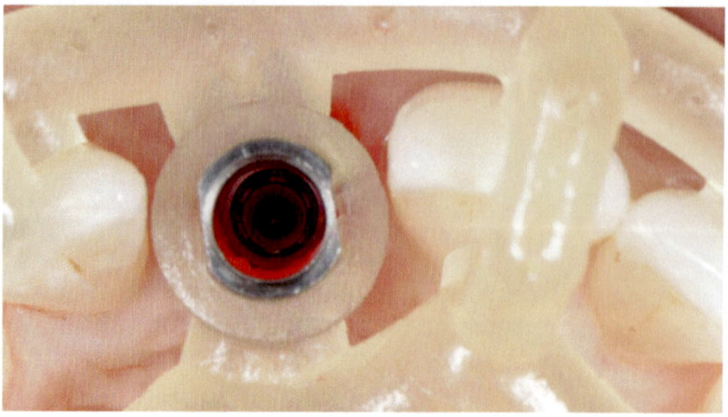

Fig. 8.6 Dental implant being placed through the surgical guide and showing the precision of the placement

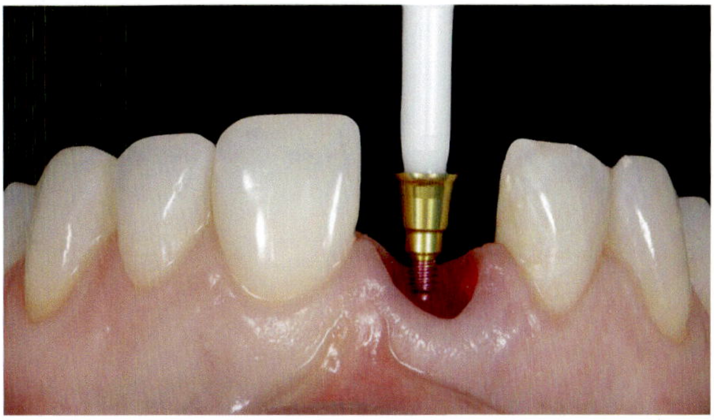

Fig. 8.7 Implant abutment placed and torqued. The abutment will not be removed and that ensures moving the platform more coronally and makes the prosthetic procedures more acccssible

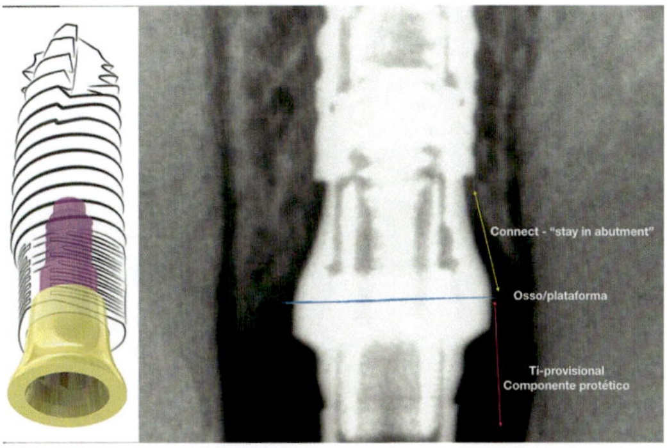

Fig. 8.8 The radiograph showing the implant and abutment. Note how the implant is placed sub-osseous, and the abutment shifts the connection higher than the bone crest

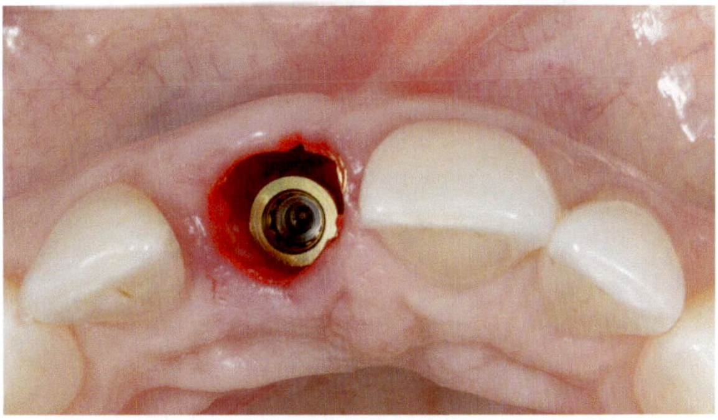

Fig. 8.9 Clinical photograph of the implant and abutment in the extraction socket

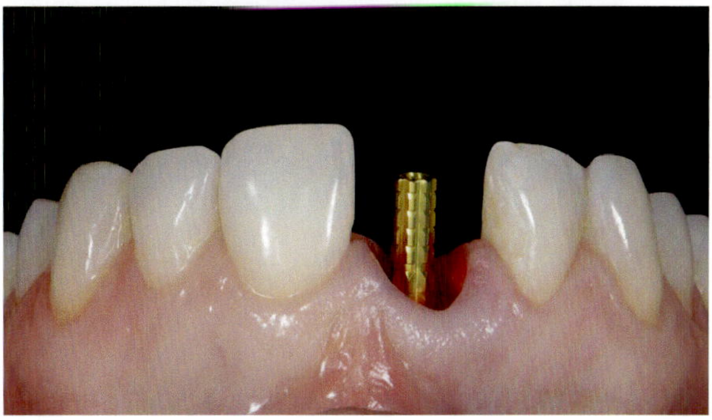

Fig. 8.10 The temporary cylinder placed on the connected abutment to start the temporizing phase

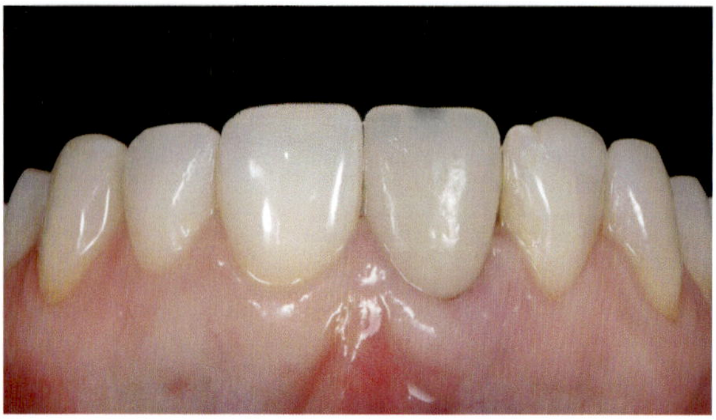

Fig. 8.11 Pre-made shell placed with wings to stabilize the placement and position

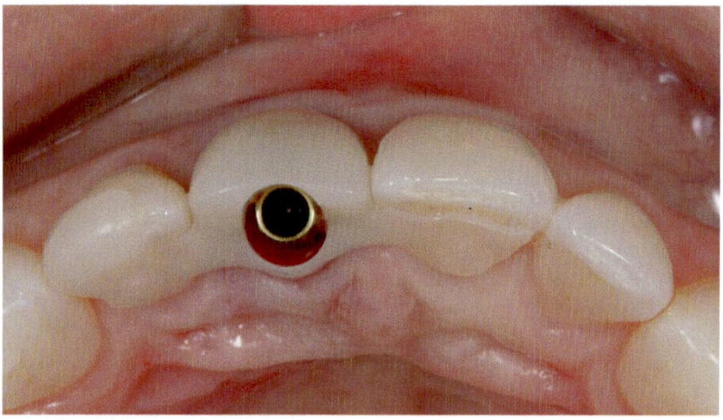

Fig. 8.12 Occlusal photograph of the shell in place; note the wings

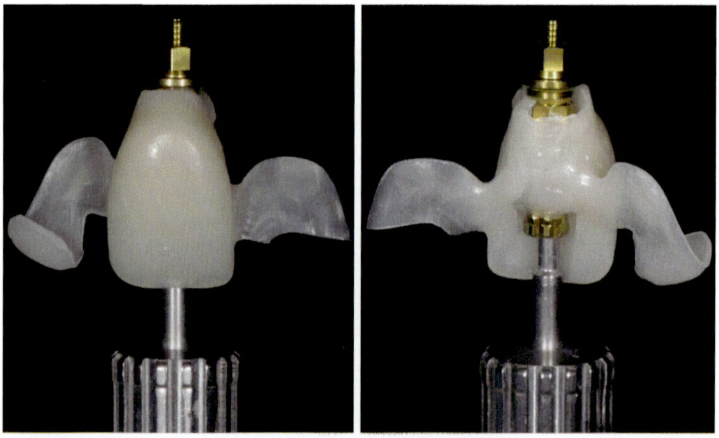

Fig. 8.13 The shell being picked up with resin. Now it is ready to be trimmed and finished

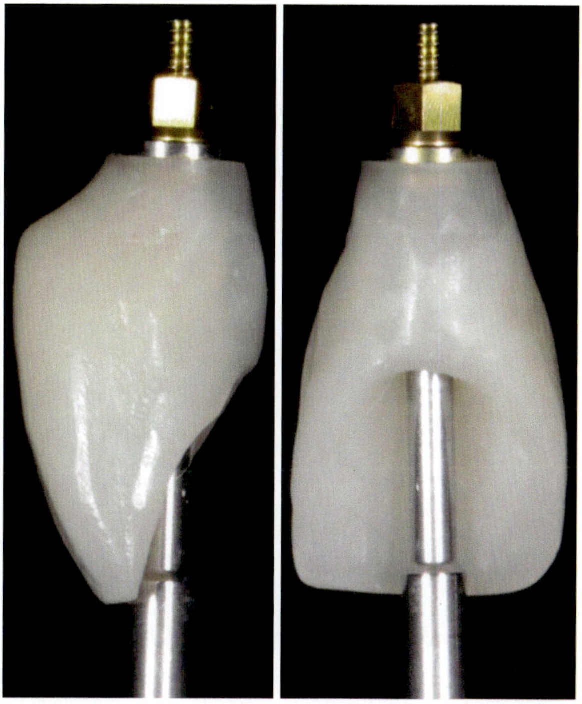

Fig. 8.14 The temporary restoration is screw retained after being finished and polished. Note the concave sub-mucosal emergence on the buccal side to allow room for the connective tissue addition

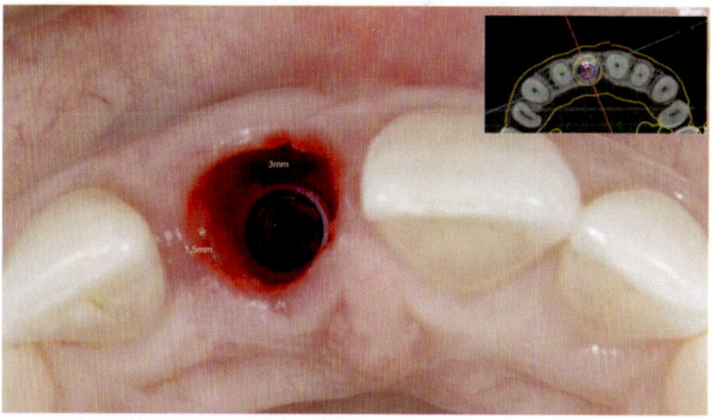

Fig. 8.15 Clinically, the space between the implant and the buccal and proximal bone

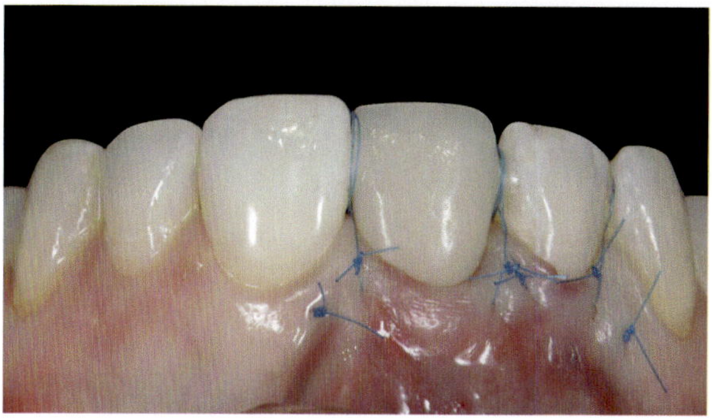

Fig. 8.16 The temporary restoration is placed, and then bone and connective tissue addition is placed in the sub-mucosal space (Fig. 8.15). Suturing is done to stabilize the tissues to allow for maximal growth around the implant in the healing period

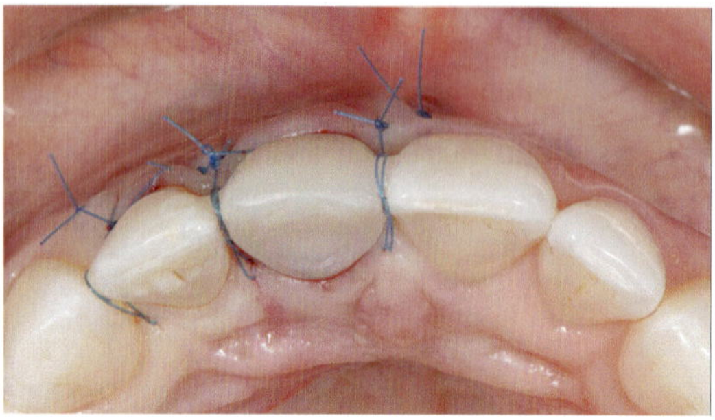

Fig. 8.17 Occlusal image of the suturing after the temporary restoration is attached

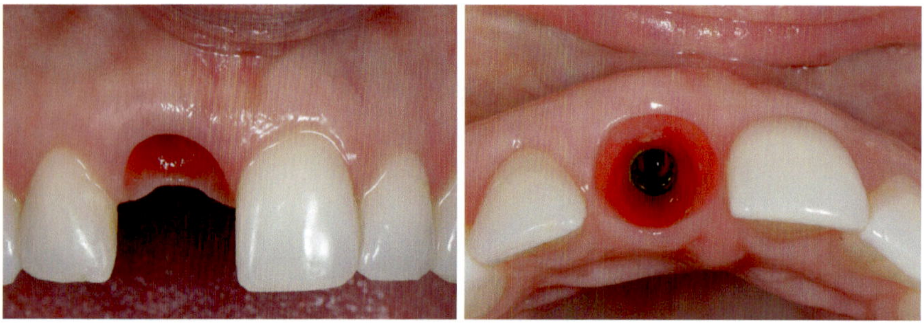

Fig. 8.18 After 4 months of healing, note the form of the sub-mucosal contours once the temporary prosthesis is removed

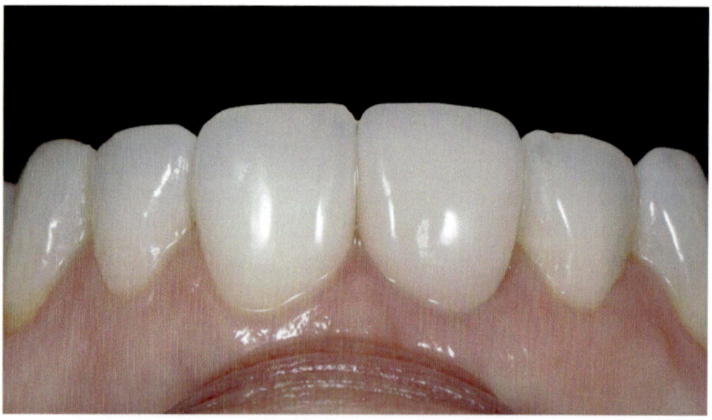

Fig. 8.19 Definitive crown is placed

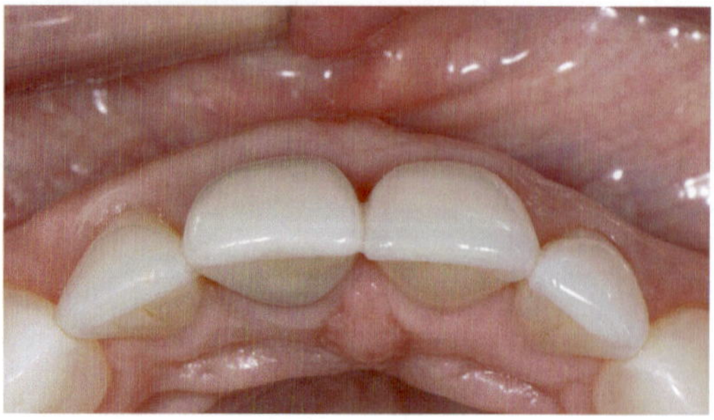

Fig. 8.20 Occlusal image. Note the similar soft tissue contour around the natural tooth and the dental implant

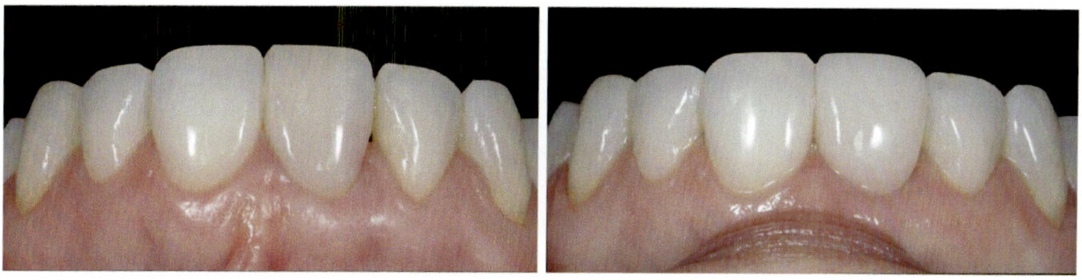

Fig. 8.21 Comparison images. On the left is the preoperative image, and on the right is the post-operative image

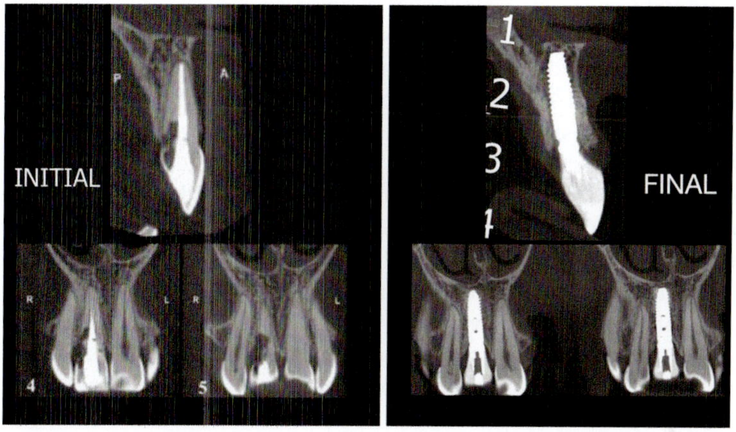

Fig. 8.22 Comparison CT scan images. On the left is the preoperative CT scan, and on the right is the post-operative CT scan images

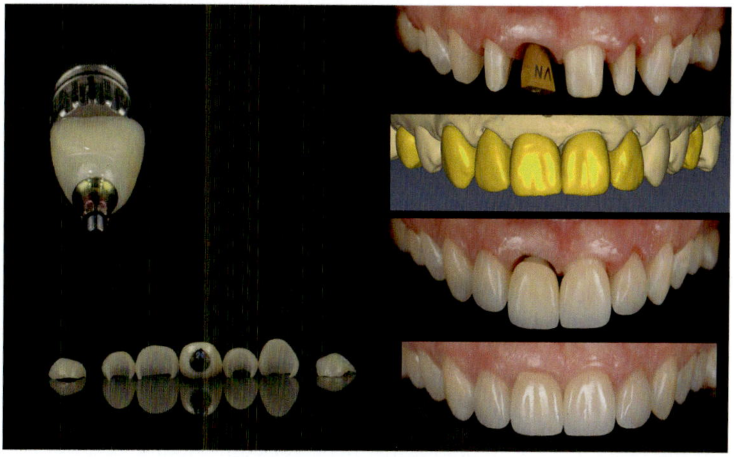

Fig. 8.23 Collage of images of the digital workflow of a dental implant and ceramic veneers. The images show steps of placing the scan body on the dental implant and teeth being prepared and ready to scan using an intra-oral scanner. Then designing the case with full monolithic material on Exocad software and then milling the definitive units using empress leucite-reinforced ceramics without the need to have a model. Teeth are just stained, glazed and polished and inserted intra-orally

8.4 Paradigm Shift in Dental Practice

The integration of these digital tools has drastically transformed the dental implant arena. A few highlights of this paradigm shift include the following:

1. Increased precision and predictability: Digital tools provide measurements and visualizations that are incredibly accurate, leading to better treatment outcomes.
2. Enhanced efficiency: Many digital tools, for example:
3. CAD/CAM systems that allow for faster treatment processes. This means that procedures that require multiple visits can often be reduced, in some situations even offering same-day restorations.
4. Improved patient experience: The use of digital tools can lead to less invasive procedures leading to reduced pain and discomfort. For example, patients benefit from having to take fewer dental impressions, experiencing less radiation exposure and generally spending less time in the dental chair which may also lead to shorter healing periods.
5. Interdisciplinary collaboration: Digital files can be easily shared among dental professionals to facilitate interaction. For instance, an orthodontist, oral surgeon and prosthodontist can work together seamlessly using shared digital data, ensuring a comprehensive treatment approach.
6. Continuous learning and adaptation: With the digital transformation, dental professionals can continuously update their skills and knowledge. This ensures that they are always at the forefront of the latest techniques and technologies, offering the best care to their patients.
7. Cost efficiency: While the initial investments in digital technology can be substantial, over time, these tools can reduce the need for physical materials that were used for manual planning and fabrication of restorations. These modernized factors can minimize clinical errors and streamlining processes.

In conclusion, the ascent of digital dentistry, particularly in the realm of dental implants, represents a significant paradigm shift. The incorporation of advanced digital tools has not only optimized clinical procedures but has also elevated the standard of care and patient experience. As technology continues to evolve, the future of dentistry lies firmly in the digital realm.

8.4.1 Digital Impressions

Digital impressions have brought in a new era of precision and efficiency to dentistry. Intra-oral scanners, such as those by CEREC (Dentsply, Sirona) or iTero (Align Technology), employ optical scanning technology to capture detailed, 3D images of the oral cavity, eliminating the need for cumbersome and often uncomfortable traditional impression materials [1]. Additionally, the recent exploration of photogrammetry in dentistry offers an exciting alternative to intra-oral scanners by using multiple 2D photographs to reconstruct a 3D model of the dental arches [2].

This has made digital impressions increasingly popular in contrast to traditional methods of dental implant impressions, which have relied on elastomeric materials. The conventional methods were time-consuming, had a risk of distortions and often required retakes [3]. The digital technologies offer enhanced accuracy, more rapid turnaround times and an overall more pleasant patient experience.

8.4.2 Intra-oral Scanners

Intra-oral scanners have significantly changed the landscape of dentistry. They use optical scanning technology to capture high-resolution digital impressions of the dental arches and surrounding oral structures.

1. Accuracy: Studies have shown that digital impressions can be more accurate than their traditional counterparts. With fewer chances for human error, and no possibility of material distortion or shrinkage, the scans provide a precise representation of the oral structures [1].
2. Efficiency: The digital process is generally faster than traditional methods, as there is no waiting time for materials to set, and in addition, the digital files can be directly sent to the laboratory without physical shipping delays [1].
3. Patient comfort: Many patients find the traditional mould-taking process uncomfortable, especially those with a gag reflex. Intra-oral scanners eliminate this discomfort, making the experience more patient-friendly [1].

When using intra-oral scanners for digital impression of dental implants, a few items should be considered:

1. When printing a cast using the scans for full-arch implant-supported prostheses, there is a method where printing models with digital analogues is one path of proceeding down a workflow. The added costs are of printing a model, the need to take a jaw registration in the traditional way of either using wax rims or mounting casts with provisional prosthesis using bite registration materials if needed.
2. When using a model-less approach, the dentist or laboratory technician will forgo the printing of a model. There are limitations using this method when making single-unit implant crowns that are screw retained and fabricated with monolithic materials such as zirconia or lithium disilicate without layering of materials. The drawback of such practice will be difficulty of shade matching because oftentimes layering is needed to properly match shades, especially in the anterior zone. Also, cementing the Ti base to zirconia or lithium disilicate can often lead to proximal contacts being open or too tight as there is tolerance when milling the restoration to the Ti base. When having a fixed partial denture (bridge), this issue can lead to further misfit of Ti bases to the restoration causing an exponential deviation of the fit between the Ti bases that are cemented without guidance that will cause a more serious misfit that can lead to de-cementation of the Ti bases, screw loosening, zirconia fracture or fixed partial denture (bridge) not fitting at all.

8.5 Full-Arch Implant Scanning

8.5.1 Rationale and Scientific Evidence

In the past decades, intra-oral scanners were meant to serve quadrant dentistry. This was related to the scanner hardware and software limitations, which made the stitching of image through the arch essentially inaccurate. Although such limitations existed in other applications such as orthodontic aligners, the precise nature of implant prosthetics has limited the intra-oral scanner use in this situation. The consensus in past days is that full-arch implant prosthetics should be deferred to the conventional implant impression techniques or should be practiced digitally only in the presence of a 3D photogrammetry system. Despite the reported accuracy of photogrammetry, its use is restricted among practitioners due to the high cost of the extra-oral scanner and the need for special scanning pegs.

The continuous improvement in the hardware and software technology for intra-oral scanners has led to a major shift in concept and application. Numerous in vitro and clinical studies have begun to support the possibility of obtaining an intra-oral (IO) scan for a full-arch restoration that can yield acceptable accuracy. Mangano et al. studied the accuracy of 12 different IO scanners in full-arch scans. They reported that among the tested scanners, many of them had an accuracy level below 40 microns of error. It is worthy to note that according to the work of Jemt et al. the accepted level of misfit for a full-arch prosthesis is equal to half turn of the classical gold screw, which is equivalent to 150 microns. In a clinical study, Cappare et al. compared conventional implant impressions versus IO scan in full-arch maxillary prosthetics. They concluded that the clinical and radiographic results suggest that IO scans can be a predictable and reliable alternative to conventional impressions in full-arch scan.

8.5.2 Scanning Strategy and Technique

The main key for a successful full-arch scan is to maintain a continuous optical tracking path for the scanner as it moves across the arch. In maxillary arches, especially with closely placed implants, the palatal topography serves as an excellent tracking path (Fig. 8.27). An s-shaped path moving from the ridge to the palate and back to the ridge allows for efficient image stitching. A difficulty can be encountered when a large inter-implant distance exists with a shallow vestibular depth.

In mandibular arches, the situation is problematic. The lack of sufficient keratinized mucosa along with the tongue and the floor-of-the-mouth movements confounds the scan and can cause tracking loss and double images. The situation is further complicated with salivary flooding and larger inter-implant distances. The key strategy for scanning the mandibular arch is to splint the scan bodies (Figs. 8.24, 8.25, 8.26 and 8.27). The aim of the splinting material is to create an optical track for the scanner. Any scannable material can be used for this purpose such as bond sticks, elastic bands or prefabricated 3D printed resin patterns. The splinting material should

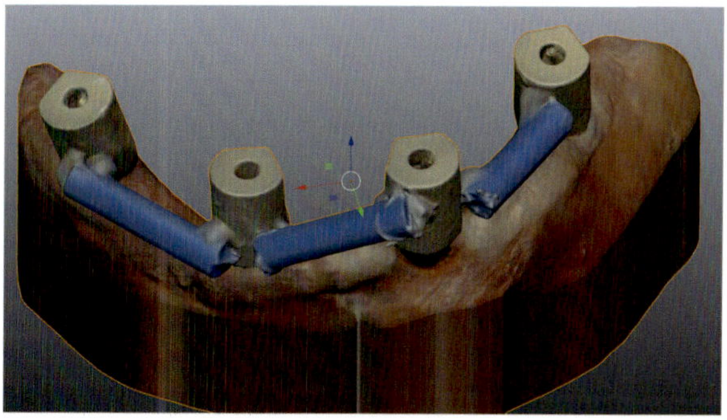

Fig. 8.24 The mandibular full-arch implants. To compensate for the scanning errors that can occur due to lack of keratinized tissue. Using plastic sticks with flowable light-cured (LC) resin allows for better optical tracking. Note that the plastic bands are placed in non-strategic locations in the scan body, allowing the top of the scan body to be free and the flat part of the scan body also to be free of any material

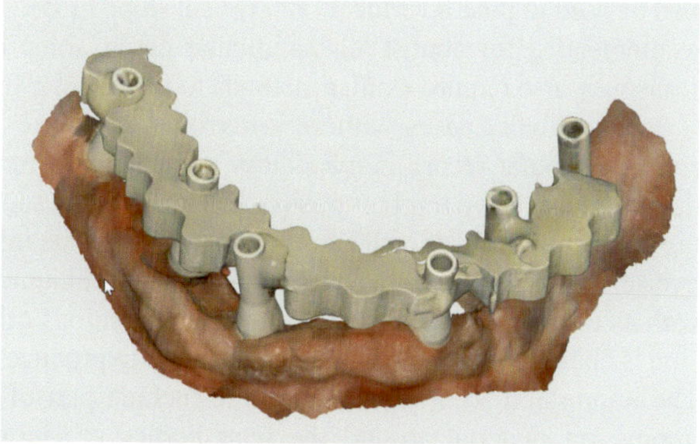

Fig. 8.25 Another method for the mandibular full-arch scan is to place a printed mesh and glue it with flowable resin to the scan bodies

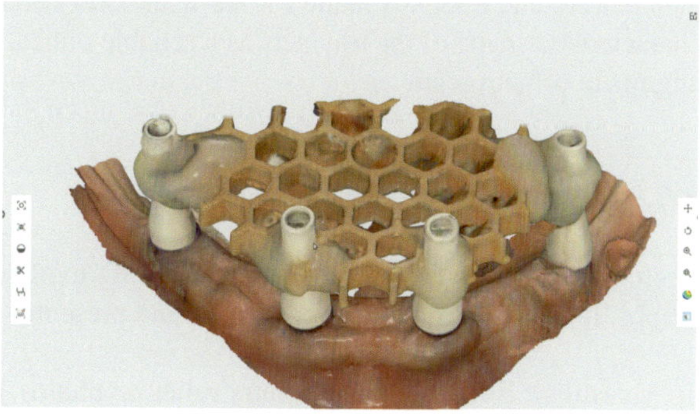

Fig. 8.26 Using a honeycomb mesh which can be scanned alone in the lab or extra-orally and then matched to the intra-oral scan

Fig. 8.27 In the maxillary arch, if there are enough implants and there is no significant distance between the implants, then splinting is not mandatory

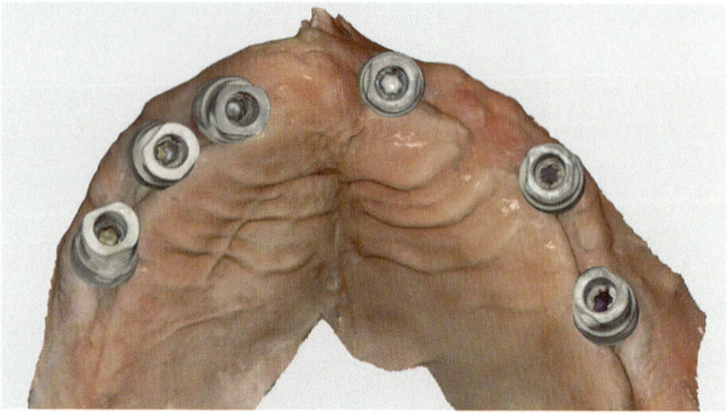

Splinting is not mandatory in maxillary arches with small inter-implant distance as the maxillary topography provides sufficient optical tracking path

be attached to a non-strategic location in the scan body. The scan body top and the characteristic axial feature, if present, should be clearly visible. Additionally, the splint material should allow for mucosal scanning beneath it. Prefabricated 3D printed resin patterns facilitate the splinting job and yield a reliable scan. They can also be used to pour a verification physical stone model. Although splinting is highly recommended for almost all mandibular cases, some difficult maxillary full-arch scans may also require similar methods to mandibular full-arch scans.

In mandibular cases with very narrow keratinized mucosa, or in cases where active vestibular record is mandatory as in over-dentures, splinting will guarantee the accuracy of the implant positions. However, in such cases, the morphology of the scanned soft tissue will be insufficient soft tissue information. For such cases, a hybrid impression scan is advocated; in this technique, a conventional impression with an elastomeric material taken of the edentulous ridge is obtained. The impression is optically scanned with the IO scanner to produce a positive soft tissue model. The impression scan should extend to include part of the tray outer surface. The impression material around the scan bodies is trimmed with scalpel or a burr (Figs. 8.28 and 8.29). The impression is reseated intra-orally after having openings in the completed impression to accommodate the scan bodies. The scan bodies are then placed, and a scan is made for the scan bodies and the tray outer surface. The characteristic shape of the tray acts as a reliable optical track and allows for proper alignment of both scans.

8.5.3 Photogrammetry in Dentistry

Photogrammetry is the process of creating 3D models using multiple 2D photographs. In dentistry, it is a newer method and presents some promising advantages.

1. Versatility: Since photogrammetry relies on photos, there is potential for capturing detailed information even in challenging areas where intra-oral scanners might face limitations [2].

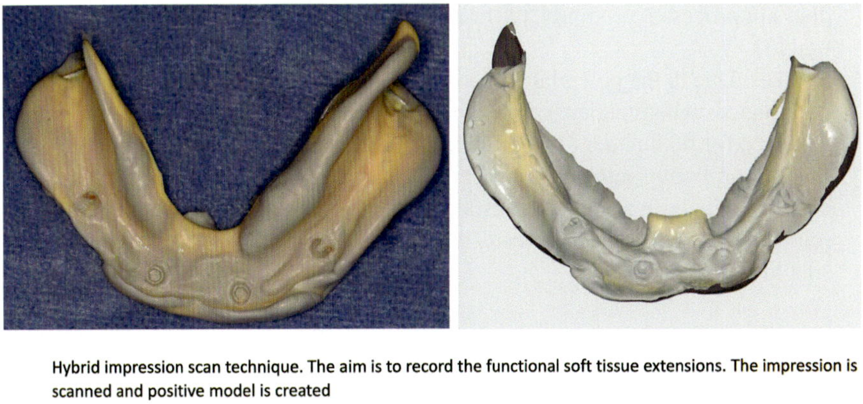

Fig. 8.28 Hybrid impression scan technique. The aim is to record the functional soft tissue borders. The impression is scanned, and a positive model is created

Fig. 8.29 Hybrid impression scan technique. The impression tray is opened to allow the scan bodies to emerge through the impression. The patient scan is made with scan bodies projecting outside the tray. The tray outer topography serves as an ideal optical track (instead of splinting of scan bodies)

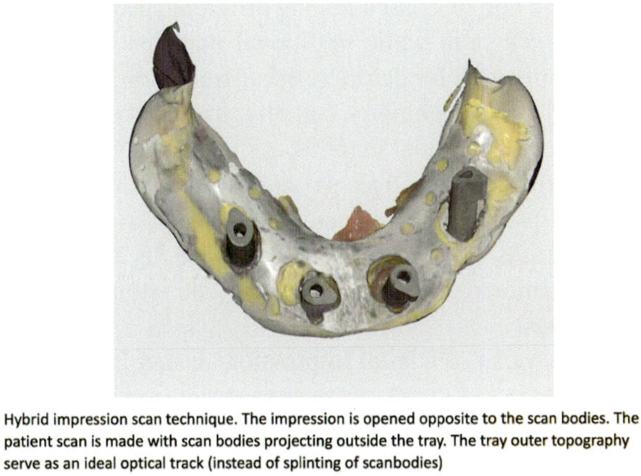

2. Integration with other digital platforms: The data obtained can be easily integrated into digital workflows, aiding in treatment planning, orthodontic analysis and prosthesis fabrication [2].

Traditional dental impressions, particularly for dental implants, typically utilize elastomeric impression materials. These materials used with an impression tray can sometimes be uncomfortable for patients and have inherent limitations:

1. Accuracy concerns: Traditional methods can introduce errors, including bubbles, pulls, drags and distortions. These can result from the material's setting characteristics, improper handling or even environmental factors [3].
2. Time-consuming: The set time for materials and the additional time required for shipping the impressions to labs and waiting for the poured casts to return can make traditional methods less efficient than digital alternatives [3].
3. Material limitations: Some elastomeric materials can undergo dimensional changes over time. If an impression is not immediately poured, or if a laboratory

does not process it promptly, the final prosthesis might not fit as accurately intra-oral [3].
4. Retakes: Due to the potential for errors with traditional impressions, there might be instances where patients need to return to retake impressions, causing inconvenience for both patient and provider requiring additional appointments [3].
5. Storage and environmental impact: Physical casts require storage space, and over time, this can accumulate, especially in busy practices. Moreover, the environmental impact of consistently using and discarding impression materials should be considered [4].

In contrast, digital impressions, whether taken with intra-oral scanners or photogrammetry, present a solution to many of these challenges. They offer immediate visualization, allowing clinicians to ensure quality at the time of scanning. Digital files can be stored indefinitely without consuming physical space; in addition, they can be sent electronically to labs instantaneously, reducing wait times. Moreover, the digital workflow encourages interdisciplinary collaboration, as files can be easily shared and discussed among different specialists.

In conclusion, while traditional impression techniques have served the dental community well for decades, the advent of digital technologies, like intra-oral scanners and photogrammetry, can offer transformative advantages in terms of accuracy, efficiency and patient comfort. As technology continues to evolve, it is anticipated that more dental practices will transition to fully digital workflows, emphasizing the value of precise, efficient and sustainable care.

Figures 8.30, 8.31, 8.32, 8.33, 8.34, 8.35, 8.36 and 8.37 show the PIC system of photogrammetry. Scan bodies can be attached to implants and/or multi-unit abutments.

Drawbacks of Digital Impressions Using Intra-oral Scanners

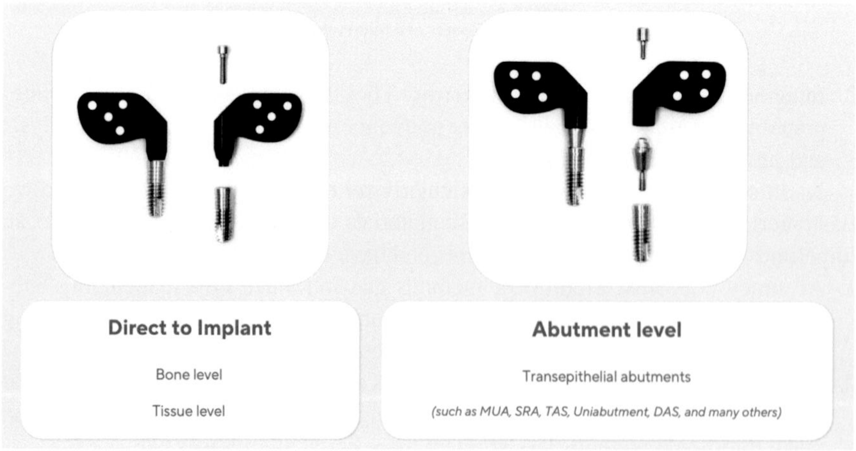

Fig. 8.30 The photogrammetry system "PIC" scan flags. Either attached to the implant or to the multi-unit abutment

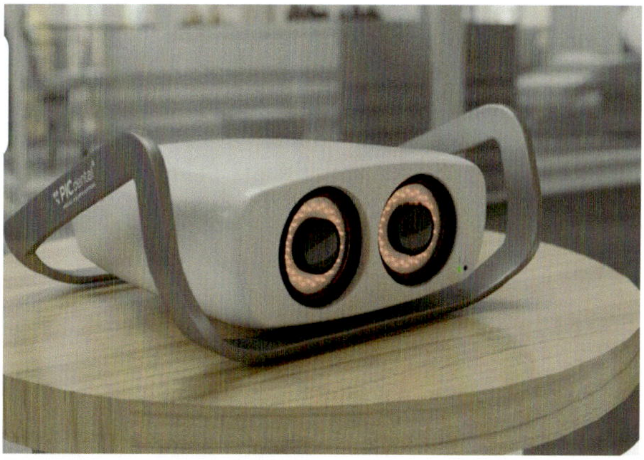

Fig. 8.31 The photogrammetric handheld device. PIC

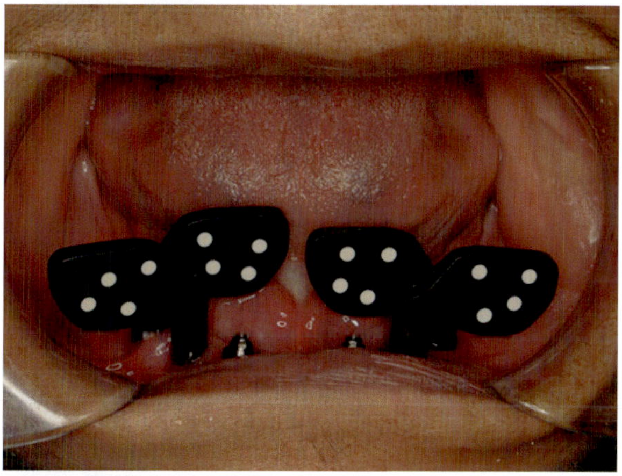

Fig. 8.32 Scan flags intra-oral placement. The flags must be placed in a way so that the device can read the dots on the flags

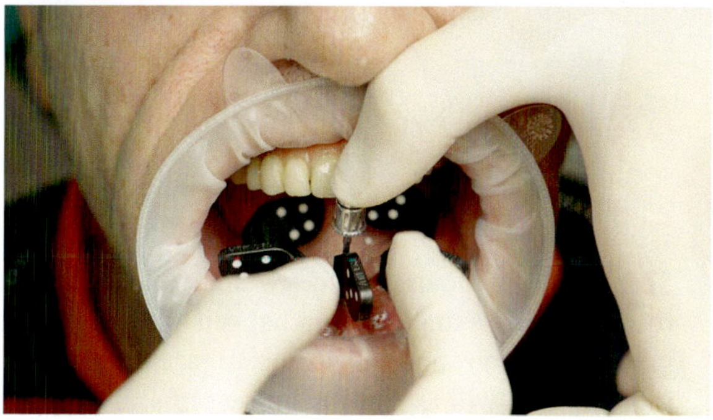

Fig. 8.33 Scan flags screwed directly to the implant system used or to the multi-unit abutment

1. Initial cost: The initial cost can be a barrier for many practices [1].
2. Learning curve: Adapting to a new technology requires a period of adjustment [5].
3. Software limitations: Some software can be limiting in terms of compatibility [6].

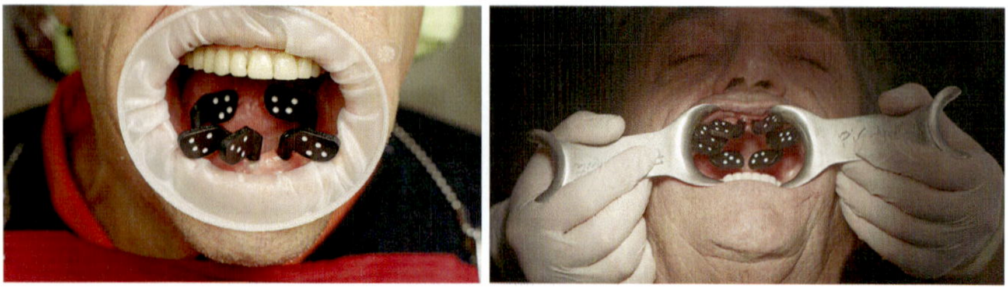

Figs. 8.34 and 8.35 Maxillary and mandibular full-arch implants. Note how the scan flags are placed to allow proper reading

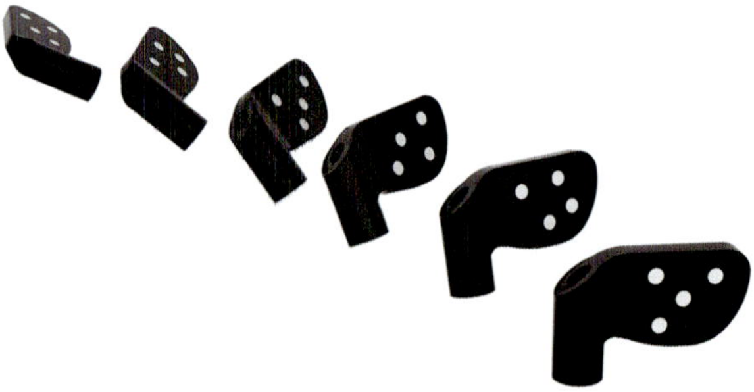

Fig. 8.36 Clear images of the scan flags with different patterns

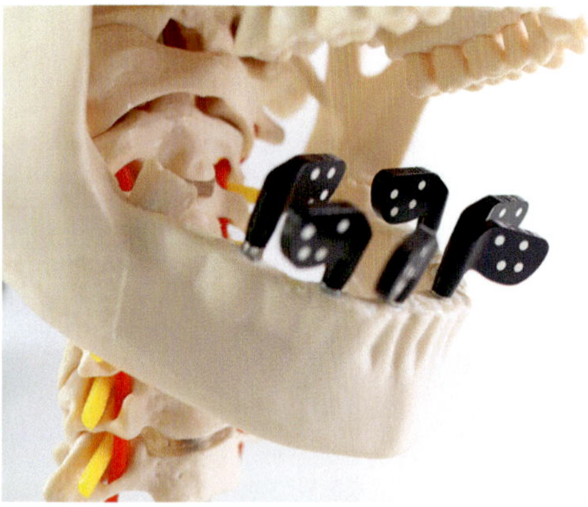

Fig. 8.37 Side view of the scan flags on the mandibular arch

4. Size and ergonomics: Manoeuvrability can be an issue with some scanners and the lag and freezing that can happen. Many software require certain computer processor speeds and memory card size and strength; less-than-ideal hardware requirements will lead to the process of scanning to stop or freeze as the processors and storage are inadequate [7].
5. Ongoing maintenance and updates**: Technology requires regular updates [8].
6. Limited field of view: Some areas might be challenging to capture due to limited mouth openings or edentulous areas can be challenging to capture [9].
   **Drawbacks of Photogrammetry in Dentistry: **

1. Accuracy in challenging areas: Photogrammetry might not always be accurate [2].
2. Photogrammetry equipment is expensive compared to intra-oral scanners, and using it is limited to full-arch restorations.
3. Equipment and set-up: Requires specific equipment set-ups [10].
4. Data processing time: Photogrammetry requires significant computational power and specific computers [11].
5. Similar to intra-oral scanners, there is the need to print models when making full-arch restorations and also the need to make bite registrations using traditional methods.
6. External factors: Results can be influenced by ambient lighting and camera quality [12].
7. Less established in dentistry: It is a newer approach in the dental field [13].

8.5.4 2D Design Series

2-Dimensional design in the digital era allows the practitioner and the patient to communicate objectively. Software with calibrated tools to accurately measure distances and assess defects such as soft tissue recessions, edentulous ridges or diastemas that may need to be corrected.

The 2-dimensional design serves to be the road map for dental treatment.

The digital design has many advantages. Figures 8.38, 8.39, 8.40, 8.41, 8.42, 8.43, 8.44, 8.45, 8.46 and 8.47 show a clinical situation demonstrating step by step the usage of 2D in a comprehensive full-arch implant treatment using smile cloud software.

1. Objectively communicate with the patient about the design and what the possible treatment modalities and tips toward a desired outcome.
2. Objectively communicate with peers and other specialists about the possible treatment modalities.
3. Design a mock-up or provisional prosthesis that will be accurate with minimal alterations in the first trial.
4. Eliminate the need for facebows or earbows to have no canting of the occlusal plane in the mock-up or the final prosthesis.
5. Choose natural tooth libraries that fit the patient's gingival architecture, smile line and facial features. The same tooth libraries chosen for the mock-up can be extracted in Standard Tessellation Language (STL) format and applied to the provisional or definitive prosthesis.
6. Choose tooth libraries that apply to the restorative space needed, for example, zenith levels, smile curves and tooth proportions. These will have an impact on the treatment planning part later in the treatment.
7. Design cases with facially driven planning that are done in real time and can be used in future steps in the same case. Positioning of the tooth shapes should be done in reference to the existing biology and face.

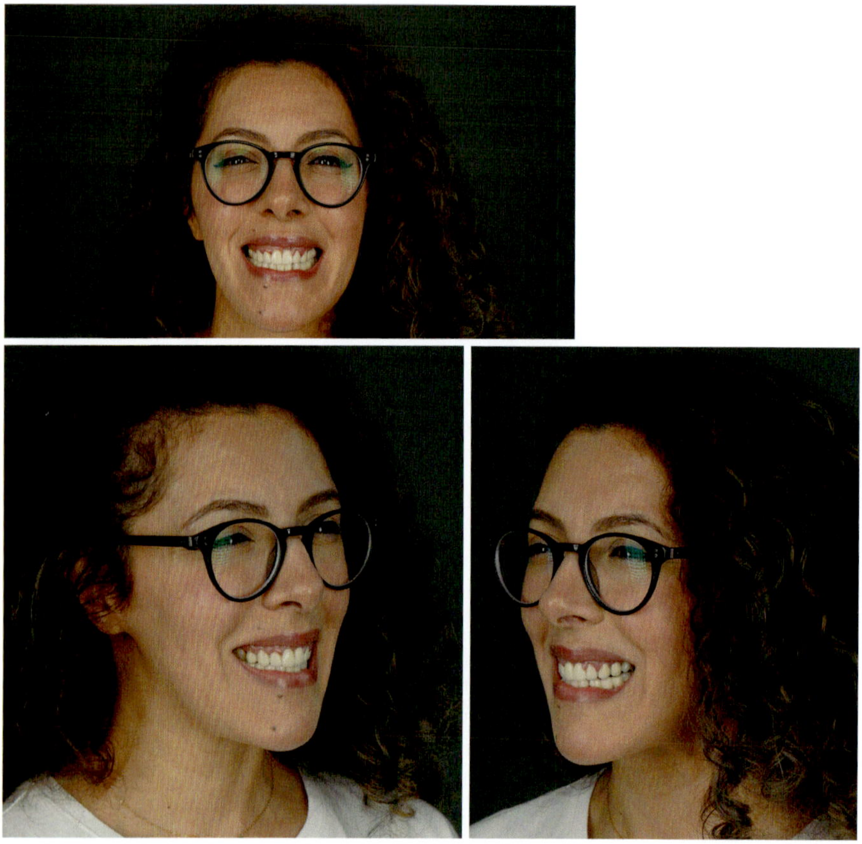

Figs. 8.38 and 8.39 Frontal and 45° images of the patient's face smiling. Note the gingival display showing her current fixed partial denture (FPD) "bridges" on her remaining teeth

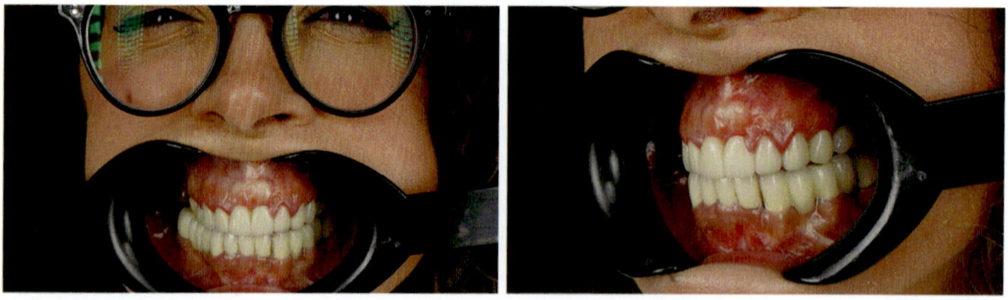

Figs. 8.40 and 8.41 Frontal and 45° images' retracted views. Note the lack of gingival health around the FPD abutments

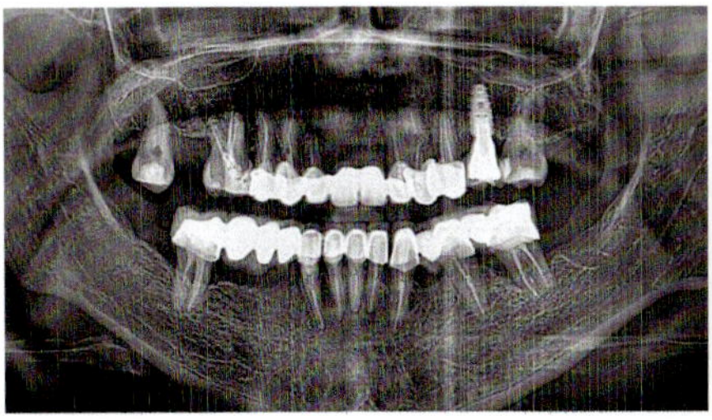

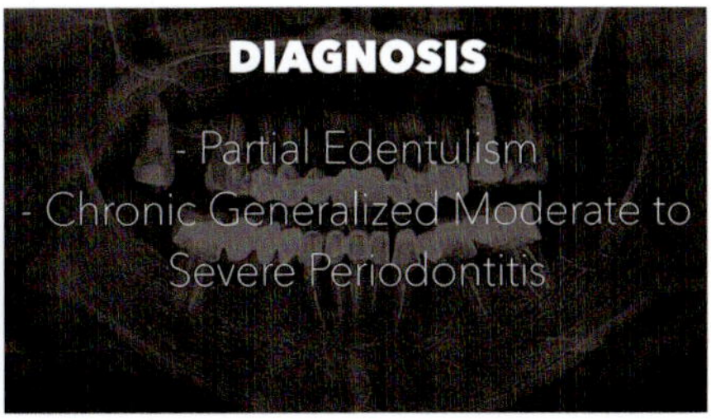

Figs. 8.42 and 8.43 Panoramic radiograph of the patient. Note the amount of bone loss around the teeth. Diagnosis is partial edentulism and chronic generalized moderate to severe periodontitis

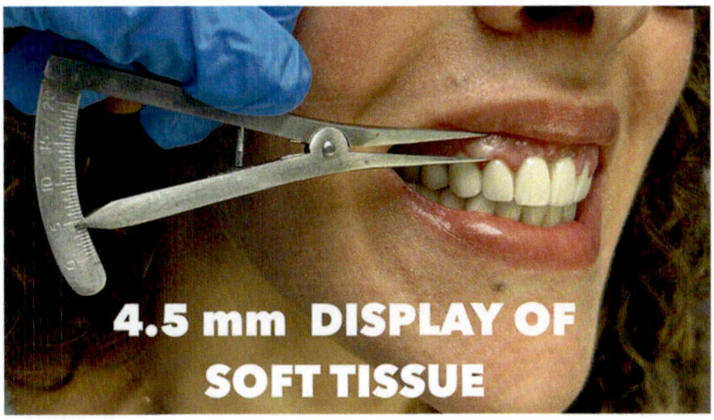

Fig. 8.44 Lateral close-up view of the patient's smiling showing with the caliper the amount of gingival display which is approximately 4.5 mm

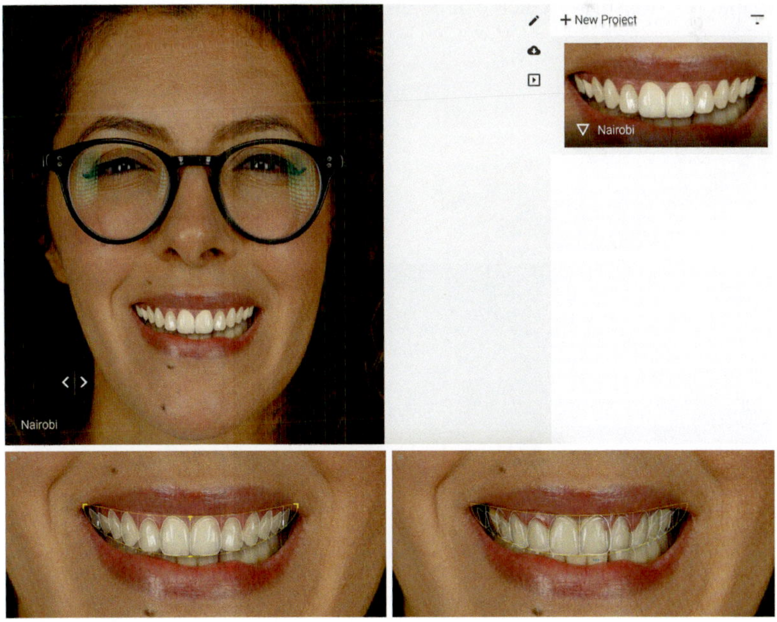

Figs. 8.45, 8.46 and 8.47 2-Dimensional smile design using software similar to smile cloud; the design serves as the road map. It is the first step to determine a plan to execute in time. In this case, the clinician and patient opted to edentulate and place dental implants in both the maxillary and mandibular arches

8.5.5 3D Design Series

One of the main advantages of the digital tools is the ability to digitalize the patient, meaning transforming each element into data and being able to analyse each data set individually.

Face and smile images can be transformed via JPEG photos or even facial scans.

Teeth and soft tissue surroundings can be scanned via IOS and transformed into STL files.

Bone and surrounding hard tissues can be scanned via CT scans and transformed into a Digital Imaging and Communications in Medicine (DICOM) file.

All these files can be morphed (blended) and meshed together to what is known as digitalizing the patient, which allows treatment planning and digital wax-ups to provide better visualization in three dimensions.

After the 2-dimensional designs are done, transform them into the 3-dimensional wax-up using the same tooth library. Export the same library chosen for the 2-dimensional design, and then set teeth up into the ideal 3D positions being able to visualize the soft tissue, hard tissue and smile simultaneously (Figs. 8.48, 8.49, 8.50, 8.51 and 8.52).

Transforming a 2-dimensional (2D) model into a 3-dimensional (3D) model offers numerous advantages, especially in the field of implant dentistry. Here are some of the key benefits of using 3D models for tooth design, bone and soft tissue visualization, and implant placement:

1. Depth perception: 3D models provide a better understanding of the depth and spatial relationships, which can be difficult to fully appreciate in 2D images.

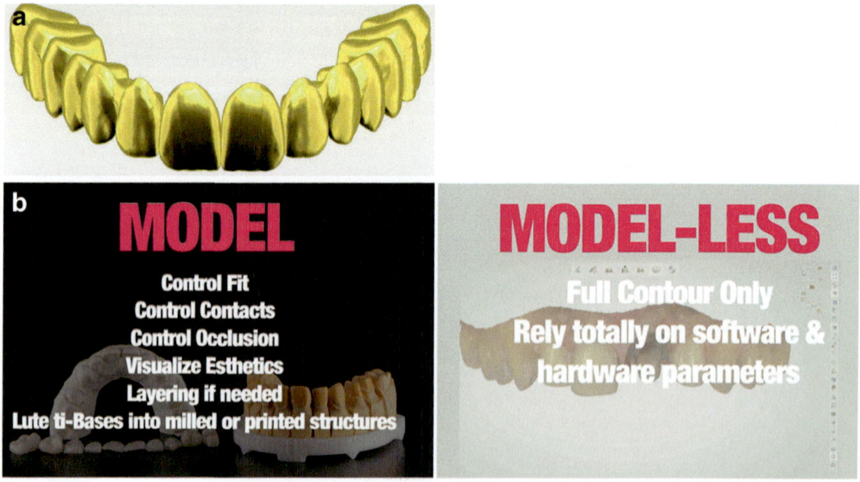

Fig. 8.48 (**a**) The library exported from the 2-dimensional design software to Exocad. The image shows the dental library exported from natural tooth algorithms and will be used to make the 3-dimensional wax-up for the case in the following steps. (**b**) Comparison of model vs. model-less properties

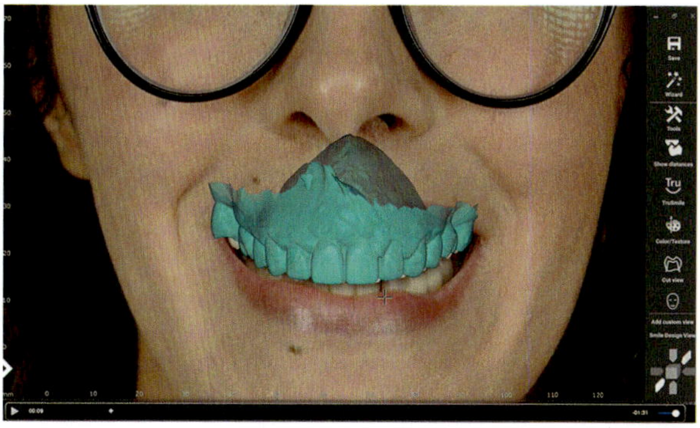

Fig. 8.49 Exocad software 3-dimensional wax-up. The beauty of this digital workflow is that you can align multiple different layers. The preoperative smile and the STL file of the patient's teeth obtained from IOS. After this, we can also align the 2-dimensional design on top. This creates a wax-up that is very precise

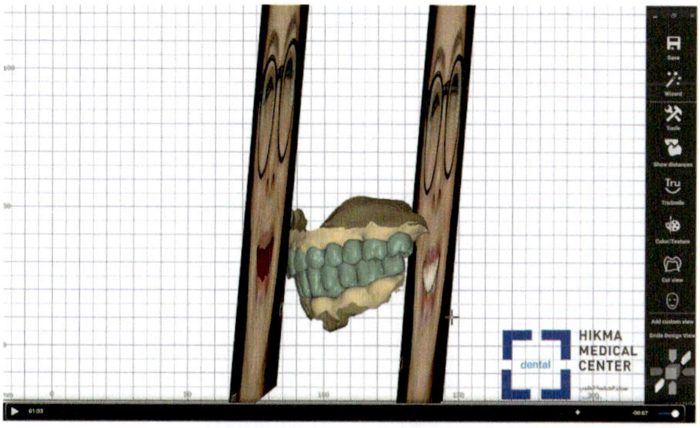

Fig. 8.50 Side view from the software showing the alignment of the different layers. Preoperative face view and STL teeth with digital wax-up

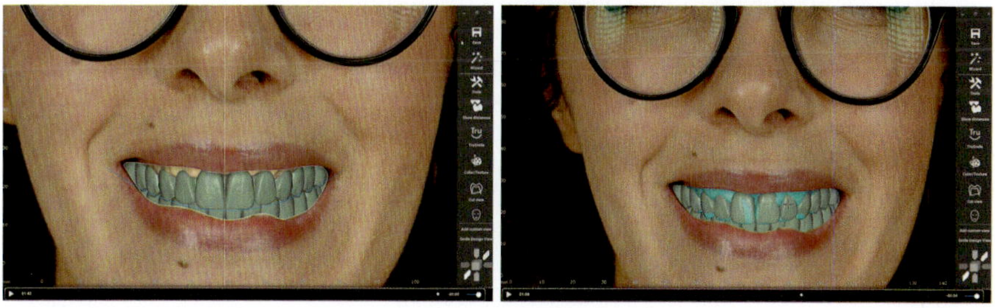

Figs. 8.51 and 8.52 Face view with the digital wax-up in green. Note the tooth set-up respecting the aesthetic parameters. Incisal edges following the lower lip curvature

2. Accurate visualization: A 3D model allows for the visualization of anatomical structures from various angles, providing a comprehensive view that can aid in treatment planning.
3. Implant positioning: The accurate representation of bone volume and density in 3D helps in determining the ideal position for implant placement, minimizing the risk of perforation or damage to vital structures.
4. Predictability: With 3D models, clinicians can simulate implant placement in preparation of the surgery, enhancing predictability and reducing errors.

5. Bone quantity and quality assessment: 3D models can provide detailed insights into bone quality and quantity, crucial for deciding on implant type, size and placement.
6. Soft tissue visualization: 3D imaging helps in understanding the thickness and contour of gingival and mucosal tissues, which is vital for aesthetic outcomes and implant health.
7. Digital planning tools: 3D models can be integrated with digital treatment planning tools, allowing for virtual implant placement, prosthetic-driven planning and fabrication of surgical guides.
8. Improved patient communication: 3D models can be an excellent tool for patient education. The 3D models can provide a clear and more intuitive understanding for the patient about the proposed treatment outcome, which can help in obtaining informed consent.
9. Integration with CAD/CAM: 3D models can be integrated with computer-aided design and computer-aided manufacturing (CAD/CAM) systems for designing and fabricating dental prosthetics, surgical guides and other appliances.
10. Reduction in surgery time: With better planning from 3D models, surgical procedures can be streamlined, reducing the overall surgery time and improving patient comfort.
11. Reduced radiation exposure: By getting a comprehensive view through a single 3D scan radiograph, there is potentially reduced need for multiple 2D image radiographs, thereby reducing cumulative radiation exposure to the patient.
12. Cost efficiency: Although the initial investment in 3D imaging technology might be significant, the reduction in errors, time savings and improved treatment outcomes can allow a cost-effective expenditure in the long run.

At this point, the treatment can be finalized, having in mind the path toward the completion of the definitive prosthesis. Export the tooth set-up or the virtual wax-up to Meshmixer software, which is a prototype design tool based on high-resolution dynamic triangle meshes. This will produce a file in the STL format to print the mock-up model (in reference to the waxed-up model).

Place the implants in the virtual world based on the wax-up dimensions.

Implant placement positions need to consider biological and anatomical parameters of aesthetics. Implants are placed in the optimal locations considering both bone volume and the desired prosthetic outcome. Implants can be placed 2–3 mm apical to the zenith of the proposed design. Also, place implants keeping in mind 1.5 mm distance from the neighbouring teeth and 3 mm from any neighbouring implant [14].

Guide production: After finalizing the virtual plan, a software is used to design surgical guides. This guide, when placed intra-orally, directs the drilling and implant placement, ensuring that the implant is placed exactly as planned. This guide is fabricated using methods such as 3D printing.

Surgical procedure: During the surgery, the guide ensures accurate positioning, depth and angulation of the implants, reducing the risk of errors and unexpected complications.

There are many versions of surgical guide designs. Mainly, they can be either tooth supported for single units or FPDs or lateral pin (bone anchored) supported for full-arch restorations. Stable support is essential to ensure proper drilling toward planned positions for implant placement. As placement is usually blind, any misplacement of the guide will exaggerate the error in the positional placement of the implant, which can lead to implants being close to vital structures or being out of the bony housing.

Surgical guides can preferably be designed to allow water cooling to reach the osteotomy site as shown in these photos. Surgical guides can also be designed with metal rings or tubes that will be glued into the guide after it is printed and cleaned; these tubes will receive the implant drills. Or another type is made with no metal ring needed as that is already incorporated into the design and calculated so that surgical burs fit the resin. The burs will have a stopper that will dictate the depth of the osteotomy site.

Precise printing technology is needed to make these guides. Moreover, the cleaning of the printed resin must be meticulously done, and special finishing burs are required to finalize the guide before it being used intra-orally. Figures 8.53, 8.54, 8.55, 8.56, 8.57, 8.58, 8.59, 8.60, 8.61, 8.62, 8.63, 8.64, 8.65, 8.66, 8.67, 8.68, 8.69, 8.70, 8.71, 8.72, 8.73, 8.74, 8.75, 8.76, 8.77 and 8.78 show the steps of aligning the CT scan to the previous STL file of teeth and soft tissue and then placing implants digitally in the most ideal prosthetic and surgical place. Print stackable guides, and fabricate an immediate-loaded prosthesis that matches the same design used in 2D and 3D designs.

Immediate fabrication and delivery post-implant placement can proceed either by scanning the intra-oral scan body and making an indirect laboratory provisional or by making a shell of the provisional crown. The shell can be milled or printed based on the 3D design, and lute it to the temporary cylinder that is screw retained to the implant.

Picking up the temporary cylinder can be done with flowable composite or acrylic resin. Shaping of the emergence profile can be subtractive or additive with acrylic resin that can be performed chair side. It is preferable to allow room for the soft tissue to heal and form by having the emergence profile concave. Often, soft tissue grafts are needed simultaneously with the implant placement.

These are the most predictable methods of immediate provisionalization.

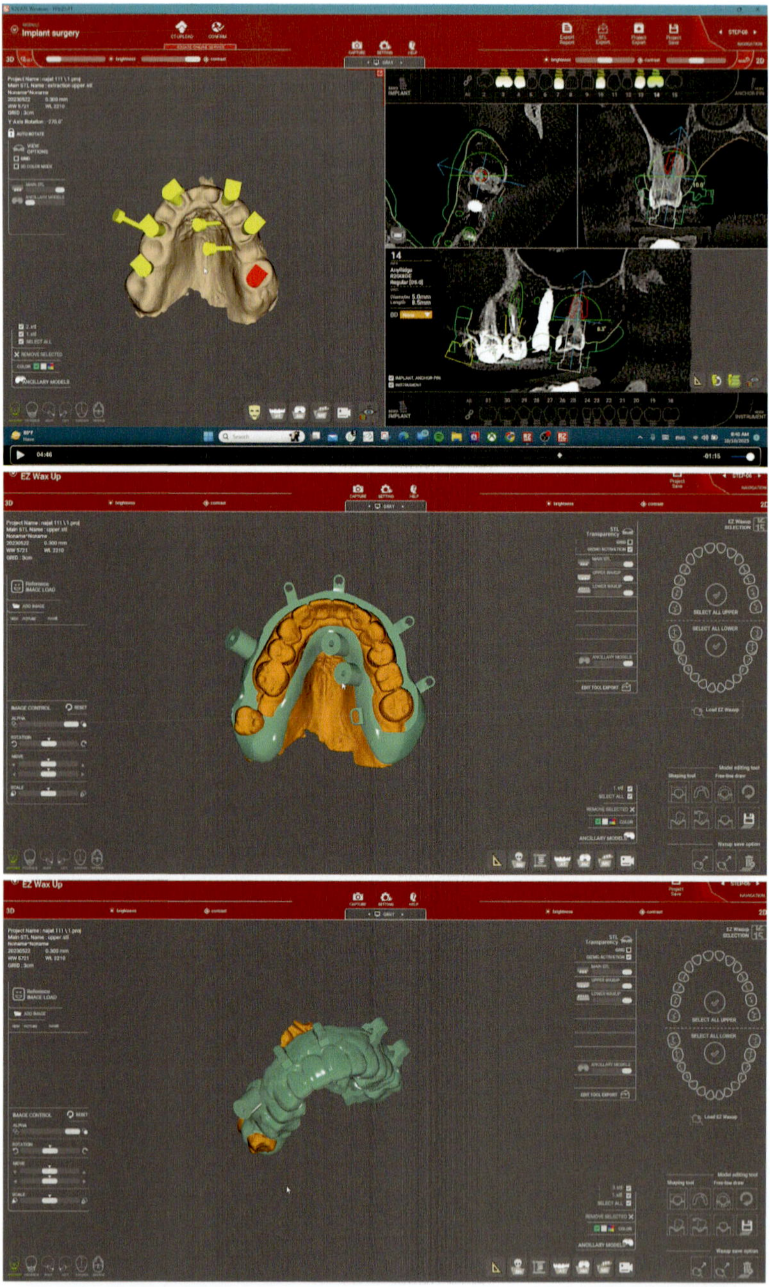

Figs. 8.53, 8.54, 8.55, 8.56, 8.57, 8.58 and 8.59 The tooth set-up is being exported to a different software (R2Gate) where the CT scan Dicom file is being aligned with the STL file. This ensures proper alignment of the bone, soft tissues, teeth and wax-up. In this step, the implant placement is being superimposed in their most optimal positions. Putting in mind that the planning is always prosthetically driven, the digital workflow allows us as clinicians to achieve that goal

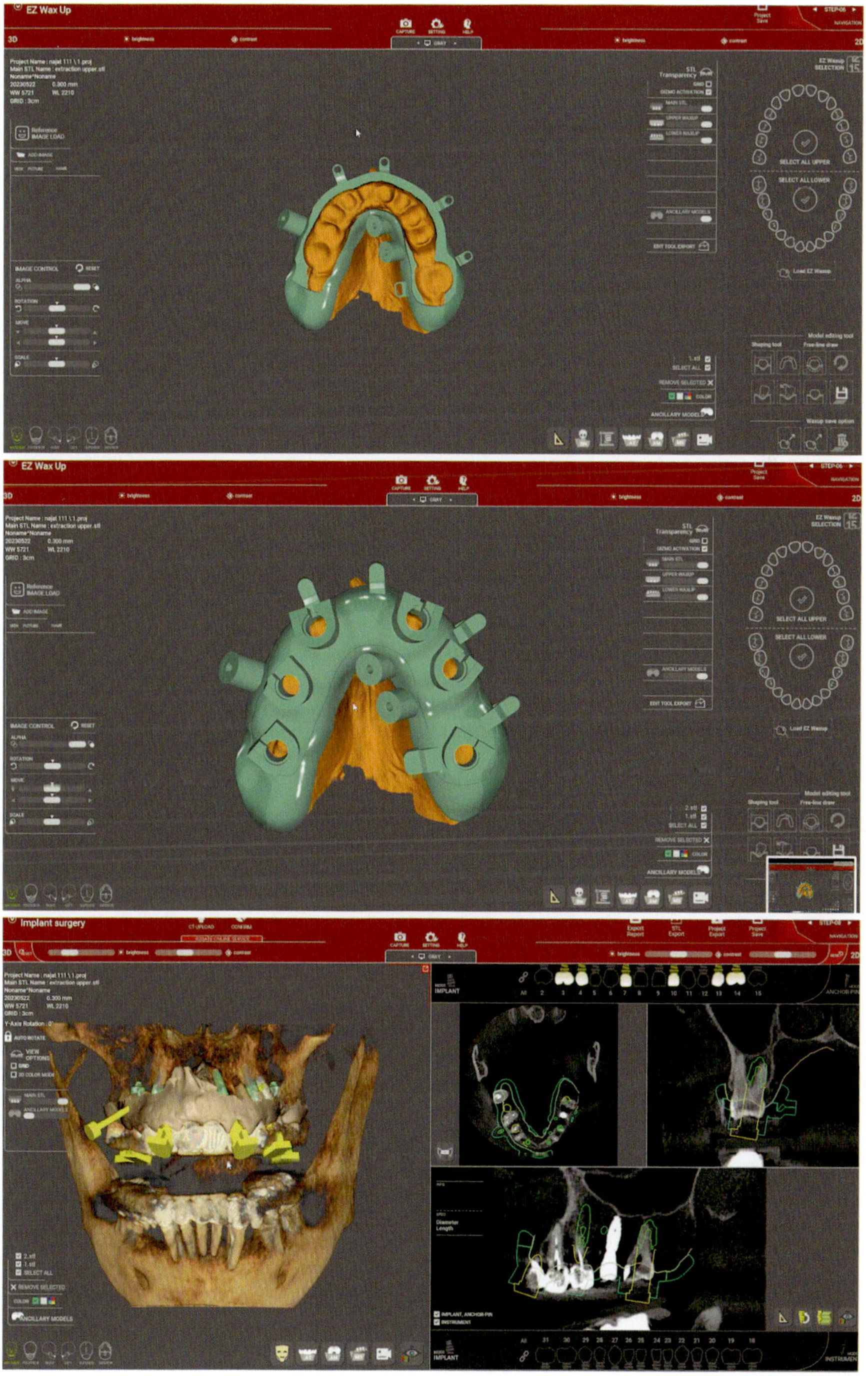

Fig. 8.53, 8.54, 8.55, 8.56, 8.57, 8.58 and 8.59 (continued)

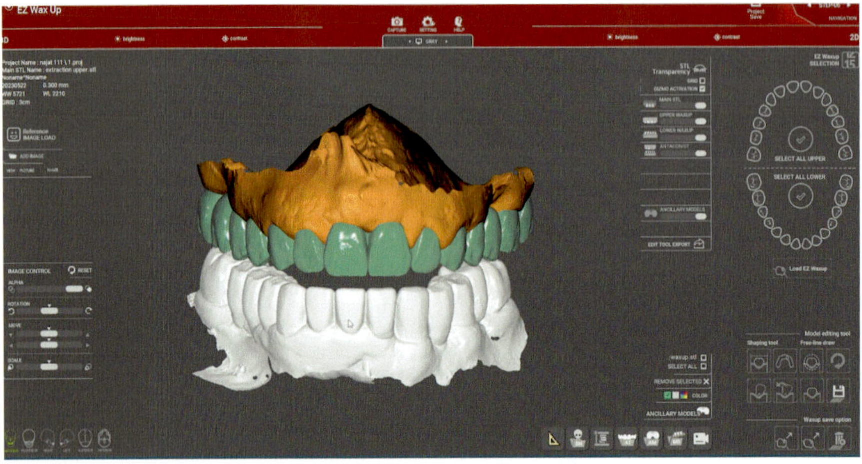

Fig. 8.53, 8.54, 8.55, 8.56, 8.57, 8.58 and 8.59 (continued)

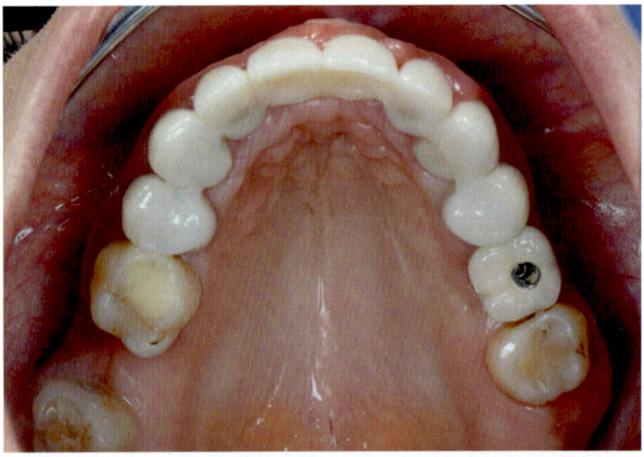

Fig. 8.60 Preoperative occlusal view of the maxillary arch

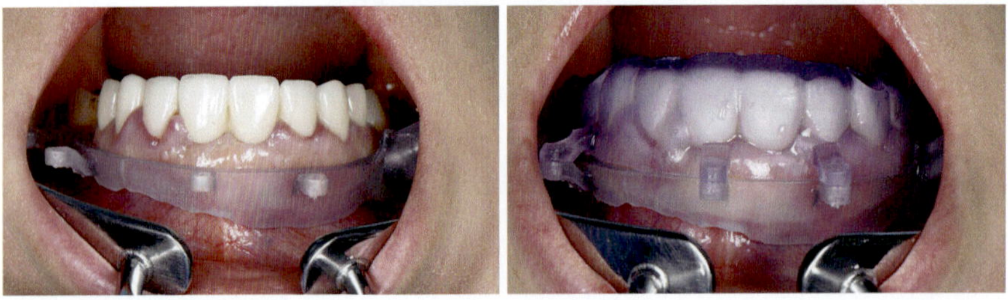

Figs. 8.61 and 8.62 Frontal view of the surgical guide made in several pieces that interdigitate using buttons or what is known as stackable guides

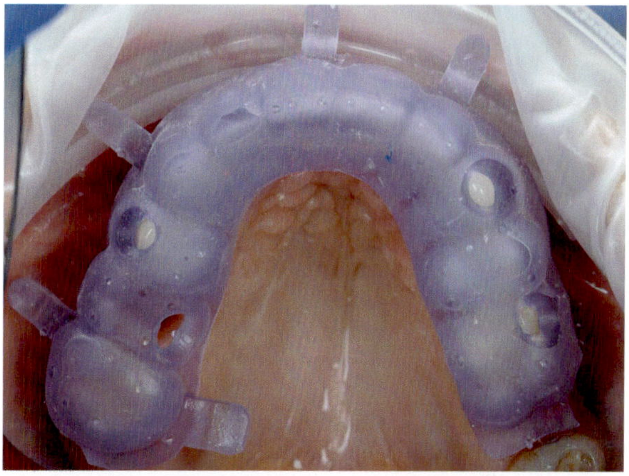

Fig. 8.63 Occlusal view of the surgical guide in place before the teeth extraction starts

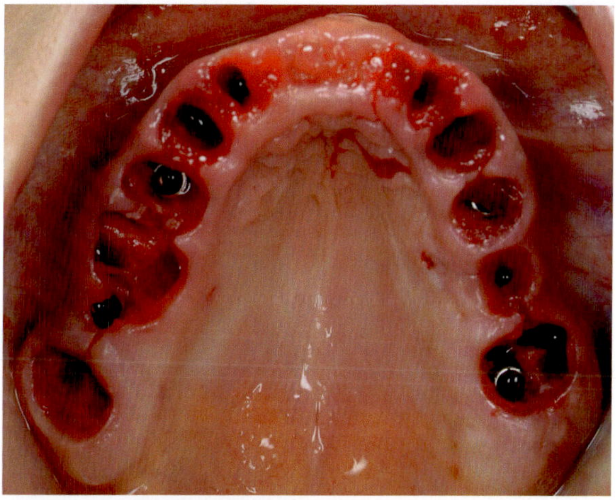

Fig. 8.64 Extraction completed, and six implants are placed

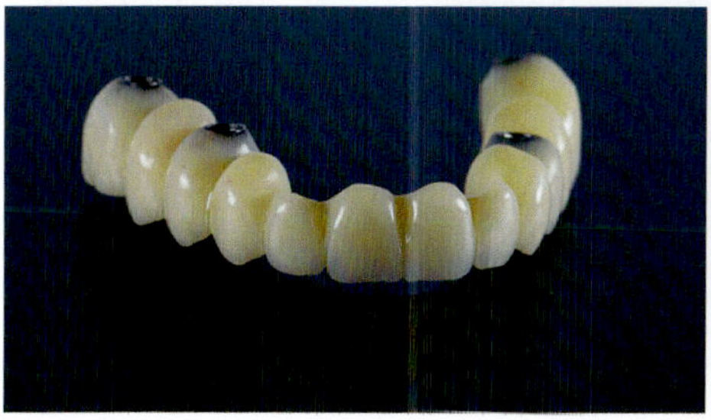

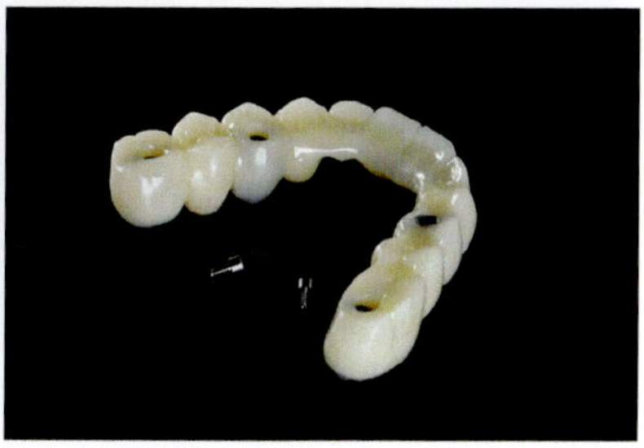

Figs. 8.65 and 8.66 Immediate load maxillary prosthesis finished and polished

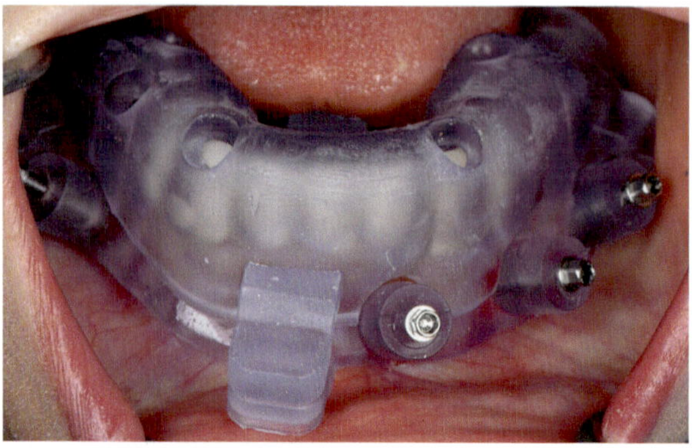

Fig. 8.67 Mandibular guides placed with the lateral stabilizing screws visible in four different positions to ensure a stable guide

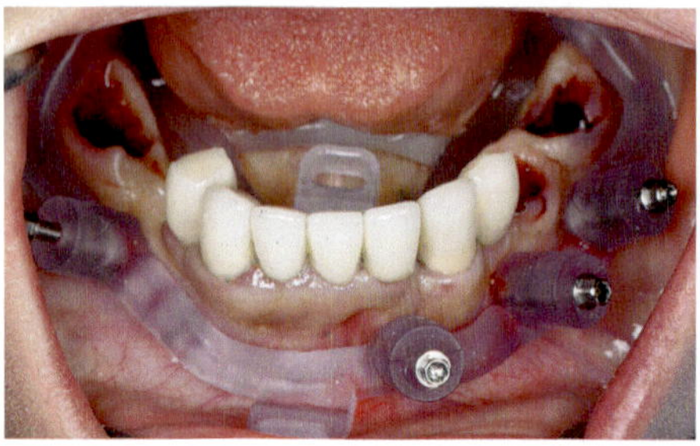

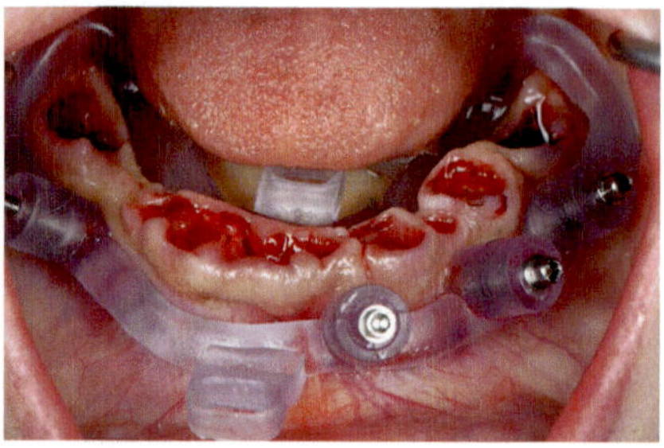

Figs. 8.68 and 8.69 Tooth extraction in process and completed

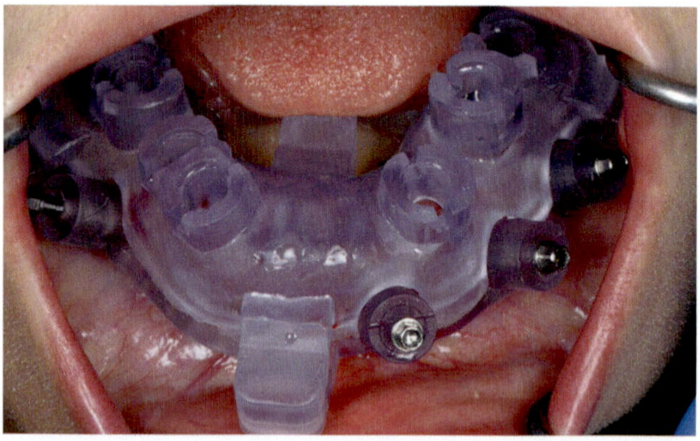

Fig. 8.70 Post-tooth extractions, the second part of the guide is stacked on the first part using button mechanisms. Now the implant-site drilling will take place

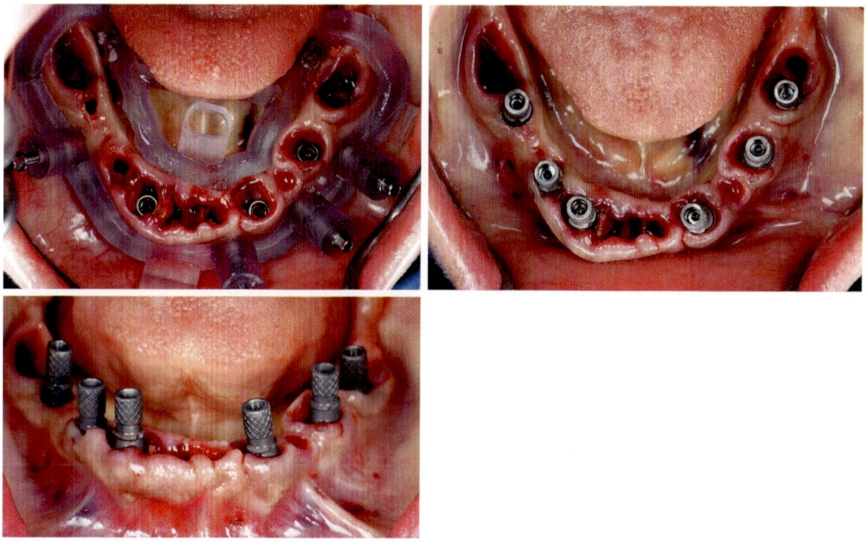

Figs. 8.71, 8.72 and 8.73 Six implants are placed, and multi-unit abutments are placed. Temporary cylinders are placed on the abutments, and then the temporary relining process starts

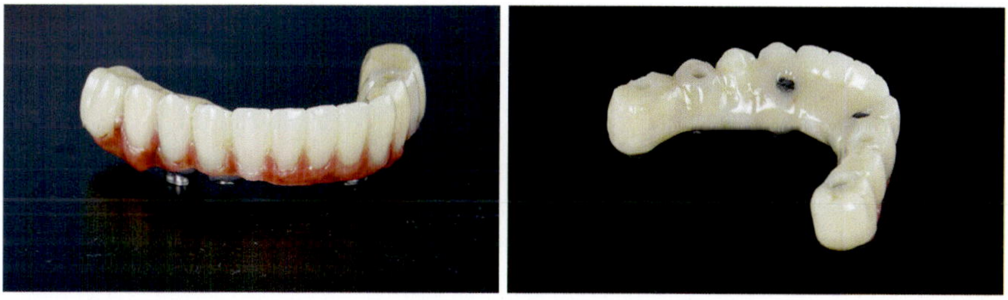

Figs. 8.74 and 8.75 Immediate load mandibular prosthesis finished and polished

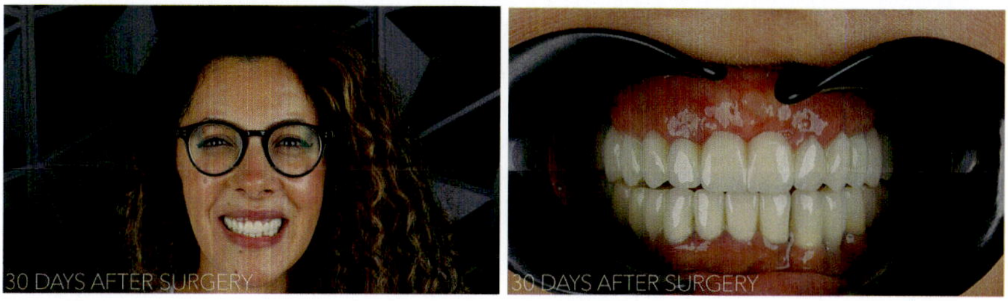

Figs. 8.76 and 8.77 Face and retracted view of the patient after 30 days of implant surgery

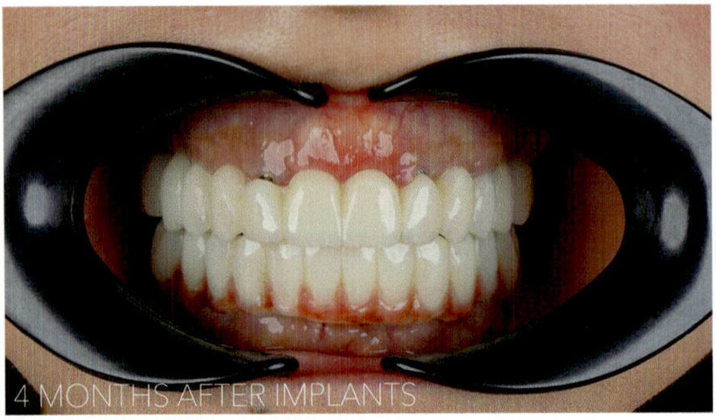

Fig. 8.78 Retracted view of the prosthesis after 4 months of the implant surgery. Note the recession that has taken place around the prosthesis, which is anticipated and will be compensated in the final stages as shown in later steps. The digital workflow allowed us to place implants and provided the patient with temporary screw-retained prostheses in a controlled and predictable fashion

8.6 Digital Workflow and the Material Selection

Once implants are osseointegrated, dental implants can be scanned using intra-oral scanners or using photogrammetry devices.

Intra-oral scanners are increasingly being used to scan dental implants. Advantages are:

1. Application: Intra-oral scanners are used to capture the position of dental implants using scan bodies that replace impression copings when making impressions. The digital impression obtained is used to manufacture the implant crown or FPD.
2. **Precision**: The precision of intra-oral scanners has greatly improved over the years. Studies have found that the accuracy of these scanners is now comparable to traditional impression techniques. The accuracy can be affected by various factors such as the scanning strategy, the scanner's resolution and the operator's experience. In general, the precision of most modern intra-oral scanners is within the range of 50–100 μm for short-span measurements, although this error might slightly increase for full-arch scans as stitching of images might decrease accuracy. Therefore, it is not advisable to use IOS for full-arch cases. Photogrammetry is the preferred device as accuracy is very high and shown to be even better than traditional impressions using pickup impression copings, a custom tray with polyvinyl siloxane (PVS) impression material.
3. Advantages over traditional impressions
   - Patient comfort: The shortcomings of conventional impression making have been discussed; there are also many advantages discussed with comfort for patients and adequate precision for short spans using IOS and photogrammetry for full-arch restorations.
   - Speed: Digital scans can be sent immediately to the dental laboratory, reducing the turnaround time for the fabrication of prostheses and eliminating the

need to pour impressions and use bite registrations, which can often be cumbersome and have the most frequent errors.
   - Digital storage: Digital impressions can be stored electronically, eliminating the need for physical storage and allowing easy sharing with other dental professionals or labs.
   - Visualization: Some intra-oral scanners come with software that can visualize the expected treatment outcome, aiding in treatment planning and patient communication.
4. Limitations
   - Learning curve: It might take time for clinicians to become adept at using intra-oral scanners, especially if they are transitioning from traditional techniques.
   - Cost: Proficient intra-oral scanners can be expensive, although the cost is expected to decrease as the technology becomes more widespread.
   - There will be added cost and time if models are required. Frequently, we need models to visualize aesthetics, control contours and layer ceramics. Printers are the preferred machines, but they are often expensive if good-quality printers and faster ones are needed. However, the printing resin is not flexible to work with, and dental technicians often need time, and a learning curve is needed to be able to control outcomes.

In digital dentistry, we often see two different types of workflows: model and model-less types.

Model dentistry is often required (Fig. 8.48b).

1. Control fit
2. Control proximal contacts
3. Control occlusion
4. Visualize aesthetics
5. Layer ceramics if needed
6. Cement or lute the Ti base into the milled or printed structure

Model-less type is when we print or mill restorations but do not have a model to fit back the units on it. That is often used for

1. Full contour "monolithic" structures where layering ceramics is not needed.

One should consider that the clinician will rely solely on the software and hardware parameters and the mouth intra-orally will serve as the final model to control and check for aesthetics, fit and contacts whether proximal or occlusal (more clearly, there are no try-ins of these restorations, and all adjustments will be performed intra-orally).

Moreover, luting Ti bases can be an issue as there is no model to fit back the structure on and control that all Ti bases are luted correctly and that the structure still has a "passive" fit.

One must consider that zirconia structures are milled in the white state and that there will be 3-dimensional changes and shrinkage that is calculated in the milling strategy and CAD file. However, we often use Ti bases to lute zirconia structures to them and that can be attributed to two main reasons:

1. The cement space is calculated to compensate for the shrinkage and possible misfit in the final sintered zirconia restoration. Figs. 8.127, 8.128 and 8.129 show the full arch milled without the Ti base.

Figures 8.131, 8.132, 8.133 and 8.134 show the Ti bases after being luted with dual-cure cement to the zirconia structures and being fitted back on the model for control of the passive fit and insertion axis of the screw-retained prosthesis.

2. Aim for the retaining screw to be seated on metal rather than zirconia which is brittle by nature, which can lead to crack propagation due to the high preload of the retaining screw and differential hardness in material properties.

Limitations: It will take time for clinicians to transition from traditional methods of impressions and casts to the use of intra-oral scanners.

- Costs can be prohibitive when making a choice for scanners, especially when the more accurate and precise scanners are chosen; in time, the costs may be reduced.
- In situations when there is a need for casts that will allow visualization of forms, for example aesthetic outcomes and layering of restorations unlike monolithic restorations, printers that will work fast and print in good dimensions and detail cost more and there need to be better printer resins that are at present very limited in physical properties.

Photogrammetry is also slowly getting more popular among full arches restored with dental implants. It is relatively fast to acquire the implant positions and accurate as many studies show that it is more accurate than analogue impressions using open tray copings that are splinted with resin and impressions taken with polyvinyl siloxane. However, photogrammetry is limited to usage for full arches; this makes it less popular and slowly growing in demand. And photogrammetry is expensive. The main objective of the device is solely locating the implant positions via locating scan flags that are connected and screwed into the implants. A soft tissue scan is required via an IOS or making an impression and then overlapping the photogrammetric scan in the CAD software. Additionally, a jaw registration is required and done manually using a wax occlusal rim with teeth set-up or using the provisional prosthesis.

8.7 Paradigm Shift in Laboratory Workflow

One of the major shifts in the laboratory workflows is incorporating the digital CAD/CAM software. The ability to overlap photographs with STL files makes designing easier, with reducing chances of errors in aesthetic parameters such as smile curve, midline deviation, occlusal cant tooth position, tooth proportions and bucco-lingual tooth positions in relation to upper and lower lips.

The use of traditional facebows to control aesthetics is not required anymore, as photographs can be taken with full face and software can align the eyes to the smile curve and occlusal plane, negating the need for facebow records (Figs 8.49, 8.50, 8.51 and 8.52).

Overlapping images of the provisional prosthesis with an implant working model can allow the technician to make corrections necessary to have a flawless design toward the definitive prosthesis without the need for trials (Fig. 8.50). The results have shown repeatedly that experience with designs of the provisional restorations that suit the patient's faces leads to definitive restorations. With experience, this allows clinicians to be more efficient in the treatment and skip steps that were deemed necessary in the traditional analogue workflow.

In addition, designing prosthesis and the flexibility of new abutment designs such as Dynamic Abutment Solutions (Lleida, Spain) [15] that are incorporated in CAD software allow deviation to the axis of the implant by up to 30° and its use in conjunction with monolithic zirconia restorations (Figs. 8.79, 8.80 and 8.81). The non-axial engagement of the retaining screw is facilitated by a screw-driver with a hexalobular driver tip that corresponds to the design of the screw head. This allows for a change in the screw access to exit the occlusal area in the posterior for allowing strength of the ceramics and the cingulum area in the anterior part for aesthetic purposes for implants placed with inclinations that would normally cause screw access to be in unsuitable positions due to the anatomy of the smaller residual ridge and limit preloads to the restoration-implant complex. In addition, pre-angled screw-retained restorations are not available in all implant systems. The dynamic abutment for CAD/CAM use is available for many systems, and for most systems, the screws can be torqued to 30 N/cm, where screw diameter is limited by the implant system, and lower torques may be mandated. Preloads on the tilted implants that are splinted are as good as non-angulated screw channels. Using these abutments together with

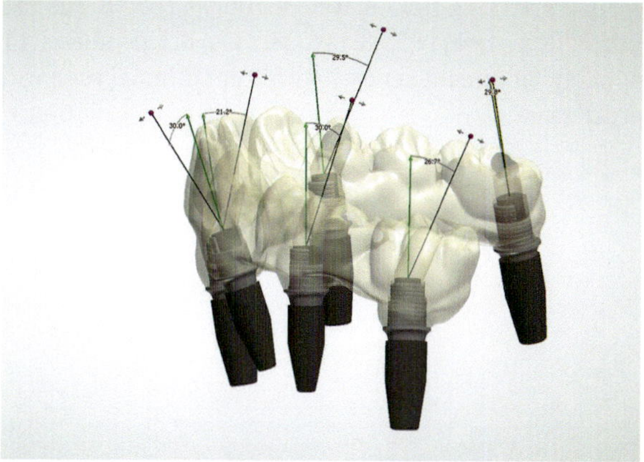

Fig. 8.79 Full arch in the CAD phase. Please note the different angles of the implants and especially in the anterior region. They are labially placed in accordance with the anatomy of the maxilla as it narrows apically

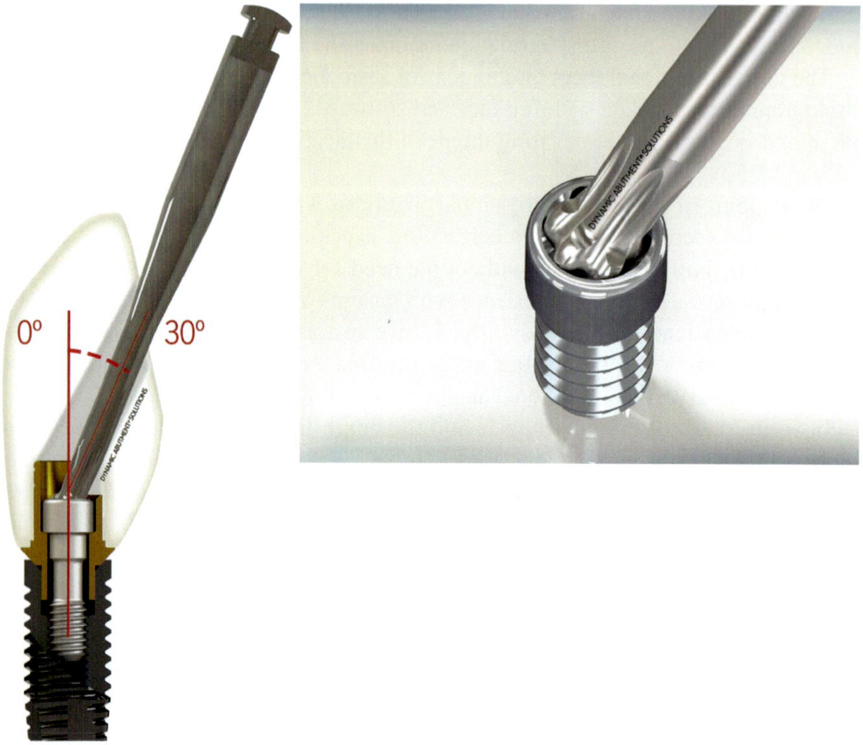

Figs. 8.80 and 8.81 The design of the screw and corresponding screwdriver allows engagement and torquing the screw up to 30 N/cm in 30° angulation. The Ti base can be luted to the zirconia suprastructure allowing the prosthesis to be screw retained. The variances in angulation to the axis of the implant are designed in the CAD software

zirconia-based restorations addresses the most common biomechanical and biologic issues mentioned above. Figures 8.82, 8.83, 8.84, 8.85, 8.86, 8.87, 8.88, 8.89, 8.90, 8.91, 8.92, 8.93, 8.94, 8.95, 8.96, 8.97, 8.98, 8.99, 8.100, 8.101, 8.102, 8.103, 8.104, 8.105, 8.106, 8.107, 8.108, 8.109, 8.110, 8.111, 8.112, 8.113, 8.114, 8.115, 8.116, 8.117, 8.118 and 8.119 show the usage of the dynamic abutment screw in different clinical scenarios of single unit to full-arch prosthesis.

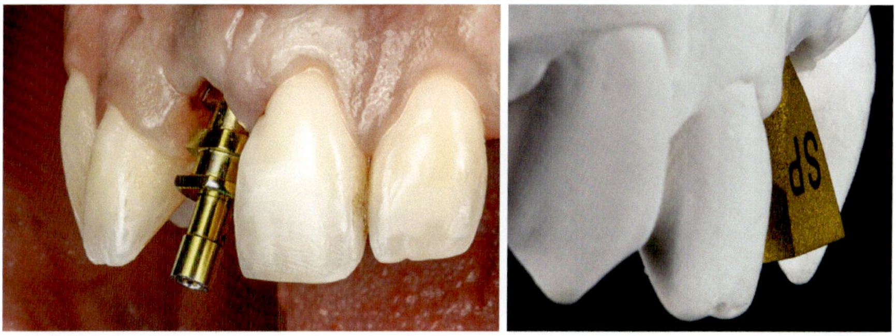

Figs. 8.82 and 8.83 Single implant placed with labial trajectory intra-oral view and on the cast with the scan body in place

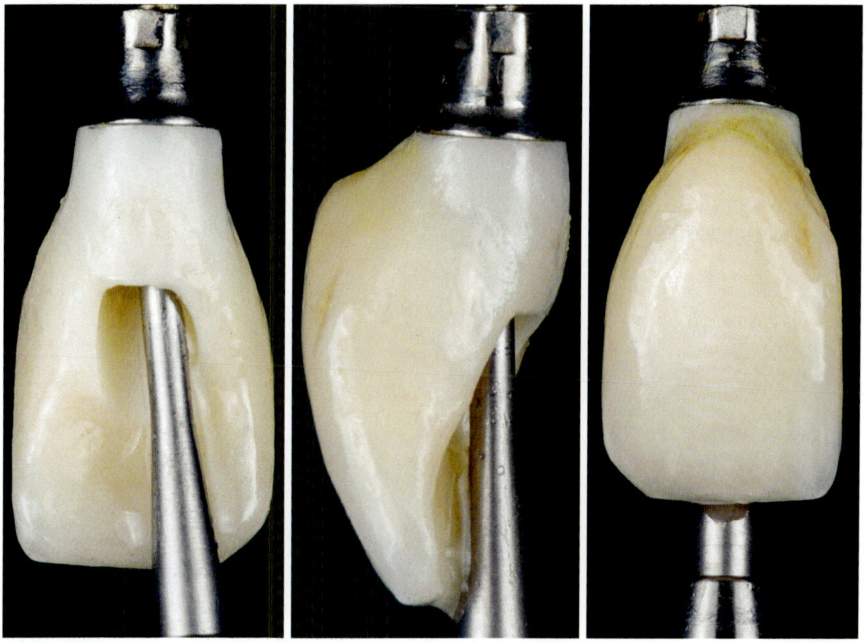

Figs. 8.84, 8.85 and 8.86 Single-implant zirconia suprastructure with the Ti base luted viewed from different aspects

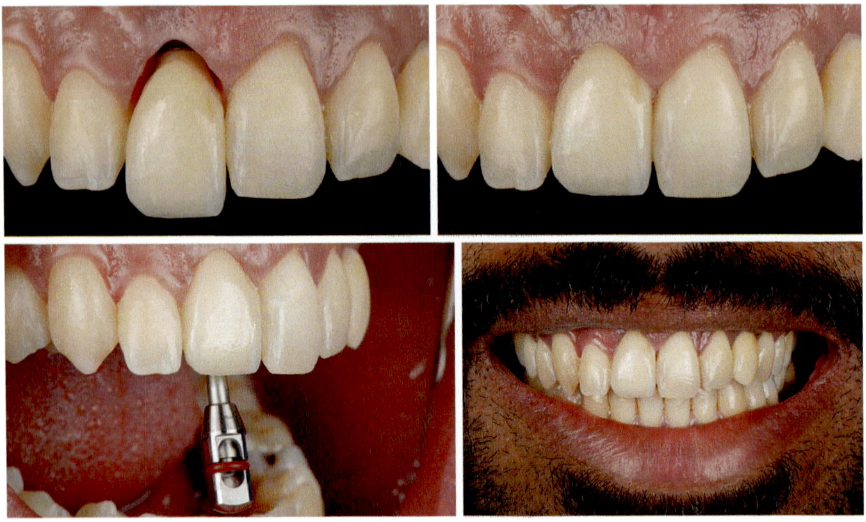

Figs. 8.87, 8.88, 8.89 and 8.90 Intra-oral views of the single implant delivered; note the change in location of screw access to the cingulum area of the restoration (Fig. 8.89)

Fig. 8.91 Radiograph of the restoration seated to the implant

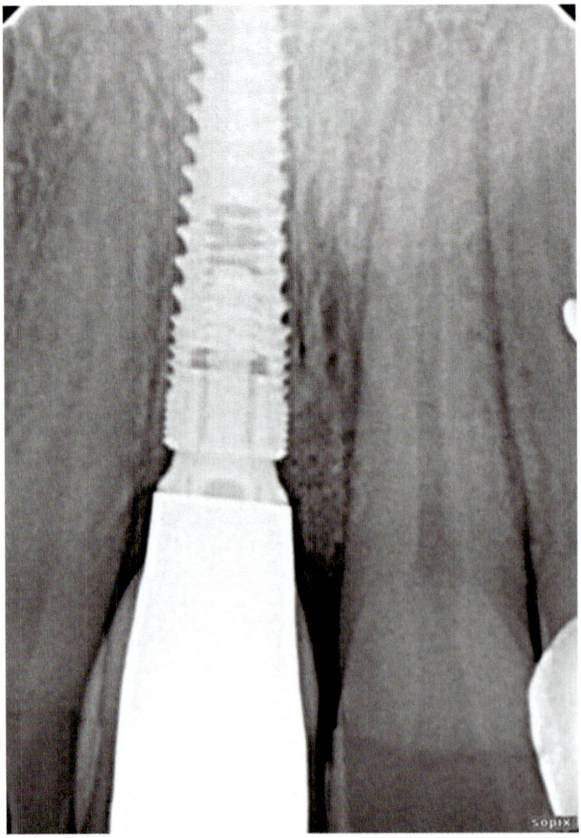

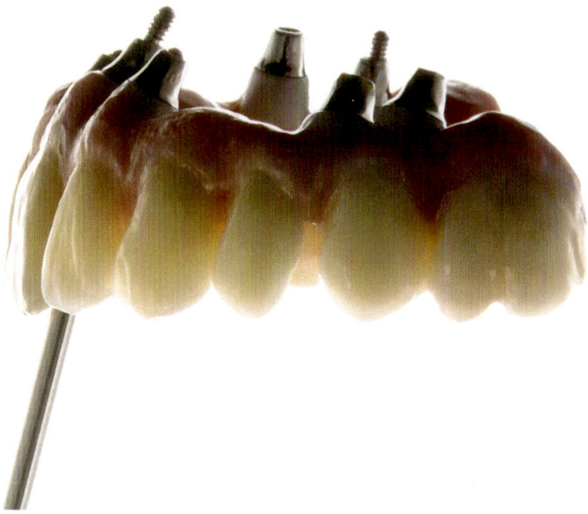

Fig. 8.92 View of extra-oral full-arch screw-retained implant-supported prosthesis. Note the differing axes of the screw access relative to the implant. The implants were placed labially due to anatomical constraints. A full contour translucent zirconia was machined with the angle changes managed during the computer-aided design (CAD) phase

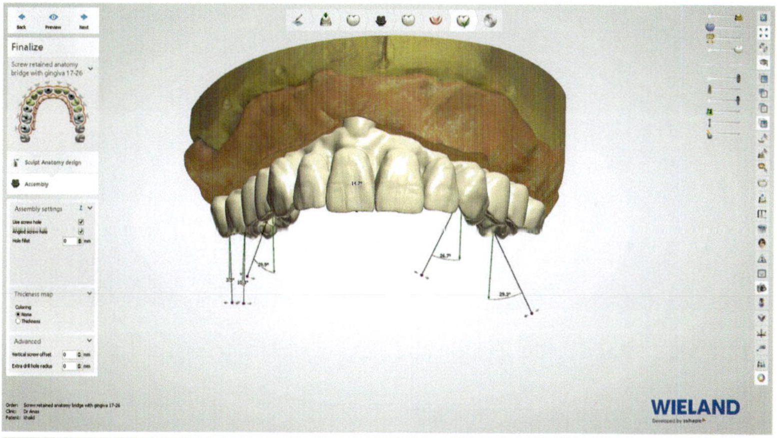

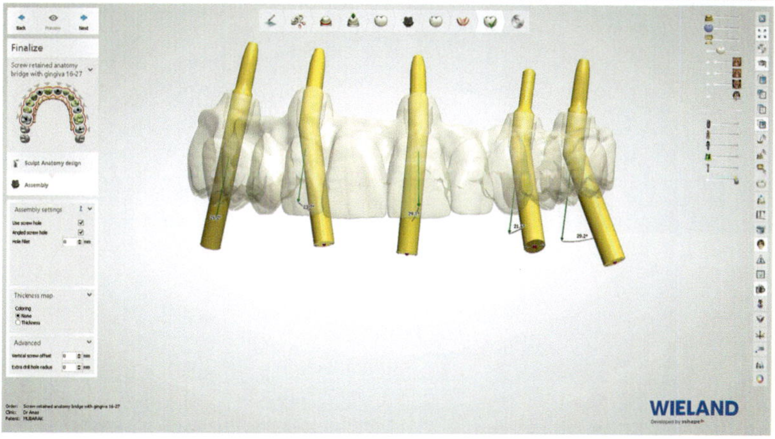

Figs. 8.93 and 8.94 Screen captures of the CAD of a full-arch restoration using the dynamic abutment and full tooth anatomy library. Note the change in the axial exit of the screw channels

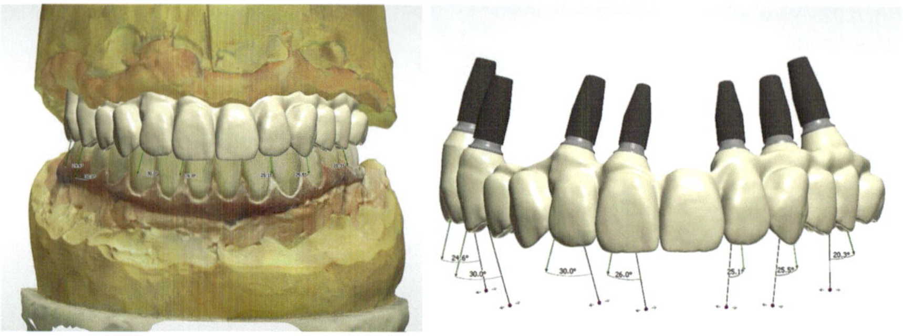

Figs. 8.95 and 8.96 The CAD phase for both the maxilla and the mandible. Full contour anatomy with cut back in areas to allow pink ceramic application to simulate soft tissues

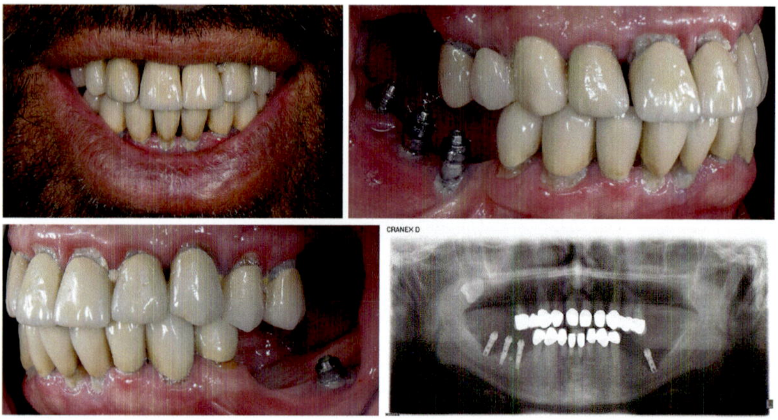

Figs. 8.97, 8.98, 8.99 and 8.100 Preoperative views of smile, intra-oral and radiograph

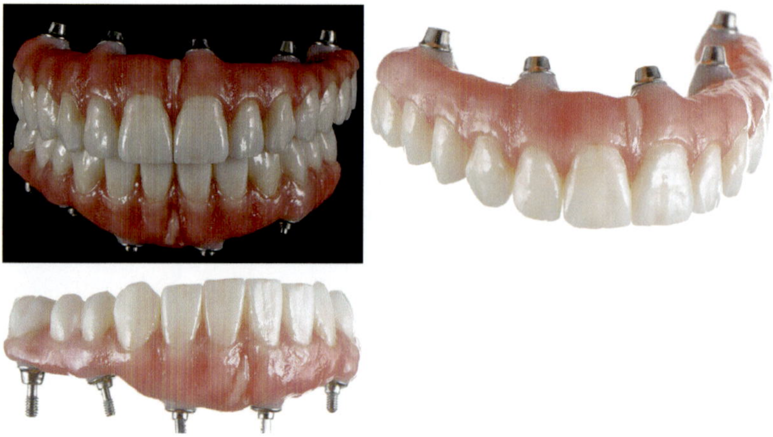

Figs. 8.101, 8.102 and 8.103 Definitive prosthesis full contour zirconia with layered pink ceramics only

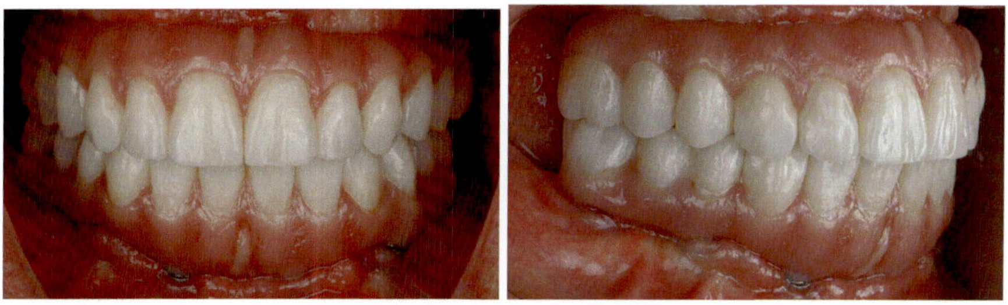

Figs. 8.104 and 8.105 Intra-oral views of the final prosthesis delivered

Fig. 8.106 Panoramic radiograph post-operatively

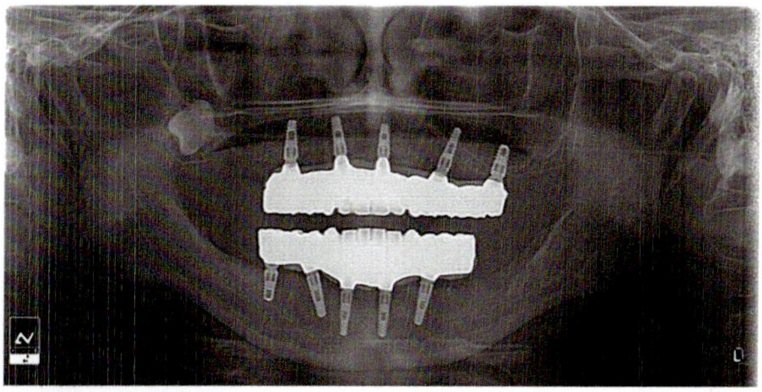

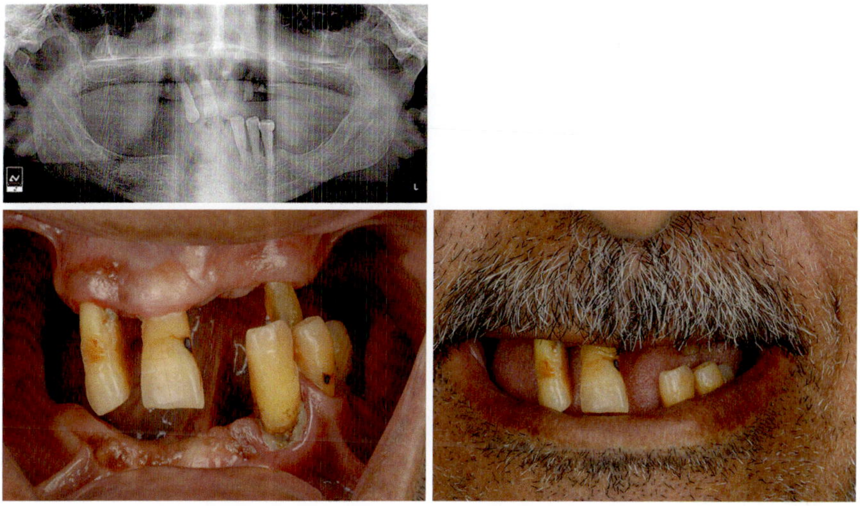

Figs. 8.107, 8.108 and 8.109 Preoperative views of the patient. Note the pneumatized sinuses and the severe bone resorption in both arches

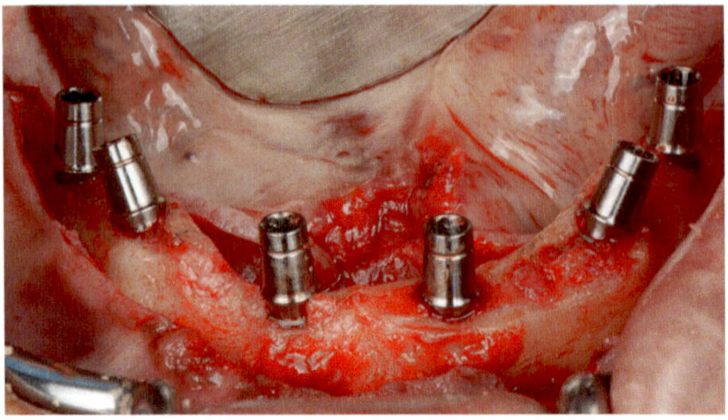

Fig. 8.110 Six implants placed with tilted implants to avoid the mental foramen and sinuses

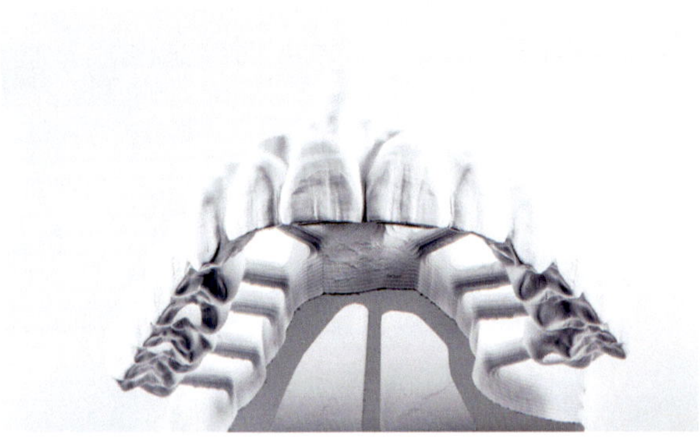

Fig. 8.111 Pre-sintered full frame zirconia. Now the frame is ready to be sintered for a 9-h cycle

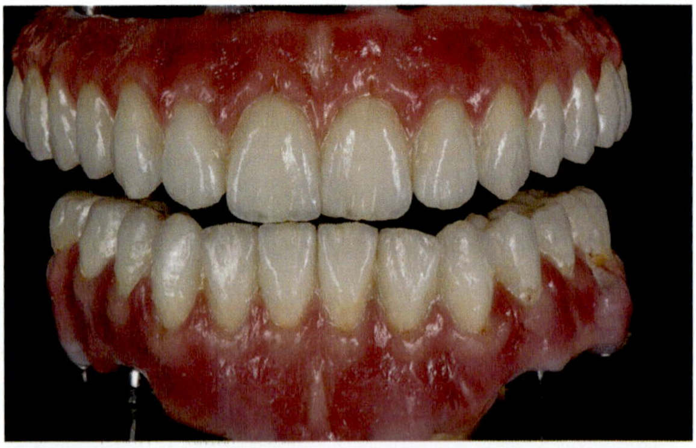

Fig. 8.112 Full contour zirconia with layered pink ceramics

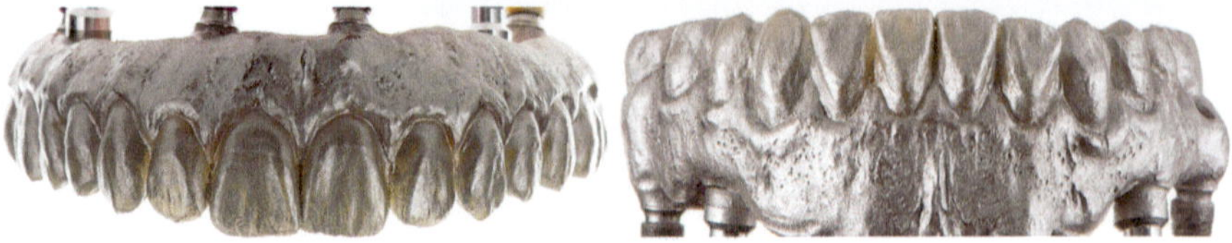

Figs. 8.113 and 8.114 Using a coating silver powder to show the detail we can obtain from milling

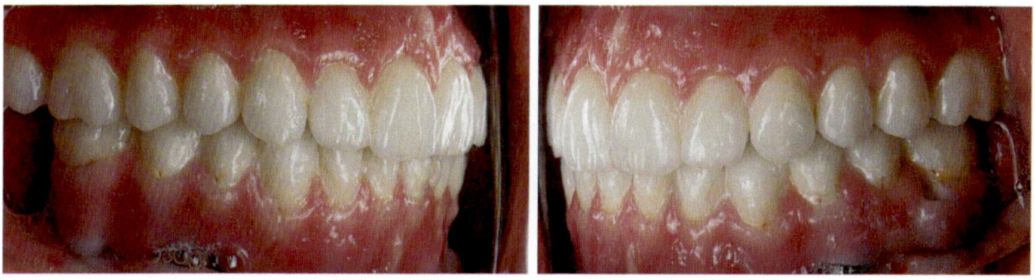

Figs. 8.115 and 8.116 Lateral views in occlusion

Figs. 8.117 and 8.118 Post-operative smile

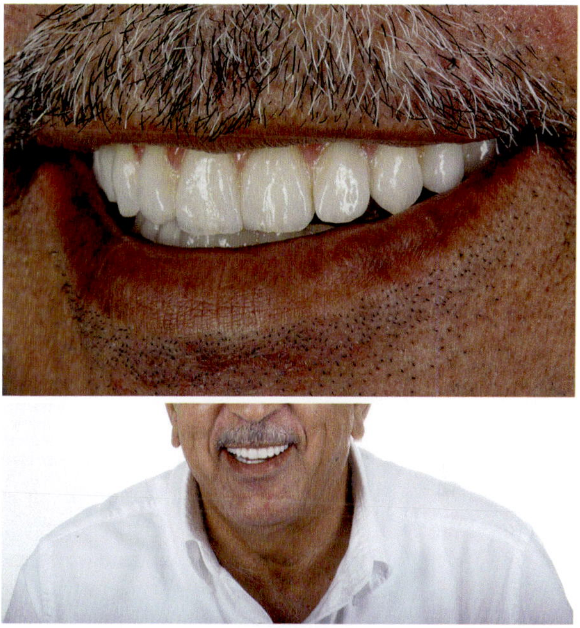

Fig. 8.119 Post-operative panoramic radiograph. Note the tilted implants avoiding the sinus and mental foramina

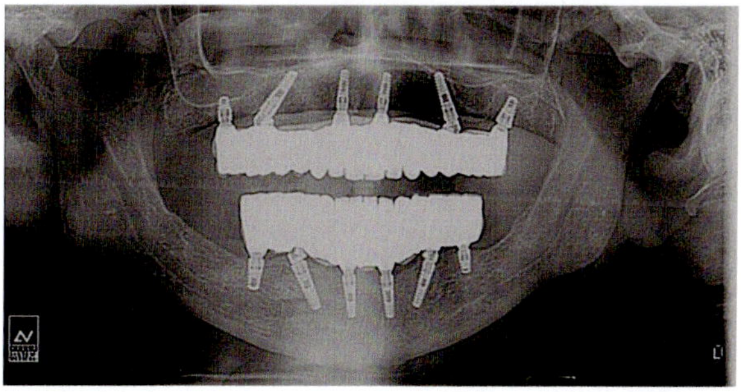

8.8 Full-Contour Zirconia for Large Rehabilitations

Zirconia exists in several allotropic forms. For fabrication of dental restorations, the most desirable form is the tetragonal allotrope, as it has the physical and optical properties to provide strength and aesthetics. The resistance to fracture that zirconia comes from a process known as transformation toughening. This process occurs because of allotropic change from the tetragonal to the monolithic form, which is 25% larger volumetrically than the tetragonal allotrope. The monolithic allotrope is the most stable form at room temperature; therefore, any energy applied to the material will cause this allotropic change, which in turn causes a volumetric change. This volumetric change in the adjacent areas of the crack prevents the crack from propagating [16, 17]. In the literature that describes the clinical use of layered zirconia restorations, chipping of the veneering porcelain has been reported to be up to 50%; this was early in the use of zirconia, and we did not have feldspathic ceramics with suitable expansion and contraction when layered and heating and cooling as zirconia does not conduct heat; the substructures were made with the same metal ceramic designs, so things have improved and changed—different designs can be used to have layered ceramics, and monolithic structures have also improved and are mechanically the most durable. However, few of the zirconia substructure frameworks have been reported to fail, and those few failures were found to be caused by poor design, largely due to insufficient bulk of material in connector areas for fixed partial dentures [18, 19].

Implant-supported reconstructions fabricated from monolithic zirconia have the potential to be very durable because the weak link of veneering porcelain is removed from any areas with occlusal function. In addition, implant-supported structures have dimensions that are usually much larger than tooth-supported restorations and allow a much larger volume of material [20, 21]. This results in eliminating areas of weakness with monolithic zirconia implant-supported screw-retained restorations. Together with excellent biocompatibility, good optical properties for tooth replacement and ease of fabrication, zirconia should be considered as an attractive material to restore dental implants. Figures 8.120, 8.121, 8.122, 8.123, 8.124, 8.125, 8.126, 8.127, 8.128, 8.129, 8.130, 8.131, 8.132, 8.133, 8.134, 8.135, 8.136, 8.137, 8.138, 8.139, 8.140, 8.141, 8.142, 8.143 and 8.144 illustrate the clinical steps of fabricating full-arch maxillary and mandibular zirconia monolithic structures with minimal layering of soft tissue analogues with pink ceramics only. Modify the pre-sintered-state zirconia, and use organic colouring to add background chroma and pigments that can simulate translucent optical illusions. Note that addition of the papillae in the maxillary arch compensates for the lack of interdental tissue because of multiple extractions. Adding pink papillae will give the freedom to change the shape of teeth to more ovoid or triangular shapes, which can satisfy patients' needs and prevent the block-like appearance of missing interdental soft tissue. However, this requires special training and skills to match the pink shade that can be technically cumbersome in many scenarios.

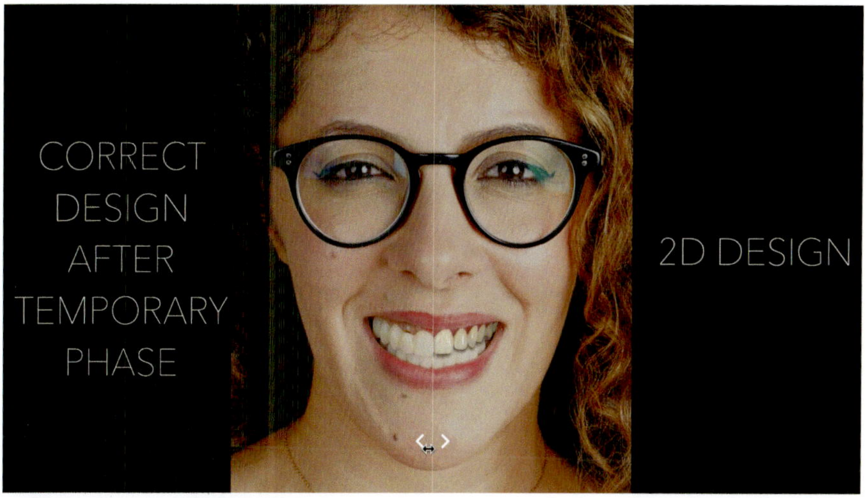

Fig. 8.120 The same case described above in the chapter. After the temporary phase is done. Now the 2-dimensional design on the photo of the temporary prosthesis to correct any minor details that need correction as the patient is now accustomed to the temporary prosthesis after 4 months. Needed corrections will be shown in the right side of the image. The incisal edges are shifted apically, and tooth shapes are being altered slightly toward more rounded edges for the laterals upon the patient's request

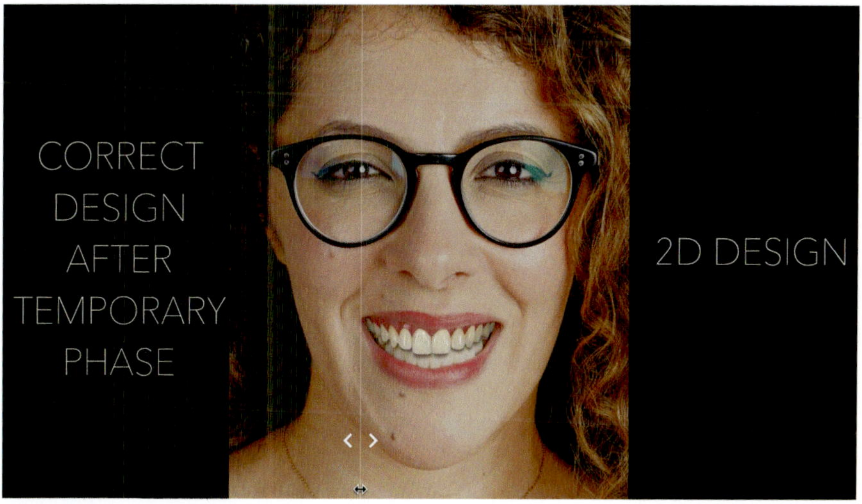

Fig. 8.121 The completed 2-dimensional design

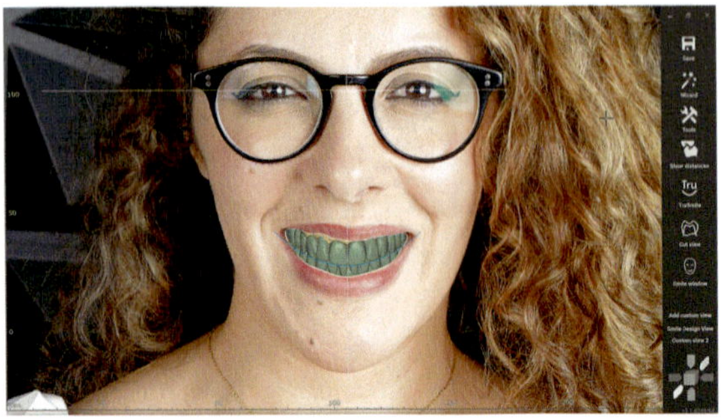

Fig. 8.122 The completed design on Exocad after being exported. This is a frontal view of the 3-dimensional design aligned on the patient's face and smile

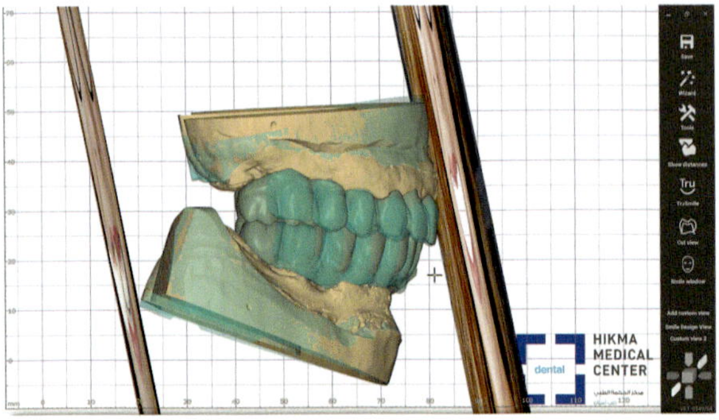

Fig. 8.123 Lateral view on Exocad showing the different layers after being aligned

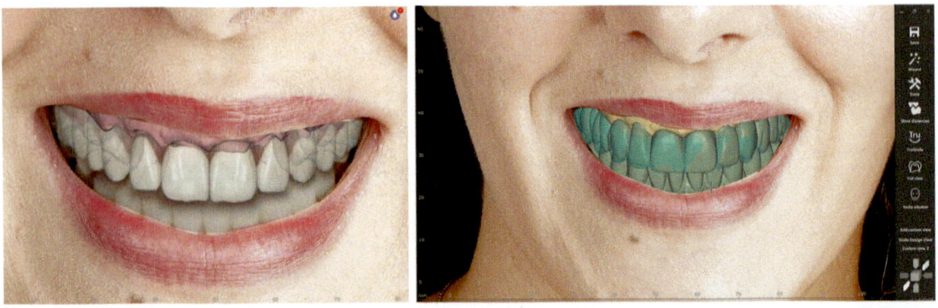

Figs. 8.124 and 8.125 Different views of the design process on Exocad setting the final tooth library on the patient's smile respecting the implant's emergence and the soft tissue profiles

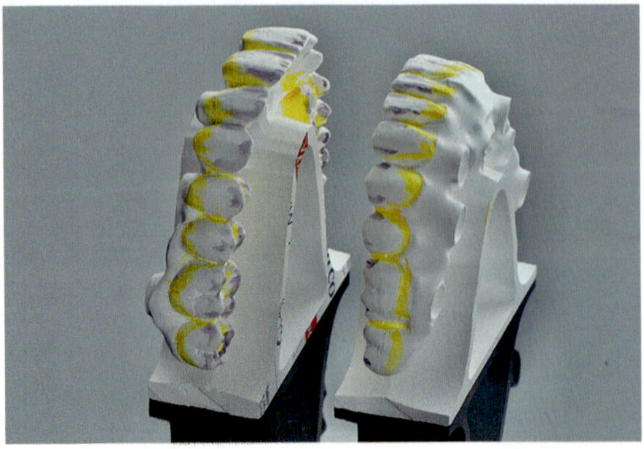

Fig. 8.126 Pre-sintered state of the upper and lower zirconia structures after being infiltrated with organic shades

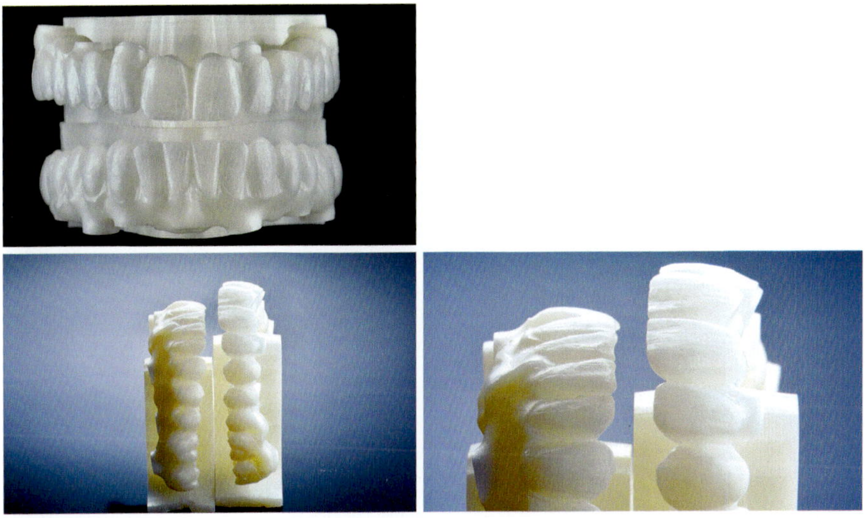

Figs. 8.127, 8.128 and 8.129 Different views of the zirconia full contour structures after sintering

Fig. 8.130 The upper model with the soft tissue scalloping

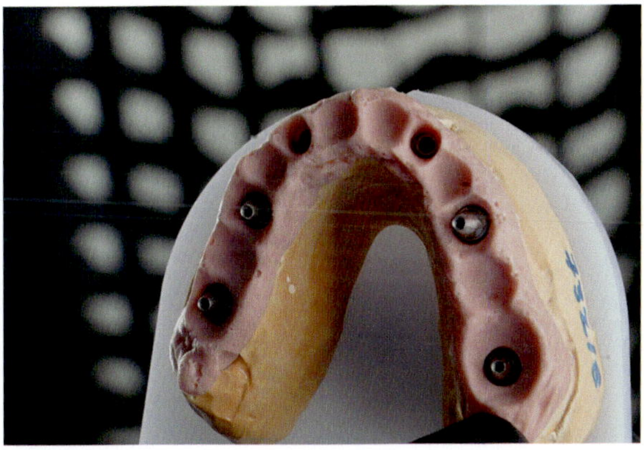

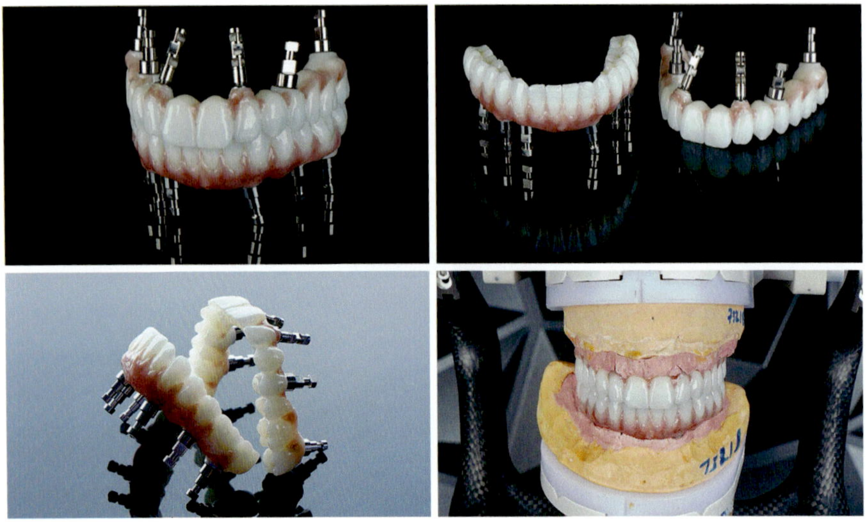

Figs. 8.131, 8.132, 8.133 and 8.134 Different views of the definitive zirconia upper and lower structures. Note the added pink papillae of the upper arch as there is a need to compensate for the loss of soft tissue due to past bone loss and history of periodontitis

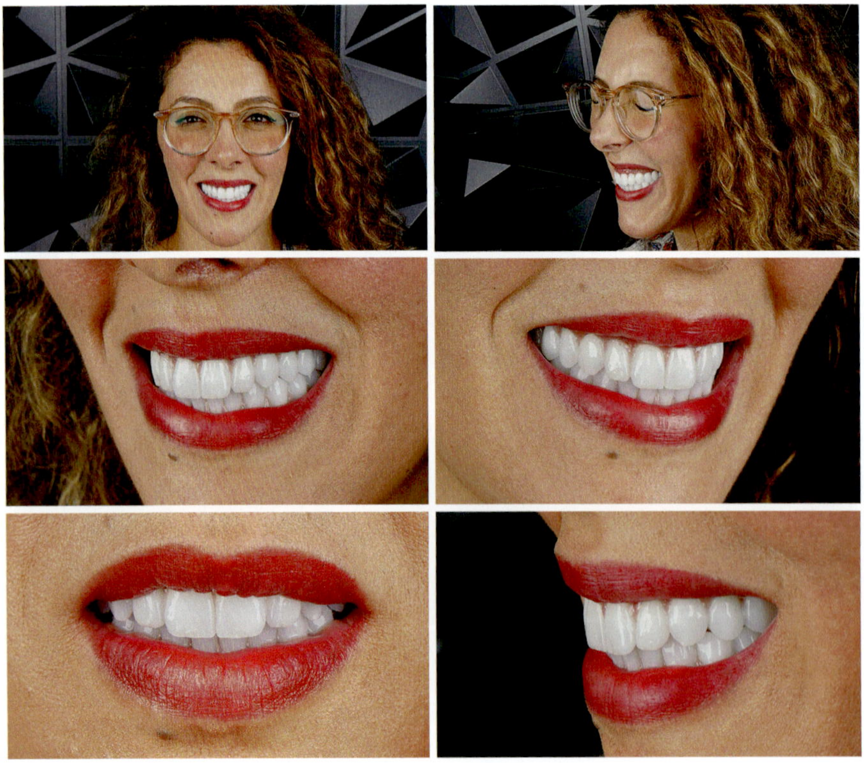

Figs. 8.135, 8.136, 8.137, 8.138, 8.139 and 8.140 Post-operative face and smile

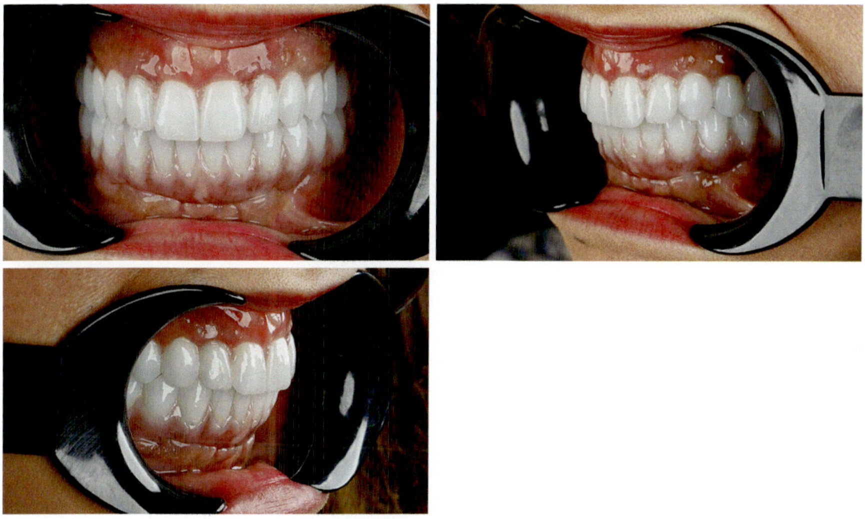

Figs. 8.141, 8.142 and 8.143 Frontal and lateral views in occlusion

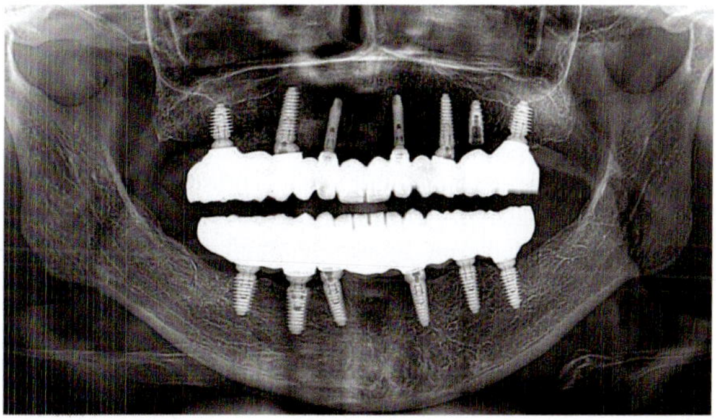

Fig. 8.144 Post-operative panoramic radiograph

References

1. Mangano F, Gandolfi A, Luongo G, Logozzo S. Intraoral scanners in dentistry: a review of the current literature. BMC Oral Health. 2017;17(1):149.
2. Revilla-León M, Özcan M. The use of photogrammetry in dental medicine: a narrative review. J Prosthodont Res. 2019.
3. Anadioti E, Aquilino SA, Gratton DG, Holloway JA, Denry IL, Thomas GW, Qian F. 3D and 2D marginal fit of pressed and CAD/CAM lithium disilicate crowns made from digital and conventional impressions. J Prosthodont. 2015;24(8):610–7.
4. Kugel G, Ferrari M. The science of bonding: from first to sixth generation. J Am Dent Assoc. 2016;137:20S–5S.
5. Ting-Shu S, Jian S. Intraoral digital impression technique: a review. J Prosthodont. 2015;24(4):313–21.
6. Joda T, Brägger U. Digital vs. conventional implant prosthetic workflows: a cost/time analysis. Clin Oral Implants Res. 2014;27(12):e185–9.

7. Ender A, Mehl A. Full arch scans: conventional versus digital impressions—an in-vitro study. Int J Comput Dent. 2015;18(4):371–82.
8. Flügge T, Schlager S, Nelson K, Nahles S, Metzger M. Precision of intraoral digital dental impressions with iTero and extraoral digitization with the iTero and a model scanner. Am J Orthod Dentofac Orthop. 2017;152(3):381–6.
9. Mehl A, Ender A, Mormann W, Attin T. Accuracy testing of a new intraoral 3D camera. Int J Comput Dent. 2009;12(1):11–28.
10. Kravitz ND, Groth C. The future of computer-aided orthodontics. Am J Orthod Dentofac Orthop. 2017;151(2):216–7.
11. Vezzetti E, Marcolin F. 3D photogrammetry using a smartphone. Procedia CIRP. 2018;75:50–5.
12. Teixeira M, Fernandes PO, Claro APN, Armada L. Comparative analysis of photogrammetry methods from UAVs in low-cost projects. ISPRS Int Arch Photogramm Remote Sens Spatial Inf Sci. 2016;41:1099–106.
13. Logozzo S, Zanetti EM, Franceschini G, Kilpelä A, Mäkynen A. Recent advances in dental optics—part I: 3D intraoral scanners for restorative dentistry. Opt Lasers Eng. 2014;54:203–21.
14. Tarnow DP, Cho SC, Wallace SS. The effect of inter-implant distance on the height of inter-implant bone crest. J Periodontol. 2000;71(4):546–9.
15. Araújo MG, Lindhe J. Dimensional ridge alterations following tooth extraction. An experimental study in the dog. J Clin Periodontol. 2005;32:212–8.
16. Kelly JR, Denry I. Stabilized zirconia as a structural ceramic: an overview. Dent Mater. 2008;24:289–98.
17. Denry I, Kelly JR. State of the art of zirconia for dental applications. Dent Mater. 2008;24:299–307.
18. Koenig V, Vanheusden AJ, Le Goff SO, Mainjot AK. Clinical risk factors related to failures with zirconia-based restorations: an up to 9-year retrospective study. J Dent. 2013;41:1164–74.
19. Guess PC, Att W, Strub JR. Zirconia in fixed implant prosthodontics. Clin Implant Dent Relat Res. 2012;14:633–45.
20. Venezia P, Torsello F, Cavalcanti R, D'Amato S. Retrospective analysis of 26 complete-arch implant-supported monolithic zirconia prostheses with feldspathic porcelain veneering limited to the facial surface. J Prosthet Dent. 2015;114:506–12.
21. Larsson C, Vult Von Steyern P. Implant-supported full-arch zirconia-based mandibular fixed dental prostheses. Eight-year results from a clinical pilot study. Acta Odontol Scand. 2013;71:1118–22.

Surgical Guidelines for Dental Implant Placement

9

Kian Kar and Erin Lee

9.1 Patient Assessment

Patient assessment should include a review of systemic health, allergies and medications to manage systemic conditions. Although there are very few absolute contraindications for implant surgery, there are several medical conditions that can influence the outcome of implant therapy. These include smoking, diabetes, obesity/hyperlipidaemia, impaired organ function, osteoporosis, hormonal disturbances, medications such as long-term corticosteroids, selective serotonin reuptake inhibitors (SSRIs) and bisphosphonates, irradiation and genetics [1–4]. Patients with self-reported allergy to penicillin exhibit higher implant failure rate [5–7].

Vitamin D deficiency is a common finding, and it is associated with a higher rate of implant failure. Dietary supplement with vitamin D for 4–6 weeks prior to implant surgery seems to establish normal levels of vitamin D in blood prior to surgical appointment [8–11].

Patient personality classification influences their suitability for complex multidisciplinary treatment. Clinicians may alter their treatment planning recommendations upon assessment of patient personality classification [12]. Some personality and psychological features such as neuroticism, extraversion, agreeableness, openness and conscientiousness might affect and predict dental satisfaction and impact daily living [13].

Clinicians should get a clear understanding as why the patient is seeking treatment with them, meaning priorities of aesthetics and/or function, and why the patient is at the current state of oral condition, meaning history of dental diseases, previously provided treatment and patient's compliance. This evaluation should

K. Kar (✉)
Advanced Periodontology, Herman Ostrow School of Dentistry, University of Southern California, Los Angeles, CA, USA

E. Lee
Private Practice, Pasadena, California, USA

W. Chee, S. Jivraj (eds.), *Treatment Planning In Implant Dentistry*, BDJ Clinician's Guides, https://doi.org/10.1007/978-3-031-68726-6_9

take into consideration the clinician's level of training, competence and management ability in achieving those expectations. Upon assessing these factors thoroughly, clinicians should decide whether they can reasonably meet patient-specific expectations within the context of the state of their dental disease. A proper informed consent that is composed can be presented and accepted by the patient prior to initiation of implant rehabilitation [14, 15].

9.2 Periodontal Examination

Patient assessment should include a comprehensive evaluation of periodontal condition to classify patients' periodontal status, including susceptibility to inflammatory periodontal diseases. Numerous studies have reported a history of severe or aggressive periodontitis to be a risk factor for peri-implant diseases [16–18]. However, animal studies, cross-sectional and longitudinal human observations as well as association studies indicate that peri-implantitis has similarities to a microbiota comparable to that of periodontitis. Periodontitis risk factors such as diabetes, smoking and poor oral hygiene seem to increase the risk for peri-implantitis. Some have argued the case for bacterial translocation from periodontitis to implant sites and suggested that by achieving periodontal health in the remaining dentition and utilizing relatively smooth abutments and implant surfaces, a reduction in bacterial translocation can be achieved [19]. With a 3-year and 5-year follow-up study, Mengel showed that oral rehabilitation with implants could be successful in partially edentulous patients treated for generalized aggressive and generalized chronic periodontitis. However, the success rate for implant therapy was 88.8% in aggressive periodontitis group compared to 100% in chronic periodontitis group [17]. Control of inflammation and mucositis is the most efficacious way to prevent progressive bone loss around dental implants [18].

9.3 Soft Tissue Phenotype

Another aspect of periodontal examination includes assessment of hard and soft tissues of edentulous sites together with adjacent teeth or teeth that need to be removed and replaced by dental implants. These include assessment of patient soft tissue phenotype around teeth and edentulous sites and evaluation of post-extraction hard and soft tissue deficiencies. Becker and Ochsenbein classified three distinct types of alveolar crest topography based on the evaluation of dry skulls: pronounced scalloped, scalloped and flat [20]. Prevailing assumption is that pronounced scalloped or scalloped bony architecture will be associated with a thinner, soft tissue phenotype. A flat bony profile would be associated with thicker, soft tissue topography with flat gingival architecture; this is usually supported by thick buccal and lingual plates of alveolar bone. A thin skeletal pattern with scalloped architecture will present with root dehiscence and fenestrations even in a healthy periodontium [20–23].

9.4 Location of Alveolar Bone Crest

It is important to establish both the attachment and crestal bone levels along with probing depth measurement of teeth planned for extraction along with teeth adjacent to implant sites. The distance from alveolar bone crest to cemento-enamel junction (CEJ) or gingival/mucosal zenith of the restorations can influence the surgical planning with needed modifications for implant placement. In natural dentition, the distance of 2 mm from bone crest to CEJ of teeth is considered normal. When the CEJ-to-bone crest distance is less than 2 mm, it is considered a high crest bone level [21] which is usually associated with thicker crestal bone and margin located crestal to CEJ [22]. Although some contradictory evidence is reported concerning the correlation between soft and hard tissue thickness, prevailing evidence supports the concept that a thicker buccal alveolar plate is present with a thick, soft tissue phenotype presentation. This is particularly beneficial when planning for procedures affecting periodontal structures such as crown lengthening, extractions and implant therapy [23]. Therefore, crestal bone height is an important consideration for implant therapy that can influence surgical planning and modifications for implant therapy. Kois described five key factors for predictable single-tooth peri-implant aesthetics. These keys include relative tooth position, form of the periodontium, biotype of the periodontium, tooth shape and position of the osseous crest [24].

The papilla height between an implant and a tooth is predominantly dependent on the clinical attachment level of the tooth. When two adjacent implants are present, interproximal tissues of adjacent implants will present with a flat architecture. With the absence of adjacent teeth, it is difficult to predict interproximal soft tissue (papillary) height and define the optimal horizontal distance between two adjacent implants restored with fixed dental prostheses [25]. Traditionally, a 3 mm distance between two implants with appropriate transmucosal depth is required to form interproximal papillae.

To reduce the risk of aesthetic failures, interproximal probing and measurement of attachment level are important and should be considered as part of periodontal evaluation of the adjacent teeth to implant sites before implant placement [26] (Fig. 9.1a–d).

Other mucogingival considerations such as amount of keratinized attached tissue and soft tissue thickness and depth are also important factors in surgical planning for implant placement [27]. Keratinized and attached tissues around implants seem to have a positive effect on plaque control and inflammation control [28, 29]. Transmucosal depth from restorative platform to mucosal zenith is critical in providing transitional room for emergence profile and support of buccal mucosa [30] (Fig. 9.2a–c). Mucosal thickness of the tissue surrounding the implant is another important consideration to provide an adequate emergence profile [31]. Deficiency in any of the mentioned parameters can be a risk factor for soft tissue complications, such as recession, inflammation and symptoms such as soft tissue tenderness to touch (Fig. 9.3).

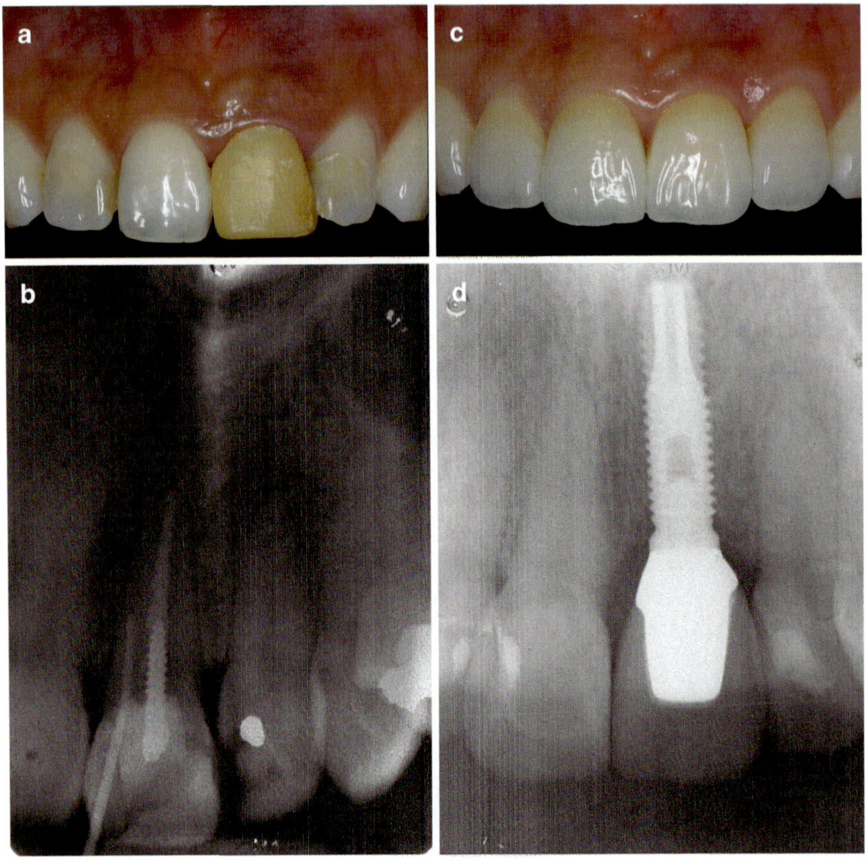

Fig. 9.1 Tooth # 9 presents with poor restorative prognosis (**a**, **b**). Probing depths are 2–3 mm with interproximal bone within 1–2 mm distance from CEJ of adjacent teeth providing a favourable support for interdental papilla following extraction and replacement with dental implant. Implant depth provides transitional space from restorative platform to gingival zenith so the soft tissue contours are supported by restoration (**c**, **d**). (Restorative treatment courtesy of Dr. James Kim Irvine, California)

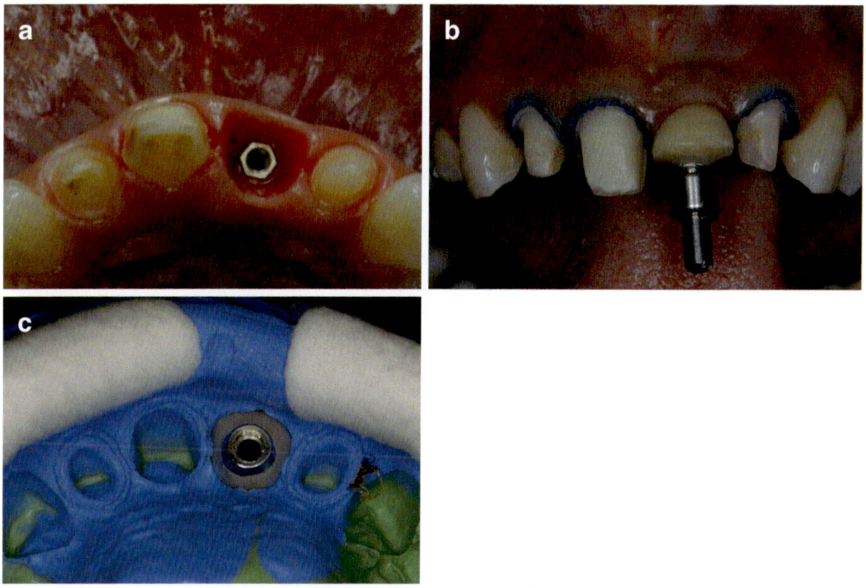

Fig. 9.2 4–5 mm of submucosal depth providing adequate transmucosal contour and mucosal support. Custom impression coping to capture soft tissue contour in final impression (**b**, **c**). (Restorative treatment courtesy of Dr. James Kim Irvine, California)

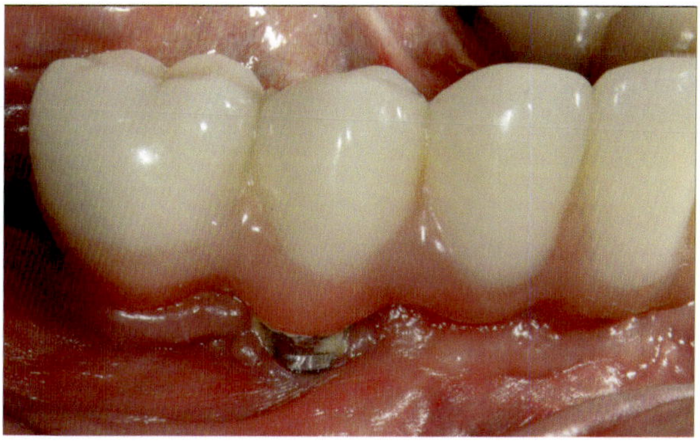

Fig. 9.3 Lack of mucosal keratinization and thickness leading to mucosal recession around dental implant

9.5 Gingival/Mucosal Display

The amount of soft tissue displayed and more importantly the proportions of tooth to gingival display and gingival/mucosal margin harmony are important considerations in implant therapy in the aesthetic zone [32]. Lip mobility and lengths influence the amount of teeth and gingival display. With a high smile line, when there is tissue loss in aesthetic zones, clinicians must weigh the risk/benefits and cost/benefits of decision-making between reconstructing lost soft and hard tissues and using prosthetic replicas of missing tissues. When using prosthetic soft tissue replicas,

Fig. 9.4 Patient presents with severe vertical overlap, gingival display and dento-alveolar extrusion causing trauma to the palatal of maxillary anterior teeth (**a**–**e**). Treatment alternatives of orthognathic and orthodontic therapy to correct malocclusion was not accepted by the patient. Patient opted for replacement of maxillary and mandibular anterior teeth with implant-supported prosthesis. Preoperative view of maxillary and mandibular arch 4 months post-extraction indicating excessive bone height due to history of dentoalveolar extrusion and the need for alveolar bone resection to provide restorative space for implant therapy (**f**, **g**, **m**). Crestal bone reduction was performed to create transmucosal restorative space according to diagnostic wax-up and surgical guide (**h**, **o**). Crestal reduction also helps with assuring soft tissue depth of more than 3 mm. Implant placement positioned in screw-retained prosthetic position (**i**, **j**, **n**, **o**). Bone scraper was used for alveolar reduction and to collect autogenous bone shavings from contour augmentation of buccal concavity and crestal dehiscence (**k**, **p**) with tension-free primary closure (**k**, **q**). Definitive restoration following initial planning to address malocclusion, function and aesthetic of maxillary and mandibular anterior teeth (**r**–**w**). Note the suitable transmucosal emergence profile corresponding to proper transmucosal depth, soft tissue thickness, prosthesis support and formation of soft tissue profile (**x**–**z**). (Surgery in collaboration with Dr. Yun Wang, Dr. Alexander Aalam and restorative treatment courtesy of Dr. Sangho Byun)

adequate apical displacement of prosthesis-mucosal interface should be considered to hide the junction of the prostheses under the lip during function and exaggerated smile. Ideally, maintenance of teeth even with compromised prognosis would be a first choice of planning in aesthetic zone; however, at times to achieve aesthetic and functional treatment goals, additional teeth may be included for strategic extractions to accommodate a reasonable outcome [33] (Fig. 9.4a–z).

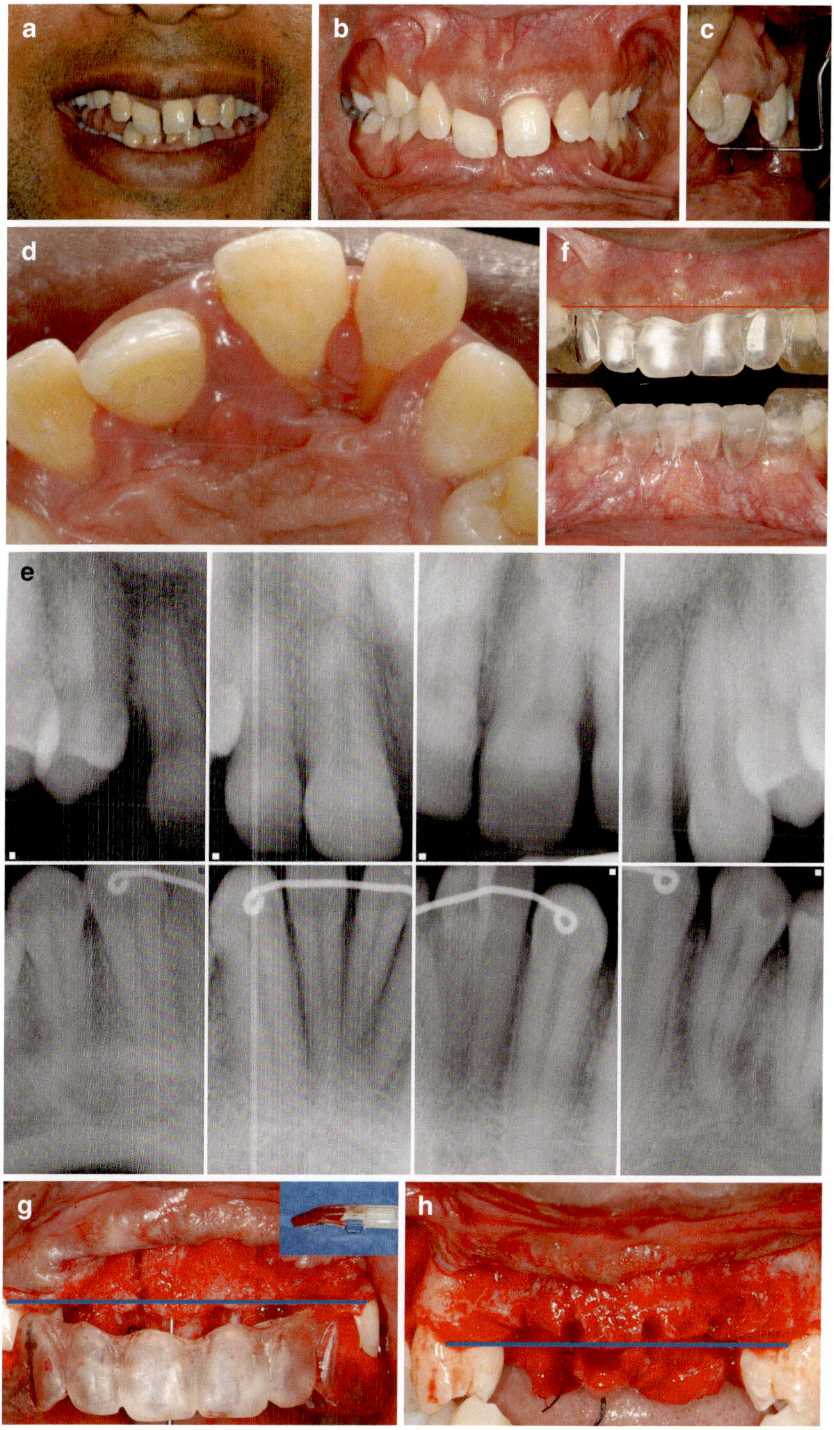
a
b
c
d
f
e
g
h

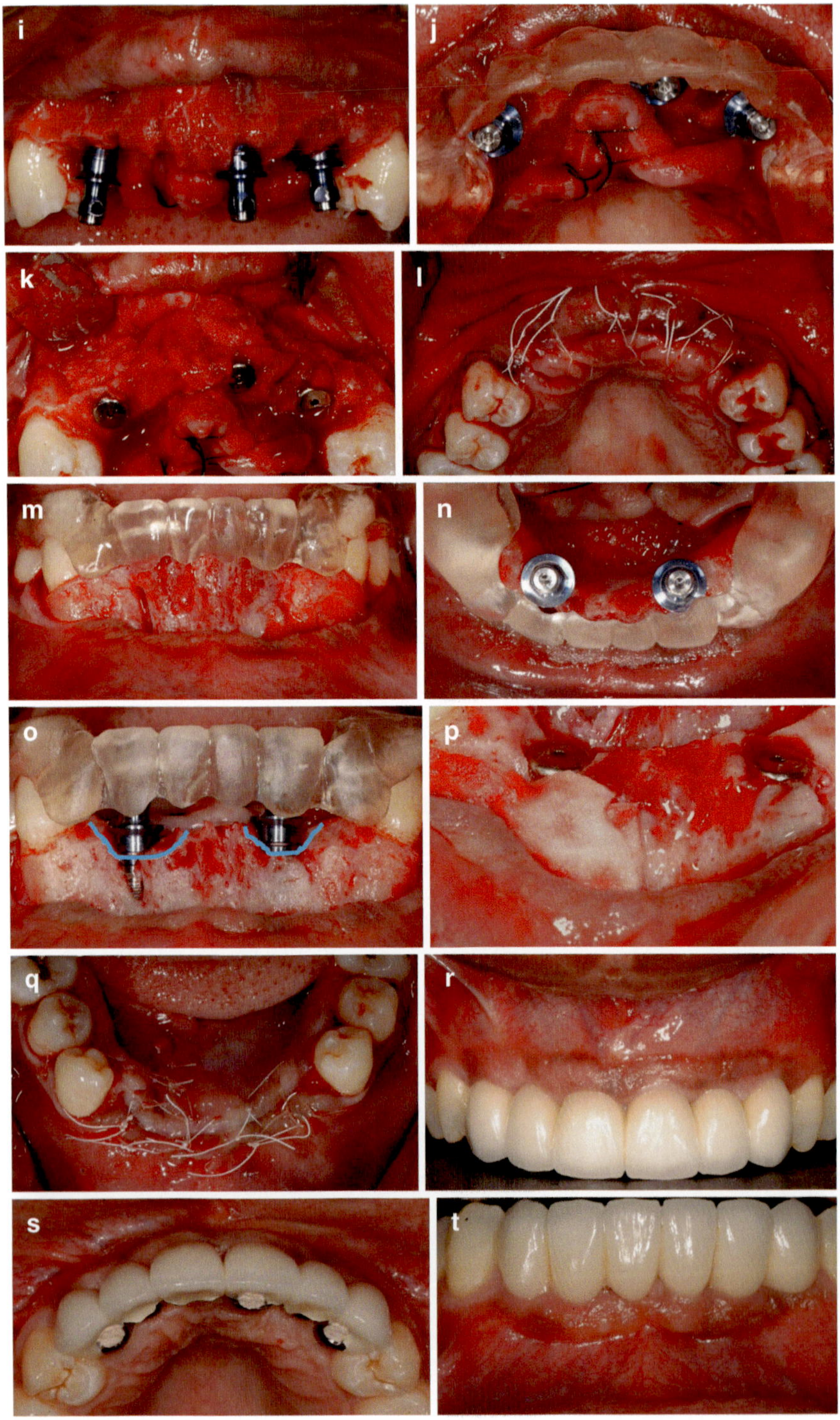

Fig. 9.4 (continued)

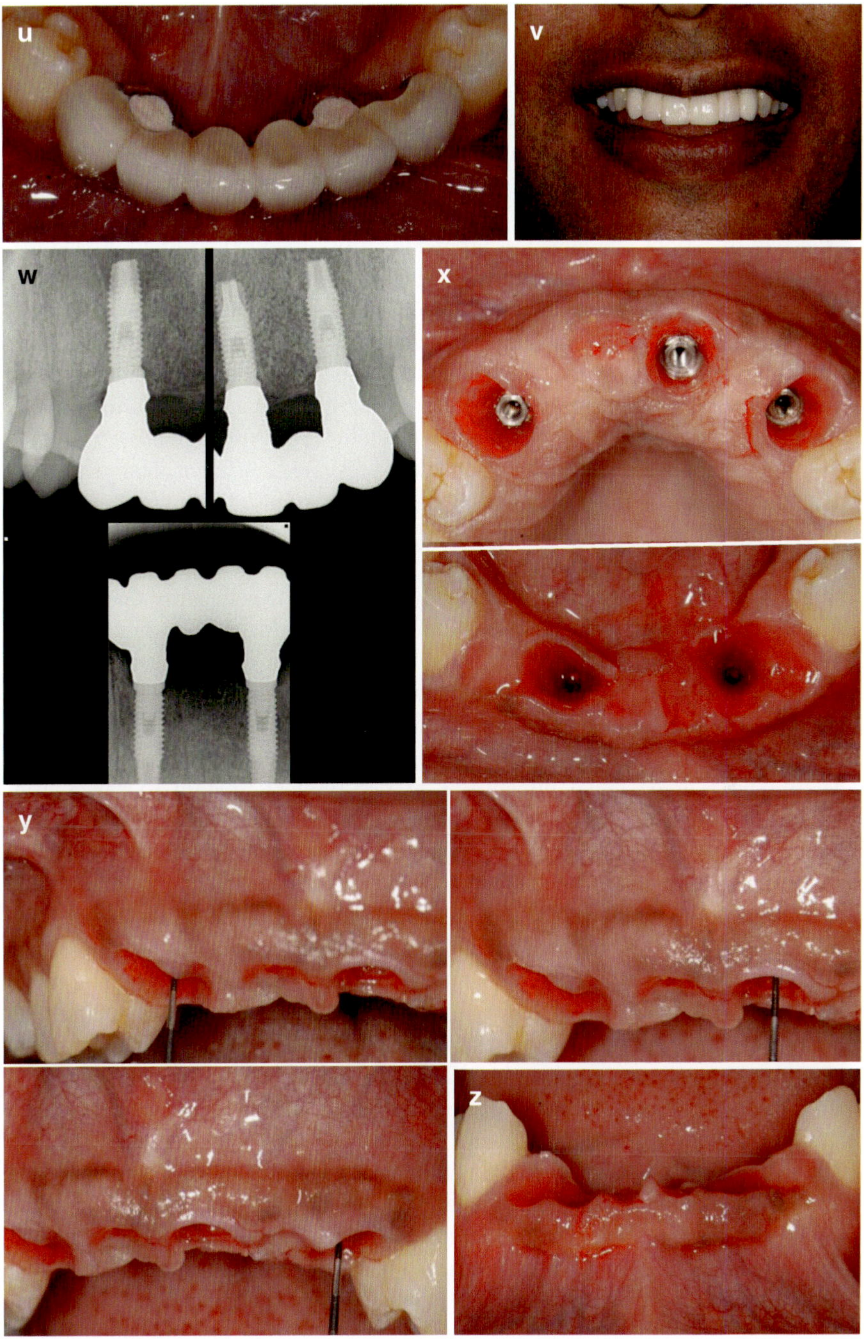

Fig. 9.4 (continued)

9.6 Emergence Profile

Post-extraction soft and hard tissue remodelling is a common observation after tooth extraction [34, 35]. Changes in ridge dimension present with varying degrees [36]. Many factors will influence the amount of ridge remodelling including soft and hard tissue phenotype, position of the root relative to the alveolar housing, prominence of the roots, remaining radicular bone thickness, presence of bony ledges and exostosis, presence of infections and bone loss around the roots, traumatic extractions and flap vs. flapless extraction [37]. Consensus is that thinner remaining facial bone, especially when beyond the apical basal bone, would have greater amount of bone remodelling leading to spontaneous soft tissue thickening in thin bone phenotype following tooth extraction. Occasionally, this thicker, soft tissue may mask bone deficiency, but nevertheless the spontaneous soft tissue thickening offers advantages for implant therapy and if needed bone augmentation procedures [38]. Although post-extraction, bone ridge remodelling cannot be completely prevented, different interventions to reduce the amount of ridge remodelling have been proposed [34]. Although these interventions can reduce the amount of dimensional changes [39], the clinical significance of these procedures in achieving a superior outcome in implant placement and aesthetic management is not well established [35, 40]. This is partly due to differences of healing process amongst individuals and tooth sites. Most studies in alveolar ridge preservation measure the outcome of the procedure comparing ridge dimensions at the time of extraction to ridge dimensions after socket healing. However, often edentulous ridge contours improve after the placement of restorative components that support the mucosa and correct ridge deficiency (Figs. 9.4r, t, x–z and 9.5a–c). The average facial dimensions of peri-implant mucosa (distance from restorative platform to gingival zenith) are slightly greater than the average dimension of the dento-gingival complex. While the buccal soft tissue contour will be primarily established by soft tissue thickness and transmucosal prosthetic support, the level of the interproximal papilla of the implant is related to the interproximal bone of the adjacent teeth and not the proximal bone level next to the implant (Figs. 9.1c, d and 9.2a). Greater peri-implant mucosal dimensions are present in the presence of a thick peri-implant biotype as compared to a thin biotype [41]. To provide running room for emergence profile, the position of the restorative platform of implant has to be 3–5 mm below the mucosal zenith [42–44].

The buccal contour of the ridge will be supported by the transmucosal prosthetic material/abutment providing soft tissue support. Considering the spontaneous soft tissue thickening post-extraction [38], in majority of cases, buccal contour of the soft tissue can be managed after spontaneous post-extraction healing without the need for any additional preservation/augmentation procedures.

Avila-Ortiz et al. [39] reported that additional guided bone regeneration (GBR) was required in 48.1% of unassisted socket healing sites and only in 11.5% of alveolar ridge preservation (ARP) sites treated with an allograft and a non-resorbable membrane. It could be argued that clinicians may consider performing augmentation procedures on the extra 37% of cases needing ridge augmentation rather than 100% of teeth needing extractions. Additional procedures increase surgical morbidity and fees. Also, use of grafting biomaterials delays socket bone healing [45, 46] and potential risk of soft tissue encapsulation and consequently soft tissue

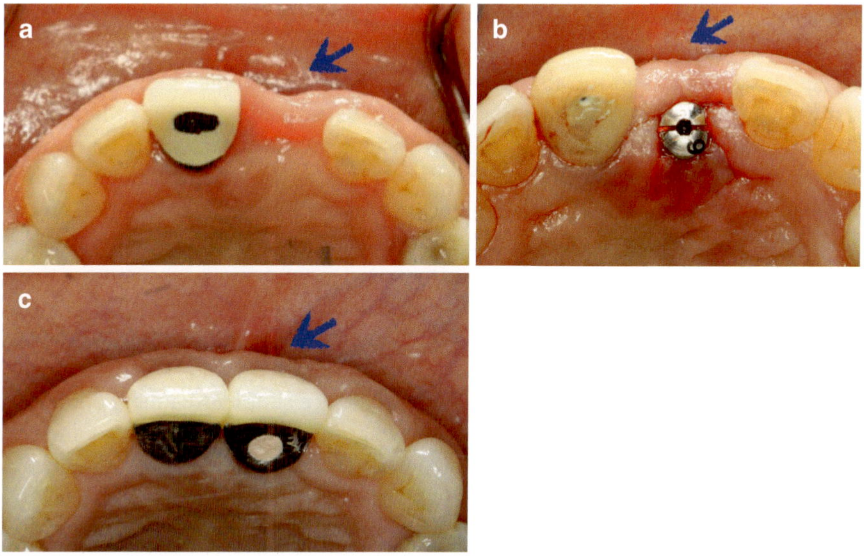

Fig. 9.5 Buccal soft tissue deficiency noted preoperatively at the site of maxillary left central incisor (**a**). At the time of uncovering, crestal incision was placed more palatal to the centre of the implant and the soft tissue was displaced to buccal correcting tissue concavity with transmucosal support of the healing abutment restoration profile. Improvement of soft tissue contour after placement of healing abutment (**b**) and restoration (**c**) supporting the buccal soft tissue without additional grafting

complications [47, 48]. Alternatively, clinicians may consider ridge preservation when site-specific or patient-specific factors may pose a higher risk for extensive bone remodelling post-extraction [49]. Considering available evidence, clinicians should weigh the risk/benefit and cost/benefit of biomaterials used for ridge preservation based on site-specific and patient-specific factors and avoid routine use of biomaterials for ridge preservation of every extraction socket.

9.7 Implant Site Development

Tooth loss can lead to significant loss of hard and soft tissue that can negatively influence the outcome of implant therapy. At times, alveolar ridge defects resulting from tooth extraction, trauma or periodontal disease often require surgical correction prior to prosthodontic reconstruction. Deficiency in hard and soft tissue can be manifested horizontally, vertically or in combination. Horizontal, vertical and combination (HVC) defect classification system is a useful tool to identify the type of needed augmentation (soft tissue, hard tissue or both), surgical techniques and predictability of outcome [50]. Correcting horizontal deficiencies is easier managed, and the outcome is more predictable. Vertical augmentation of soft and especially hard tissue is very challenging and with high potential of complications [51]. Performing multiple surgical augmentation procedures (considering the surgical trauma, treatment time, expenses) must be weighed carefully against alternatives of bony resection techniques and reconstruction with soft tissue analogues [52].

9.8 Vertical Bone Deficiency

Vertical loss of hard and soft tissues poses a challenge in implant dentistry. Loss of vertical height in the anterior maxilla will affect the aesthetic outcome of treatment. Loss of vertical height in posterior sextants poses anatomical challenges for implant therapy including proximity to the maxillary sinus floor and mandibular inferior alveolar nerve canal. Multiple surgical techniques for vertical augmentation procedures have been proposed with varying success such as GBR, onlay block grafting and distraction osteogenesis. Surgical techniques to compensate for loss of vertical heights are very challenging and unpredictable and can have multiple surgical interventions, increased treatment time and cost, difficulty in providing interim prostheses and treatment morbidity [51]. Compensating lost hard and soft tissues with either fixed or removable prosthetic replicas provides a simpler treatment option for managing vertical hard and soft tissue loss. Other treatment strategies may include use of short implants [53–55] or extra-alveolar implant devices such as zygomatic, pterygoid and transnasal implants [56–58]. However, these surgical approaches may pose elevated surgical risk, long-term management of peri-implant tissue health and post-surgical morbidity. The long-term effectiveness of these surgical approaches needs to be substantiated with further studies [59–62].

9.9 Horizontal Bone Deficiency

Horizontal loss of soft and hard tissues is more easily managed with various surgical techniques such as block grafts, GBR, ridge expansion/split and use of narrow-diameter implants [51, 63–65]. Most ridge deficiencies are a combination of vertical and horizontal loss where the predominant deficiency is in the horizontal dimension (Fig. 9.6b). Although the surgical techniques can more predictably correct horizontal deficiencies, a thorough assessment of the ridge deficiency relative to anticipated prosthetic plan is

Fig. 9.6 Maxillary right central incisor is planned for implant placement for cantilever FPD replacing maxillary right central and lateral incisors. Lateral incisor with previous RCT, post and core and weak tooth structure with poor restorative prognosis. Restorative plan is for implant placement at the site of right central incisor and replace # right central and lateral incisors with cantilever implant-supported FPD (**a**). Diagnostic wax-up and radiographic/surgical guide fabrication for CBCT evaluation reveal thin buccal-lingual dimension (**b**). Although thicker bone is observed at the apical portion of the site, resection of crestal bone to achieve thickness will create unfavourable biomechanical forces and create height limitation due to proximity to nasal floor. Post-operative CBCT after block graft harvested from ramus and external oblique ridge showing buccal-lingual bone gain (**c**). Clinical appearance of block graft healing after 4 months (**d**, **e**). Crestal reduction to provide 3–4 mm transmucosal space for restorative contouring (**f**, **g**). Implant placement in prosthetically driven screw-retained position with 4 mm of restorative space for transmucosal transition to proposed gingival zenith of the right central incisor (**h**, **i**). Implant healing and confirmation of integration 3 months after placement (**j**), maxillary right lateral incisor with poor restorative prognosis, removal of right lateral incisor and soft tissue graft to maintain ridge thickness and delivery of implant cantilever implant-supported provisional restoration (**k**, **l**). Definitive implant-supported cantilever FPD restoration 10 years post-loading and radiographic imaging showing stability of peri-implant hard and soft tissues (**m**–**o**). (Restorative dentistry courtesy of Dr. Winston Chee)

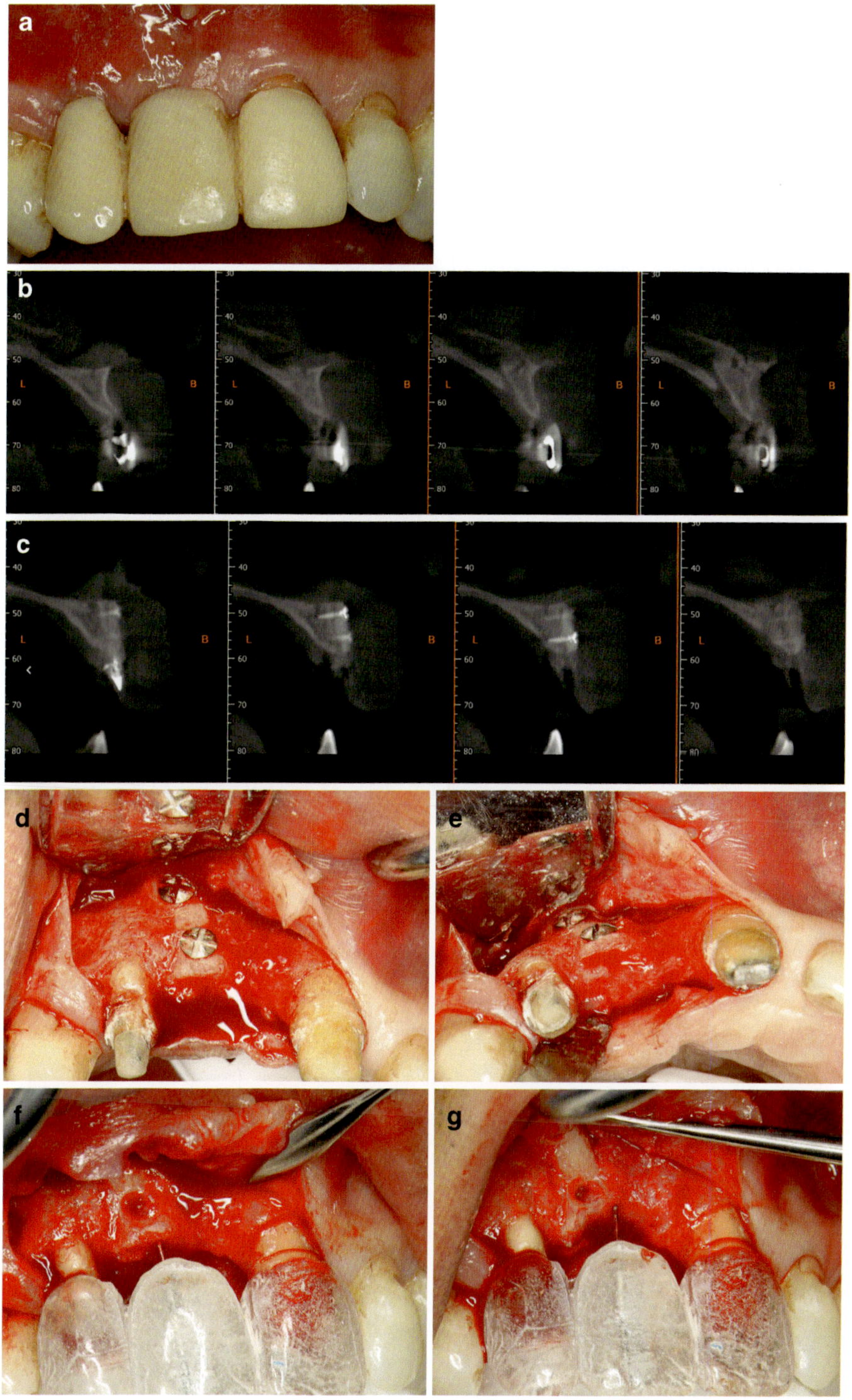

(continued)

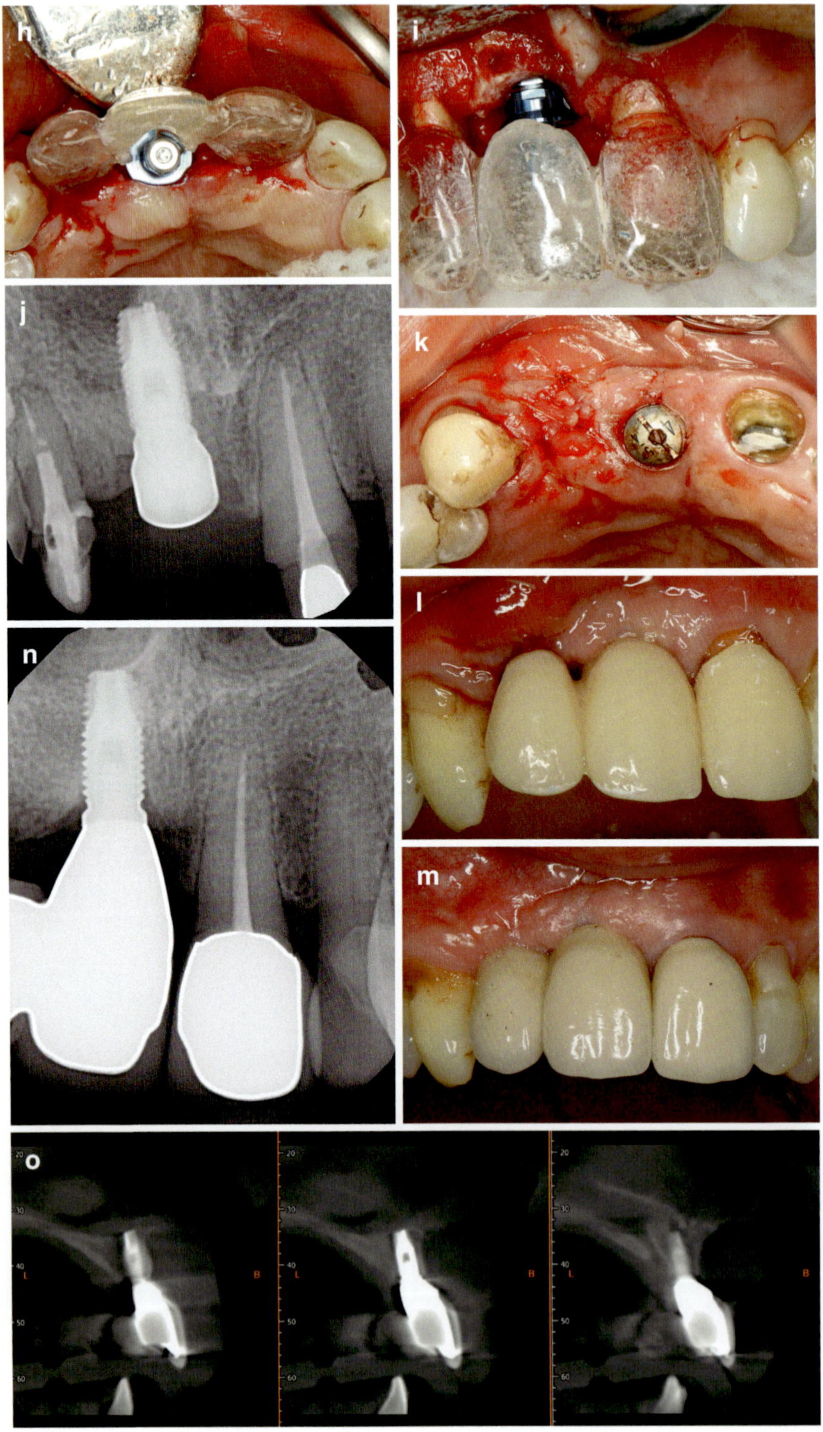

Fig. 9.6 (continued)

critical. In many cases, although grafting procedures can improve the horizontal deficiency, there still may be a need to reduce vertical height when there is a lack of restorative space. In other circumstances, there is vertical deficiency present regardless of horizontal deficiency. In these circumstances, the decision to correct horizontal deficiency should be carefully weighed versus ridge reduction for implant placement to be in thicker bone in the apical area. If there is a plan to use pink prosthetics, a resective solution to achieve adequate thickness is often a better solution than using bone augmentation. However, there are limitations to resection; large vertical resections can create more biomechanical prosthetic problems such as cantilever forces or bulk of restorative material. Additionally, anatomical limitations such as location of infra-alveolar canal, floor of the nose or jaw concavities may limit resection and drive the decision to augmentation rather than resection (Fig. 9.6c–e).

9.10 Maxillary Sinus Elevation

Proximity of sinus floor to implant site will require elevation of sinus floor to accommodate space for implant placement. Sinus elevation can be performed through vertical or lateral approaches. The decision of vertical or lateral approach to sinus elevation is dependent on variables such as remaining crestal bone, anatomy of the sinus wall such as slopes, thickness of the bony walls, intra-antral anatomy such as septum or medial-apical angle or clinician's technical skills [66, 67]. Remaining crestal residual bone is the determining factor for the need and techniques of sinus elevation. Residual bone is calculated from the planned position of the restorative platform of the implant rather than crest of the bone. Depending on the emergence profile, crestal reduction or sub-crestal placement may be indicated. In general, vertical sinus elevation is more indicated when 2–3 mm of elevation is intended. When more than 3 mm of sinus elevation is intended, a lateral approach to sinus elevation may be more prudent. When less than 3 mm of residual bone is available, a staged approach for implant placement with bone healing time of 6–9 months may be more prudent. When 3–5 mm or more of residual bone height is available, simultaneous implant placement with sinus lift and bone grafting may be considered [68–70] (Table 9.1). Risk factors for

Table 9.1 Suggestion for sinus augmentation for implant placement in posterior maxilla

Residual bone	9 mm and more	5–8 mm	3–4 mm	Less than 3 mm
Sinus augmentation technique	No sinus elevation, (consider 8 mm length implants)	Vertical approach	Lateral approach with simultaneous implant placement	Lateral approach with delayed implant placement
Healing time	12 weeks	12–16 weeks	6 months for loading	6 months for sinus augmentation and 12–16 weeks for implant placement

Residual bone is calculated from planned position of the restorative platform of the implant rather than crest of the bone. Depending on emergence profile crestal reduction or sub crestal placement may be indicated for emergence profile sinus elevation should be taken into considerations, such as history of chronic sinusitis, pathological conditions of the sinus, lack of ostium patency and sinus anatomy. Alternatives to sinus elevation such as use of short implants, tuberosity or pterygoid placement, fixed partial denture (FPD) restorations and no treatment should be considered when sinus elevation poses significant surgical risk [71, 72].

9.11 Posterior Mandible

The posterior mandible presents with anatomical features that can influence surgical placement of dental implants. One such limitation is the location of the inferior alveolar canal and mental foramen within the body of the mandible. There is individual variability in the path and apical-coronal location of the canal and mental foramen. Post-extraction bone remodelling and vertical loss of alveolar bone in molar and premolar regions of the mandible can lead to proximity of implant sites to inferior alveolar canal causing difficulty for implant placement. With the mental foramen, limiting depth and length of planned implants is similarly a hindrance. It is important to visualize these anatomical structures with radiographic examinations including peri-apical and panoramic and ideally with cone beam computed tomography (CBCT) to ensure adequate bone height for implant placement and to prevent nerve damage and neurosensory complications. This often limits implant placement to short implants [55, 73, 74]. Alternative options are the nerve transposition procedure, which has a high morbidity and rate of nerve damage, or to consider distal cantilevering of the prosthesis off implants placed mesial to the foramina [75, 76].

9.12 Contour Augmentation

Localized ridge defects may be augmented at the time of implant placement to improve emergence profiles and/or to increase bone thickness around implants. Use of both soft and hard tissue augmentation techniques has been advocated for contour augmentation. The main goal of contour augmentation is not to add supporting bone for osseointegration but mostly to increase hard and/or soft tissue thickness around the implants (Fig. 9.13j, l, m). These defects tend to be concavity defects in apical-coronal, mesial distal or a combination of both. They tend to be self-containing and very amenable to particulate grafting with autogenous or biomaterial sources [77–81].

Although these procedures can improve aesthetics and ridge contour outcome, the clinician must weigh the risk/benefit and cost/benefit factors of different techniques and biomaterials. Excessive overbulking of the ridge may have negative consequences such as increased surgical trauma, reduction of vestibular depth and mucogingival deficiencies. Also, when slow-resorbing materials are used for space maintenance properties, there is a higher chance of biomaterial encapsulation, soft tissue inflammation and soft tissue granulation and inflammation [47, 48, 82, 83].

Increase of soft tissue thickness through soft tissue augmentation procedures seems to provide a stable outcome when the goal is contour augmentation. However, in the presence of bony dehiscence around implant, use of bone grafting materials (autogenous and/or non-autogenous) might be more prudent (Fig. 9.4i, k, o, p).

9.13 Restorative and Surgical Space

Space management for rehabilitation with dental implant prosthesis is one of the most important aspects of treatment planning. Occlusal wear and/or over-eruption of teeth can create occlusal interferences and reduce the inter-occlusal space required for implant-supported restorations.

In many cases, individuals experiencing advanced periodontitis, characterized by significant attachment loss and posterior teeth loss, display noticeable drifting of posterior teeth and flaring of anterior teeth, indicative of pathological teeth migration. This pathological migration contributes to an unstable occlusal scheme, ultimately resulting in the loss of vertical dimension due to insufficient posterior support. Consequently, this scenario frequently leads to a shortage of restorative space for reconstructive therapy.

The lack of adequate restorative space is a significant factor contributing to biomechanical, mechanical as well as aesthetic failure of implant restorations. Therefore, it is crucial to identify patients' parafunctional habits leading to restorative space issues, as that can significantly impact the outcome and longevity of planned reconstructions, choice of restorative materials, prosthetic design and biomechanical complications.

A comprehensive examination should assess not only the periodontal support of the remaining and opposing dentition but also the occlusal scheme, including guidance in lateral and protrusive movements, vertical and horizontal overlap and available restorative space. A detailed risk/benefit and cost/benefit analysis is important to identify different modalities of treatment to achieve the required restorative space, which may include orthodontic intrusion, tooth reduction, increase of vertical dimension, extraction/resection or a combination of these different modalities.

9.14 Restorative Considerations of Adjacent Teeth

Implant surgeons should have a good understanding of restorative treatment needs of teeth adjacent to the implant site. Teeth with guarded to poor prognosis should be evaluated carefully for their strategic value and how they may complicate future treatment next to implant sites. Compromised teeth with a poor prognosis are often used during initial phases to support a fixed interim prosthesis that can prevent loading when augmentation procedures are indicated, while implant-site healing progresses and importantly allows patients to transition from a tooth- to implant-supported reconstruction.

When adjacent teeth are planned to be maintained, special considerations should be made to the location of the gingival zenith of the adjacent teeth. If occlusal wear or short clinical crowns are present, the surgeon must take note of the future location of those gingival zeniths when deciding the depth of implant placement. The restorative platform of implant must be deep enough to accommodate the apical relocation of the gingival level of adjacent teeth. If surgical crown lengthening is indicated both with and without restoration, it would be best to perform the surgery prior to implant placement (Fig. 9.7a, c, f, g).

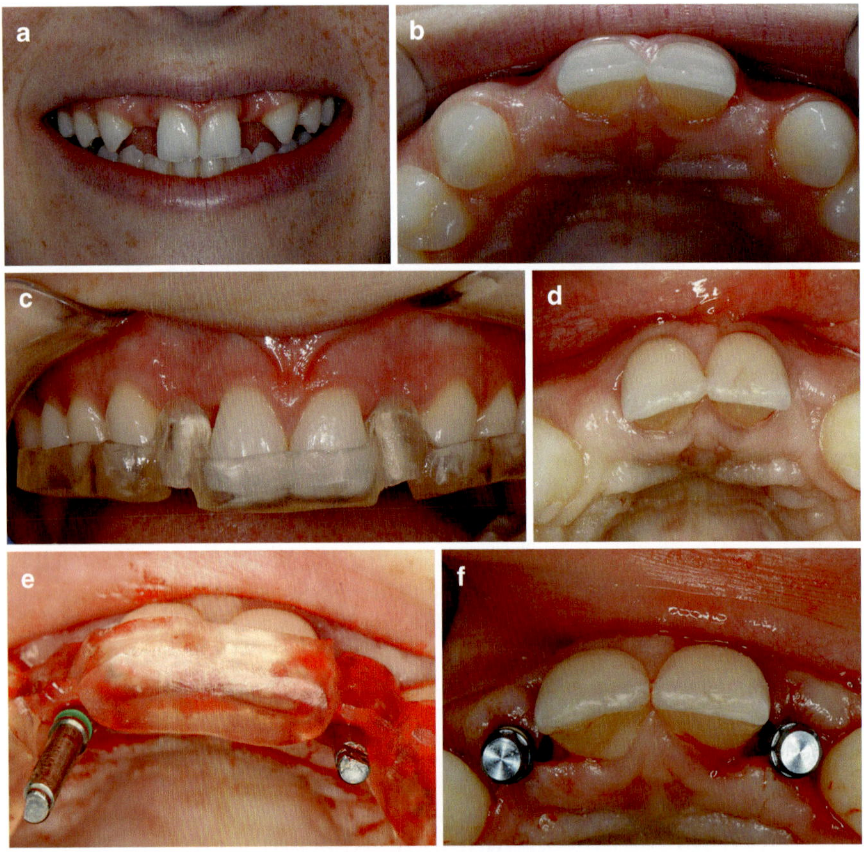

Fig. 9.7 Patient reports with congenitally missing lateral incisors and altered passive eruption post-orthodontic treatment for teeth realignment and to provide restorative space for lateral incisors. Horizontal ridge deficiency present at the site of # 7 and 10 requires hard and soft tissue ridge augmentation for implant therapy. Patient has a restorative treatment plan for veneer restoration to manage aesthetics of maxillary anterior teeth (**a**, **b**). Following diagnostic wax-up, hard and soft tissue ridge augmentation for lateral incisors was performed. Aesthetic crown lengthening was performed for anatomical tooth exposure to achieve favourable height-to-width ratio of maxillary anterior teeth (**c**, **d**). Implants were placed in screw-retained position according to diagnostic wax-up and surgical guide with 4–5 mm submucosal depth for restorative emergence profile (**e**, **f**, **h**). Depth of the implant is corresponding to gingival zenith of the future restoration according to diagnostic wax-up and surgical guide (**j**). Facial and smile views upon initial delivery underscoring the restorative and harmony of soft tissue zenith on maxillary anterior teeth. Five-year follow-up shows health and stability of peri-implant hard and soft tissues (**k**–**m**). (Restorative treatment courtesy of Dr. George Cho)

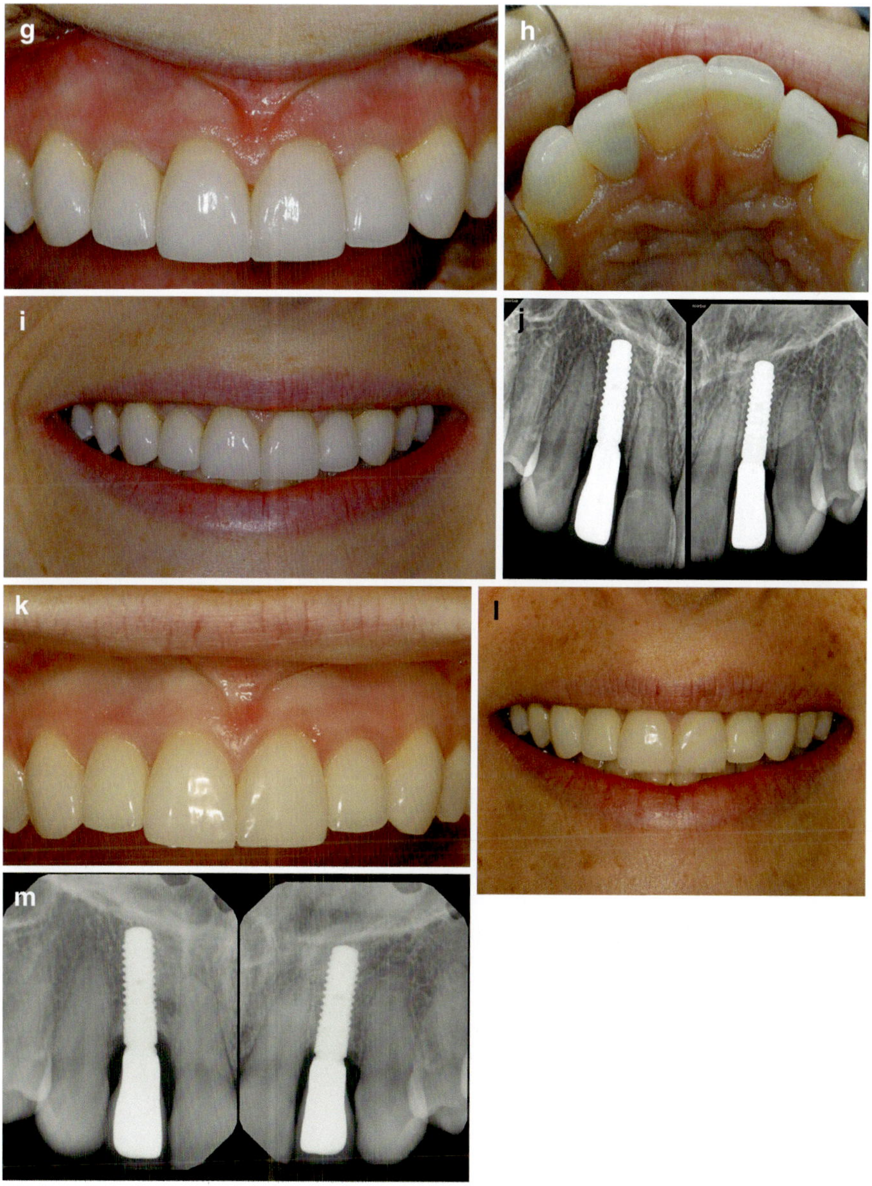

Fig. 9.7 Continued

9.15 Orthodontic Consideration for Implant-Site Development

Orthodontic therapy can improve the outcome of implant therapy by providing space distribution for restorations, creating space between roots for implant placement, soft and hard tissue augmentation for implant sites and gingival/mucosal alignment.

Orthodontic eruption of teeth planned for extraction and replacement can provide soft and hard tissue height to correct soft and hard tissue deficiencies prior to implant therapy [84, 85] (Fig. 9.8a–g). Up-righting of tilted teeth with orthodontic

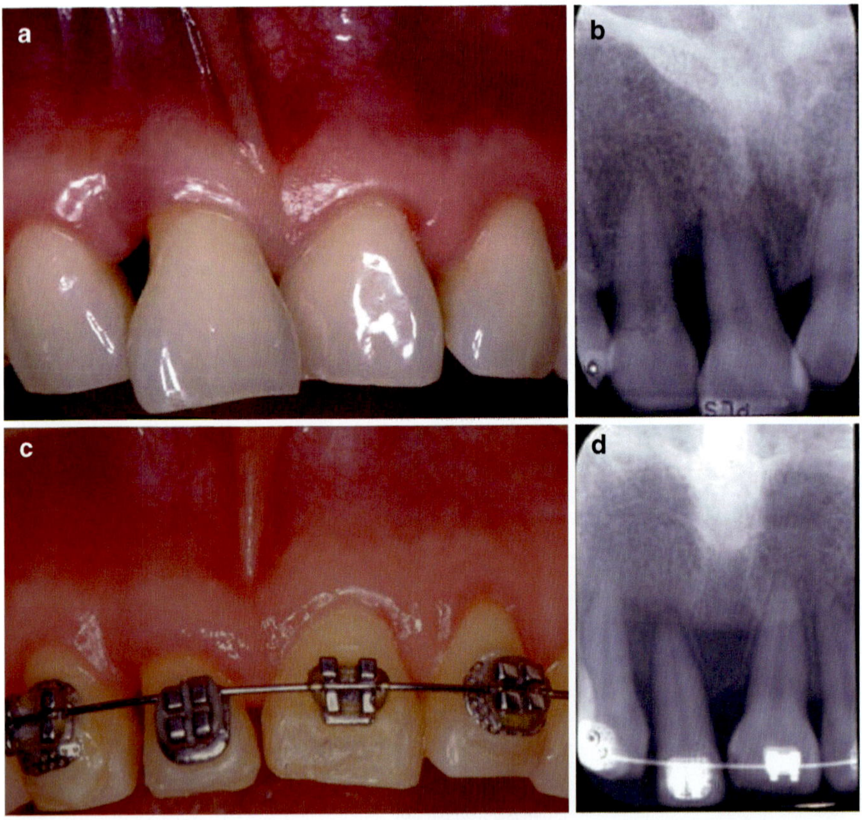

Fig. 9.8 Patient presents with soft and hard tissue deficiency on the distal area of maxillary right central incisor subsequent to advanced periodontitis and periodontal therapy. Patient presents with aesthetic concerns seeking to improve maxillary anterior aesthetic. Central incisors also present with teeth mispositioning rotation, occlusal wear and midline discrepancy (**a**, **b**). Orthodontic therapy for extrusion of maxillary right central incisor and realigning of central incisors. Occlusal reduction of maxillary right central incisor to provide room for extrusion, and coronal movement of apex and correction of distal soft tissue and hard tissue bony defect is evident (**c**, **d**). Definitive implant-supported restoration of right and labial veneer of left central incisor restorations to correct wear and midline (**e**, **f**) with radiographic follow-up to evaluate stability of crestal bone 10 years post-treatment (**g**). (Restorative treatment courtesy of Dr. Nick Nguyen)

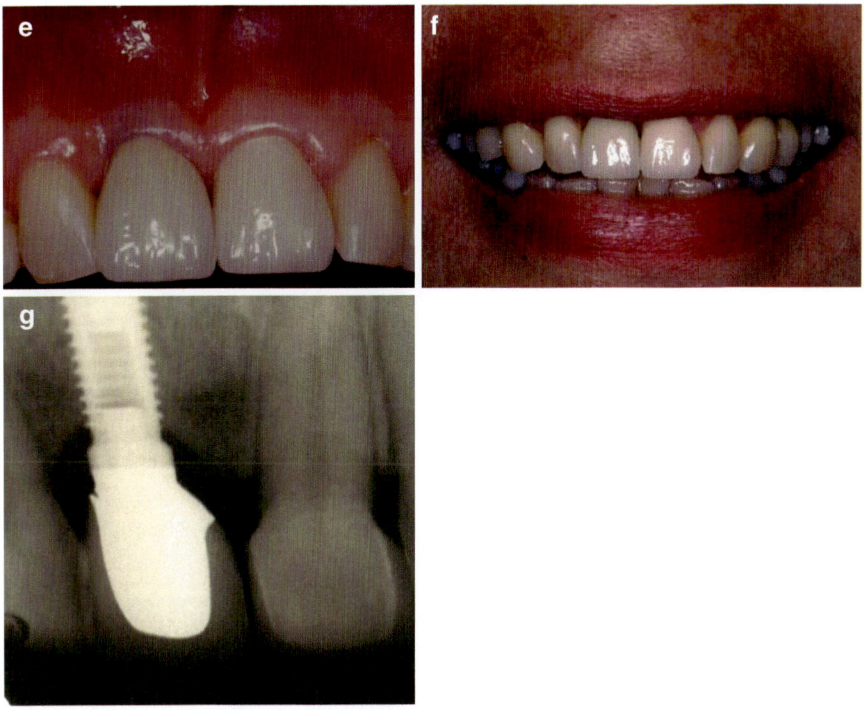

Fig. 9.8 (continued)

therapy can make implant placement and restorative space management feasible (Fig. 9.9a–g). Space distribution will provide the correct mesial-distal space for restorations, and alignment of the roots will provide needed space for implant placement (Fig. 9.10a–j). In most cases, the placement of implant is typically postponed until the completion of orthodontic tooth movement. However, there are instances where implants can be strategically positioned by adapting their placement to align with the definitive positions of teeth outlined with diagnostic teeth set-up. In such cases, the implants can serve as an anchorage for tooth movement. This approach necessitates a comprehensive evaluation and meticulous planning of space distribution, fostering collaboration amongst restorative, orthodontic, periodontic and implant surgical disciplines [86].

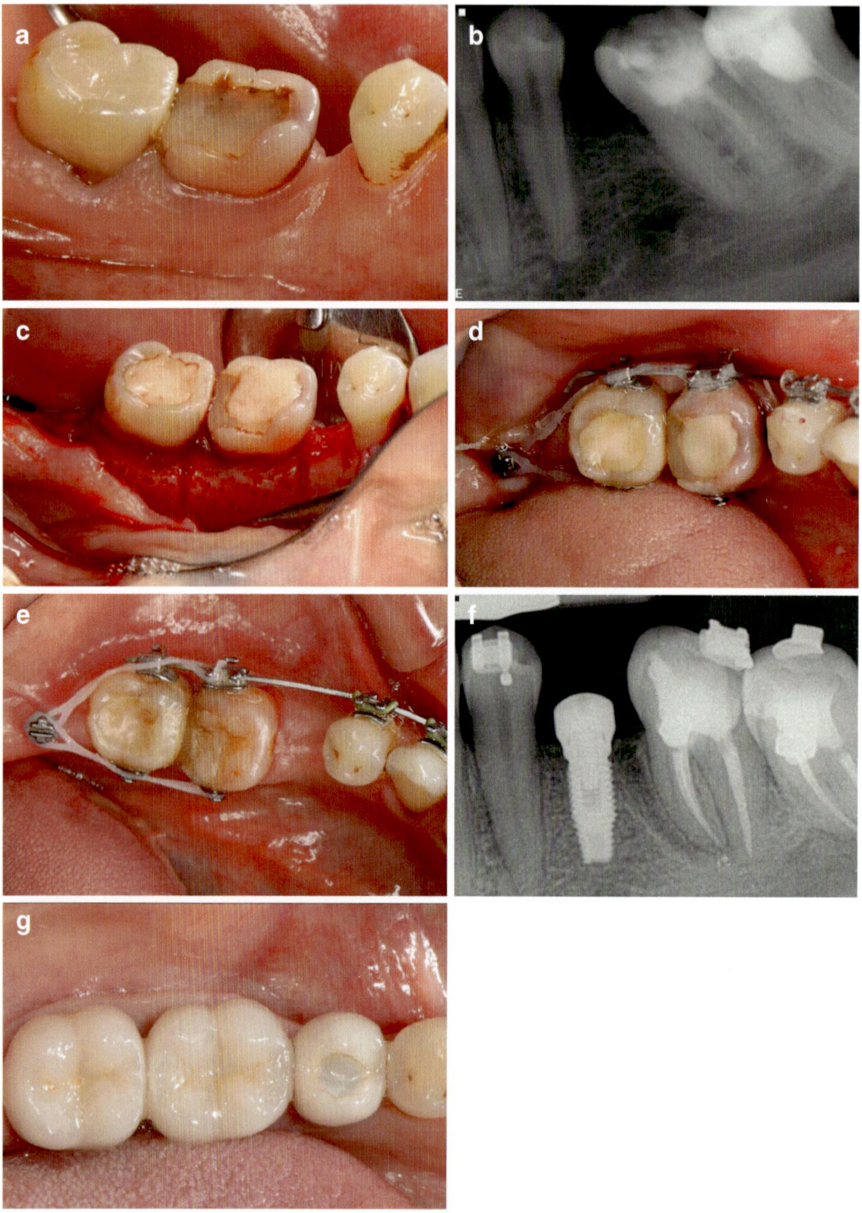

Fig. 9.9 Mandibular left second premolar with limited restorative space for implant-supported restoration (**a**, **b**). Molar up-righting of mandibular left first and second molar to accommodate space for implant-supported prosthesis. Periodontally accelerated osteogenic orthodontic (PAOO) treatment and temporary anchorage device (TAD) were employed to assist with orthodontic treatment (**c**–**e**). 4 months after tooth movement, sufficient space was available for implant placement and implant-supported restoration (**f**, **g**). (Orthodontic and surgical treatment in collaboration with Dr. Maria Galvan, restorative treatment courtesy of Dr. Cheryl Park)

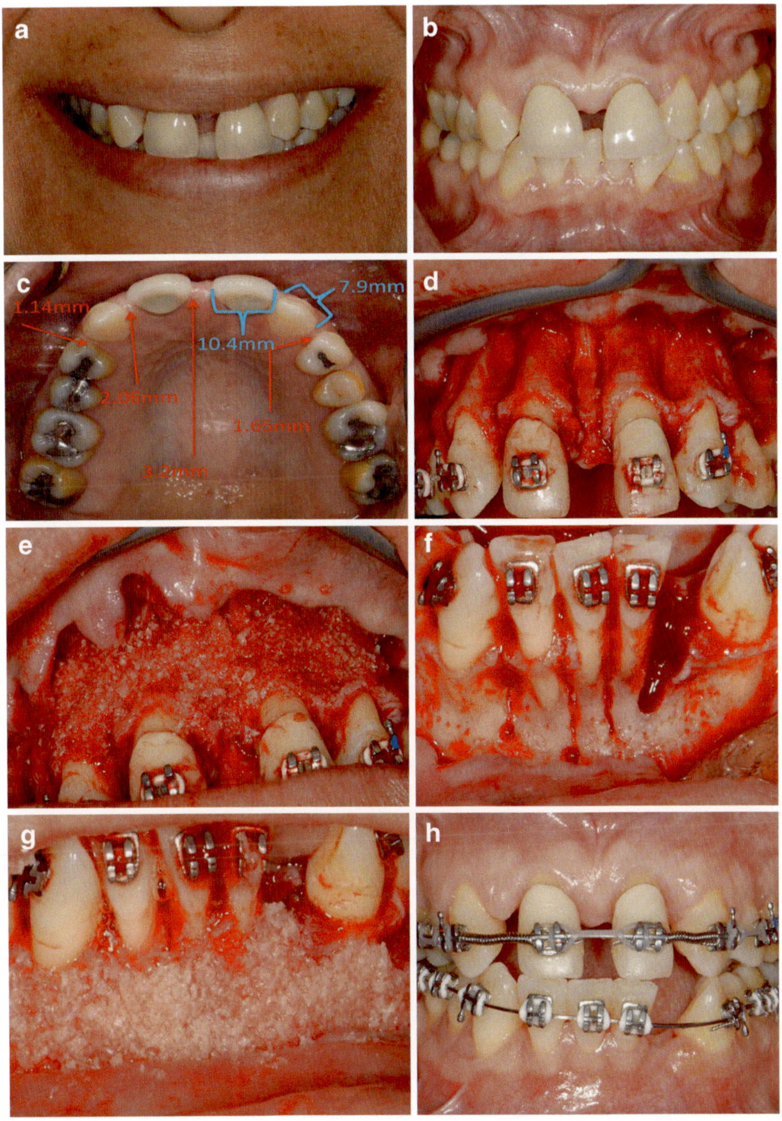

Fig. 9.10 Patient presents with concerns about maxillary anterior aesthetic and interproximal spacing. Patient presents with missing lateral incisors, over-contoured restoration of maxillary incisors and crowding of mandibular anterior teeth. Orthodontic treatment was planned for space distribution and to align teeth with a favourable restorative position providing space for replacement of lateral incisors with implant-supported restoration (**a**–**c**). PAOO to facilitate orthodontic movement and to thicken the phenotype for orthodontic tooth movement. Corticectomy cuts with half round bur and piezoelectric surgery. Autogenous bone particles harvested from exostosis and external oblique ridge with bone scraper mixed with allograft to increase volume to increase bone thickness (**d**–**g**). Orthodontic treatment progresses in 6–9 months (**h**, **i**). Treatment completed with full-coverage restoration of central incisors, implant-supported restoration of lateral incisors and orthodontic realignment of mandibular anterior. (Surgery in collaboration with Dr. Yun Wang, orthodontic treatment courtesy Dr. Ryan Hungate, restorative treatment courtesy of Dr. Sangho Byun)

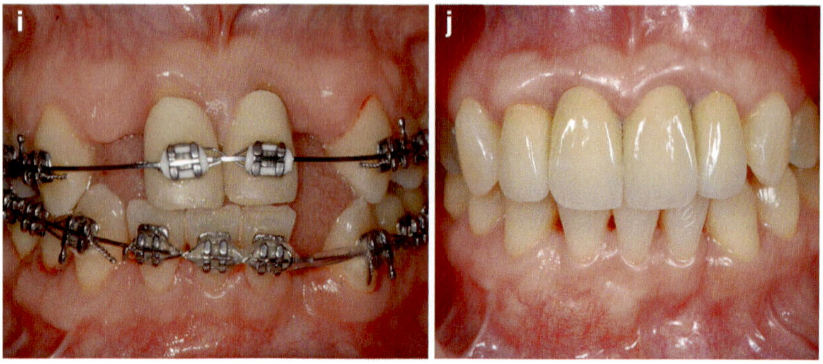

Fig. 9.10 (continued)

9.16 Radiographic Examination

Radiographic evaluation is an integral part of implant therapy planning. Traditional periapical and interproximal radiographs will provide information about bone level, mesio-distal angulation of adjacent teeth and interdental space of implant site, vertical height of the remaining bone and possible endodontic pathologies. Panoramic radiographs will provide additional information about anatomic structures near implant sites with an overall view of the dentition. Clinicians need to be cognizant of the distortions associated with peri-apical and panoramic radiograph when evaluating information presented with two-dimensional radiographs. Cone beam computerized tomography provides much more detailed and life-size information about the anatomy of the site of interest. As the use of CBCT technology becomes more commonplace, it is important to utilize imaging with consideration of risk/benefit and cost/benefit. Indiscriminate use of CBCT is not prudent as it presents with higher level of radiation to the patient. This can lead to accumulative dose of radiation when a person presents with multiple treatment needs. Sequencing of treatment and imaging is an important consideration to reduce the amount of radiation exposure. Decisions for different radiographic imaging should be made after a thorough clinical assessment of the site; at times, when all anatomical and risk factors can be accounted for, a simple periapical radiograph may be adequate for placement of implants. However, the most accurate information for implant planning can be obtained through CBCT imaging; this information is critical for risk assessment of implant therapy. These include assessment of remaining alveolar bone height and width, location of inferior alveolar nerve canal and mental foramen, residual crestal bone and sinus anatomy, patency of sinus ostium, presence of bony concavities or deficiencies of the implant site, location of the roots relative to basal bone prior to extraction and assessment of bone quality/density [87–89]. Contemporary CBCT images will provide a panoramic view of the arches, which has a lot more accuracy together with the advantages of three-dimensional assessment. The amount of radiation

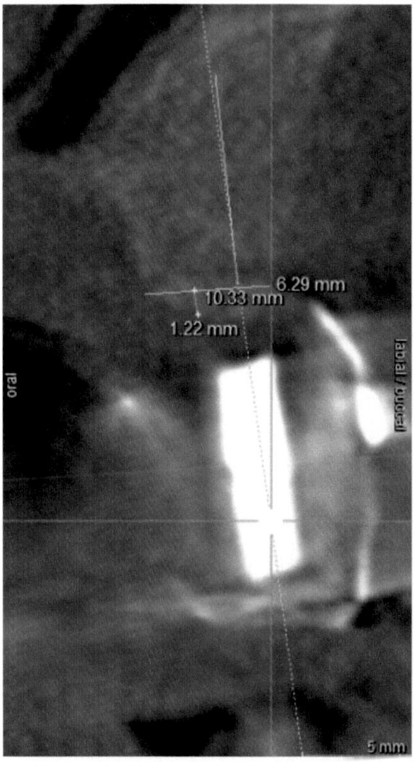

Fig. 9.11 CBCT with resection guide. Surgical guide with radiographic marker indication apical extension of the guide and the need for alveolar resection to provide restorative space for prosthesis

exposure of a full-mouth CBCT is about 3–6 times higher than digital panoramic radiograph [90]. Ideally, CBCT is captured after diagnostic wax-up and restorative planning; once the desired locations of implants have been determined, a radiographic guide is fabricated with radiographic markers indicating contours of desired restoration and reference of a needed resection to accommodate restorative treatment (Fig. 9.11). However, considering the amount of additional information obtained from CBCT, use of a two-dimensional panoramic radiograph may not be as useful as a diagnostic radiograph.

9.17 Surgical Planning for Implant Placement

CBCT radiography captured with radiographic guides is utilized to formulate the surgical plan and the need for any needed modifications to implant sites. Mesial-distal, buccal-lingual and apical-coronal position of the implant can be evaluated and planned. Surgical planning can be implemented using conventional analogue or guided surgery protocols. Subsequently, radiographic guides will be converted to surgical guides transferring the restorative and surgical planning information to execute the surgical plan (Fig. 9.7c, e). Guided surgery protocols can help to expedite predetermined osteotomy with good accuracy, yet they can present challenges and shortcomings. To manage these shortcomings, clinician's competency in performing analogue surgery is essential. Some of these limitations to use guided surgery systems include limited inter-occlusal space, need for surgical modification of implant site, overheating during osteotomy and inaccuracy in implant position due to inaccuracy in data capture or manufacturing of the guides [91].

Mesial-distal, buccal-lingual and apical-coronal position of the implant will have an impact on restorative treatment and long-term outcome of implant therapy. Precise placement of the implant in all three dimensions will not only provide easier and predictable restorative treatment but also reduces the long-term biological and mechanical complication of implant therapy [92–98]. The most common mistake in surgical placement of implants seems to be the depth and buccal-lingual trajectory of the implant. Mistakes in both planes will confound the problem and restorative solution to the problem (Fig. 9.12a–d). Most proper surgical placement when screw-retained restorations are planned for calls for depths of 3–5 mm in apical-coronal dimension and buccal-lingual trajectory to cingulum of anterior teeth and central groove of posterior teeth aiming the functional cusps of the opposing dentition (Figs. 9.4s, 9.7h and 9.9g). Deviation from these guidelines may require the use of custom abutments and cement-retained restorations, angled abutments and angulated screw channels. Poorly placed implants may require removal and replacement with corrected restorative trajectory. All these solutions can complicate and compromise treatment outcomes in the long term. Therefore, any anticipated deviation from proper restorative position should be anticipated, and different alternatives for treatment should be discussed with the restorative provider and patient to reduce complications in patient management.

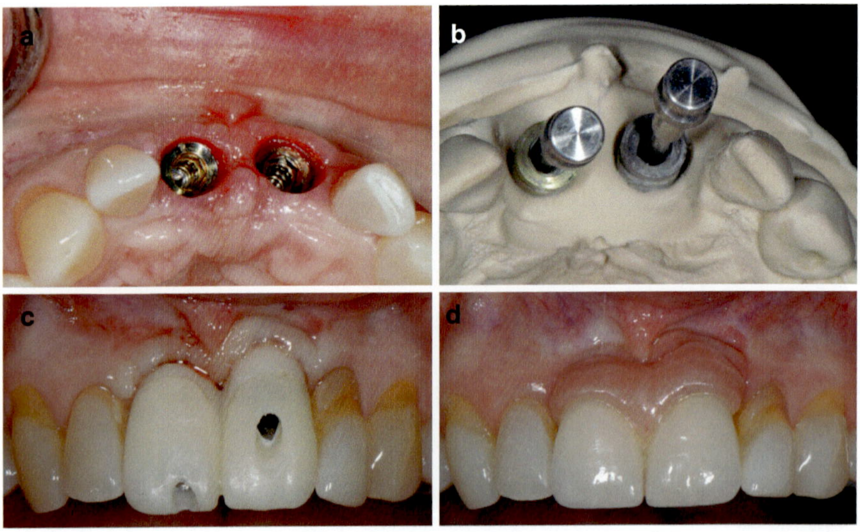

Fig. 9.12 Central incisor implants were placed too far coronal and too far facial creating a difficult transmucosal transition room. Prosthetic pink was used to mask deficiencies in soft tissue. Patient social lip line does not display a full contour of restorations. (Courtesy of Dr. Winston Chee)

9.18 Implant-Site Osteotomy and Modification for Implant Placement

Different implant systems have different protocols for osteotomy preparation for implant placement. In general, the final diameter of the osteotomy is smaller than implant diameter to provide implant stability. Bone quality can influence surgical protocol for implant osteotomy. Classification by Lekholm and Zarb for quantity and quality is helpful to decide for surgical modifications of the osteotomy site that can be utilized by tactile sensation of the clinicians during osteotomy site preparation [99, 100]. In type 1 bone, almost the entire site is composed of homogenous compact bone; this calls for wider osteotomy (final osteotomy to be less than 1 mm different from implant diameter) with full counter sink and use of bone tap to reduce insertion torque. In type 2 bone, a thick layer of compact bone surrounds a core of dense trabecular bone; this type of bone calls for countersink and wider osteotomy (final osteotomy to be less than 1 mm different from implant diameter); bone tap may not be indicated for self-tap implants. In type 3 bone, a thin layer of cortical bone surrounds a core of relatively dense trabecular bone of favourable strengths. This type of bone calls for minimal countersink with smaller diameter of osteotomy (with final osteotomy 1 mm or more, smaller than final diameter of implant). In type 4 bone, a thin layer of cortical bone surrounds a core of low-density trabecular bone. When placing implants in type 4 bone, osteotomy modification techniques may be considered to improve primary stability. This may include osseo-densification techniques using burs or osteotome [101, 102], implant site under preparation (final osteotomy to be more than 1 mm smaller than the diameter of the implant) and more engaging implant thread designs [103, 104]. To achieve primary stability in type 4 bone, minimal or no countersink should be considered. Excessive vibration during osteotomy, changes in the path of osteotomy and lack of drill stability during sequential widening of the osteotomy can lead to widened osteotomy and lack of primary stability, especially in softer type 3 and 4 bones.

9.19 Crestal Bone Modification

Post-extraction remodelling of bone will often lead to uneven crestal bone that may need flattening for implant placement. Removal of thin crestal portion of the residual bone at the implant site will help to provide more soft tissue depth providing a more favourable transmucosal running room for implant-supported prosthesis. Flattening of the bone will also allow to level off lingual/buccal slope of the bone at the extraction site providing thicker apical bone to surround the implant that can help with the stability of the crestal bone [27, 105] (Figs. 9.13 and 9.14). Crestal bone modification also provides the adequate implant depth placement for transmucosal transition from implant diameter to tooth diameter, especially on posterior teeth, and provides adequate soft tissue support with transmucosal restorative components (Figs. 9.1c, 9.2, 9.4r, t, x–z, 9.13).

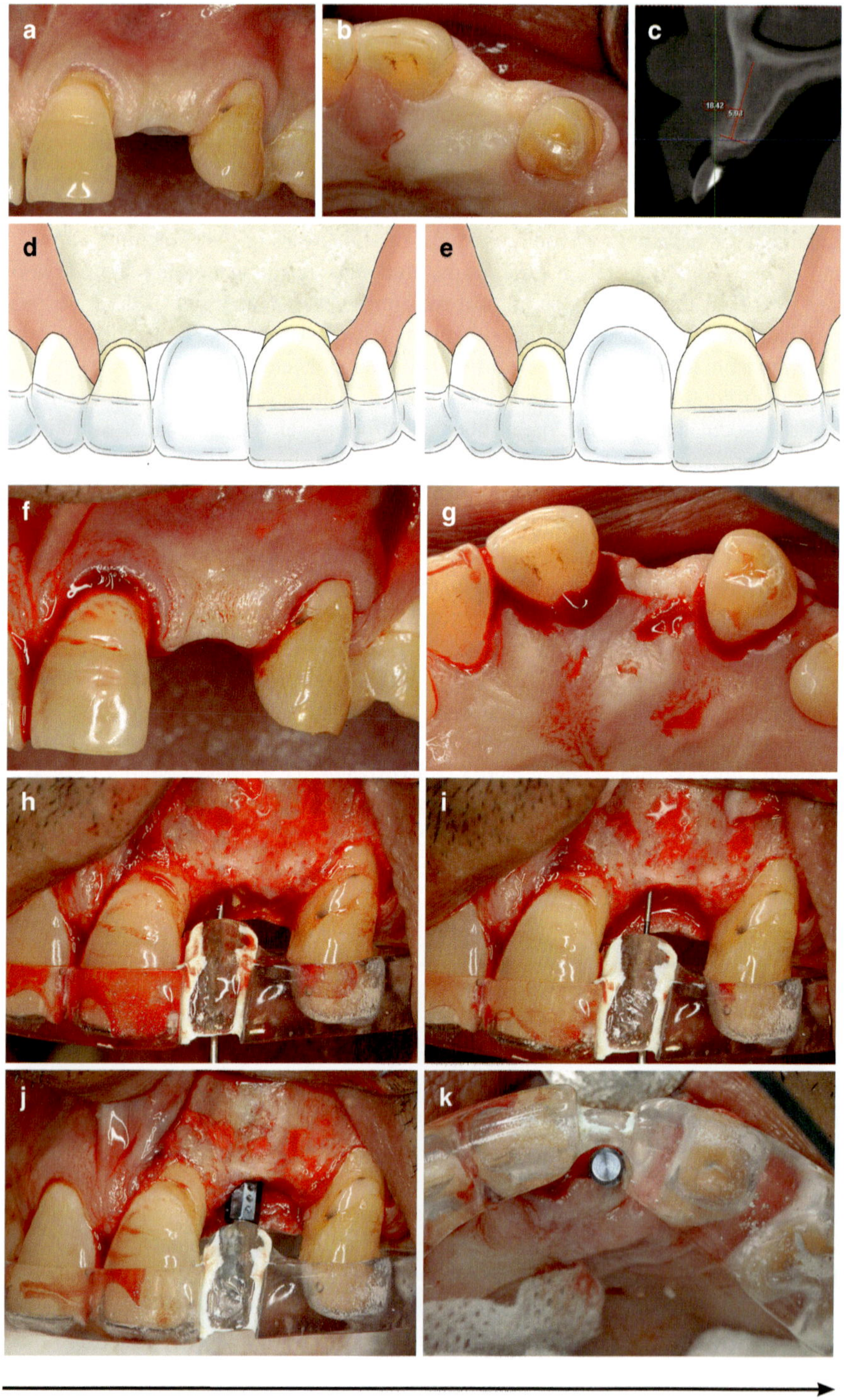
a
b
c
d
e
f
g
h
i
j
k

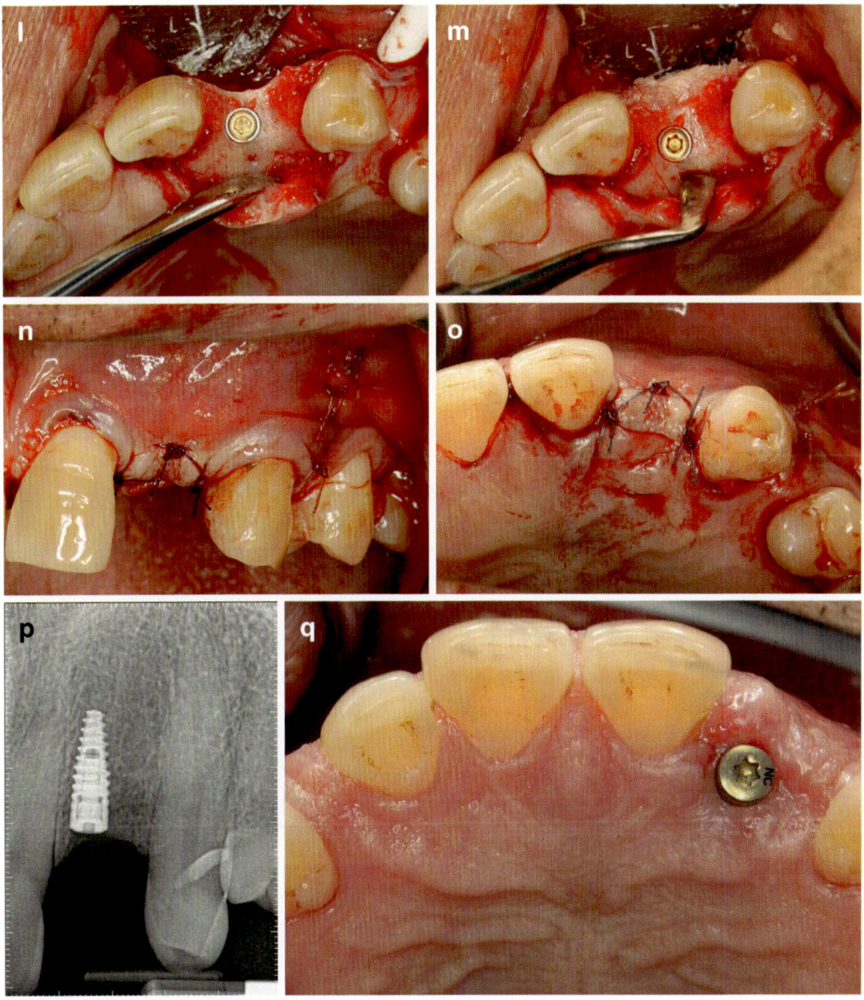

Fig. 9.13 Maxillary left lateral incisor is planned for implant placement. Restorative plan is to restore the tooth maintaining a diastema between lateral incisor and cuspid, mimicking the patient's original condition prior to loss of lateral incisor. Site presents with buccal horizontal ridge concavity (**a**, **b**). CBCT evaluation of the implant site with radiographic marker reveals the need for crestal ridge modification to provide 4 mm of transmucosal space for emergence profile (**c**). Diagram illustrating crestal reduction plan (**d**, **e**). Crestal incision performed with papillary preservation design to maintain thickness of papilla (**f**, **g**). Placement of surgical guide shows less than 2 mm of space for transmucosal transition (**h**). Reduction of the edentulous ridge was completed in a scalloped manner to provide 4 mm of transmucosal space to allow for restorative contouring and transmucosal soft tissue moulding (**i**). Implant was placed in a screw-retained position confirming 3-dimensional position through surgical guide (**j**, **k**). Simultaneous contour grafting was completed using autogenous bone shavings from the crestal reduction site mixed with cortico-cancellous mineralized and demineralized allograft (**l**, **m**). Tension-free flap closure with IMPRS technique (see Fig. 9.15) to maintain the height of the adjacent papillae. Uncovering of the implants was completed after 4 months of healing. An increase in ridge width and improvement of buccal concavity can be observed after contour grafting and support from healing abutment after uncovering (**q**). (Surgery in collaboration with Dr. Erin Lee. Diagrams courtesy of Dr. Erin Lee)

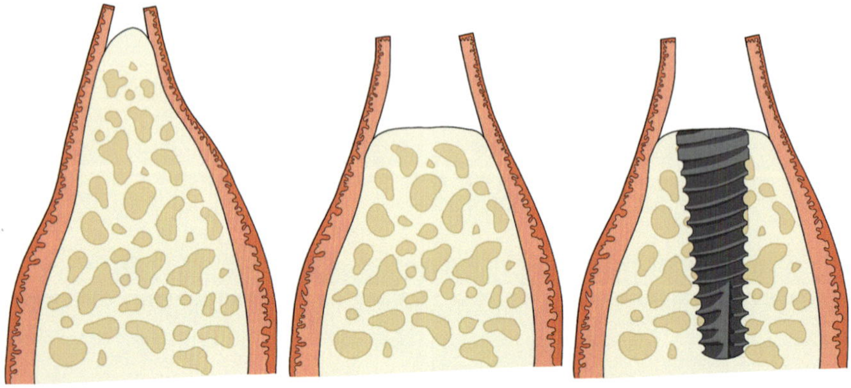

Fig. 9.14 Flattening of the bone will allow to level off lingual/buccal slope of the bone at the extraction site to house the implant on thicker apical bone and increased transmucosal space for adequate emergence profile and greater soft tissue thickness. (Courtesy of Dr. Erin Lee)

9.20 Flap Design

The primary purpose of mucosal/gingival flap is to provide surgical access for implant placement. At times, implant placement can be achieved through a transmucosal access to alveolar bone when there is no needed modification to alveolar bone crest or soft tissue profile. There is no difference in survival rates and marginal bone levels compared with the conventional flap approach [106]. However, flap access for implant surgery provides numerous advantages for surgical placement of the implant. One important factor for flap access is that a full-thickness flap will allow for visual assessment of bone healing and any deformities such as soft tissue invagination to osteotomy site, presence of loose bone graft particles and soft tissue-encapsulated bone graft materials that can potentially influence soft tissue health around implant restorations. A second factor is that a full-thickness flap will provide the ability to modify implant sites to improve hard and soft tissue thickness and profile around implants. Care must be given to minimize scarring and soft tissue shrinkage when elevating mucoperiosteal flap specially with the presence of thin tissue and highly scalloped gingival zenith and pointed interproximal papillae. To reduce unwanted soft tissue changes and scarring, a novel incision design and suturing technique, namely internal mattress papillary retention suture (IMPRS), is proposed. This technique allows for a full retention of papillary thickness and closure with internal mattress sutures to hike up the papillae while providing the seal of incision line with one suture knot. This technique for interproximal tissue and vertical release is illustrated in Figs. 9.15a–c and 9.16.

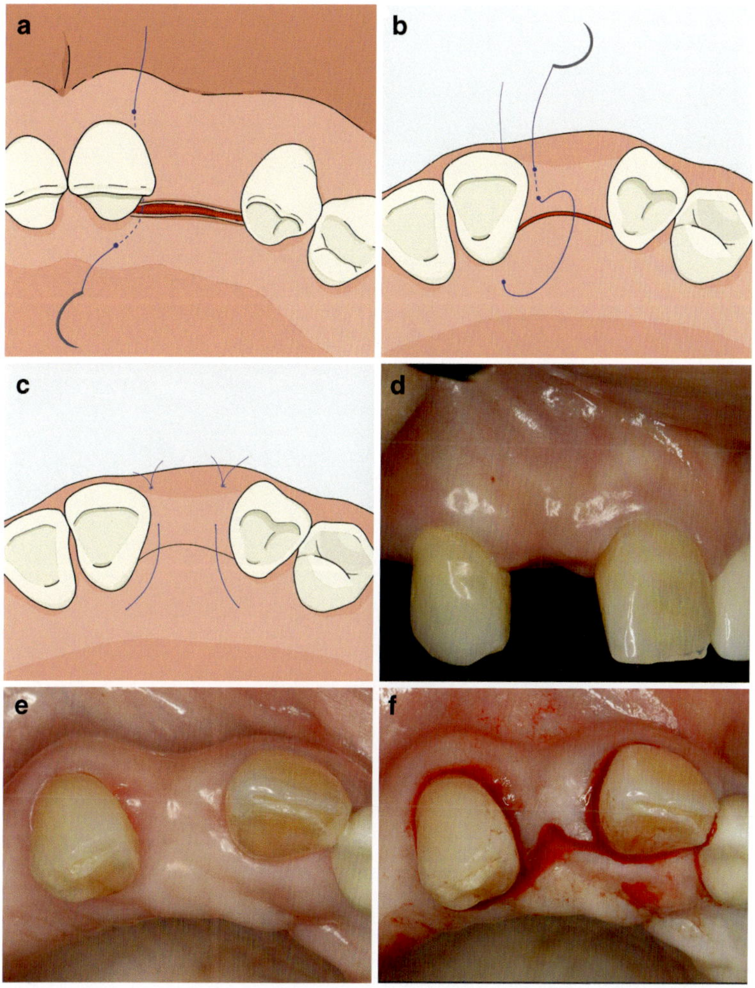

Fig. 9.15 Internal mattress papillary preservation suture (IMPRS) for closure of crestal incision access of edentulous ridge. Crestal incision is made from palatal line angle of adjacent teeth to preserve the full thickness of the papillary tissue and extend over the ridge following the crestal curve of the bone in a C-shaped design (**a**). Initial buccal suture purchase close to MGJ of adjacent tooth to keep the tension of the vector towards the tooth. Suture line is extended under the flap, and the second purchase is from inside to a palatal flap close to the tooth (**a**). Third purchase is over the incision line apical to the tip of the papilla from outside-in exiting coronal to initial bite to produce an internal mattress vector to the tissue next to the tooth and providing a seal over incision line (**b**, **c**). Clinical case demonstrating IMPRS for crestal closure. Maxillary right lateral site planned for implant placement (**d**, **c**). Papillary preservation incision from palatal line angles curved over crestal bone maintaining full thickness of papilla in buccal flap (**f**, **g**). Full-thickness flap and implant placement in prosthetically driven placement for screw-retained position (**h**, **i**). Flap closure with IMPRS technique providing vertical mattress on mesial and distal with simultaneous seal of crestal incision with vertical mattress tie (**j**, **k**). Soft tissue healing 2 weeks (**i**, **m**) and 5 months (**n**, **o**) post-operatively. No change of papillary height and no soft collapse are observed. Preservation of full papillary thickness and IMPRS technique helped to preserve the height and volume of the interproximal tissue. (Surgery in collaboration with Dr. Jane Law and diagrams courtesy of Dr. Erin Lee)

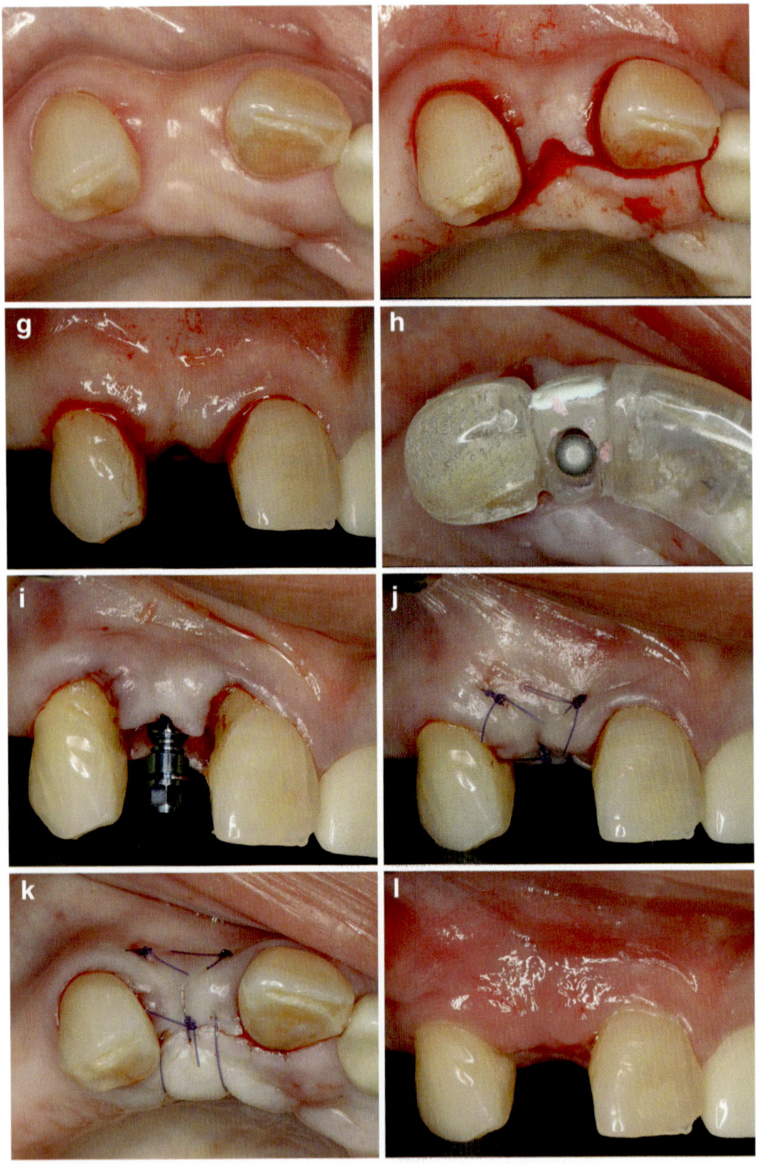

Fig. 9.15 (continued)

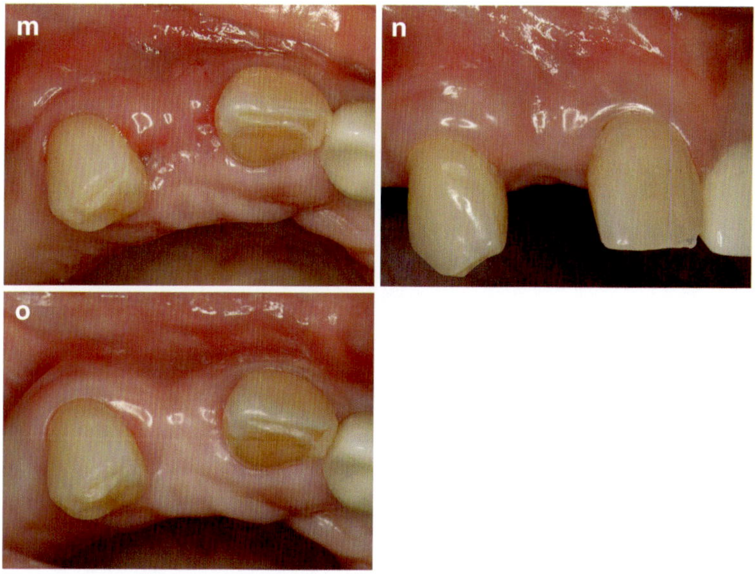

Fig. 9.15 (continued)

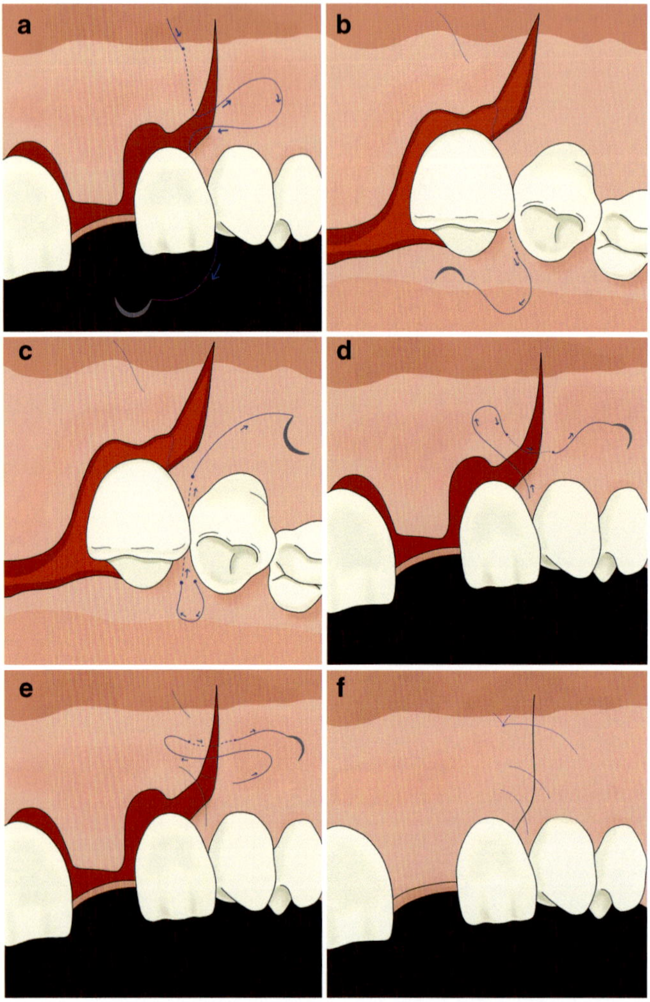

Fig. 9.16 Internal mattress papillary preservation suture (IMPRS) for closure of vertical releasing incision. Incision is made on distal line angle perpendicular to the edge of the sulcus with a hockey stick design to keep thick edges at the incision line and to preserve the full thickness of the papillary tissue; crestal incision performed same way as described in Fig. 9.15 (**a**). Initial buccal suture purchase is close to or apical to MGJ of the movable flap. Suture line is extended under the flap underneath of the papilla and exits the palatal tissue inside out (**b**). Second purchase is from outside into palatal papilla exiting from the base of the buccal coronal to incision line. This technique disburses the tension of the suture to the thicker palatal tissue rather than fragile edges of the incision line (**c**). Third purchase is close to the edge of the flap approximating the flap to papilla. The suture extends underneath the attached tissue approximating the two edges of the flap. Fourth purchase is apical to the third and coronal to the first purchase on the movable tissue and extends under the flap to the attached tissue creating a continuous loop over the incision line. If needed, another loop can be introduced for better approximation of the edges of the flap (**d**, **e**). Knot is placed at the apical bites pulling the edges of the flap in a vertical mattress fashion providing coronal advancement and seal of the incision line (**f**). Clinical example of IMPRS vertical closure suture at the day of the surgery (**g**) providing tension-free closure at the edges of the flap, at two weeks post-op (**h**) and 5 months post-op (**i**). (Surgery in collaboration with Dr. Leah Andriasian and diagrams courtesy of Dr. Erin Lee)

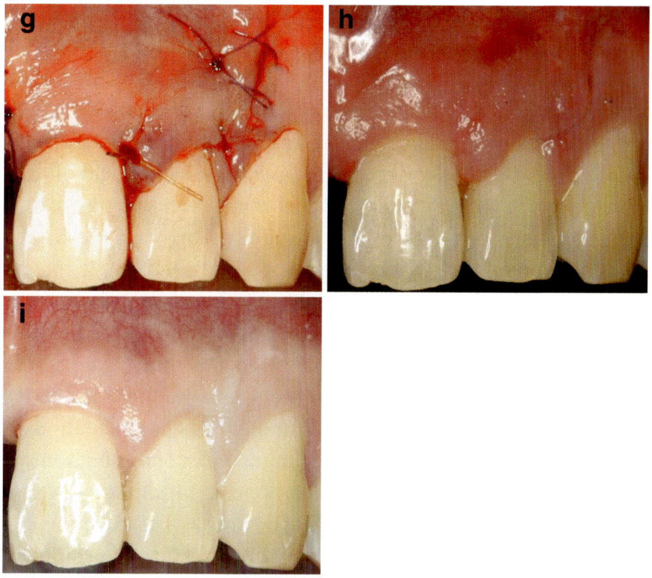

Fig. 9.16 (continued)

9.21 Timing of Placement

When considering replacement of teeth with dental implants, several factors need to be considered. When edentulous spaces are present, consideration must be made for the need of bone and/or soft tissue augmentation. Implant placement at the time of augmentation has the advantage of shortening timing of the surgical phase and number of surgical procedures. However, it is critical for clinicians to assess a risk/benefit analysis of combining augmentation procedures at the time of implant placement vs. a staged approach. Topography and containment of the defect are an important factor in deciding staged approach and at times will provide a better predictability in treatment outcome. Utilizing classification systems for the extent and shape of the horizontal and vertical defects can provide guidelines in the decision-making process for ridge augmentation [50].

When planning for implant surgery to replace an existing compromised tooth, there are four approaches that can be considered for replacement as described by Buser et al. It includes simultaneous placement at the time of extraction, early placement with soft tissue healing (4–8 weeks post-extraction), early placement with partial bone healing (12–16 weeks post-extortion) and late implant placement (more than 6 months of healing) [107]. Immediate implant placement in the aesthetic zone carries a risk of soft tissue complications [108, 109]. When optimal conditions present with a presence of thick buccal bone (more than 1 mm), simultaneous strategy along with possible bone and soft tissue grafting is suggested. Grafting techniques may be utilized often to compensate for the potential of soft tissue recession after immediate implant placement [110–112]. However, the success and aesthetic outcome of immediate implant placement is highly dependent on case selection and clinician's expertise [113]. Conversely, in the absence of buccal bone excessive post-extraction, bone remodelling is anticipated resulting in soft tissue shrinkage and recession around the implant restoration. When post-extraction remodelling can be anticipated by experienced clinicians, staged approach for implant placements is more predictable. Soft tissue thickness increases after tooth extraction improving flap manipulation and closure during augmentation procedure. Majority of the time when remaining bone allows for proper restoratively driven placement and stability, an early placement approach (4–8 weeks post-extraction) with simultaneous augmentation procedure or "contour grafting" is utilized. Alternatively, if initial defect presentation will not allow proper positioning on the implant in remaining bone, then additional waiting period is recommended for partial bone healing (12–16 weeks) before implant placement. However, if an implant cannot be stabilized in proper restorative position during early placement protocol, a staged bone augmentation approach is recommended, building the bone with a block or particulate graft and membrane using fixation screws for stability. Implant placement is then delayed until after 4–6 months of healing. At that point, the choice between a one-stage approach (exposed healing abutment or immediate loading with a provisional restoration) and a buried two-stage approach can be considered based on primary stability and placement of provisional restorations. Delayed placement approach (more than 6-month post-extraction healing) with or without staged ridge preservation will be the least desirable approach for treatment and should be considered when patient management considerations are present or when site-specific reasons such as large apical bone lesions do not provide sufficient bone volume to stabilize the implant with immediate or early implant placement protocols [107, 114, 115]. It is of the author's opinion that based on the review of available evidence from all practical purposes, the early placement with partial bone healing seems to be the most favourable surgical protocol. This approach can ensure a more predictable placement and stability in a prosthetically driven position, less potential soft tissue complications and a better soft tissue quality and quantity to manage any needed hard and soft tissue augmentation [116]. Also, through early placement protocol, the clinician will decide for the need of augmentation procedures on a case-by-case basis rather than frequent augmentation procedures advocated with immediate or delayed protocols.

9.22 Loading Protocols

Loading protocols of implants are considered as immediate (within 48 h), early (6 weeks) and delayed (more than 3 months). Overall, most studies do not report a clinically important difference in prosthesis failure, implant failure or bone loss associated with different loading times of implants [117, 118]. An important parameter to consider in immediate loading is the implant insertion torque and primary stability; implants with torque less than 30 ncm or 60–65 ISQ pose a higher risk of failure for immediate loading [119, 120]. This can pose a patient management challenge as the actual insertion torque cannot be known prior to implant placement, making it challenging to plan and execute immediate loading. One of the main advantages of immediate loading of dental implants is shortening the number of treatment appointments and efficacy in prosthetic rehabilitation [121]. This advantage must be weighed against the potential risk of implant failure or potential prosthetic complications during the provisional phase. Full-arch implant-supported provisional restorations have high risk for fracture and may require frequent repair creating patient management challenges as well as additional financial cost to the patient and/or practitioner [122]. Also, there is contrary evidence that immediate loading could be a risk factor for early implant failure and crestal bone loss compared to implants with delayed loading [123–125]. Additionally, immediately loaded single implants have lower survival rates with a five times higher risk when compared with delayed loading [126]. The discrepancy between success rate reports of immediate load and delayed loading can be related to influence of case selection, stringent treatment protocols and follow-ups that may not necessarily correspond to daily practice [127] and also observations from under-power studies with limited number of implants [122]. An important parameter to consider in immediate loading is the implant insertion torque and primary stability; implants with torque less than 30 ncm and 60–65 ISQ pose a higher risk of failure for immediate loading [119, 120]. This can pose a patient management challenge as the actual insertion torque cannot be known prior to implant placement, making it challenging to plan and execute immediate loading. It is of the author's opinion that the decision for immediate loading of implants must be made in the context of risk/benefits and cost/benefits. Although immediate loading by itself does not reduce the overall treatment time, it can provide a more efficient and patient-friendly transitional prosthesis. Patient selection is an important factor for the success of immediate loading. It is important to consider practitioner experience, patient-specific and site-specific factors such as patient's systemic health, biomechanical forces, presence of extraction sockets and need for ridge modification when deciding on immediate loading to reduce the overall risk of treatment.

9.23 Submerged vs. Non-submerged Implant Surgery

Another factor in surgical placement of implants is the decision for submerged or non-submerged implant placement. Most available data do not allude to differences in failure rate or crestal bone loss between two different surgical protocols [128, 129]. On the contrary, some systematic reviews point to slight increase in failure rate with non-submerged protocol [130]. It is important to consider that the lack difference between the two protocols is applicable when there is higher insertion torque of more than 20 ncm; non-submerged implants with low insertion torque of less than 20 ncm can exhibit 30-fold increased odds of failure [131]. In addition to the consideration of insertion torque and primary stability, the decision to undertake a submerged protocol may be related to the use of interim removable partial denture restoration or consideration of implant site development at the time of implant placement.

9.24 Surgical Discharge and Prosthetic Phase

Confirmation of implant integration is a clinical assessment based on the absence of symptoms and radiographic assessment of peri-implant bone around implant with a pressure test/torque test. Soft tissue health of the implant is determined by lack of clinical inflammation, bleeding on probing and probing depth measurements [132]. It is important to consider that probing depth around implant is the outcome of the location of restorative platform to the mucosal margin. Location of the mucosal margin is influenced by soft tissue thickness, presence or absence of adjacent teeth, and restorative contours and emergence profile. In general, probing depths are less reliable around peri-implant tissues than around teeth in the assessment of health [133, 134]. Presence of restorations and their emergence contours hinder the accuracy of probing depth measurements and correlation to alveolar bone; therefore, removal of prosthesis will help in better correlation of pocket depth to alveolar bone level [135]. Therefore, a final assessment of probing depth prior to placement of prosthesis is important to evaluate and correlate the health of the tissue to radiographic bone level around implants.

References

1. Dawson DR 3rd, Jasper S. Key systemic and environmental risk factors for implant failure. Dent Clin N Am. 2015;59(1):25–39.
2. da Rocha Costa Coelho T, Almeida de Azevedo R, Borges Maia WW, Nunes Dos Santos J, Ramos Cury P. Evaluation of the association of early implant failure with local, environmental, and systemic factors: a retrospective study. J Oral Maxillofac Surg. 2021;79(6):1237–45.
3. Jung RE, Al-Nawas B, Araujo M, et al. Group 1 ITI consensus report: the influence of implant length and design and medications on clinical and patient-reported outcomes. Clin Oral Implants Res. 2018;29(Suppl 16):69–77.
4. Chrcanovic BR, Kisch J, Albrektsson T, Wennerberg A. Is the intake of selective serotonin reuptake inhibitors associated with an increased risk of dental implant failure? Int J Oral Maxillofac Surg. 2017;46(6):782–8.
5. Edibam NR, Lorenzo-Pouso AI, Caponio VCA. Self-reported allergy to penicillin and clindamycin administration may be risk factors for dental implant failure: a systematic review, meta-analysis and delabeling protocol. Clin Oral Implants Res. 2023;34(7):651–61.
6. Zahra B, Nicholas B, Geoffrey R, et al. Dental implant failure rates in patients with self-reported allergy to penicillin. Clin Implant Dent Relat Res. 2022;24(3):301–6.
7. Salomó-Coll O, Lozano-Carrascal N, Lázaro-Abdulkarim A, et al. Do penicillin-allergic patients present a higher rate of implant failure? Int J Oral Maxillofac Implants. 2018;33(6):1390–5.
8. Nastri L, Moretti A, Migliaccio S, et al. Do dietary supplements and nutraceuticals have effects on dental implant osseointegration? A scoping review. Nutrients. 2020;12(1):268.

9. Choukroun J, Khoury G, Khoury F, et al. Two neglected biologic risk factors in bone grafting and implantology: high low-density lipoprotein cholesterol and low serum vitamin D. J Oral Implantol. 2014;40(1):110–4.
10. Waskiewicz K, Oth O, Kochan N, Evrard L. Risk factors generally neglected in oral surgery and implantology: the high LDL-cholesterol and the insufficient level of vitamin D. Rev Med Brux. 2018;39(2):70–7.
11. Paz A, Stanley M, Mangano FG, Miron RJ. Vitamin D deficiency and early implant failure: outcomes from a pre-surgical supplementation program on vitamin D levels and antioxidant scores. Oral Health Prev Dent. 2021;19(1):495–502.
12. Gamer S, Tuch R, Garcia LT. M. M. House mental classification revisited: intersection of particular patient types and particular dentist's needs. J Prosthet Dent. 2003;89(3):297–302.
13. AlZarea BK. Randomized controlled clinical investigation on the association between personality profiles and the impacts of two types of maxillary anterior implant-supported crown restorations on daily living and dental satisfaction. Clin Implant Dent Relat Res. 2019;21(4):602–12.
14. Evasic RW. Special report: evaluating the benefit-risk of dental implants provides informed consent. 1. Establishing the basic requirements for a standard of care in implant dentistry. J Oral Implantol. 1991;17(4):384–9.
15. Hajivassiliou EC, Hajivassiliou CA. Informed consent in primary dental care: patients' understanding and satisfaction with the consent process. Br Dent J. 2015;219(5):221–4.
16. Garber DBU. Restoration driven implant placement with restoration generated site development. Compend Contin Educ Dent. 1995;16:796–804.
17. Mengel R, Schröder T, Flores-de-Jacoby L. Osseointegrated implants in patients treated for generalized chronic periodontitis and generalized aggressive periodontitis: 3- and 5-year results of a prospective long-term study. J Periodontol. 2001;72(8):977–89.
18. Jepsen S, Berglundh T, Genco R, et al. Primary prevention of peri-implantitis: managing peri-implant mucositis. J Clin Periodontol. 2015;42(Suppl 16):S152–7.
19. Quirynen M, De Soete M, van Steenberghe D. Infectious risks for oral implants: a review of the literature. Clin Oral Implants Res. 2002;13(1):1–19.
20. Becker W, Ochsenbein C, Tibbetts L, Becker BE. Alveolar bone anatomic profiles as measured from dry skulls. Clinical ramifications. J Clin Periodontol. 1997;24(10):727–31.
21. Kois J. Altering gingival levels: the restorative connection. Part 1: biologic variables. J Esthet Dent. 1994;6:3–9.
22. Coslet JG, Vanarsdall R, Weisgold A. Diagnosis and classification of delayed passive eruption of the dentogingival junction in the adult. Alpha Omegan. 1977;70(3):24–8.
23. Shafizadeh M, Amid R, Tehranchi A, Motamedian SR. Evaluation of the association between gingival phenotype and alveolar bone thickness: a systematic review and meta-analysis. Arch Oral Biol. 2022;133:105287.
24. Kois JC. Predictable single-tooth peri-implant esthetics: five diagnostic keys. Compend Contin Educ Dent. 2004;25(11):895–6. 98, 900 passim; quiz 06–7.
25. Jung RE, Heitz-Mayfield L, Schwarz F. Evidence-based knowledge on the aesthetics and maintenance of peri-implant soft tissues: Osteology Foundation Consensus Report Part 3—Aesthetics of peri-implant soft tissues. Clin Oral Implants Res. 2018;29(Suppl 15):14–7.
26. Roccuzzo M, Roccuzzo A, Ramanuskaite A. Papilla height in relation to the distance between bone crest and interproximal contact point at single-tooth implants: a systematic review. Clin Oral Implants Res. 2018;29(Suppl 15):50–61.
27. Linkevicius T, Puisys A, Steigmann M, Vindasiute E, Linkeviciene L. Influence of vertical soft tissue thickness on crestal bone changes around implants with platform switching: a comparative clinical study. Clin Implant Dent Relat Res. 2015;17(6):1228–36.
28. Schwarz F, Becker J, Civale S, et al. Influence of the width of keratinized tissue on the development and resolution of experimental peri-implant mucositis lesions in humans. Clin Oral Implants Res. 2018;29(6):576–82.

29. Roccuzzo M, Grasso G, Dalmasso P. Keratinized mucosa around implants in partially edentulous posterior mandible: 10-year results of a prospective comparative study. Clin Oral Implants Res. 2016;27(4):491–6.
30. Chee WW. Treatment planning and soft-tissue management for optimal implant esthetics: a prosthodontic perspective. J Calif Dent Assoc. 2003;31(7):559–63.
31. Wang II, Barootchi S, Tavelli L, Wang HL. The peri-implant phenotype and implant esthetic complications. Contemporary overview. J Esthet Restor Dent. 2021;33(1):212–23.
32. Bidra AS. Three-dimensional esthetic analysis in treatment planning for implant-supported fixed prosthesis in the edentulous maxilla: review of the esthetics literature. J Esthet Restor Dent. 2011;23(4):219–36.
33. Moshaverinia A, Kar K, Chee WW. Treatment planning decisions: implant placement versus preserving natural teeth. J Calif Dent Assoc. 2014;42(12):859–68.
34. Jung RE, Ioannidis A, Hämmerle CHF, Thoma DS. Alveolar ridge preservation in the esthetic zone. Periodontology 2000. 2018;77(1):165–75.
35. Atieh MA, Alsabeeha NH, Payne AG, et al. Interventions for replacing missing teeth: alveolar ridge preservation techniques for dental implant site development. Cochrane Database Syst Rev. 2015;2015(5):Cd010176.
36. Tan WL, Wong TL, Wong MC, Lang NP. A systematic review of post-extractional alveolar hard and soft tissue dimensional changes in humans. Clin Oral Implants Res. 2012;23(Suppl 5):1–21.
37. Berglundh T, Armitage G, Araujo MG, et al. Peri-implant diseases and conditions: consensus report of workgroup 4 of the 2017 World Workshop on the Classification of Periodontal and Peri-implant Diseases and Conditions. J Clin Periodontol. 2018;45(Suppl 20):S286–s91.
38. Chappuis V, Engel O, Shahim K, et al. Soft tissue alterations in esthetic postextraction sites: a 3-dimensional analysis. J Dent Res. 2015;94(9 Suppl):187s–93s.
39. Avila-Ortiz G, Gubler M, Romero-Bustillos M, et al. Efficacy of alveolar ridge preservation: a randomized controlled trial. J Dent Res. 2020;99(4):402–9.
40. Mardas N, Trullenque-Eriksson A, MacBeth N, Petrie A, Donos N. Does ridge preservation following tooth extraction improve implant treatment outcomes: a systematic review: group 4: therapeutic concepts and methods. Clin Oral Implants Res. 2015;26(Suppl 11):180–201.
41. Kan JY, Rungcharassaeng K, Umezu K, Kois JC. Dimensions of peri-implant mucosa: an evaluation of maxillary anterior single implants in humans. J Periodontol. 2003;74(4):557–62.
42. Chee WW, Nowzari H, Kaneko L. Esthetic replacement of the anterior tooth with an implant-supported restoration. J Calif Dent Assoc. 1997;25(12):860–5.
43. Neale D, Chee WW. Development of implant soft tissue emergence profile: a technique. J Prosthet Dent. 1994;71(4):364–8.
44. Sadan A, Blatz MB, Salinas TJ, Block MS. Single-implant restorations: a contemporary approach for achieving a predictable outcome. J Oral Maxillofac Surg. 2004;62(9 Suppl 2):73–81.
45. Hämmerle CH, Chiantella GC, Karring T, Lang NP. The effect of a deproteinized bovine bone mineral on bone regeneration around titanium dental implants. Clin Oral Implants Res. 1998;9(3):151–62.
46. Araújo M, Linder E, Wennström J, Lindhe J. The influence of Bio-Oss Collagen on healing of an extraction socket: an experimental study in the dog. Int J Periodontics Restor Dent. 2008;28(2):123–35.
47. Rodriguez AE, Nowzari H. The long-term risks and complications of bovine-derived xenografts: a case series. J Indian Soc Periodontol. 2019;23(5):487–92.
48. Nowzari H, Teoh C, Rodriguez AE. The migration of the bovine-derived xenograft particles: a case series. J Indian Soc Periodontol. 2022;26(2):178–85.
49. Mardas N, Macbeth N, Donos N, Jung RE, Zuercher AN. Is alveolar ridge preservation an overtreatment? Periodontology 2000. 2023;93:289.
50. Wang HL, Al-Shammari K. HVC ridge deficiency classification: a therapeutically oriented classification. Int J Periodontics Restor Dent. 2002;22(4):335–43.

51. Jepsen S, Schwarz F, Cordaro L, et al. Regeneration of alveolar ridge defects. Consensus report of group 4 of the 15th European Workshop on Periodontology on Bone Regeneration. J Clin Periodontol. 2019;46(Suppl 21):277–86.
52. Singh V, Bhagol A, Ashwin V. Controversies in the dental implant treatment planning for anterior maxillary aesthetic zone—a review. Natl J Maxillofac Surg. 2023;14(1):3–8.
53. Palacios JAV, Garcia JJ, Caramês JMM, Quirynen M, da Silva Marques DN. Short implants versus bone grafting and standard-length implants placement: a systematic review. Clin Oral Investig. 2018;22(1):69–80.
54. Nisand D, Picard N, Rocchietta I. Short implants compared to implants in vertically augmented bone: a systematic review. Clin Oral Implants Res. 2015;26(Suppl 11):170–9.
55. Esposito M, Buti J, Barausse C, et al. Short implants versus longer implants in vertically augmented atrophic mandibles: a systematic review of randomised controlled trials with a 5-year post-loading follow-up. Int J Oral Implantol (Berl). 2019;12(3):267–80.
56. Almeida PHT, Cacciacane SH, Arcazas JA. Extra-long transnasal implants as alternative for Quad Zygoma: case report. Ann Med Surg (Lond). 2021;68:102635.
57. Rosenstein J, Dym H. Zygomatic implants: a solution for the atrophic maxilla: 2021 update. Dent Clin N Am. 2021;65(1):229–39.
58. Aalam AA, Krivitsky-Aalam A, Kurtzman GM, Mahesh L. The severely atrophic maxilla: decision making with zygomatic and pterygoid dental implants. J Oral Biol Craniofac Res. 2023;13(2):202–6.
59. Chrcanovic BR, Abreu MH. Survival and complications of zygomatic implants: a systematic review. Oral Maxillofac Surg. 2013;17(2):81–93.
60. Chrcanovic BR, Albrektsson T, Wennerberg A. Survival and complications of zygomatic implants: an updated systematic review. J Oral Maxillofac Surg. 2016;74(10):1949–64.
61. Dawood A, Kalavresos N. Management of extraoral complications in a patient treated with four zygomatic implants. Int J Oral Maxillofac Implants. 2017;32(4):893–6.
62. Lan K, Wang F, Huang W, Davó R, Wu Y. Quad zygomatic implants: a systematic review and meta-analysis on survival and complications. Int J Oral Maxillofac Implants. 2021;36(1):21–9.
63. Starch-Jensen T, Becktor JP. Maxillary alveolar ridge expansion with split-crest technique compared with lateral ridge augmentation with autogenous bone block graft: a systematic review. J Oral Maxillofac Res. 2019;10(4):e2.
64. Javed F, Romanos GE. Role of implant diameter on long-term survival of dental implants placed in posterior maxilla: a systematic review. Clin Oral Investig. 2015;19(1):1–10.
65. González-Valls G, Roca-Millan E, Céspedes-Sánchez JM, et al. Narrow diameter dental implants as an alternative treatment for atrophic alveolar ridges. Systematic review and meta-analysis. Materials (Basel). 2021;14(12):3234.
66. Testori T, Weinstein T, Taschieri S, Wallace SS. Risk factors in lateral window sinus elevation surgery. Periodontology 2000. 2019;81(1):91–123.
67. Leung M, Alghamdi R, Guallart IF, et al. Patient-related risk factors for maxillary sinus augmentation procedures: a systematic literature review. Int J Periodontics Restor Dent. 2021;41(3):e121–e28.
68. Esposito M, Grusovin MG, Rees J, et al. Effectiveness of sinus lift procedures for dental implant rehabilitation: a Cochrane systematic review. Eur J Oral Implantol. 2010;3(1):7–26.
69. Molina A, Sanz-Sánchez I, Sanz-Martín I, Ortiz-Vigón A, Sanz M. Complications in sinus lifting procedures: classification and management. Periodontology 2000. 2022;88(1):103–15.
70. Ting M, Rice JG, Braid SM, Lee CYS, Suzuki JB. Maxillary sinus augmentation for dental implant rehabilitation of the edentulous ridge: a comprehensive overview of systematic reviews. Implant Dent. 2017;26(3):438–64.
71. Tonetti MS, Hämmerle CH. Advances in bone augmentation to enable dental implant placement: Consensus Report of the Sixth European Workshop on Periodontology. J Clin Periodontol. 2008;35(8 Suppl):168–72.
72. Chan HL, Wang HL. Sinus pathology and anatomy in relation to complications in lateral window sinus augmentation. Implant Dent. 2011;20(6):406–12.

73. Thoma DS, Cha JK, Jung UW. Treatment concepts for the posterior maxilla and mandible: short implants versus long implants in augmented bone. J Periodontal Implant Sci. 2017;47(1):2–12.
74. Sáenz-Ravello G, Ossandón-Zúñiga B, Muñoz-Meza V, et al. Short implants compared to regular dental implants after bone augmentation in the atrophic posterior mandible: umbrella review and meta-analysis of success outcomes. Int J Implant Dent. 2023;9(1):18.
75. Kablan F, Abu-Sobeh A, Lorean A, Levin L. Spontaneous mandibular fracture as a complication of inferior alveolar nerve transposition and placement of endosseous dental implants in the atrophic mandible: a review of the literature and a report of two cases and their nonsurgical conservative management. Quintessence Int. 2020;51(3):230–7.
76. Allavéna J, Nicot R, Majoufre C, Schlund M. Inferior alveolar nerve repositioning surgical techniques and outcomes—a systematic review. J Stomatol Oral Maxillofac Surg. 2023;125(1):101631.
77. Jensen SS, Bosshardt DD, Gruber R, Buser D. Long-term stability of contour augmentation in the esthetic zone: histologic and histomorphometric evaluation of 12 human biopsies 14–80 months after augmentation. J Periodontol. 2014;85(11):1549–56.
78. DeGroot BS, Villar CC, Mealey BL, et al. Osseous healing around immediate implants placed using contour augmentation: a prospective case series. Int J Periodontics Restor Dent. 2017;37(6):883–91.
79. Chappuis V, Rahman L, Buser R, et al. Effectiveness of contour augmentation with guided bone regeneration: 10-year results. J Dent Res. 2018;97(3):266–74.
80. Tsai YL, Tsao JP, Wang CL, et al. Stability of contour augmentation of implant-supported single crowns in the esthetic zone: 1-year cone-beam computed tomography results of a comparative, randomized, prospective, two-center clinical study using two different bone grafting techniques in early implant placement. J Periodontol. 2022;93(11):1661–70.
81. Artzi Z, Renert U, Pirc M, Netanely E, Thoma DS. Contour changes following implant placement and concomitant soft tissue augmentation applying a volume-stable collagen matrix. Int J Periodontics Restor Dent. 2022;42(4):515–22.
82. Bannister SR, Powell CA. Foreign body reaction to anorganic bovine bone and autogenous bone with platelet-rich plasma in guided bone regeneration. J Periodontol. 2008;79(6):1116–20.
83. Galindo-Moreno P, Hernández-Cortés P, Mesa F, et al. Slow resorption of anorganic bovine bone by osteoclasts in maxillary sinus augmentation. Clin Implant Dent Relat Res. 2013;15(6):858–66.
84. Salama H, Salama M. The role of orthodontic extrusive remodeling in the enhancement of soft and hard tissue profiles prior to implant placement: a systematic approach to the management of extraction site defects. Int J Periodontics Restor Dent. 1993;13(4):312–33.
85. Uribe F, Taylor T, Shafer D, Nanda R. A novel approach for implant site development through root tipping. Am J Orthod Dentofac Orthop. 2010;138(5):649–55.
86. Smalley WM. Implants for tooth movement: determining implant location and orientation. J Esthet Dent. 1995;7(2):62–72.
87. Jacobs R, Salmon B, Codari M, Hassan B, Bornstein MM. Cone beam computed tomography in implant dentistry: recommendations for clinical use. BMC Oral Health. 2018;18(1):88.
88. Benavides E, Rios HF, Ganz SD, et al. Use of cone beam computed tomography in implant dentistry: the International Congress of Oral Implantologists consensus report. Implant Dent. 2012;21(2):78–86.
89. Rios HF, Borgnakke WS, Benavides E. The use of cone-beam computed tomography in management of patients requiring dental implants: an American Academy of Periodontology Best Evidence Review. J Periodontol. 2017;88(10):946–59.
90. Signorelli L, Patcas R, Peltomäki T, Schätzle M. Radiation dose of cone-beam computed tomography compared to conventional radiographs in orthodontics. J Orofac Orthop. 2016;77(1):9–15.
91. Tatakis DN, Chien HH, Parashis AO. Guided implant surgery risks and their prevention. Periodontology 2000. 2019;81(1):194–208.

92. Katafuchi M, Weinstein BF, Leroux BG, Chen YW, Daubert DM. Restoration contour is a risk indicator for peri-implantitis: a cross-sectional radiographic analysis. J Clin Periodontol. 2018;45(2):225–32.
93. Romandini M, Pedrinaci I, Lima C, et al. Prevalence and risk/protective indicators of buccal soft tissue dehiscence around dental implants. J Clin Periodontol. 2021;48(3):455–63.
94. Romanos GE, Delgado-Ruiz R, Sculean A. Concepts for prevention of complications in implant therapy. Periodontology 2000. 2019;81(1):7–17.
95. Roccuzzo A, Imber JC, Salvi GE, Roccuzzo M. Peri-implantitis as the consequence of errors in implant therapy. Periodontology 2000. 2023;92(1):350–61.
96. Serino G, Hultin K. Peri-implant disease and prosthetic risk indicators: a literature review. Implant Dent. 2019;28(2):125–37.
97. Ng KT, Fan M, Leung MC, Fokas G, Mattheos N. Peri-implant inflammation and marginal bone level changes around dental implants in relation to proximity with and bone level of adjacent teeth. Aust Dent J. 2018;63(4):467–77.
98. Staubli N, Walter C, Schmidt JC, Weiger R, Zitzmann NU. Excess cement and the risk of peri-implant disease—a systematic review. Clin Oral Implants Res. 2017;28(10):1278–90.
99. Lekholm UZG. Patient selection and preparation. Tissue integrated prostheses: osseointegration in clinical dentistry. Chicago: Quintessence; 1985.
100. Linck GK, Ferreira GM, De Oliveira RC, et al. The influence of tactile perception on classification of bone tissue at dental implant insertion. Clin Implant Dent Relat Res. 2016;18(3):601–8.
101. Potdukhe SS, Iyer JM, Nadgere JB. Evaluation of implant stability and increase in bone height in indirect sinus lift done with the osseodensification and osteotome technique: a systematic review and meta-analysis. J Prosthet Dent. 2023.
102. Inchingolo AD, Inchingolo AM, Bordea IR, et al. The effectiveness of osseodensification drilling protocol for implant site osteotomy: a systematic review of the literature and meta-analysis. Materials (Basel). 2021;14(5):1147.
103. Heimes D, Becker P, Pabst A, et al. How does dental implant macrogeometry affect primary implant stability? A narrative review. Int J Implant Dent. 2023;9(1):20.
104. Yu X, Chang C, Guo W, et al. Primary implant stability based on alternative site preparation techniques: a systematic review and meta-analysis. Clin Implant Dent Relat Res. 2022;24(5):580–90.
105. Giannobile WV, Jung RE, Schwarz F. Evidence-based knowledge on the aesthetics and maintenance of peri-implant soft tissues: Osteology Foundation Consensus Report Part 1—Effects of soft tissue augmentation procedures on the maintenance of peri-implant soft tissue health. Clin Oral Implants Res. 2018;29(Suppl 15):7–10.
106. Lin GH, Chan HL, Bashutski JD, Oh TJ, Wang HL. The effect of flapless surgery on implant survival and marginal bone level: a systematic review and meta-analysis. J Periodontol. 2014;85(5):e91–103.
107. Buser D, Chappuis V, Belser UC, Chen S. Implant placement post extraction in esthetic single tooth sites: when immediate, when early, when late? Periodontology 2000. 2017;73(1):84–102.
108. Tonetti MS, Cortellini P, Graziani F, et al. Immediate versus delayed implant placement after anterior single tooth extraction: the timing randomized controlled clinical trial. J Clin Periodontol. 2017;44(2):215–24.
109. Chen ST, Buser D. Esthetic outcomes following immediate and early implant placement in the anterior maxilla—a systematic review. Int J Oral Maxillofac Implants. 2014;29(Suppl):186–215.
110. Seyssens L, De Lat L, Cosyn J. Immediate implant placement with or without connective tissue graft: a systematic review and meta-analysis. J Clin Periodontol. 2021;48(2):284–301.
111. Seyssens L, Eeckhout C, Cosyn J. Immediate implant placement with or without socket grafting: a systematic review and meta-analysis. Clin Implant Dent Relat Res. 2022;24(3):339–51.
112. Thoma DS, Cosyn J, Fickl S, et al. Soft tissue management at implants: summary and consensus statements of group 2. The 6th EAO Consensus Conference 2021. Clin Oral Implants Res. 2021;31(Suppl 21):174–80.

113. Cosyn J, Blanco J. EAO position paper: immediate implant placement: managing hard and soft tissue stability from diagnosis to prosthetic treatment. Int J Prosthodont. 2023;36(5):533–45.
114. Buser D, Wittneben J, Bornstein MM, et al. Stability of contour augmentation and esthetic outcomes of implant-supported single crowns in the esthetic zone: 3-year results of a prospective study with early implant placement postextraction. J Periodontol. 2011;82(3):342–9.
115. Tonetti MS, Jung RE, Avila-Ortiz G, et al. Management of the extraction socket and timing of implant placement: consensus report and clinical recommendations of group 3 of the XV European Workshop in Periodontology. J Clin Periodontol. 2019;46(Suppl 21):183–94.
116. Bassir SH, El Kholy K, Chen CY, Lee KH, Intini G. Outcome of early dental implant placement versus other dental implant placement protocols: a systematic review and meta-analysis. J Periodontol. 2019;90(5):493–506.
117. Donos N, Asche NV, Akbar AN, et al. Impact of timing of dental implant placement and loading: summary and consensus statements of group 1—The 6th EAO Consensus Conference 2021. Clin Oral Implants Res. 2021;32(Suppl 21):85–92.
118. Esposito M, Grusovin MG, Maghaireh H, Worthington HV. Interventions for replacing missing teeth: different times for loading dental implants. Cochrane Database Syst Rev. 2013;2013(3):Cd003878.
119. Ottoni JM, Oliveira ZF, Mansini R, Cabral AM. Correlation between placement torque and survival of single-tooth implants. Int J Oral Maxillofac Implants. 2005;20(5):769–76.
120. Benic GI, Mir-Mari J, Hämmerle CH. Loading protocols for single-implant crowns: a systematic review and meta-analysis. Int J Oral Maxillofac Implants. 2014;29(Suppl):222–38.
121. Chee W, Jivraj S. Efficiency of immediately loaded mandibular full-arch implant restorations. Clin Implant Dent Relat Res. 2003;5(1):52–6.
122. De Bruyn H, Raes S, Ostman PO, Cosyn J. Immediate loading in partially and completely edentulous jaws: a review of the literature with clinical guidelines. Periodontology 2000. 2014;66(1):153–87.
123. Pardal-Peláez B, Flores-Fraile J, Pardal-Refoyo JL, Montero J. Implant loss and crestal bone loss in immediate versus delayed load in edentulous mandibles: a systematic review and meta-analysis. J Prosthet Dent. 2021;125(3):437–44.
124. Chen J, Cai M, Yang J, Aldhohrah T, Wang Y. Immediate versus early or conventional loading dental implants with fixed prostheses: a systematic review and meta-analysis of randomized controlled clinical trials. J Prosthet Dent. 2019;122(6):516–36.
125. Sanz-Sánchez I, Sanz-Martín I, Figuero E, Sanz M. Clinical efficacy of immediate implant loading protocols compared to conventional loading depending on the type of the restoration: a systematic review. Clin Oral Implants Res. 2015;26(8):964–82.
126. Atieh MA, Atieh AH, Payne AG, Duncan WJ. Immediate loading with single implant crowns: a systematic review and meta-analysis. Int J Prosthodont. 2009;22(4):378–87.
127. Ganeles J, Wismeijer D. Early and immediately restored and loaded dental implants for single-tooth and partial-arch applications. Int J Oral Maxillofac Implants. 2004;19(Suppl):92–102.
128. Cecchinato D, Olsson C, Lindhe J. Submerged or non-submerged healing of endosseous implants to be used in the rehabilitation of partially dentate patients. J Clin Periodontol. 2004;31(4):299–308.
129. Weber HP, Crohin CC, Fiorellini JP. A 5-year prospective clinical and radiographic study of non-submerged dental implants. Clin Oral Implants Res. 2000;11(2):144–53.
130. Troiano G, Lo Russo L, Canullo L, et al. Early and late implant failure of submerged versus non-submerged implant healing: a systematic review, meta-analysis and trial sequential analysis. J Clin Periodontol. 2018;45(5):613–23.
131. Liu Q, Yang J, Wang R, Yuan L, Yu K. Dental implant failure rates with low insertion torque with a nonsubmerged surgical approach: a retrospective clinical study. Clin Implant Dent Relat Res. 2023;25(1):118–23.
132. Renvert S, Persson GR, Pirih FQ, Camargo PM. Peri-implant health, peri-implant mucositis, and peri-implantitis: case definitions and diagnostic considerations. J Periodontol. 2018;89(Suppl 1):S304–s12.

133. Mombelli A, Mühle T, Brägger U, Lang NP, Bürgin WB. Comparison of periodontal and peri-implant probing by depth-force pattern analysis. Clin Oral Implants Res. 1997;8(6):448–54.
134. Ramanauskaite A, Obreja K, Schwarz F, et al. Reliability of probing depth assessments at healthy implant sites and natural teeth. Clin Oral Investig. 2023;27(6):2533–45.
135. Serino G, Turri A, Lang NP. Probing at implants with peri-implantitis and its relation to clinical peri-implant bone loss. Clin Oral Implants Res. 2013;24(1):91–5.

Susceptibility of Peri-implantitis with Dental Implants

10

Monitoring Health and Disease Around Implants: How to Monitor and When to Treat

Jean-Pierre Albouy

10.1 Clinical Diagnosis

10.1.1 Periodontal Health and Disease Diagnosis

Health around teeth is characterized by "the absence of bleeding on probing, erythema and oedema and patient's symptoms" whether or not the patient has lost clinical attachment in the past or not. Furthermore, gingivitis is the situation in which signs of inflammation are visible without any attachment loss, while periodontal diseases will present signs of inflammation associated with loss of periodontal attachment. The discriminating factor for the clinical diagnosis of disease is inflammation, while radiographs are limited to the assessment of bone levels [1].

Figures 10.1, 10.2 and 10.3: Periodontal health—gingivitis—periodontitis.

10.2 Peri-implant Health and Disease Diagnosis

Similarly, health around implants is defined by the "absence of erythema, bleeding on probing, swelling or suppuration".

Healthy peri-implant tissue probing does not induce bleeding but is usually more prone to bleeding than around teeth. Peri-implant mucositis will present smooth reddish tissues with signs of inflammation; probing will induce bleeding and will usually be deeper. At times, tissue tightness might prevent the probe from penetrating.

There is much less information disseminated to help clinicians with developing a suitable treatment plan and post-treatment maintenance of implant-supported restorations delivered.

J.-P. Albouy (✉)
Adams School of Dentistry, University of North Carolina, Chapel Hill, NC, USA

W. Chee, S. Jivraj (eds.), *Treatment Planning In Implant Dentistry*, BDJ Clinician's Guides, https://doi.org/10.1007/978-3-031-68726-6_10

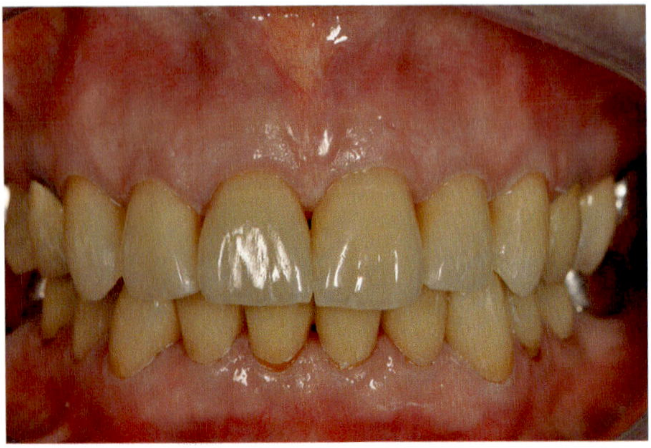

Fig. 10.1 Periodontal health demonstrating absence of bleeding, erythema and oedema

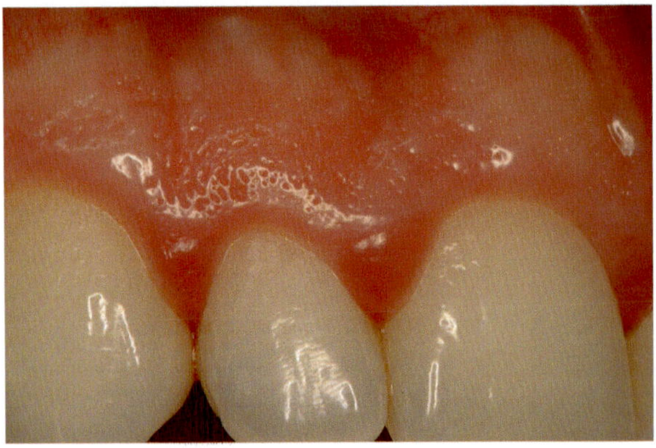

Fig. 10.2 Gingivitis demonstrating erythema, oedema and bleeding when probing

Peri-implantitis is defined by the clinical signs of inflammation, "bleeding on probing, or suppuration, increased probing depths and/or recession of the mucosal margin in addition to radiographic bone loss" for which previous radiographs can be utilized when available [2].

Figures 10.4, 10.5, 10.6: Peri-implant health—peri-implant mucositis—peri-implantitis.

10.3 Prevalence and Treatment of Peri-implant Mucositis

Peri-implant experimental human mucositis has been shown to induce statistically significant higher levels of inflammation measured via crevicular fluid level of matrix metalloproteinase-8 (MMP-8) when compared to gingivitis [3]. In this study, the peri-implant mucositis is reversible once oral hygiene measures are reinstated, but a period of more than 3 weeks is needed to return back to baseline levels.

Professional and patient-administered plaque control is the standard of care in the management of peri-implant mucositis [4].

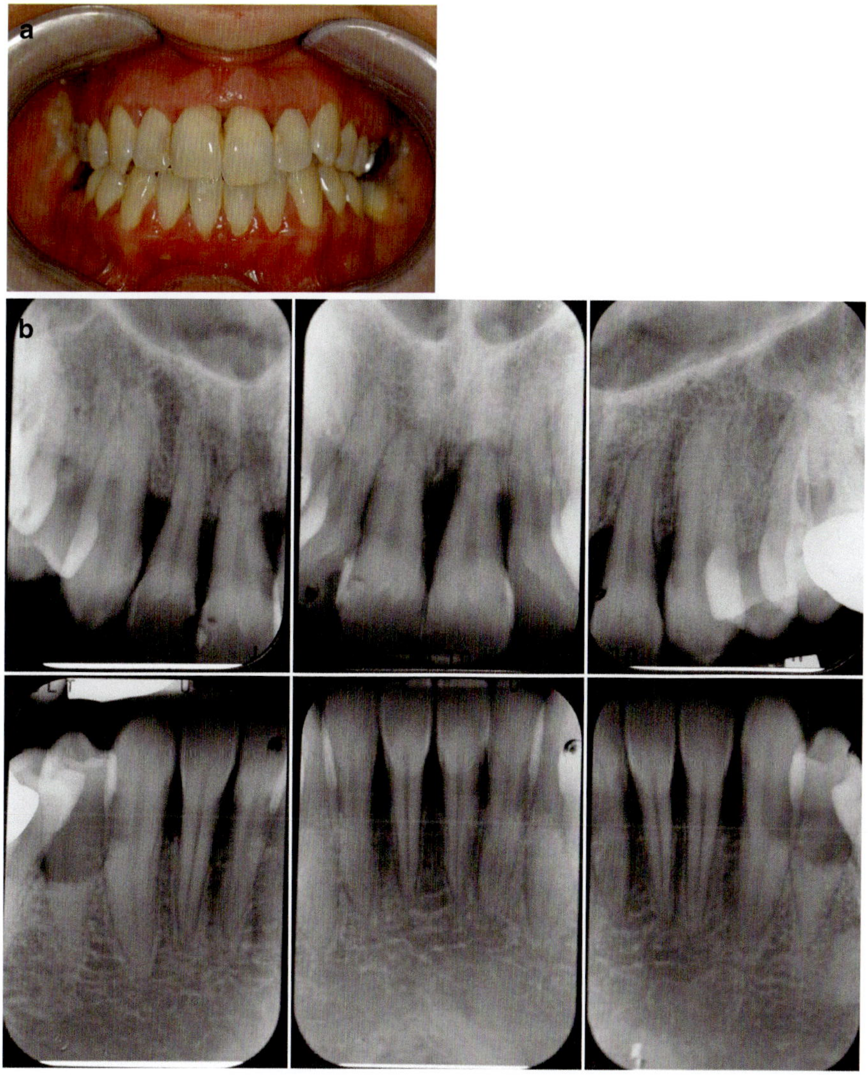

Fig. 10.3 (**a**) Periodontitis clinical aspect of a 30-year-old patient demonstrating severe oedema, loss of attachment and bleeding when probing. (**b**) Periodontitis radiographic aspect of the same patient demonstrating advanced loss of attachment

Peri-implant mucositis is a risk factor for the development of peri-implantitis when not controlled by supportive peri-implant care (SPIC); it should be addressed with appropriate measures. Finally, professional and patient-administered mechanical plaque control was found to be an effective preventive measure; the use of antiseptics, antibiotics in local and systemic forms and air-abrasive devices were also implemented [5]. However, professionally delivered chemical agents and specific mechanical or physical interventions, as adjuncts to submarginal instrumentation,

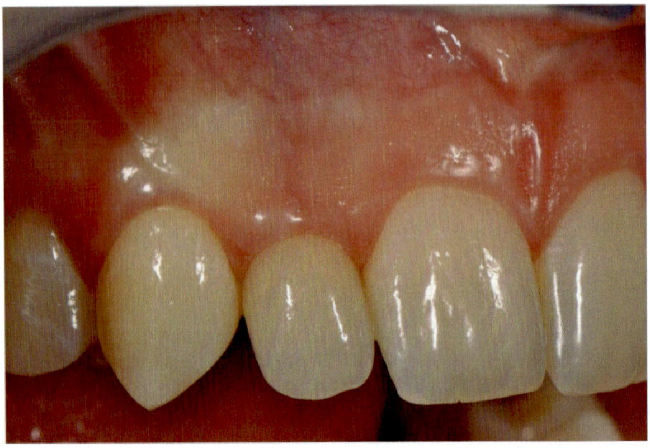

Fig. 10.4 Peri-implant health. Implant-supported restoration site #7 demonstrating absence of bleeding, erythema and oedema

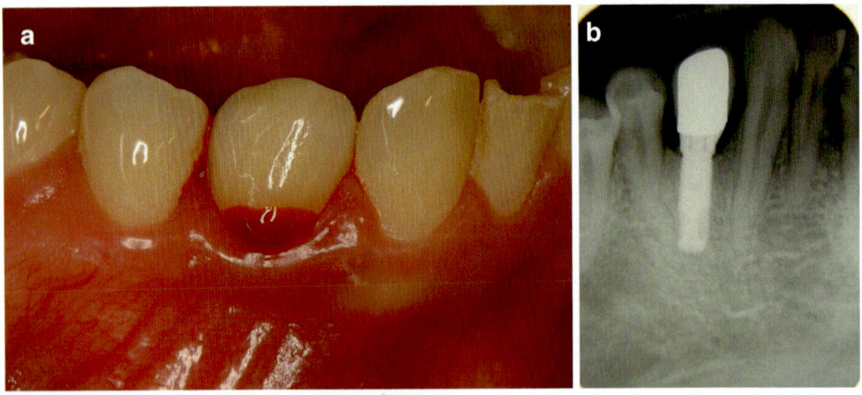

Fig. 10.5 (**a**) Peri-implant mucositis clinical aspect of a 25-year-old patient demonstrating erythema, oedema and bleeding immediately after probing. (**b**) Peri-implant mucositis radiographic aspect of the same 25-year-old patient demonstrating no radiographic loss of attachment as the present bone level is physiologic and related to establishment of biological width

have not proven significant effectiveness in the clinical parameters of peri-implant mucositis [6].

Patient's interventions have proven to provide significant improvements to peri-implant clinical parameters when used in addition to submarginal instrumentation [4, 7]. Finally, interventions to control smoking and diabetes have been demonstrated to improve periodontal health and peri-implant health [8, 9] (Fig. 10.7).

10.3.1 Peri-implantitis vs. Periodontitis

Experimental canine peri-implantitis and periodontitis have been historically compared [10–12]. Experimental peri-implantitis has been found to progress faster than periodontitis at a statistically significant level for marginal bone loss [13]. This

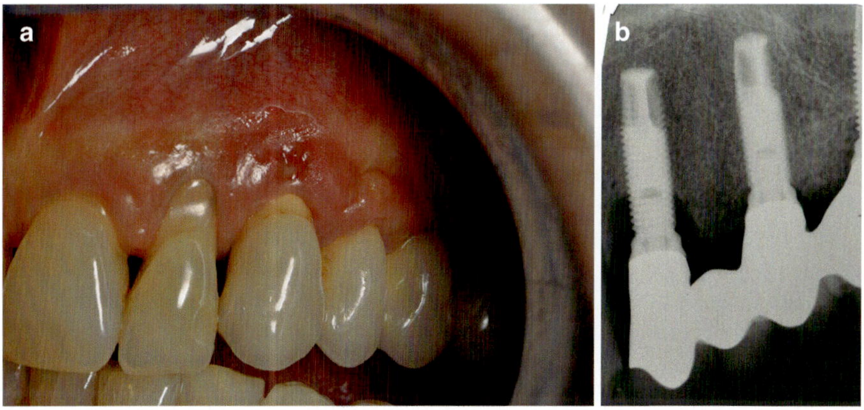

Fig. 10.6 (**a**) Peri-implantitis clinical aspect of a 60-year-old patient with an implant-supported fixed partial denture from 11 to 15, on three implants, 11, 13 and 15, demonstrating severe oedema, loss of attachment, bleeding on probing and a fistula. (**b**) Peri-implantitis radiographic aspect of the same 60-year-old patient with an implant-supported fixed partial denture from 11 to 15, on three implants, 11, 13 and 15, demonstrating loss of attachment on implant 11 indicating peri-implantitis at that site, while no loss of attachment at implant 13

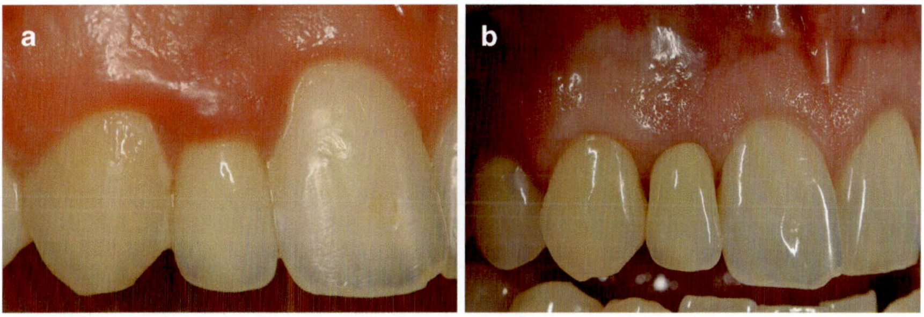

Fig. 10.7 (**a**) Peri-implant mucositis on implant #7 for a 25-year-old patient demonstrating the presence of plaque, erythema and oedema. (**b**) 10 Years post-non-surgical treatment of the same site on the same patient presenting without plaque and with no erythema, no oedema and no bleeding on probing, therefore healthy tissues around the adjacent teeth and implant #7

finding has also been confirmed on humans with an inflammatory lesion found to be twice as large around implants than around teeth, a difference which was statistically significant [14].

10.3.2 Prevalence and Risk Factors for Peri-implantitis

Prevalence and risk factors for peri-implantitis have been evaluated in numerous studies including a national randomized database, various university cohorts and private practices [15–21].

Case definitions vary, but numerous large cohort studies report prevalence of peri-implantitis ranging from 1 to 47% of patients, with meta-analysis-weighted means of 20–22% making it an undeniable clinical reality [22, 23].

In a 10-year retrospective human study, smoking and periodontitis were found to be risk factors for the colonization of periodontal bacterial species, which may play a role in peri-implant inflammation [24].

It was also demonstrated that periodontitis patients presented higher prevalence of peri-implantitis when supportive periodontal therapy was not implemented [25].

Numerous therapeutic approaches have been envisioned to treat peri-implantitis. To mimic the treatment of periodontitis, initial attempts were non-surgical but were found not to be successful [26, 27]. Furthermore, when considering non-surgical procedures, implant surface decontamination or chemical decontamination in addition to subgingival instrumentation is inconclusive at this time [28, 29].

Various antimicrobial adjunctive medications in the non-surgical treatment were also shown to be limited in efficacy except systemic antibiotics in deep sites [30].

Evidences reported above, demonstrate that surgical treatment remains the standard of care for peri-implantitis.

Primary treatment objectives for peri-implantitis are reduction in bleeding on probing and pocket depth, and secondary outcome is gain of marginal bone levels with minimal recessions.

Experts for the XVIII European workshop on Periodontology: Evidence-based guidelines for peri-implant therapy have performed meta-analyses on numerous surgical treatment protocols. Treatments are generally based on access flap and pocket elimination, which were found to reduce probing depths and bleeding on probing and marginally improve marginal bone levels [31].

Studies have compared reconstructive procedures against access flap procedures with similar pocket reduction and bleeding on probing outcomes [31, 32]. A limited four-study meta-analysis has demonstrated slightly more favourable outcomes for marginal bone levels and recessions with reconstructive surgery [32, 33].

Finally, a review of supportive care post-peri-implantitis treatment demonstrated 24–100% of peri-implant tissue stability emphasizing the need for professional care after treatment [34] as demonstrated by stable peri-implantitis treatments in Figs. 10.8 and 10.9 (Tables 10.1, 10.2, 10.3 and 10.4).

10.4 Supportive Peri-implant Care and Supportive Periodontal Therapy (SPT)

Supportive peri-implant care (SPIC) and supportive periodontal therapy (SPT) can be considered the essential monitoring tools to prevent and intercept diseases with the evaluation of patient's level risk factors and their interventions (Tables 10.1 and 10.2) but also local risk factors and their possible interventions (Table 10.3 and 10.4). SPIC and SPT are summarized according to patients' risks levels in Table 10.5.

Low-risk patients who present with low plaque index (25%), high degree of compliance, no local risk factors and no systemic risk factors may receive SPIC or SPT once a year.

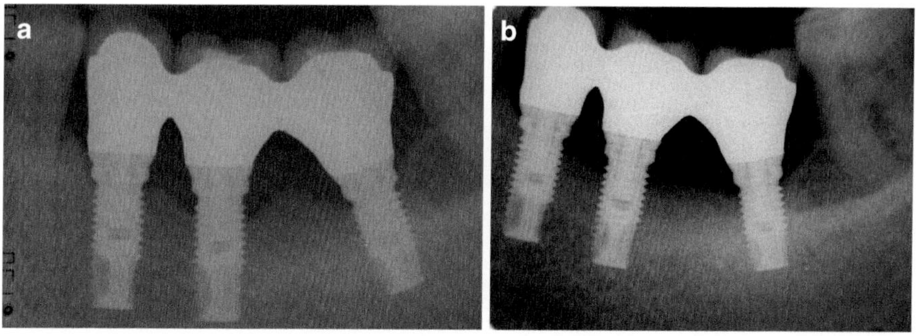

Fig. 10.8 (**a**) Pre-op periapical radiograph prior to access flap osseous recontouring treatment of peri-implantitis. (**b**) 5-Year post-op periapical radiographs. Marginal bone levels remained stable for at least 5 years at all implants

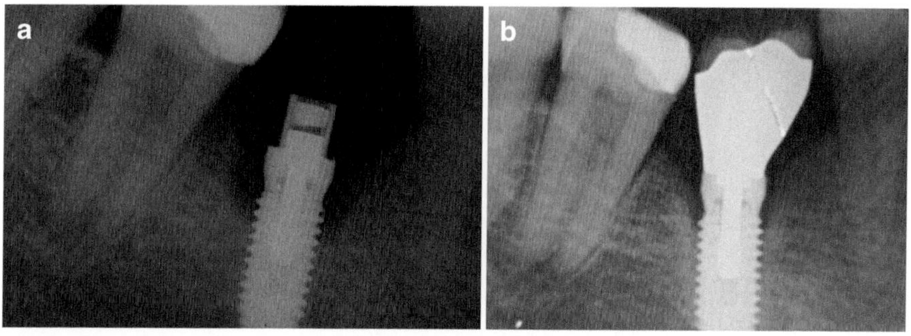

Fig. 10.9 (**a**) Pre-op periapical radiograph prior to regenerative treatment of a peri-implantitis. (**b**) 10-Year post-op periapical radiographs. Regenerative procedure was successful at maintaining marginal bone level gains up to 10 years after the surgical treatment

Medium-risk patients who present with uncontrolled plaque and bleeding indexes >25%, irregular compliance, one local risk factor and one systemic risk factor could be seen every 6 months for SPIC and/or SPT.

High-risk patients who present with inadequate oral hygiene >25%, several local risk factors and several systemic risk factors should be seen every 3–4 months.

When BOP becomes positive and pocket depth increases >6 mm, indicating a peri-implant mucositis, a periapical radiograph should be taken to evaluate marginal bone level and diagnose or rule out peri-implantitis.

Interventions guidelines according to the various peri-implant tissues diagnosis are summarized in Table 10.6.

10.5 Delaying Implant Placement (DIP)

Preventive interventions in a population can reduce all oral health pathologies, from loss of attachment to caries and edentulism, and increase the lifespan of natural dentitions in all age groups [35]. Prevention-oriented patient-centred care is core to the ideal of equating teeth lifespan to patient's lifespan. In this context, providers

Table 10.1 Patient risk factors for peri-implant health

Patient factors affecting long-term peri-implant health						
Local risk factors			Systemic risk factors			
Plaque control	Bleeding index	SPIC compliance	History of periodontal disease	Four or more implants	Smoking	Diabetes

Table 10.2 Interventions on risk factors

Interventions on patient factors to improve long-term peri-implant health					
Intervention on local risk factors			Systemic risk factors		
Patient education	Improve oral hygiene	Lower PI and BI	Periodontal supportive therapy	Smoking cessation	Glycaemic control

may sequence dental interventions, from least invasive, prevention, to most invasive, extractions, to prolong the natural dentition's lifespan and its function for as long as possible.

"Delaying implant placement" (DIP) proposes to utilize dental implants as late as possible in the life of the patient. A critical objective here is to delay peri-implant mucositis, peri-implantitis and management of these complications. High-periodontal-risk individuals, especially younger ones will benefit most from this prevention-centered approach. Furthermore, the ankylotic nature of implants seems to be an essential factor in the occurrence of inter-proximal contact openings between natural teeth and implants, which seem to be also associated with peri-implant mucositis, peri-implantitis and secondary caries [36, 37].

DIP as a concept hopes to lengthen lifespans of dentitions that may incorporate both teeth and implants; patients and practitioners both should make an effort toward preventive care of periodontal and peri-implant diseases. Studies have demonstrated that implants delivered to the elderly population are similarly successful to younger populations. However, with the long-term data that is available, patients who are susceptible to periodontal disease are also prone to developing peri-implant disease; as stated earlier in this chapter, control of the peri-implant disease is more difficult than managing periodontal disease. This susceptibility should be understood, and as populations live longer, proper care and management of the natural dentition can delay the placement of implants which will extend the function and aesthetics of the dentition and contribute to the quality of life [38, 39].

Globally, increasing populations have access to dental implants, patients' lifespan increases, dental trauma is still prevalent, occlusal stability is a critical factor of oral rehabilitations, disease control is unevenly distributed in populations and the need for complex oral rehabilitations does leave ample growth and space for dental implants to remain essential in our armamentarium.

Table 10.3 Local risk factors to consider

Local factors affecting long-term peri-implant health					
Inadequate access to oral hygiene			Abutment implant connection		
Over-contours	Excess cement	Absence of keratinized mucosa	Poor fit	Short abutments	Materials other than titanium

Table 10.4 Interventions on local risk factors

Corrections of local factors affecting long-term peri-implant health					
Inadequate access to oral hygiene			Abutment implant connection		
Educate patient and eliminate over-contours	Use screw-retained reconstructions	Surgically improve mucosal thickness if possible	Use machined titanium components	Use 2 mm abutments	Use only materials and procedures recommended by the manufacturers

Table 10.5 SPIC and patient risk levels

SPIC and/or SPT frequency according to risk levels: low risk–medium risk–high risk					
Low-risk patients	Frequency	Medium-risk patients	Frequency	High-risk patients	Frequency
No systemic risk factor No local risk factor PI BI <25% Good compliance	Once a year	One systemic risk factor No local risk factor PI BI >25% Irregular compliance	Every 6 months	Two or more systemic risk factors One or more local risk factor PI BI >25% Poor compliance	Every 3–4 months

10.6 Conclusion

Ubiquitous dental implant utilizations in the past four decades have provided ample success, yet clinicians should propose a novel approach to health and diseases around these implants. Practitioners and patients must be cognizant of existing and future challenges associated with the host's immune response specially at implants.

Our objectives were to define health and diseases around implants but also to relate these pathologies to periodontal disease which is already well known and for which treatment protocols are established. Furthermore, we wanted to establish the preventive concept of delaying implant placement in the patient's life.

We have established the parallel in clinical diagnoses, monitoring and treatment of inflammatory lesions around teeth and implants. Similitudes should not blind us on the fact that peri-implantitis seems more aggressive than periodontitis and that non-surgical treatment's efficacy is poor. Furthermore, the history of periodontitis is a clear risk factor to peri-implantitis. It is evident that the host is central to the clinical picture of any biofilm-mediated immune response. For these reasons, one can understand that extracting teeth in a patient with high periodontal risk level will not

Table 10.6 Summary guidelines of interventions based on diagnosis

SPIC according to peri-implant diagnosis: health–mucositis–peri-implantitis				
Health	Supra- and sub-marginal biofilm removal	Non-surgical sub-marginal instrumentation	Surgical procedures	Secondary prevention
Primary prevention of peri-implant mucositis BI and PI Oral hygiene instructions	**Yes** **Professional mechanical plaque removal (PMPR)**	No	No	No
Peri-implant mucositis	**Supra- and sub-marginal biofilm removal**	**Non-surgical sub-marginal instrumentation**	**Surgical procedures**	**Secondary prevention**
Mucositis treatment Primary prevention of peri-implantitis BI, PI Specific oral hygiene instructions	**Yes** **PMPR** Possible professional adjunctive therapies Possible home adjunctive therapies	**Yes if tissues allow access**	No	**Yes to maintain peri-implant health post-treatment** **To prevent peri-implantitis**
Peri-implantitis	**Supra- and sub-marginal biofilm removal**	**Non-surgical sub-marginal instrumentation**	**Surgical procedures**	**Secondary prevention**
Peri-implantitis treatment BI, PI Specific oral hygiene instructions	Yes PMPR For initial treatment To prepare for surgery	Yes Use of adjunctive therapies if possible To prepare for surgery	Yes Access flap/resective/regenerative procedures Adjunctive therapies if possible	Yes to maintain peri-implant health post-treatment

eliminate its susceptibility. In fact, implants will provide an ideal biofilm substrate for the most susceptible hosts to respond in a more pathogenic fashion.

The concept of delaying implant placement in patients which are highly susceptible to periodontal disease could provide the following advantages: It would override the idea that extracting the teeth will solve all the patients' dental problems. It would allow further evaluation of patient motivation and compliance and to improve patient education. It would push further in the patient's life the moment of implant installation and therefore implant complications which are time dependent. It would strengthen the decision of extracting the teeth when the time finally comes.

References

1. Chapple ILC, Mealey BL, Van Dyke TE, et al. Periodontal health and gingival diseases and conditions on an intact and a reduced periodontium: consensus report of workgroup 1 of the 2017 World Workshop on the Classification of Periodontal and Peri-Implant Diseases and Conditions. J Clin Periodontol. 2018;45(Suppl 20):S68–77.
2. Berglundh T, Armitage G, Araujo MG, et al. Peri-implant diseases and conditions: consensus report of workgroup 4 of the 2017 World Workshop on the Classification of Periodontal and Peri-Implant Diseases and Conditions. J Clin Periodontol. 2018;45(Suppl 20):S286–91.
3. Salvi GE, Aglietta M, Eick S, Sculean A, Lang NP, Ramseier CA. Reversibility of experimental peri-implant mucositis compared with experimental gingivitis in humans. Clin Oral Implants Res. 2012;23:182–90.
4. Salvi GE, Ramseier CA. Efficacy of patient-administered mechanical and/or chemical plaque control protocols in the management of peri-implant mucositis. A systematic review. J Clin Periodontol. 2015;42(Suppl 16):S187–201.
5. Jepsen S, Berglundh T, Genco R, et al. Primary prevention of peri-implantitis: managing peri-implant mucositis. J Clin Periodontol. 2015;42(Suppl 16):S152–7.
6. Dommisch H, Hoedke D, Valles C, Vilarrasa J, Jepsen S, Pascual La Rocca A. Efficacy of professionally administered chemical agents as an adjunctive treatment to sub-marginal instrumentation during the therapy of peri-implant mucositis. J Clin Periodontol. 2022;50:146–60. https://doi.org/10.1111/jcpe.13747.
7. Gennai S, Bollain J, Ambrosio N, Marruganti C, Graziani F, Figuero E. Efficacy of adjunctive measures in peri-implant mucositis. A systematic review and meta-analysis. J Clin Periodontol. 2023;50(Suppl 26):161–87.
8. Ramseier CA, Woelber JP, Kitzmann J, Detzen L, Carra MC, Bouchard P. Impact of risk factor control interventions for smoking cessation and promotion of healthy lifestyles in patients with periodontitis: a systematic review. J Clin Periodontol. 2020;47(Suppl 22):90–106.
9. Carra MC, Blanc-Sylvestre N, Courtet A, Bouchard P. Primordial and primary prevention of peri-implant diseases: a systematic review and meta-analysis. J Clin Periodontol. 2023;50:77–112. https://doi.org/10.1111/jcpe.13790.
10. Lindhe J, Berglundh T, Ericsson I, Liljenberg B, Marinello C. Experimental breakdown of peri-implant and periodontal tissues. A study in the beagle dog. Clin Oral Implants Res. 1992;3:9–16.
11. Berglundh T, Lindhe J, Marinello C, Ericsson I, Liljenberg B. Soft tissue reaction to de novo plaque formation on implants and teeth. An experimental study in the dog. Clin Oral Implants Res. 1992;3:1–8.
12. Ericsson I, Berglundh T, Marinello C, Liljenberg B, Lindhe J. Long-standing plaque and gingivitis at implants and teeth in the dog. Clin Oral Implants Res. 1992;3:99–103.
13. Carcuac O, Abrahamsson I, Albouy J-P, Linder E, Larsson L, Berglundh T. Experimental periodontitis and peri-implantitis in dogs. Clin Oral Implants Res. 2013;24:363–71.
14. Carcuac O, Berglundh T. Composition of human peri-implantitis and periodontitis lesions. J Dent Res. 2014;93:1083–8.
15. Fransson C, Lekholm U, Jemt T, Berglundh T. Prevalence of subjects with progressive bone loss at implants. Clin Oral Implants Res. 2005;16:440–6.
16. Derks J, Schaller D, Håkansson J, Wennström JL, Tomasi C, Berglundh T. Effectiveness of implant therapy analyzed in a Swedish population: prevalence of peri-implantitis. J Dent Res. 2016;95:43–9.
17. Vignoletti F, Di Domenico GL, Di Martino M, Montero E, de Sanctis M. Prevalence and risk indicators of peri-implantitis in a sample of university-based dental patients in Italy: a cross-sectional study. J Clin Periodontol. 2019;46:597–605.
18. Romandini M, Lima C, Pedrinaci I, Araoz A, Soldini MC, Sanz M. Prevalence and risk/protective indicators of peri-implant diseases: a university-representative cross-sectional study. Clin Oral Implants Res. 2021;32:112–22.

19. Romandini M, Pedrinaci I, Lima C, Soldini MC, Araoz A, Sanz M. Prevalence and risk/protective indicators of buccal soft tissue dehiscence around dental implants. J Clin Periodontol. 2021;48:455–63.
20. Koldsland OC, Scheie AA, Aass AM. Prevalence of peri-implantitis related to severity of the disease with different degrees of bone loss. J Periodontol. 2010;81:231–8.
21. Mir-Mari J, Mir-Orfila P, Figueiredo R, Valmaseda-Castellón E, Gay-Escoda C. Prevalence of peri-implant diseases. A cross-sectional study based on a private practice environment. J Clin Periodontol. 2012;39:490–4.
22. Mombelli A, Müller N, Cionca N. The epidemiology of peri-implantitis. Clin Oral Implants Res. 2012;23(Suppl 6):67–76.
23. Derks J, Tomasi C. Peri-implant health and disease. A systematic review of current epidemiology. J Clin Periodontol. 2015;42(Suppl 16):S158–71.
24. Eick S, Ramseier CA, Rothenberger K, Brägger U, Buser D, Salvi GE. Microbiota at teeth and implants in partially edentulous patients. A 10-year retrospective study. Clin Oral Implants Res. 2016;27:218–25.
25. Pjetursson BE, Helbling C, Weber H-P, et al. Peri-implantitis susceptibility as it relates to periodontal therapy and supportive care. Clin Oral Implants Res. 2012;23:888–94.
26. Renvert S, Samuelsson E, Lindahl C, Persson GR. Mechanical non-surgical treatment of peri-implantitis: a double-blind randomized longitudinal clinical study. I: Clinical results. J Clin Periodontol. 2009;36:604–9.
27. Persson GR, Samuelsson E, Lindahl C, Renvert S. Mechanical non-surgical treatment of peri-implantitis: a single-blinded randomized longitudinal clinical study. II. Microbiological results. J Clin Periodontol. 2010;37:563–73.
28. Cosgarea R, Roccuzzo A, Jepsen K, Sculean A, Jepsen S, Salvi GE. Efficacy of mechanical/physical approaches for implant surface decontamination in non-surgical submarginal instrumentation of peri-implantitis. A systematic review. J Clin Periodontol. 2022;50:188–211. https://doi.org/10.1111/jcpe.13762.
29. de Waal YCM, Winning L, Stavropoulos A, Polyzois I. Efficacy of chemical approaches for implant surface decontamination in conjunction with sub-marginal instrumentation, in the non-surgical treatment of peri-implantitis: a systematic review. J Clin Periodontol. 2023;50(Suppl 26):212–23.
30. Liñares A, Sanz-Sánchez I, Dopico J, Molina A, Blanco J, Montero E. Efficacy of adjunctive measures in the non-surgical treatment of peri-implantitis: a systematic review. J Clin Periodontol. 2023;50(Suppl 26):224–43.
31. Karlsson K, Trullenque-Eriksson A, Tomasi C, Derks J. Efficacy of access flap and pocket elimination procedures in the management of peri-implantitis: a systematic review and meta-analysis. J Clin Periodontol. 2023;50(Suppl 26):244–84.
32. Derks J, Ortiz-Vigón A, Guerrero A, et al. Reconstructive surgical therapy of peri-implantitis: a multicenter randomized controlled clinical trial. Clin Oral Implants Res. 2022;33:921–44.
33. Donos N, Calciolari E, Ghuman M, Baccini M, Sousa V, Nibali L. The efficacy of bone reconstructive therapies in the management of peri-implantitis. A systematic review and meta-analysis. J Clin Periodontol. 2023;50:285–316. https://doi.org/10.1111/jcpe.13775.
34. Stiesch M, Grischke J, Schaefer P, Heitz-Mayfield LJA. Supportive care for the prevention of disease recurrence/progression following peri-implantitis treatment: a systematic review. J Clin Periodontol. 2023;50(Suppl 26):113–34.
35. Hugoson A, Koch G, Göthberg C, et al. Oral health of individuals aged 3–80 years in Jönköping, Sweden during 30 years (1973–2003). II. Review of clinical and radiographic findings. Swed Dent J. 2005;29:139–55.
36. Sheba M, Floriani F, Nimmo A, Ercoli C, Hosney S. Interproximal contact loss between implant restorations and adjacent natural teeth: a systematic review and meta-analysis. J Prosthodont. 2024;33:313–23.
37. Latimer JM, Gharpure AS, Kahng HJ, Aljofi FE, Daubert DM. Interproximal open contacts between implant restorations and adjacent natural teeth as a risk-indicator for peri-implant disease—a cross-sectional study. Clin Oral Implants Res. 2021;32:598–607.

38. Engfors I, Ortorp A, Jemt T. Fixed implant-supported prostheses in elderly patients: a 5-year retrospective study of 133 edentulous patients older than 79 years. Clin Implant Dent Relat Res. 2004;6:190–8.
39. de Baat C. Success of dental implants in elderly people—a literature review. Gerodontology. 2000;17:45–8.

11 Transitioning Patients from a Failing Dentition to Implant-Supported Restorations

Cheryl Park, Saj Jivraj, and Winston Chee

Today's patients have high expectations regarding aesthetics, and providing functional restorations alone may not be sufficient to satisfy many of them. With heightened aesthetic expectations, it becomes imperative that the restorative dentist understand the patient's desires and expectations prior to embarking upon any irreversible therapy. Moreover, emphasis should be placed on diagnosis and treatment planning because in most situations the proper diagnosis will dictate the appropriate treatment plan. Inadequately planned treatment and inadequately informed patients, even when well executed, will result in less-than-ideal treatment satisfaction.

The functional and aesthetic replacement of missing teeth with dental implants remains a complex task under most conditions. With comprehensive treatment planning and proper surgical and restorative protocols, more predictable results can be achieved. With this in mind, transitioning a patient from teeth- to implant-supported restorations becomes even more difficult as precise planning will now include timing of extractions, method of retaining fixed provisional restorations, manipulation of remaining teeth to enhance implant receptor sites and many other issues. Patient's preference is almost always to have a fixed prosthesis during this transition. The rationale for fixed transitional prostheses suits both the patient and the clinician.

C. Park (✉) · W. Chee
Advanced Prosthodontics, Herman Ostrow School of Dentistry, University of Southern California, Los Angeles, CA, USA

S. Jivraj
Private Practice, Anacapa Dental Art Institute, Oxnard, CA, USA

W. Chee, S. Jivraj (eds.), *Treatment Planning In Implant Dentistry*, BDJ Clinician's Guides, https://doi.org/10.1007/978-3-031-68726-6_11

Patient management with a fixed prosthesis has the advantages of elimination of the discomfort experienced with a removable prosthesis due to impingement of the mucosa, psychological advantage of having a fixed restoration during integration of the implants, preventing transmucosal loading of the implants and not interfering with any grafting procedures. The clinician also benefits by decreased chair time, unscheduled visits and reduced maintenance of the provisional prosthesis.

One disadvantage of using a fixed prosthesis in transition is the additional cost involved. However, in patients embarking upon already costly and lengthy therapy, the additional cost for comfort and convenience outweighs the social embarrassment of wearing a removable prosthesis.

The practitioner should consider the following questions in determining the choice of interim prosthesis for the patient:

1. Which choices of interim prostheses does the given situation allow?
2. Does the chosen method of interim prosthesis meet the patient's aesthetic and functional expectations?
3. Does this method of interim prosthesis give the clinician and the surgeon flexibility in modification throughout the implant treatment?
4. Is the method of interim prosthesis favourable for allowing the most optimal healing conditions for the hard and soft tissue grafts as well as the implant?
5. Does the method of interim prosthesis facilitate ease of transitioning to the definitive restoration?
6. Does the method of interim prosthesis facilitate transferring any references toward the definitive phase of treatment?

When answering question #1 above, the clinical scenario may include compromised teeth that may limit the choice of a fixed interim prosthesis. Another cofactor to consider when deciding which teeth to maintain for support and retention of the interim prosthesis is whether the remaining teeth will positionally occupy optimal implant positions. If the tooth positions interfere with optimal implant placement, the fixed tooth-supported interim option may not be viable since the less-than-ideal implant position may have long-term repercussions. In this scenario, if clinical circumstances allow, thought should be given to immediate loading. This strategy will provide ideal implant positioning as well as a fixed transitional prosthesis. If immediate loading is not a consideration and ideal implant positioning is not possible with the existing teeth, alternative methods of provisionalization must be discussed and understood by the patient. The patient and clinician must understand that all clinical situations cannot be transitioned in a fixed provisional restoration.

With these considerations in mind, there are several different approaches to the interim prosthesis options when transitioning a failing dentition to implant-supported restorations. Following are the interim prosthesis methods that will be discussed:

1. Removable prostheses (interim partial denture, immediate complete denture, Essix retainer)

2. Bonded interim options (resin-bonded FPD, orthodontic retainer with attached pontic)
3. Interim fixed partial denture (FPD using strategic abutments)
4. Provisional implants (to retain an overdenture or to support an interim fixed partial denture)
5. Immediately loaded implant-supported interim prosthesis
6. No interim prosthesis

11.1 Removable Interim Options

Removable interim prostheses such as complete dentures or interim resin partial dentures are options in transitioning a failing dentition to an implant-supported restorations. Some benefits to the removable options are the ease of interim prosthesis insertion, removal and modifications such as relines [1]. Conversely, removable options come with a number of drawbacks such as mucosal coverage, tissue discomfort or inflammation, inadequate or reduced retention, speech impediment, poor retention and inadequate aesthetics or patient dissatisfaction [2–4]. Thus, when clinicians consider these major drawbacks with the removable prostheses, the fixed interim prosthesis as a transitional restoration becomes more appealing to both the clinician and the patient.

This patient presentation in Fig. 11.1 illustrates the value of a removable provisional in treatment planning. This 28-year-old female presented with congenitally missing lateral incisors. These edentulous spaces had been restored previously with resin-bonded fixed partial dentures, which had not provided a successful outcome. The patient also felt that the maxillary central incisors were narrow and requested a more dominant appearance.

Clinical and radiographic examination indicated a number of issues which could be corrected to improve the overall aesthetics. These included relative tooth dimensions, prosthetic replacement of the lateral incisors, colour and smile symmetry. To confirm that the analysis matched the perceptions of the patient, a diagnostic wax pattern was formed, and an acrylic resin template of the wax pattern fabricated. This template served to communicate the desired result to the patient. Approval from the patient was sought and obtained, and then the treatment plan was formulated and put into action. Radiographic examination also revealed inadequate inter-radicular space for placement of the implants without damaging the adjacent teeth, and computed tomography revealed inadequate bucco-lingual osseous dimensions for insertion of implants (Fig. 11.1b, c).

A treatment plan was formulated which included communication between the orthodontist, surgeon and prosthodontist. The first phase of treatment included orthodontic therapy to provide sufficient inter-radicular place for the placement of implants (Fig. 11.1d). It was communicated to the patient that following orthodontic therapy, the incisal edges of teeth #8 and #9 (maxillary right central and left central incisors) would be irregular and as a result would require restoration. From a practical perspective while orthodontics was being completed, an interim removable

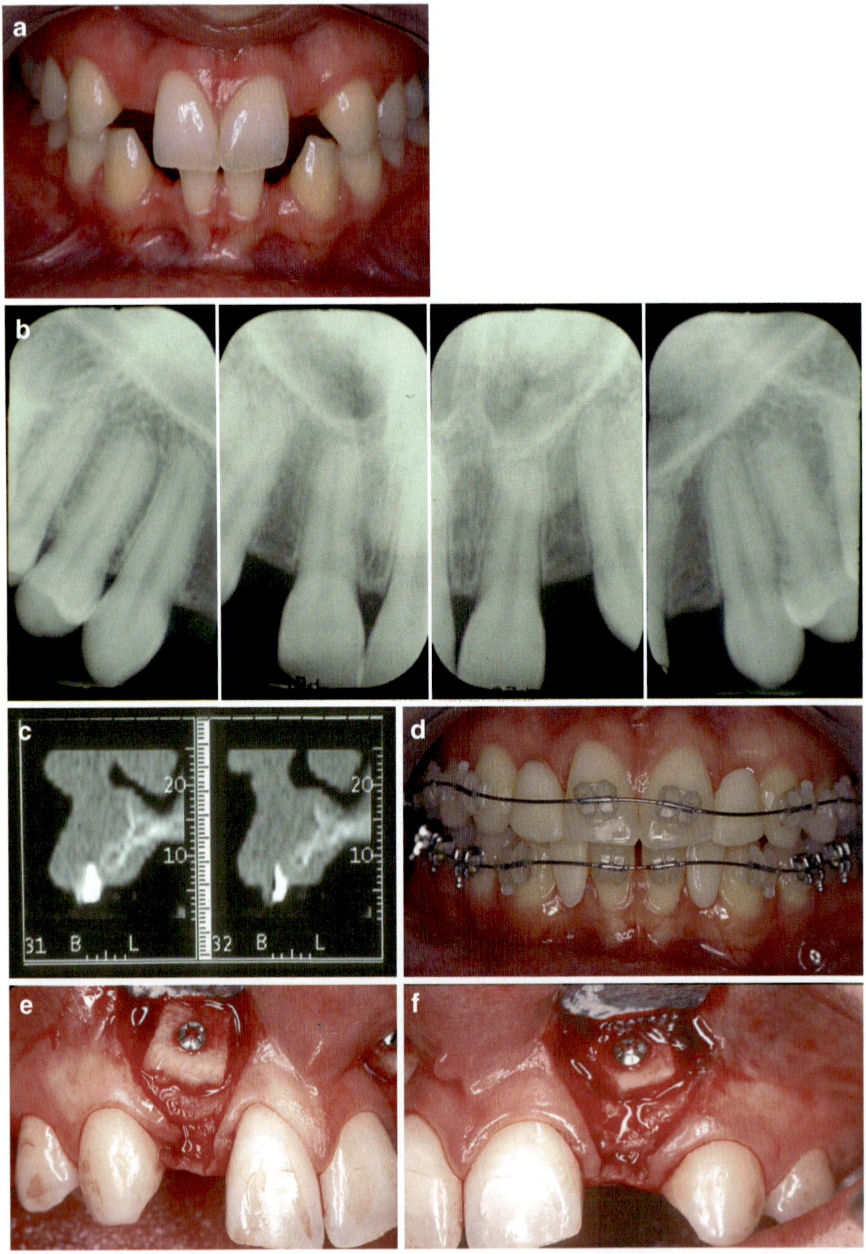

Fig. 11.1 (**a**) Anterior view of congenitally missing maxillary lateral incisors. (**b**) Radiographs indicated insufficient space for implant placement. (**c**) Sagittal view of computed tomography showing insufficient bone to accept implants. (**d**) Anterior view of removable prostheses while orthodontic tooth movement progresses. (**e**, **f**) Block grafts are placed to accommodate implant placement. (**g**, **h**) Definitive restorations are completed

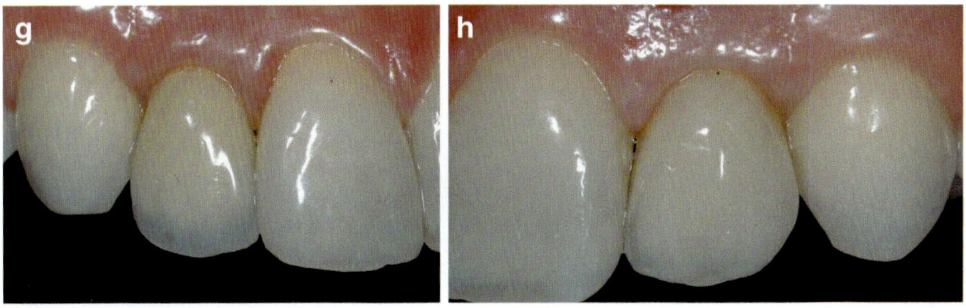

Fig. 11.1 (continued)

partial denture was provided. This allowed the orthodontist to shape the proportions of the teeth to align with the restorative plan. A removable restoration in this regard is convenient to use and easy to insert and remove and allows the orthodontist to physically measure the mesiodistal spaces. Following orthodontic therapy, an autogenous bone graft was performed to restore the osseous volume in the regions of teeth #7 and #10 (maxillary lateral incisors). Bone was harvested from the mandibular symphysis (Fig. 11.1e, f).

To attain the optimal morphology of the prosthetic restorations, accurate three-dimensional positioning of the implant fixtures is critical. A diagnostic wax-up was completed and used to fabricate a surgical template which served to communicate the implant position to the surgeon. The mesiodistal positioning of the implant required at least 1.5 mm of clearance from the adjacent teeth. This clearance was necessary to develop and maintain the integrity of the papilla. Bucco-lingually, the implants were placed for screw-retained restorations with the screw access holes emerging from the cingulum of the definitive restorations. Apico-coronally, the fixtures were placed 3 mm apical to the adjacent CEJ; this allowed for adequate transition from the cross section of the implant to the natural contours of the replacement tooth. An implant-level impression was obtained immediately after implant insertion. This impression was used to fabricate provisional restorations which were delivered after uncovering the implant (at stage II) to develop appropriate soft tissue contours.

After preparation of the maxillary central incisors for porcelain veneers, the implant provisional restorations were used as impression copings and incorporated into the impression. A soft tissue cast poured was against the provisional restoration to provide a good replication of soft tissue (see Chap. 5). Provisional restorations were provided for the patient, and definitive restorations were fabricated (Fig. 11.1g, h).

The definitive restorations satisfied the functional and aesthetic goal of treatment. This was a result of coordinated efforts between the surgeon, orthodontist, prosthodontist and laboratory technician. Restoration of tooth position and optimal bone volume was essential to ensure that only minor adjustments were required at the time of implant placement. Careful observation of the chronology of treatment

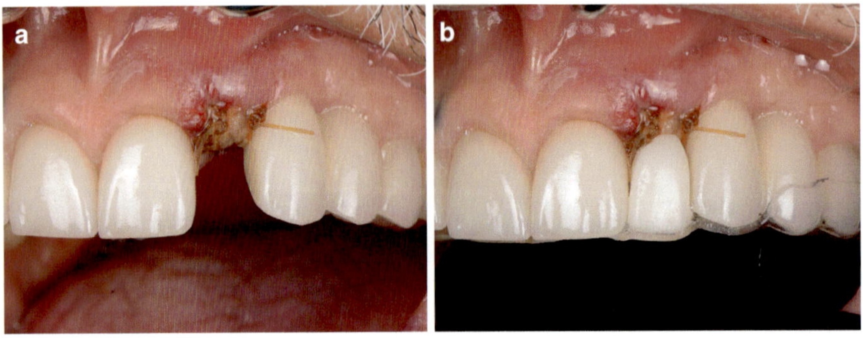

Fig. 11.2 (**a**) Maxillary left lateral incisor extracted due to failing dentition. (**b**) Modified Essix retainer design using PMMA pontic tooth and minimal Essix retainer coverage over aesthetic area

stages and constant communication between the allied specialists ensured an optimal aesthetic and functional outcome (Fig. 11.1a–h).

The Essix retainer is a clear plastic device that fits over teeth and can be removed when needed; when teeth are missing, tooth-coloured acrylic can be attached to the clear plastic. While Essix retainers may not be as aesthetic or functional as compared to interim fixed partial dentures, it is a useful method to replace missing dentition to provide aesthetics. This type of restoration avoids drawbacks such as mucosal coverage, tissue discomfort or inflammation, inadequate retention, reduced function and impeding speech that presents with interim partial dentures. Essix retainers have advantages such as ease of fabrication, provision of aesthetics and no mucosal coverage and are often well accepted by patients [5–7]. Figure 11.2a, b shows extracted tooth #10 (maxillary left lateral incisor) and a modified Essix retainer design with pontic #10 made of polymethyl methacrylate (PMMA) and minimal facial coverage of the clear plastic in the aesthetic area. This modified design may be readily accepted by patients due to better aesthetics than the traditional Essix design.

11.2 Bonded Interim Options

Bonded restorations have allowed the clinician to develop a plethora of techniques that allow fixed transitional restorations during implant therapy. The literature is quite clear in that resin-bonded fixed partial dentures (FPDs) have achieved clinical success over time and there are indications for their use as definitive restorations [1, 8, 9]. Resin-bonded FPDs have also been an option for replacement of missing teeth in growing adolescent patients or when implant restorations are contraindicated [10, 11]. During implant treatment, interim resin-bonded FPDs may be fabricated by using polymethyl methacrylate or composite resin on a base metal substructure. When treatment planning implant-supported restorations, adhesively retained FPDs are a useful tool. They can be bonded to a single abutment tooth. Advantages are that the implant is not loaded, the patient has the convenience of a fixed prosthesis and no tooth structure is removed from the abutment tooth. As with any other options of interim prosthesis, resin-bonded FPDs have several limitations. Resin-bonded FPDs are retained by bonding to the lingual surface of the adjacent tooth, and this can create an inconvenience when removal and reinsertion are needed to facilitate surgical phases of the patient treatment. For example, the interim resin-bonded bridge must be removed to facilitate surgical implant placement and replaced after implant placement by the clinician. When implant placement is coordinated with a surgical specialist, the timing of removal and replacement of the interim resin-bonded restoration can be a problematic issue that can become a drawback to this choice of interim prosthesis.

The following example will illustrate the utility of resin-bonded FPDs used as a transitional restoration. Patient presented with mobile mandibular central deciduous incisors and was seeking an implant-supported solution. On clinical and radiographic examination, it was deemed that these teeth were of poor prognosis and treatment was planned for implant-supported restorations. The patient's request was to be transitioned in fixed restorations. On clinical evaluation, immediate restoration at the time of placement was ruled out as an option. Use of conventional FPDs in preparing adjacent teeth as abutments was also ruled out since the adjacent teeth were sound and restoration free. A resin-bonded base metal FPD with acrylic employing two wings was selected. The rational for this type of provisional was that it was easily removed and replaced and strong enough to withstand the forces of mastication. Conventional impressions were made, and a resin-bonded FPD was fabricated in the laboratory. On the day of surgery, the teeth were removed, dental implants were placed and simultaneous grafting was performed. The interim resin-bonded FPD was delivered utilizing a resin luting agent 24 h post-surgery. The implants were allowed to heal. Impressions were made of the integrated implants to fabricate acrylic provisionals to sculpt the tissue. Once the patient was satisfied with the aesthetics, the soft tissue information was transferred to the laboratory and definitive screw-retained zirconia restoration was fabricated (Fig. 11.3a–j).

Teeth may also be attached via an orthodontic wire if the patient has had the tooth extruded for implant site development or is currently going through orthodontics (Fig. 11.4). The prosthetic tooth can provide minimal compression to surgical areas. The clinician must provide an anti-rotational element to keep the pontic stable. These types of interim restorations are only options in particular clinical presentations having no more than one or two missing teeth in the anterior region [12–14]. Similar drawbacks exist when retaining pontic teeth for missing dentition with orthodontic wires on brackets. The wires and pontic attached to the orthodontic brackets must be removed each time as access is required to the edentulous ridge to facilitate treatment of the implant site [15, 16].

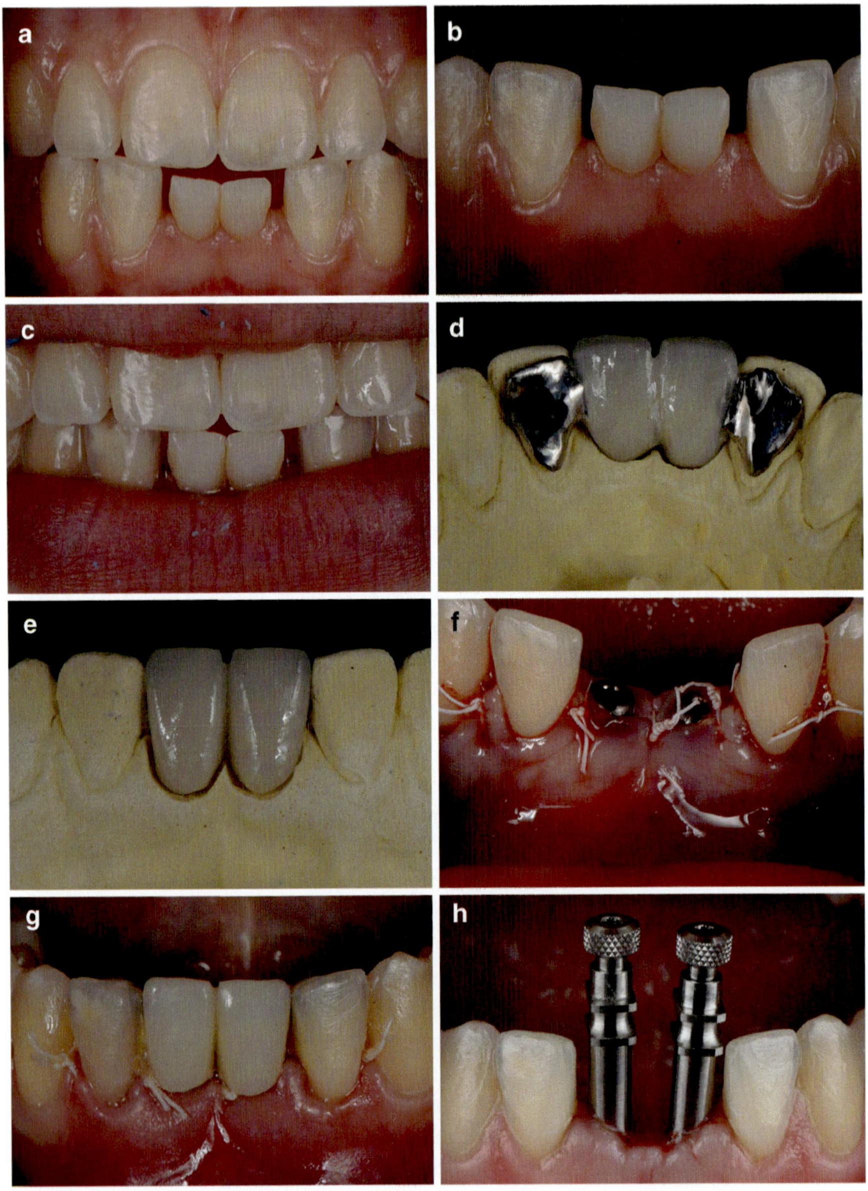

Fig. 11.3 (**a**) Patient presented with mobile deciduous mandibular central incisors. (**b**) Deciduous mandibular central incisors showing mesiodistal spacing. (**c**) Smile view. (**d**) Base metal resin-bonded bridge was fabricated as a provisional. (**e**) Resin-bonded bridge used to delineate the depth of implant placement. (**f**) Implant placement and soft tissue grafting performed. (**g**) Resin-bonded bridge bonded. No contact with healing abutments. (**h**) Impressions of integrated implants. (**i**) Polymethylmethacrylate provisionals to sculpt gingiva. (**j**) Definitive zirconia screw-retained restorations

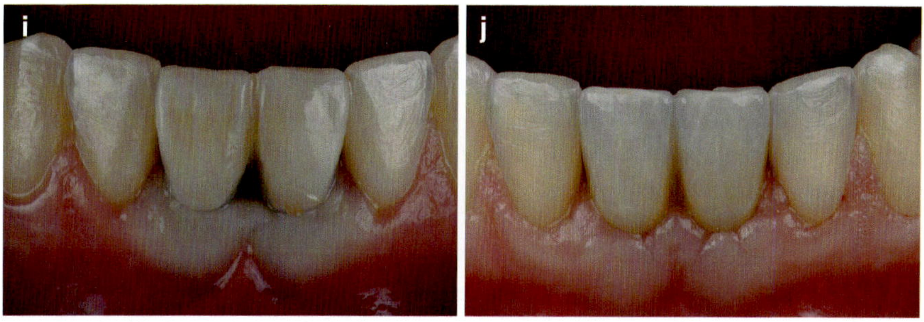

Fig. 11.3 (continued)

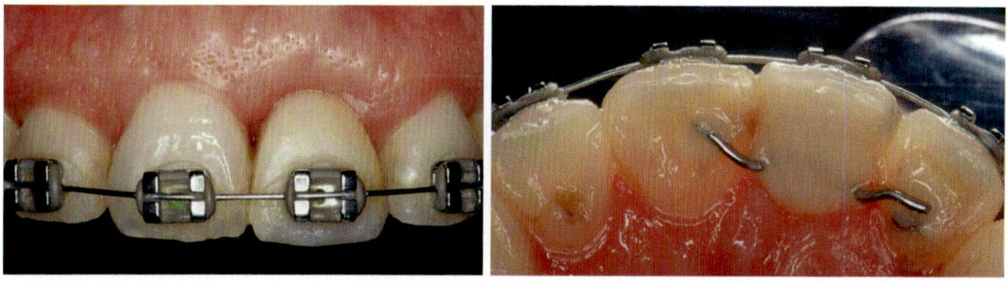

Fig. 11.4 Prosthetic tooth attached to orthodontic brackets in the region of #21. (Photo courtesy of Dr. Alex Chung)

11.3 Use of Strategic Abutments for Interim Fixed Partial Dentures (FPDs)

When there is an opportunity for planning a tooth-borne fixed partial denture as an interim prosthesis, it is considered the most aesthetically and functionally sound option for meeting the patient's expectations together with facilitating implant treatment. In most cases, the tooth-borne transitional fixed partial denture provides the clinician with flexibility in modification such as adding or removing from the apical surface of the pontic to facilitate minimal pressure post-surgery or to add material to the apical areas of the pontics to minimize the gap during the soft tissue healing throughout implant treatment [17–20]. However, there are drawbacks such as the higher biologic cost of preparing the abutment teeth if initially unrestored abutment teeth are to be retained in the final outcome [17]. Another drawback may be the possible difficulties in managing the fixed interim partial denture for the surgical team if the implant surgeon compares the ease of removing a removable prosthesis versus removing the fixed interim prosthesis cemented to abutment teeth to facilitate surgery and then having to recement the transitional prosthesis after a surgical procedure. Often, the patient's restorative provider will not be chairside during surgical procedures. There are, however, surgical providers who are adept in removing and recementing fixed provisional restorations, and of course there are many who provide both the surgical and restorative procedures.

The advantage to the fixed interim prosthesis option is an undisturbed healing post-surgical procedure in the pontic sites. Since the functional demands are borne by abutments that support the transitional FPD, the surgical site is free from pressure or physical irritation during the healing phase. This will allow the most undisturbed wound-healing environment and comfort for the patient [19, 20]. In addition with grafting procedures, the tooth-supported interim prosthesis significantly reduces any movement of the graft; this will provide the best stability of the graft leading to the best outcome. A 38-year-old female patient presented with a terminal maxillary dentition (Fig. 11.5a, b). Her health history was compromised by uncontrolled diabetes. She had desired implant-supported restorations and wanted to be transitioned with a fixed restoration. Risks and benefits were explained to the patient, and she was deemed not to be a candidate for full-arch immediate loading on implants. In this clinical scenario, the maxillary canines and first molars would be preserved. Since the patient had requested to be transitioned in a fixed restoration, these teeth would be used as abutments during the healing phase when grafting and implants would be completed and left undisturbed. The disadvantage of this approach was that four teeth had to be prepared to retain a fixed provisional restoration. The patient was scanned, and a shell provisional was milled in the laboratory. On the day of surgery, maxillary premolars and incisors were extracted, implants were placed and simultaneous grafting was performed. The provisional was relined on the preparations with the pontic site designed not to impinge on the grafted tissues. Once implants had integrated, a second set of provisionals were fabricated. These were a combination of tooth- and implant-supported provisionals. The provisionals were used to sculpt the soft tissue and convey the aesthetics to the patient. Once all parameters had been satisfied, zirconia restorations were fabricated. Single units were used for the teeth and splinted FPDs for the implants (Fig. 11.5a–j).

In addition to being able to secure provisional restorations, an additional benefit of preserving teeth during the integration phase is to be able to support a surgical guide. The abutment teeth can serve as indices for surgical guides to accurately position implants that will lead to restoratively driven implant positions downstream in the workflow. Once the abutment teeth have finished serving its function and implants can be utilized, the abutment teeth can be easily extracted (Fig. 11.6a–d).

Another benefit gained with a fixed interim provisional is that when the time comes to load the implant post-integration, one can transition the fixed tooth-borne prosthesis to implant-supported provisional by connecting the provisional indexed on abutment teeth by attaching temporary restorative cylinders on the implants in

Fig. 11.5 (**a**) Patient presented with a periodontally terminal maxillary dentition. (**b**) Smile and intra-oral view demonstrating teeth position and soft tissue levels. (**c**) Shell provisionals fabricated in the laboratory. (**d**) PMMA shell provisional to be relined at the time of surgery. (**e**) Day of surgery teeth prepared, implants placed, grafting performed and provisional relined. (**f**) 48-h Post-operative appointment. Soft tissue levels are not ideal. (**g**) Post-integration. Implant- and tooth-supported provisionals. (**h**) Soft tissue sculpting. (**i**) Screw-retained splinted zirconia restorations. Single-unit zirconia restorations on teeth. (**j**) Intra-oral and smile view of definitive zirconia restorations

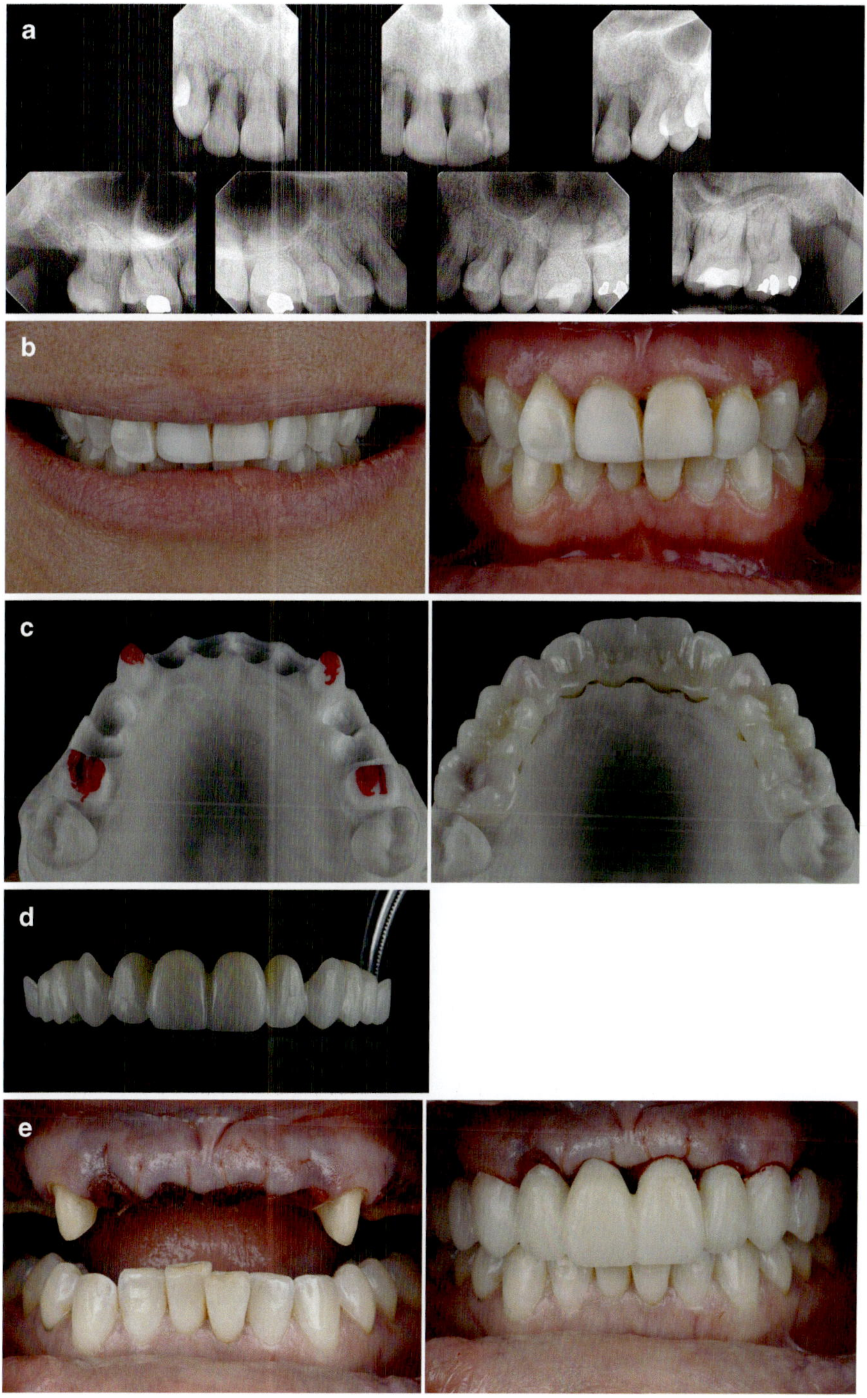

(continued)

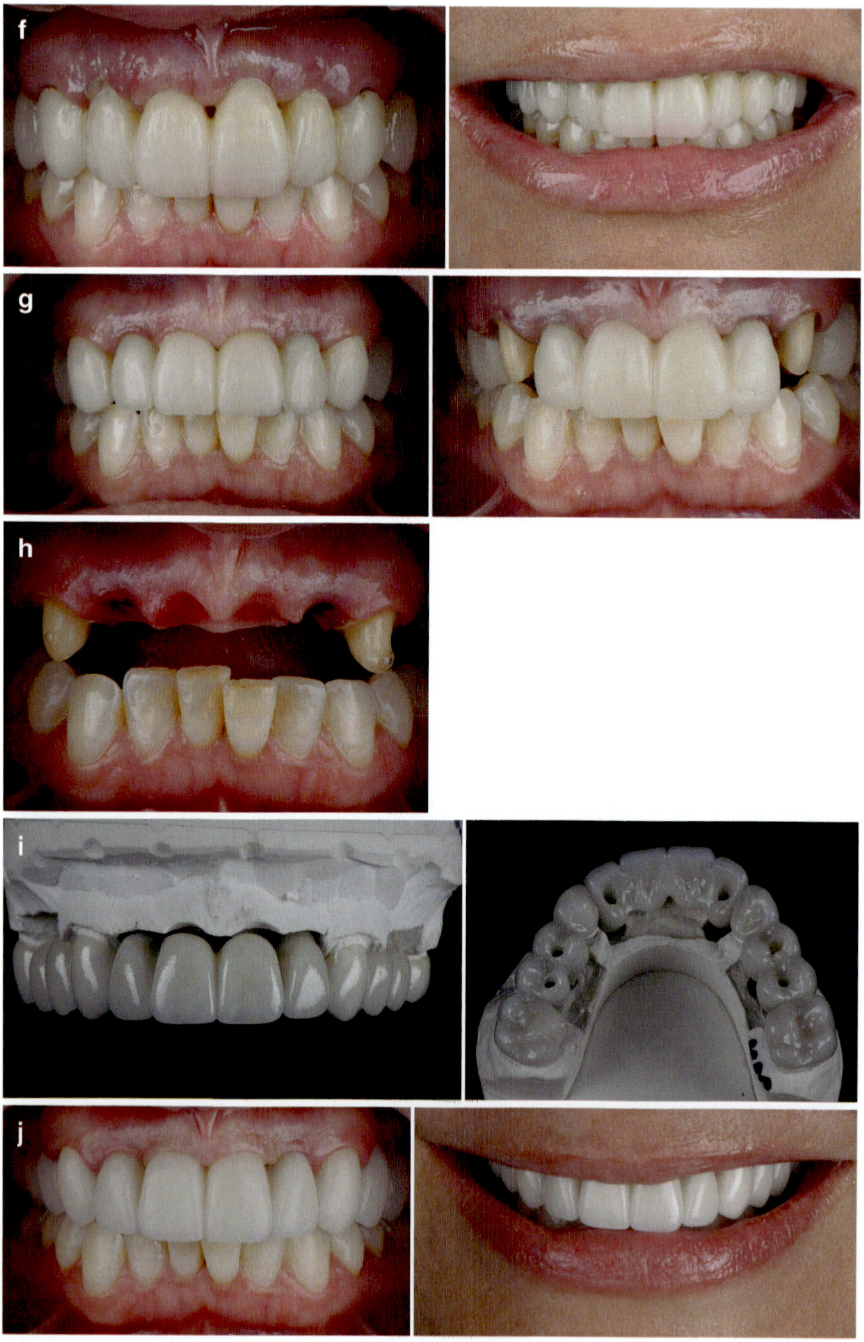

Fig. 11.5 (continued)

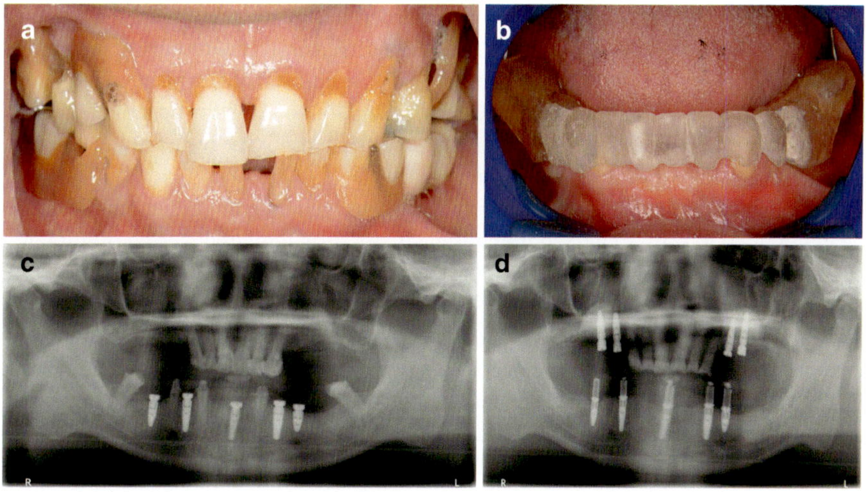

Fig. 11.6 (**a**) Patient with failing dentition due to corrosive tooth wear and bruxism. (**b**) Mandibular surgical stent indexed over retained abutment teeth. (**c**) Panoramic radiograph showing implants placed around strategically retained teeth. (**d**) Panoramic radiograph after extraction of the strategic abutment teeth and delivery of mandibular complete-arch implant provisional restoration

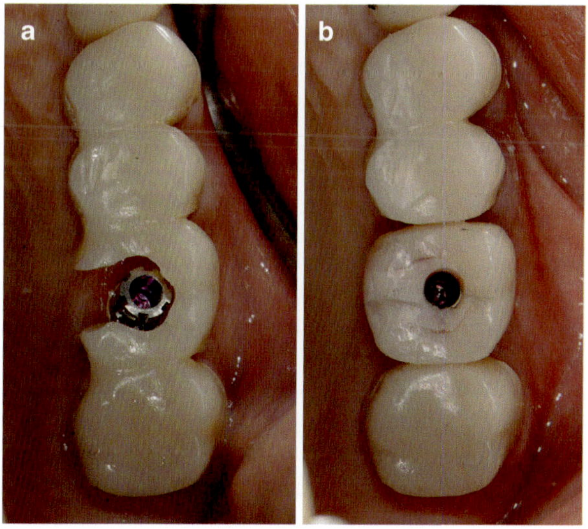

Fig. 11.7 (**a**) Pontic of fixed partial denture provisional restoration on teeth #24, 25 and 26 is modified to connect the position of implant #26. (**b**) #26 implant provisional has been separated from tooth-borne provisional fixed partial denture

the positions of pontics of the provisional FPD (Fig. 11.7a, b). This procedure can be referred to as "jumping" the tooth-borne provisional to implant-supported provisional; this process can be applied to partially edentulous or fully edentulous situations if abutment teeth are present and can serve as a reliable index for this procedure. With a removable interim prosthesis, "jumping" procedures can also be performed, however, with less precision due to dependence on mucosal support. Currently, in preparation for this procedure, a computer-aided design/computer-aided manufacturing (CAD/CAM) approach can be taken where CAD of the initially utilized provisional can be milled with spaces on the occluso-lingual area, which would allow for connection of the temporary implant cylinders to the milled provisional without the clinician having to locate the positions of the temporary restorative cylinders and then manually modify the provisional.

In considering the use of the existing abutment teeth, the abutment teeth need to be maintained to support a fixed transitional restoration until uncovering of implants that successfully integrate. Some abutment teeth require additional steps such as endodontic treatment, large build-ups and temporary post and cores to support the fixed transitional restoration. The clinician must account for the cost and time of these procedures and verify the benefits outweighing the risks. There could be additional time and cost considerations due to emergency breakage of the compromised abutments, extraction and tissue healing, which may have some delays in progressing toward the delivery of definitive restorations. Additionally, this may cause tissue changes especially due to remodelling of extraction sites of the abutment teeth in the aesthetic zone. One can try to eliminate these risks by choosing abutments toward non-aesthetic zones or discussing the cost-time and risk-benefits of fixed interim option vs. removable option to the patient. Patients will have different demands that will allow the clinician's determination of the decision to choose the interim restoration. After all, the patient will understand that if remaining abutments allow a fixed transitional prosthesis, this will provide them the most "transparent" transition to definitive restorations. This type of transitional restoration provides the closest representation of aesthetics and function to the definitive restorations supported with implants. Clinicians should disclose all benefits, risks, costs and treatment time to the patient.

It is recommended that if the fixed partial denture provisional on abutment teeth were to be maintained for more than 2 months, ideally the provisional should be recemented with temporary cement every 2 months to prevent any decay or to mitigate cement washout. Occlusal stability during initial delivery of the provisional restorations and throughout the waiting period is another critical factor in minimizing unscheduled visits due to decemented provisional restorations.

11.4 Provisional Implants

When there are no reliable abutment teeth for fixed interim restorations and the patient is not a candidate for immediate loading, provisional implants may be used. Clinicians can utilize provisional implants to support a fixed interim prosthesis or even utilize the provisional implants as overdenture retention for an interim removable prosthesis [21–24]. These narrow provisional implants require planning for their placement, and the clinician must evaluate the availability of bone to receive these additional implants. As described earlier with teeth as support for transitional prostheses, the actual implant positions should take precedence over available bone to house the provisional implants. Although using these provisional implants may

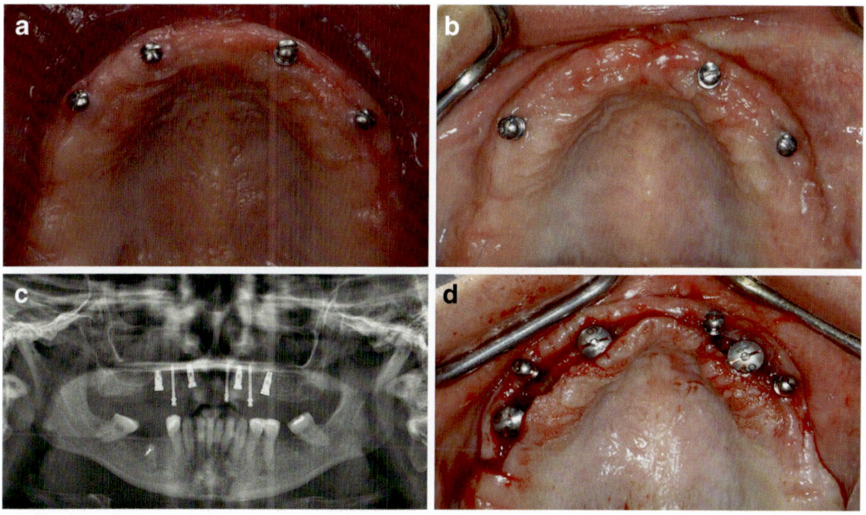

Fig. 11.8 (**a**) Interim transitional implants to serve as overdenture retention during implant treatment (Courtesy of Dr. Alexis Pawlak). (**b**) Unexpected failure of one transitional implant; remaining transitional implants still allow retention for overdenture (Courtesy of Dr. Alexis Pawlak). (**c**) Implant placement between transitional implants, transition implants are to serve as overdenture retention until implant uncovering (Courtesy of Dr. Alexis Pawlak). (**d**) On the day of uncovering of implants, transitional implants are used to pick up the position of the uncovered implants onto the denture and convert the overdenture to implant-supported restoration (Courtesy of Dr. Alexis Pawlak)

seem to be the perfect solution as a support for transitional prostheses, clinicians must be ready to manage the possible failures of the temporary implants before definitive implants are ready for loading, space taken up by the temporary implants that may interfere with definitive implant positions and high risk of mechanical complications with high-function patients. There are instances where a provisional implant fails, causing the transitional prosthesis to be modified during healing of the definitive implants. Therefore, when provisionalization relies on provisional implants, clinician must have an alternative way of provisionalization prepared and must prepare the patient for these risks. In Fig. 11.8b, one of the provisional implants failed during treatment; however, due to three provisional implants remaining, the interim overdenture option was not compromised during implant healing (Fig. 11.8a–d).

Another useful role of temporary implants is that they may serve as reliable references for implant planning either with a conventional surgical guide or with a computer-aided surgical guide (Fig. 11.9a–e) [21–24]. Certain temporary implant systems offer impression-making components as well as temporary cylinders that may expand the role of temporary implants (Fig. 11.10a–e).

After the interim provisional stage, temporary implants may be removed during the implant uncovering visit or at a later visit when a fixed provisional on implants is ready to be delivered.

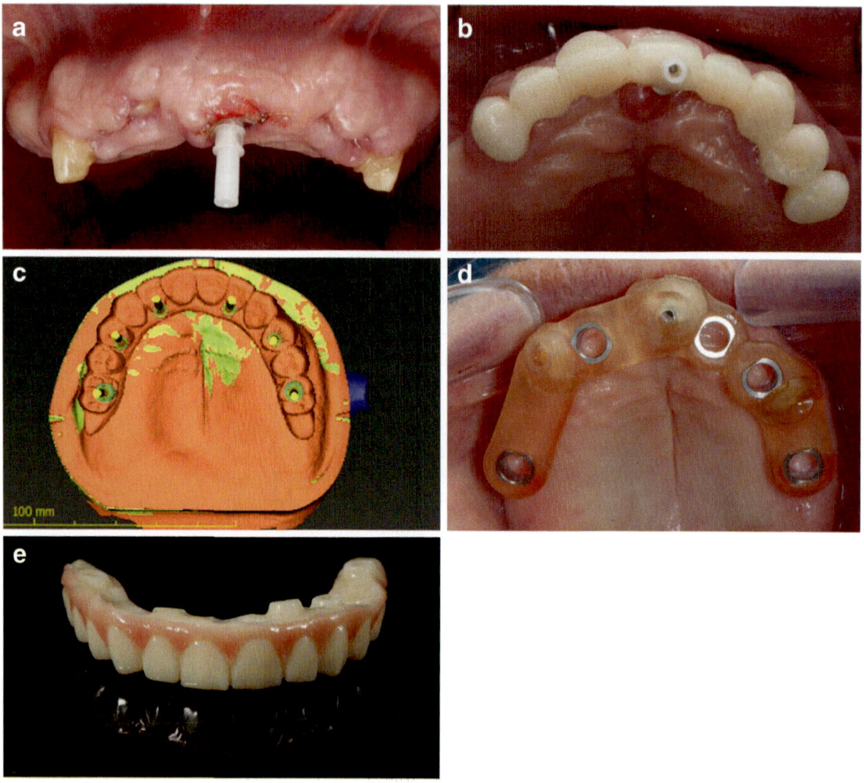

Fig. 11.9 (**a**) Transitional implant in maxillary anterior position with temporary cylinder (Courtesy of Dr. Chen Chen). (**b**) Transitional implant temporary cylinder is connected with tooth-borne provisional restoration to offer additional support (Courtesy of Dr. Chen Chen). (**c**) Guided implant position planning using abutment teeth and transition implant as references (Courtesy of Dr. Chen Chen). (**d**) Guided surgical guide resting on the transitional implant and two abutment teeth shown in Fig. 13a (Courtesy of Dr. Chen Chen). (**e**) Milled maxillary provisional restoration prior to implant placement based on computer-aided designing of guided surgical planning with preplanned opening for picking up implants after placement (Courtesy of Dr. Chen Chen)

11.5 Immediately Loaded Interim Prostheses

The term immediate loading does not have an established universal definition.

Two variables exist when one attempts to define immediate loading [25]:

1. The acceptable time interval between implant placement and prosthetic loading
2. The type of forces exerted on the implant and prosthesis

Immediate loading can be utilized as an alternative fixed interim solution before the definitive implant-supported restorations in both single and full-arch clinical scenarios in an immediate loading [26, 27]. This option of immediate implant

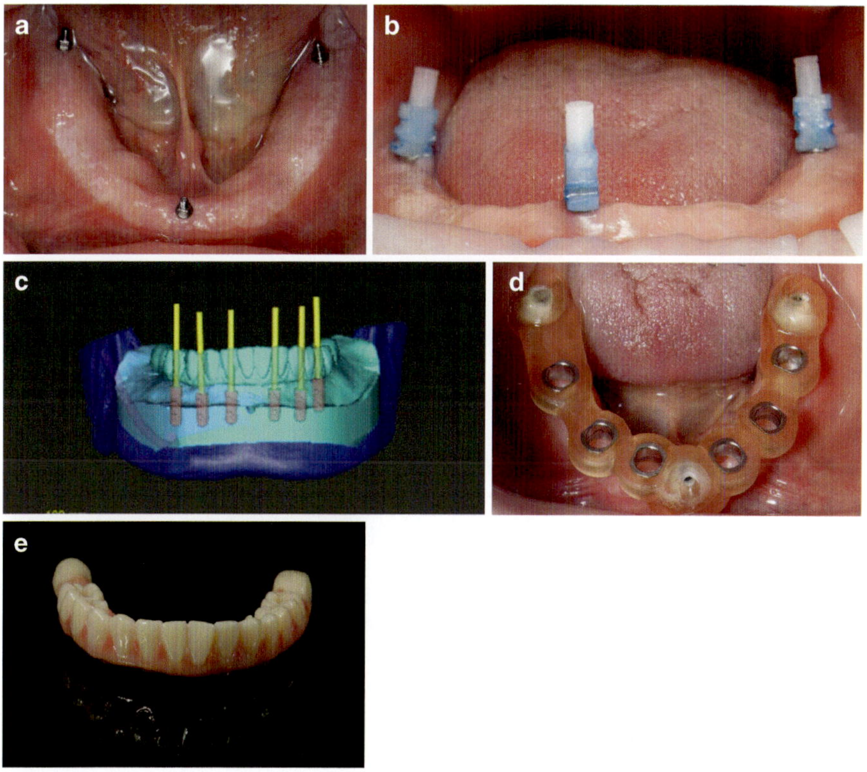

Fig. 11.10 (**a**) Transitional implants in the mandible to serve as reference for guided surgery (Courtesy of Dr. Chen Chen). (**b**) Impression coping on transitional implants. (**c**) Guided implant position planning using transition implants from Fig. 14a as references (Courtesy of Dr. Chen Chen). (**d**) Guided surgical guide indexed on the transitional implants shown in Fig. 14a (Courtesy of Dr. Chen Chen). (**e**) Milled mandibular provisional restoration prior to implant placement based on computer-aided designing of guided surgical planning with preplanned opening for picking up implants after placement (Courtesy of Dr. Chen Chen)

provisionalization has gained popularity with the advantage of providing the patient immediate function and aesthetics via provisional restorations on implants [28–30]. Immediate loading has been proven to be more efficient in number of visits required to receive an implant-supported provisional restoration. When choosing the patient suitable for immediate loading of implants, the clinician should consider the occlusal force from the opposing dentition of prosthesis as well as the surgeon's experience, which may influence the overall success rate of the immediately loaded implants [29, 31, 32]. An additional benefit to this option is the elimination of a second-stage uncovering procedure which may be attractive to patients.

However, this option does come with a higher risk in testing the functional boundaries of newly placed implants [33, 34]. When weighing the risks and benefits of delayed versus immediate loading of the implants, clinicians must consider each patient's situation for immediate loading. Some factors that are favourable or unfavourable should be evaluated, for example, the quality and quantity of the bony anatomy, patient's systemic health and forces from opposing dentition. Any compromise to the ideal presentation of bony anatomy, health and magnitude of forces can cause unpredictable loss of immediately loaded implants [25–27, 33].

There are technical aspects that the clinician has to be well versed with the immediate loading technique [22, 25, 35, 36]. Clinicians must be aware of the technical steps and components involved in immediate loading of the placed implants [37].

When discussing the sequence of wound healing during implant placement, one can divide the stability of the implant into mechanical stability followed by biologic stability. Primary stability of implants after placement is a mechanical stability within its surrounding bone. This mechanical stability of the implant starts to decrease with the healing process where osteocyte turnover takes place before laying down bone to develop biologic stability of the implant [38–40]. Immediately loading an interim provisional prosthesis would challenge the wound-healing process before the biologic stability is established; therefore, initial insertion torque of 35–50 Ncm is of importance when considering immediate loading to ensure that loading is performed on mechanically (primary stability) stable implants [41–43].

Not only biological risks are present with this option, but there are also typically more restorative components to be utilized as we often provide the restoration on an abutment level for immediately loaded provisional restorations. This may pose additional mechanical challenge or component costs to the clinician. Lastly, considerations of patient inconvenience may play a role in deciding to take this option because the immediate loading by the restorative clinician cannot be done "immediately" if referring out to a surgical colleague for implant surgery. However, since delivering the provisional within 48 h of the implant placement is still considered as "immediate" loading, clinicians may be able to facilitate a second-day immediate loading after the first day of implant placement [44].

11.5.1 Single-Tooth Immediate Load

When considering immediate loading of a single tooth in the aesthetic zone, a number of parameters must be observed to yield an optimal result (Fig. 11.11a–j).

The considerations below are preferable, but there are no absolutes. These include but are not limited to:

(a) Infection-free site or minimally infected tissues that can be removed with curettes.
(b) Intact buccal bone that is less than 3 mm below the free gingival margin.
(c) High crestal interproximal bone.
(d) Sufficient quantity and quality of bone to allow adequate primary stability of 35 Ncm.
(e) No excessive occlusal forces and posterior support present. The tooth should not be in centric or eccentric occlusion.

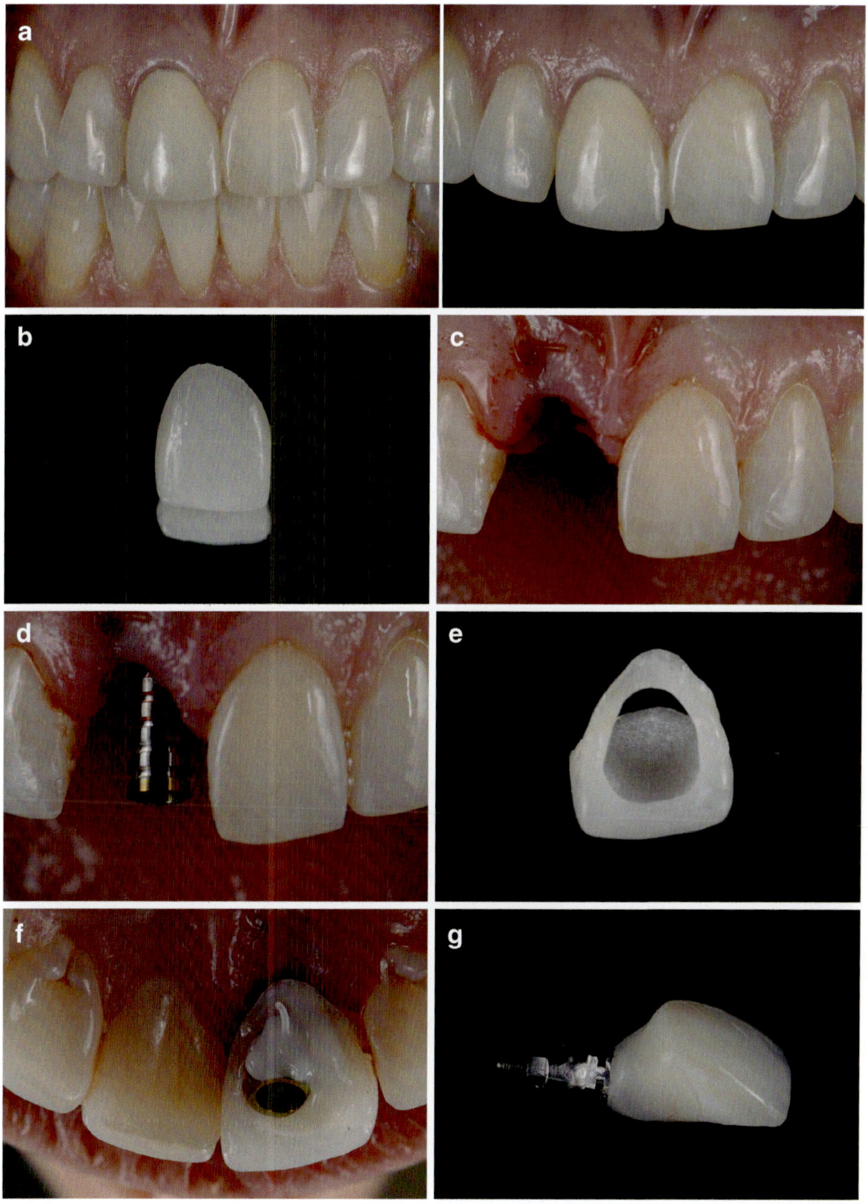

Fig. 11.11 (**a**) Preoperative situation of failing tooth #11 (maxillary right central incisor). (**b**) Shell provisional fabricated. (**c**) Tooth extracted and dental implant placed. (**d**) Engaging temporary cylinder connected to fixture. (**e**) Hole made in the palatal aspect of shell provisional. (**f**) Pickup of provisional intra-orally utilizing flowable composite. (**g**) Back fill of provisional, finished, contoured and polished. (**h**) Delivery of provisional, occlusion relieved, interproximal contacts relived. Subgingival under-contoured to provide excess tissue which will be shaped during healing. (**i**) Definitive screw-retained zirconia restorations. (**j**) Pre- and post-restoration illustrating aesthetic tooth and gingival contours

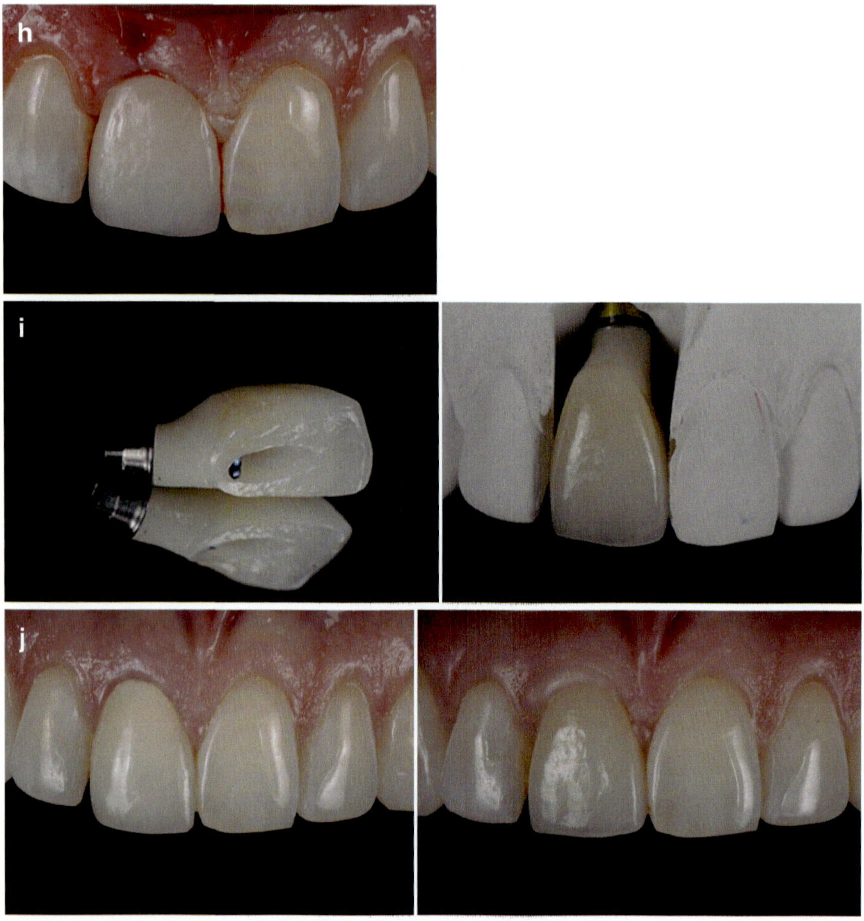

Fig. 11.11 (continued)

(f) Minimal micromovements—interproximal contacts between the adjacent teeth should be relieved.

11.5.2 Full-Arch Immediate Loading

Given that implant initial stability has been attained, the main clinical factor that influences successful immediate loading treatment is the design of the immediately delivered interim full-arch restoration. The clear majority of these types of full-arch restorations are screw-retained in design and cross-arch splinted.

There are a number of prosthetic considerations that must be understood prior to embarking upon the immediate load process. Meticulous attention to detail is required for the process to be successful. An important prerequisite for predictable healing is the absence of micro-motion. Favourable loading conditions can be achieved by splinting the implants together immediately after placement. For practicality, full-arch implant restorations are loaded at abutment level. This allows a more efficient clinical procedure, and micro-motion at the bone-implant interface is limited, thus facilitating the healing process (Fig. 11.12a–k).

The interim prosthesis should satisfy the following requirements:

(a) Cross-arch stabilization with a screw-retained rigid prosthesis with no cantilevers
(b) No premature occlusal contacts
(c) No interferences in lateral excursion
(d) Minimal vertical and horizontal overlap
(e) An occlusal scheme which protects the implants most at risk

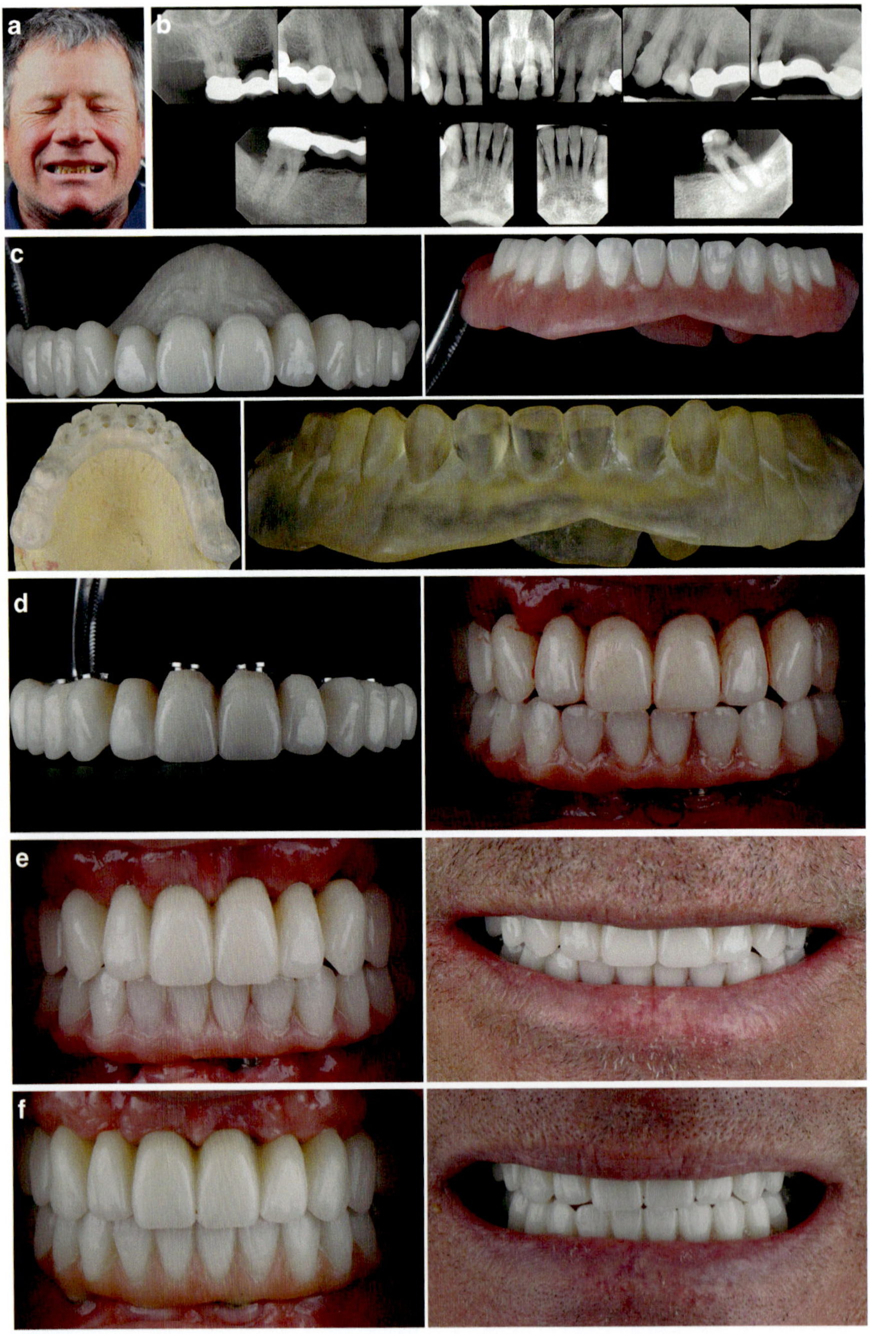

Fig. 11.12 (**a**) Pre-op smile, patient showing hesitation in smiling. (**b**) Full-mouth periapical radiographs showing bone loss. (**c**) Provisionals and surgical guides fabricated from an intra-oral scan. (**d**) Implants placed, day of immediate loading of maxillary and mandibular arch. (**e**) One week post-op of immediate-load provisional restorations. (**f**) Additional set of provisional restorations fabricated to optimize aesthetics, phonetics and soft tissue contact. (**g**) Minimally layered zirconia restorations. (**h**) Day of delivery of definitive zirconia restorations. (**i**) Pre- and post-op of implant rehabilitation. (**j**) Panoramic radiograph. (**k**) Post-op facial view of patient

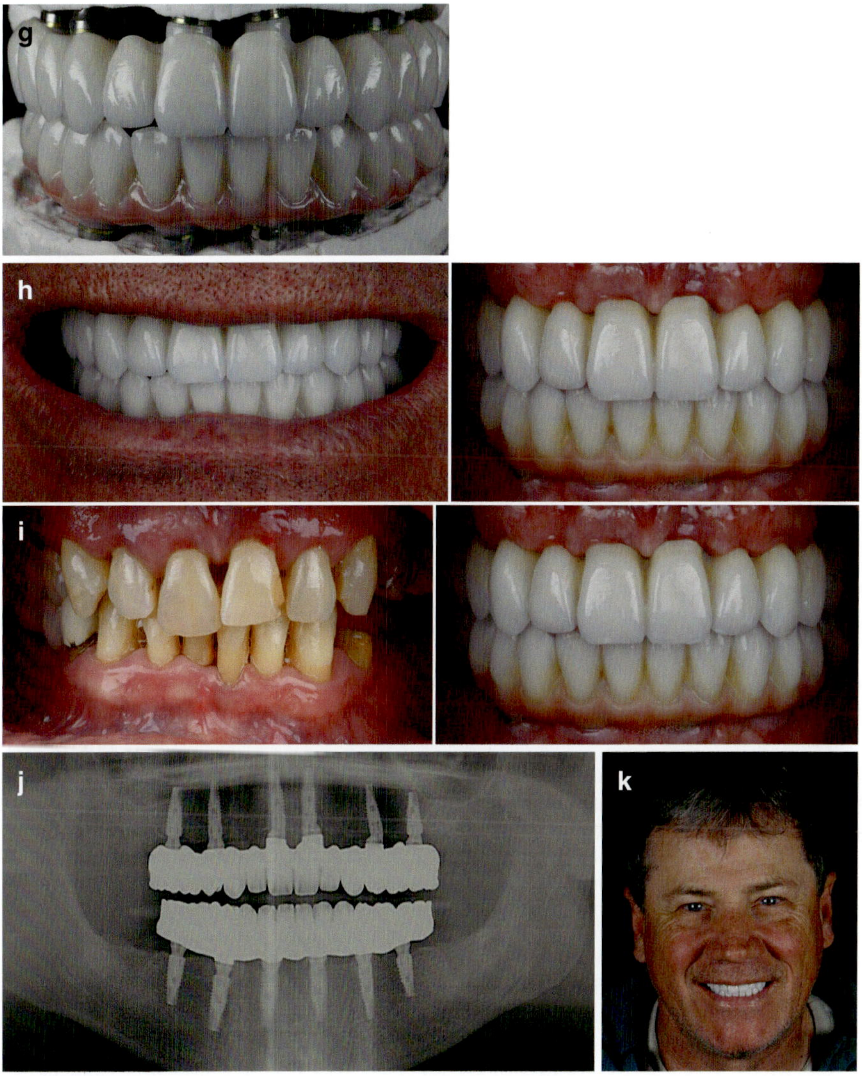

Fig. 11.12 (continued)

11.6 No Interim Prosthesis

A last option to take into consideration is the option not to replace the missing tooth or teeth until the implants are successfully integrated. This can be considered conventional loading since the clinician is waiting to load the implant after 3–6 months of implant placement [44]. As one can imagine for multiple missing teeth, patients are less likely to opt for this option due to functional and aesthetic challenges this poses; however, in some clinical scenarios, where severely worn and supra-erupted teeth as well as large mandibular tori exist, either immediately loaded provisional or no provisional may be considered. In case of an immediately loaded provisional, the patient should be informed, especially when they show signs of bruxism, that there will be additional risks for immediately loaded implants. When considering no replacement of teeth during interim phase, it is important to understand that this option does not ultimately protect the surgical site from functional trauma as the opposing dentition or prosthesis may cause inevitable functional trauma or irritation to the surgical site.

11.7 Summary

This chapter has offered and compared various options of interim prostheses during transitioning a failing dentition to implant-supported restoration. While many options of provisionalization exist, a provisional fixed partial denture that is supported by teeth, temporary implants or immediately placed implants provides the most "transparent" transition toward implant-supported restoration. After perusing this chapter, one should be able to clearly weigh the risks, costs and benefits of each interim provisional type and narrow down to the viable options for an individual clinical scenario. When needing to find the answer, the best starting point is for one to know which questions they are wanting to solve; therefore, starting with the set of guided question list presented in the beginning of this chapter will be beneficial.

References

1. Cortes AR, Cortes DN, No-Cortes J, Arita ES. Transition from failing dentition to full-arch fixed implant-supported prosthesis with a staged approach using removable partial dentures: a case series. J Prosthodont. 2014;23(4):328–32.
2. Cho SC, Shetty S, Froum S, Elian N, Tarnow D. Fixed and removable provisional options for patients undergoing implant treatment. Compend Contin Educ Dent. 2007;28:604–8.
3. Jivraj S, Chee W. Transitioning patients from teeth to implants. Br Dent J. 2006;201:699–708.
4. Sheridan JJ, McMinn R, LeDoux W. Essix thermosealed appliances: various orthodontic uses. J Clin Orthod. 1995;29:108–13.
5. Simon DG. Securing pontics in an Essix retainer. J Clin Orthod. 2011;45:384.
6. Moskowitz EM, Sheridan JJ, Celenza F Jr, Tovilo K, Muñoz AM, Essix appliances. Provisional anterior prosthesis for pre and post implant patients. N Y State Dent J. 1997;63(4):32–5.
7. Zinner ID, Panno FV, Pines MS, Small SA. First-stage fixed provisional restorations for implant prosthodontics. J Prosthodont. 1993;2(4):228–32.
8. Zoidis P, Papathanasiou I. Modified PEEK resin-bonded fixed dental prosthesis as an interim restoration after implant placement. J Prosthet Dent. 2016;116(5):637–41.
9. Myers ML, Caughman WF. Provisional treatment for resin-bonded fixed partial dentures. Quintessence Int. 1994;25(7):465–9.
10. Zitzmann NU, Özcan M, Scherrer SS, Bühler JM, Weiger R, Krastl G. Resin-bonded restorations: a strategy for managing anterior tooth loss in adolescence. J Prosthet Dent. 2015;113(4):270–6.
11. Prathyusha P, Jyoti S, Kaul RB, Sethi N. Maryland bridge: an interim prosthesis for tooth replacement in adolescents. Int J Clin Pediatr Dent. 2011;4(2):135–8.
12. Rochette AL. Attachment of a splint to enamel of lower anterior teeth. J Prosthet Dent. 1973;30:418–23.

13. Creugers NHJ, Van't Hof MA. An analysis of clinical studies on resin bonded bridges. J Dent Res. 1993;72:1244–8.
14. Kern M, Passia N, Sasse M, Yazigi C. Ten-year outcome of zirconia ceramic cantilever resin-bonded fixed dental prostheses and the influence of the reasons for missing incisors. J Dent. 2017;65:51–5.
15. Carmichael RP, Sándor GK. Dental implants, growth of the jaws, and determination of skeletal maturity. Atlas Oral Maxillofac Surg Clin N Am. 2008;16(1):1–9.
16. Op Heij DG, Opdebeeck H, van Steenberghe D, Quirynen M. Age as compromising factor for implant insertion. Periodontology 2000. 2003;33:172–84.
17. Jivraj S, Reshad M, Chee WW. Transitioning patients from teeth to implants utilizing fixed restorations. J Calif Dent Assoc. 2008;36(8):599–606.
18. Drew HJ, Alnassar T, Gluck K, Rynar JE. Considerations for a staged approach in implant dentistry. Quintessence Int. 2012;43(1):29–36.
19. Cordaro L, Torsello F, Ercoli C, Gallucci G. Transition from failing dentition to a fixed implant-supported restoration: a staged approach. Int J Periodontics Restor Dent. 2007;27(5):481–7.
20. Chronopoulos V, Kourtis S, Katsikeris N, Nagy W. Tooth- and tissue-supported provisional restorations for the treatment of patients with extended edentulous spans. J Esthet Restor Dent. 2009;21(1):7–18.
21. Aalam AA, Reshad M, Chee WW, Nowzari H. Surgical template stabilization with transitional implants in the treatment of the edentulous mandible: a technical note. Int J Oral Maxillofac Implant. 2005;20:462–5.
22. Wu AY, Chee W. Use of 3 transitional implants as stabilization aid for predictable immediate loading of implants in the edentulous mandible. Quintessence Int. 2006;37(8):627–31.
23. Krennmair G, Krainhöfner M, Weinländer M, Piehslinger E. Provisional implants for immediate restoration of partially edentulous jaws: a clinical study. Int J Oral Maxillofac Implants. 2008;23(4):717–25.
24. Petrungaro PS, Windmiller N. Using transitional implants during the healing phase of implant reconstruction. Gen Dent. 2001;49:46–51.
25. Attard NJ, Zarb GA. Immediate and early implant loading protocols: a literature review of clinical studies. J Prosthet Dent. 2005;94(3):242–58.
26. Esposito M, Grusovin MG, Willings M, Coulthard P, Worthington HV. The effectiveness of immediate, early, and conventional loading of dental implants: a Cochrane systematic review of randomized controlled clinical trials. Int J Oral Maxillofac Implants. 2007;22(6):893–904.
27. Galli F, Capelli M, Zuffetti F, Testori T, Esposito M. Immediate non-occlusal vs. early loading of dental implants in partially edentulous patients: a multicentre randomized clinical trial. Peri-implant bone and soft-tissue levels. Clin Oral Implants Res. 2008;19(6):546–52.
28. Schnitman PA, Wohrle PS, Rubenstein JE. Immediate fixed interim prostheses supported by two-stage threaded implants: methodology and results. Int J Oral Implantol. 1990;16:96–105.
29. Chiapasco M, Gatti C, Rossi E, Haeflige W, Markwaldel TH. Implant-retained mandibular overdentures with immediate loading. Clin Oral Implants Res. 1997;8(1):48–57.
30. Aalam AA, Nowzari H, Krivitsky A. Functional restoration of implants on the day of surgical placement in the fully edentulous mandible: a case series. Clin Implant Dent Relat Res. 2005;7(1):10–6.
31. Chee W, Jivraj S. Efficiency of immediately loaded mandibular full-arch implant restorations. Clin Implant Dent Relat Res. 2003;5(1):52–6.
32. Schnitman PA, Wöhrle PS, Rubenstein JE, DaSilva JD, Wang NH. Ten-year results for Brånemark implants immediately loaded with fixed prostheses at implant placement. Int J Oral Maxillofac Implants. 1997;12(4):495–503.
33. Szmukler-Moncler S, Piattelli A, Favero GA, Dubruille JH. Considerations preliminary to the application of early and immediate loading protocols in dental implantology. Clin Oral Implants Res. 2000;11(1):12–25.
34. Degidi M, Nardi D, Piattelli A. A comparison between immediate loading and immediate restoration in cases of partial posterior mandibular edentulism: a 3-year randomized clinical trial. Clin Oral Implants Res. 2010;21(7):682–7.

35. Bergkvist G, Nilner K, Sahlholm S, Karlsson U, Lindh C. Immediate loading of implants in the edentulous maxilla: use of an interim fixed prosthesis followed by a permanent fixed prosthesis: a 32-month prospective radiological and clinical study. Clin Implant Dent Relat Res. 2009;11(1):1–10.
36. Jaffin RA, Kumar A, Berman CL. Immediate loading of dental implants in the completely edentulous maxilla: a clinical report. Int J Oral Maxillofac Implants. 2004;19(5):721–30.
37. Froum S, Emtiaz S, Bloom MJ, et al. The use of transitional implants for immediate fixed temporary prostheses in cases of implant restorations. Pract Periodontics Aesthet Dent. 1998;10(6):737–46.
38. Raghavendra S, Wood MC, Taylor TD. Early wound healing around endosseous implants: a review of the literature. Int J Oral Maxillofac Implants. 2005;20(3):425–31.
39. Charatchaiwanna A, Rojsiraphisa T, Aunmeungtong W, Reichart PA, Khongkhunthian P. Mathematical equations for dental implant stability patterns during the osseointegration period, based on previous resonance frequency analysis studies. Clin Implant Dent Relat Res. 2019;21(5):1028–40.
40. De Smet E, Duyck J, Vander Sloten J, Jacobs R, Naert I. Timing of loading—immediate, early, or delayed—in the outcome of implants in the edentulous mandible: a prospective clinical trial. Int J Oral Maxillofac Implants. 2007;22(4):580–94.
41. Tarnow DP, Emtiaz S, Classi A. Immediate loading of threaded implants at stage 1 surgery in edentulous arches: ten consecutive case reports with 1- to 5-year data. Int J Oral Maxillofac Implants. 1997;12(3):319–24.
42. Derbabian K, Simonian K. Immediate loading dental implants: overview and rationale. J Calif Dent Assoc. 2005;33(4):337–41.
43. Brunski JB. Avoid pitfalls of overloading and micromotion of intraosseous implants. Dent Implantol Update. 1993;4(10):77–81.
44. Cochran DL, Morton D, Weber HP. Consensus statements and recommended clinical procedures regarding loading protocols for endosseous dental implants. Int J Oral Maxillofac Implants. 2004;19(suppl):109–13.

Treatment Planning Posterior Sextants 12

Winston Chee and Saj Jivraj

Replacing missing teeth in posterior sextants with implants may consider factors with different priorities compared to dental implants used to restore missing anterior teeth or rather in "aesthetic zones".

This chapter considers appearances of implant-supported restorations in posterior sextants that are in "aesthetic zone" where restorations are visible when patients smile or speak. In some situations, patients will accept compromises where restorations on implants may not mimic the appearance of natural dentition. This occurs when severe remodelling of supporting bone may have taken place post-extraction or due to trauma; some patients will accept deviations from ideal appearing restorations; this acceptance also reduces additional procedures such as hard and soft tissue grafts to improve aesthetic outcomes.

Biomechanical issues will usually be the priority when restoring posterior sextants; however, issues of aesthetics may dominate in aesthetic zones. In general, biomechanical issues considered will be the number of implants, distribution of implants and materials selected. Aesthetic issues will dictate precise placement of implants to allow the implant-supported restorations to integrate with the existing teeth as seamlessly as possible.

Current literature reports that success rates of posterior implants are high with over 90% success rates over 10 years [1, 2]. Whenever a replacement of posterior teeth is indicated, implants are often the first choice to consider; implants are conservative to remaining teeth and provide support independently from tooth and mucosa [3]. Implant-supported restorations can also be repaired or modified without affecting remaining teeth especially when screw retained, removal and

W. Chee (✉)
Advanced Prosthodontics, Herman Ostrow School of Dentistry, University of Southern California, Los Angeles, CA, USA

S. Jivraj
Private Practice, Anacapa Dental Art Institute, Oxnard, CA, USA

W. Chee, S. Jivraj (eds.), *Treatment Planning In Implant Dentistry*, BDJ Clinician's Guides, https://doi.org/10.1007/978-3-031-68726-6_12

replacement of the restoration or connecting existing implants to additional implants can be easily executed [4–7].

With respect to function, more opposing tooth units will improve the masticatory process; these opposing units will reduce loading to remaining dentition. These additional units, as mentioned before, can provide aesthetics when patients display teeth further posterior.

Newer materials and methods include the use of digital planning and manufacture, together with the use of more durable materials that are available and gaining use to fabricate restorations. In the past, when metal ceramic restorations were very prone to chipping and fracture, this was a common occurrence leading to a costly repair. Using monolithic restorations made with zirconia, which is one of the newer materials, has reduced this complication significantly. When better aesthetics is required, modified cut-back designs can significantly reduce any chipping of layered porcelain [8–11]. The newer materials and technologies will be presented in more detail in other chapters of this book to discuss in detail CAD/CAM (Chap. 8).

12.1 Aesthetic Considerations

In the aesthetic zone, sufficient space is required to allow the restorative dentist to fabricate restorations which are harmonious with the adjacent teeth. Some factors that will help to determine space requirements will entail (1) mesio-distal spacing, (2) occlusal-gingival spacing and (3) depth of implant to allow development of the contour.

12.1.1 Mesio-distal

When the restoration of the posterior sextant is within the aesthetic zone, there should be suitable mesio-distal space to allow a similar resemblance to a tooth; firstly, there must be sufficient mesio-distal inter-radicular space to allow placement of an implant, and there should be at least 1 mm of bone between the implant and tooth root. Too close a proximity can cause loss of interproximal bone when any insult such as inflammation can be detrimental; a thicker septum of bone will be more resistant to bone loss [12, 13].

On average, the mesio-distal spacing should be about 7 mm for premolars and 10.5 mm for molars. For the restoration to have sufficient room to have similar mesio-distal dimensions of a tooth space between adjacent teeth if the dimensions presented differ too much, in more severe situations, orthodontic movement may be required to accommodate the implant and restoration and in less severe situations enameloplasty can suffice (Figs. 12.1, 12.2, 12.3 and 12.4).

The following guidelines should be used when selecting implant size and evaluating mesio-distal space for implant placement to accommodate the dimensions of the restoration:

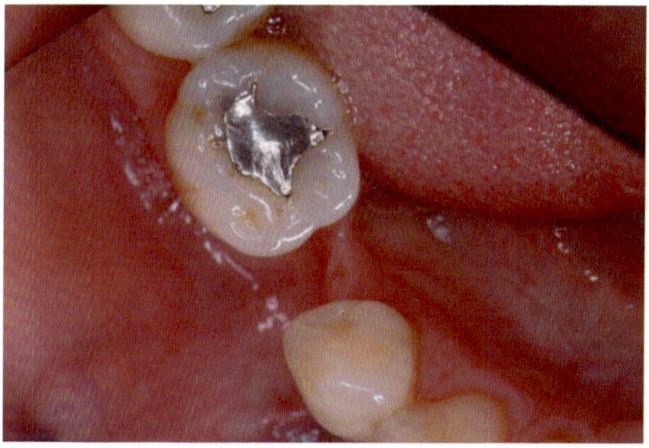

Fig. 12.1 Occlusal view of reduced mesio-distal spacing

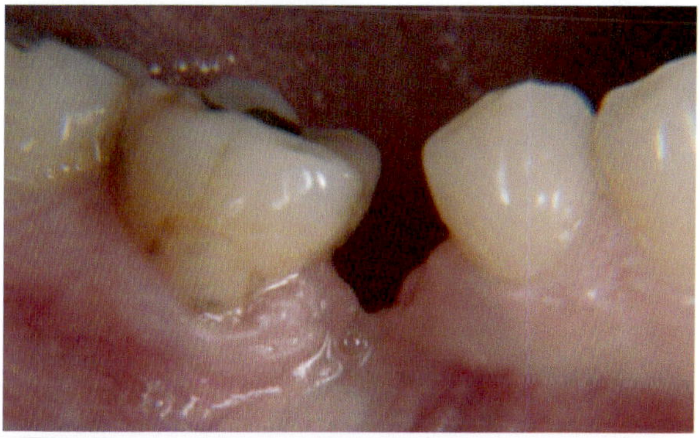

Fig. 12.2 Lateral view of the reduced mesio-distal space

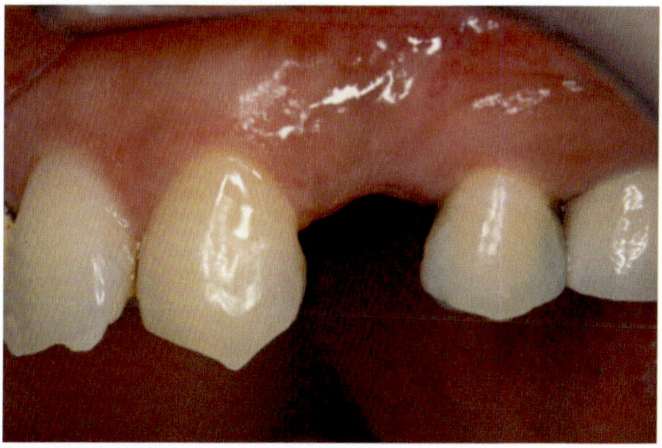

Fig. 12.3 Lateral view of adequate mesio-distal space

1. The implant should be at least 1.5 mm away from the tooth roots.
2. The implant should be at least 3 mm away from an adjacent implant.
3. A wider diameter implant should be selected for molar teeth if anatomy allows (Figs. 12.5, 12.6 and 12.7).

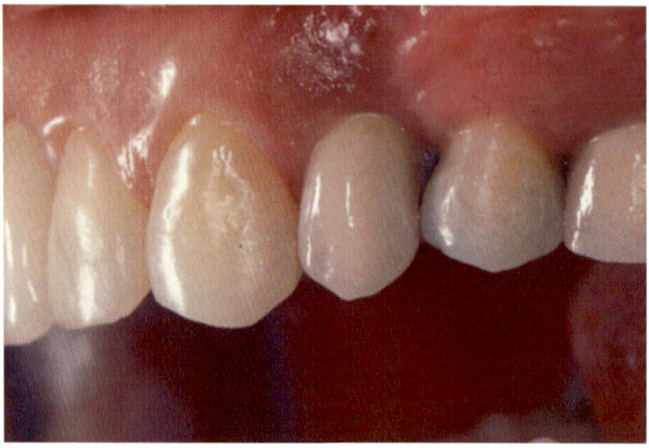

Fig. 12.4 Implant-supported restoration restoring space in Fig. 12.3

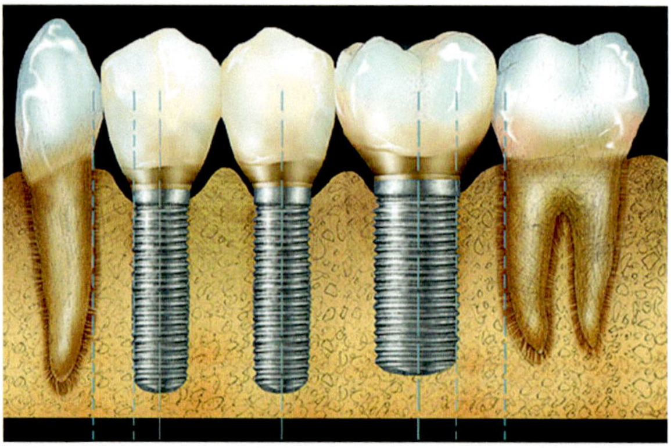

Fig. 12.5 Illustration of ideal spacing of implants

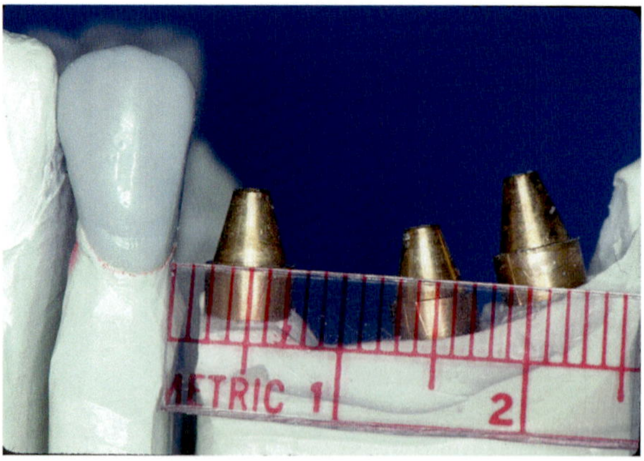

Fig. 12.6 Image of distribution of implants mesio-distally with implant approximately 1.5 mm from root and 3 mm apart from additional implant

At least 6 mm of bone buccolingually is required for placement of a 4 mm diameter implant and 7 mm for a wider diameter 5 mm implant. The implants should be placed so that the projection facilitates the screw access to be positioned towards the centre of the occlusal surface. In the chapter discussing screw vs. cemented

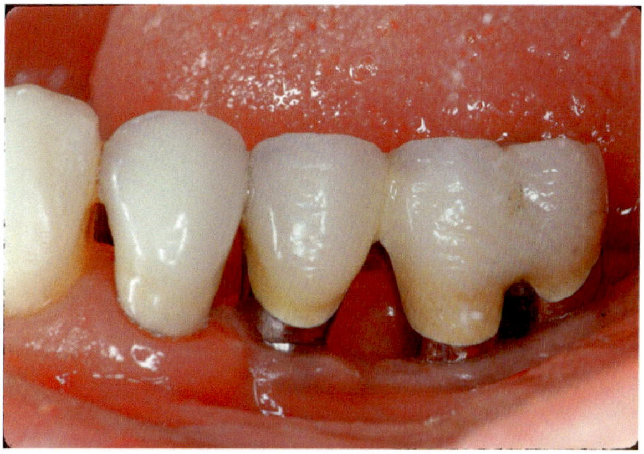

Fig. 12.7 Lateral view of implants with sufficient spacing of the implants in relation to tooth and other implants

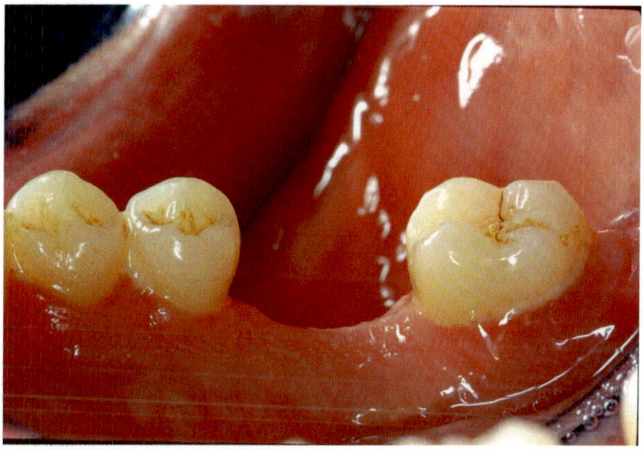

Fig. 12.8 Image showing adequate mesio-distal space for a molar

restorations, this topic will be expanded; current technology will allow the screw access to be shifted up to 30° from the axis of the implant; this will accommodate the bony anatomy presented and reduce the need for grafting of the site. It is still preferable that implant placement should be guided with a surgical guide to ideally position the implant. Clinicians need to be familiar with the type of implant being used to confirm that these components to alter the screw access are available. It should be avoided to fabricate cement abutments and then to cement retain the restorations; again, the shortcomings of cement-retained restorations will be described in Chap. 3.

Based on the above restorative space in the mesial-distal dimension when spaces are bounded by teeth, ideal dimensions for implants and restorations will depend on sufficient bony anatomy to receive an implant; for example, a 4 mm diameter implant can be placed for a molar; in this situation, the implant is placed more apically to accommodate the transition of implant platform to exit the profile of the molar (Figs. 12.8, 12.9, 12.10 and 12.11).

Multiple missing teeth in a bounded space will dictate tooth replacements; in this situation (Fig. 12.12), a premolar and molar will suitably fit spatially and will be restored with a 4 mm diameter implant that can be used for a premolar and a 5 mm

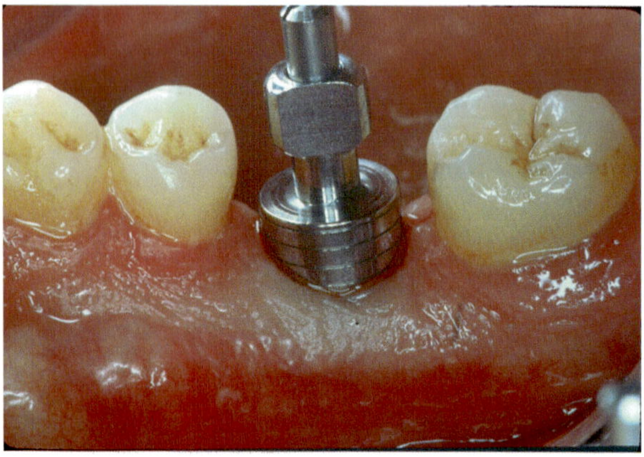

Fig. 12.9 Image of widened impression coping to accommodate soft tissue contours from implant platform to exit profile

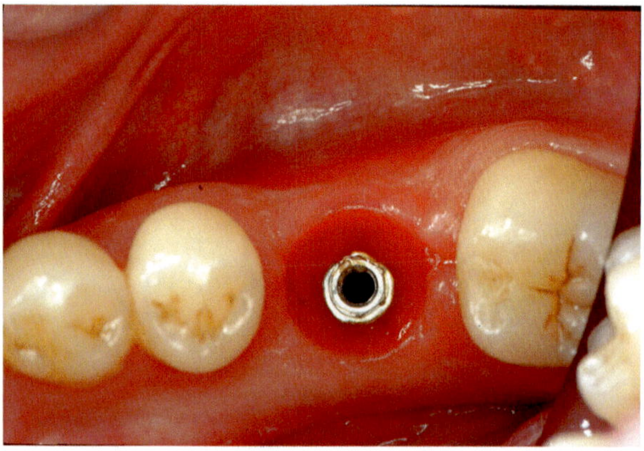

Fig. 12.10 Occlusal view shows soft tissue contours from 4 mm implant platform to exit profile that is facilitated by placing the implant more apically

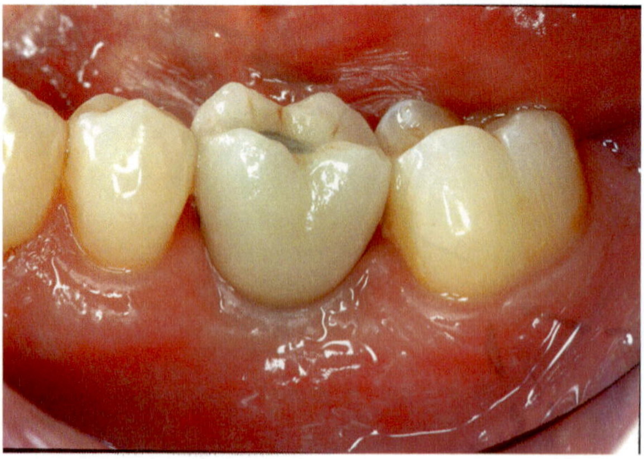

Fig. 12.11 Restoration has adequate soft tissues to mimic molars as closely as possible

diameter implant for a molar. This allows the depths of the implants to be equal and can accommodate gradual submucosal contours from the implant platforms to the exit profile (Figs. 12.12, 12.13, 12.14, 12.15, 12.16 and 12.17).

When implants are misplaced, aesthetics can be affected adversely; for example, when implants are placed with increased spacing from adjacent teeth, in the aesthetic zones, a less-than-ideal outcome will present (Figs. 12.18, 12.19 and 12.20).

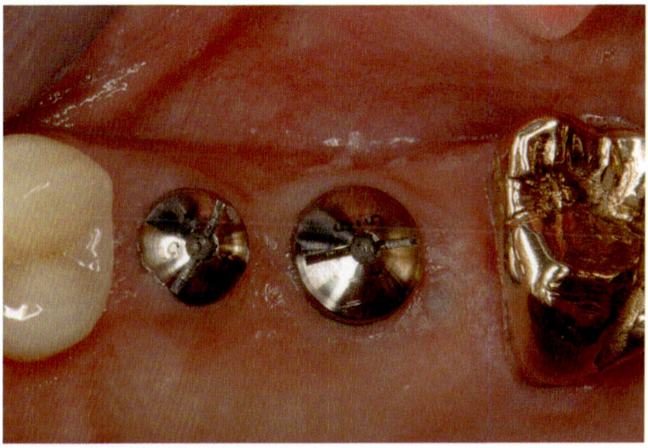

Fig. 12.12 Occlusal view of implants with differing diameters for the respective restorations (Figs. 12.12, 12.13, 12.14, 12.15, 12.16 and 12.17 courtesy of Dr. George Cho)

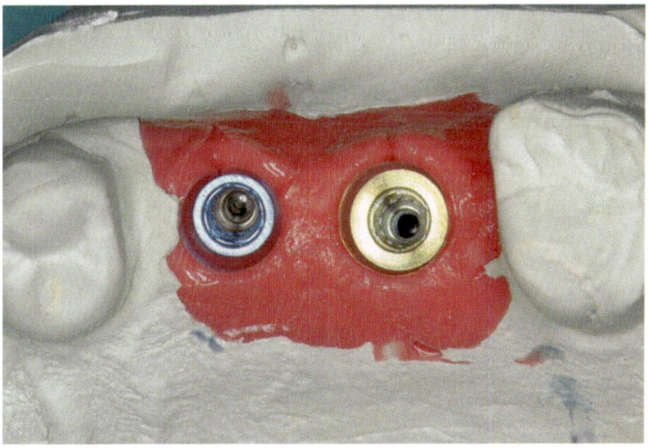

Fig. 12.13 View from occlusal perspective of the soft tissue cast with implant analogues on the cast

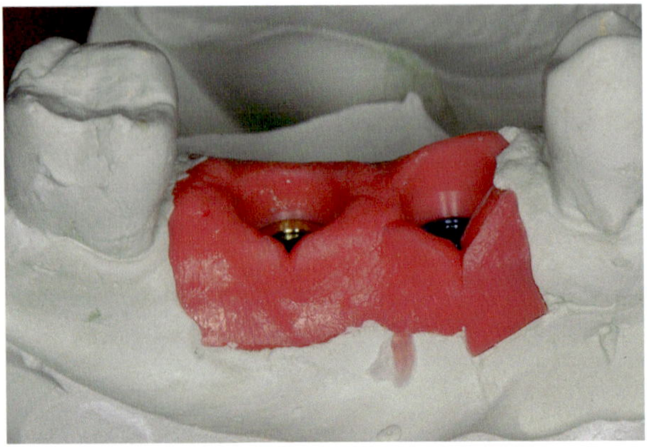

Fig. 12.14 View from lateral perspective of the soft tissue cast with implant analogues on the cast

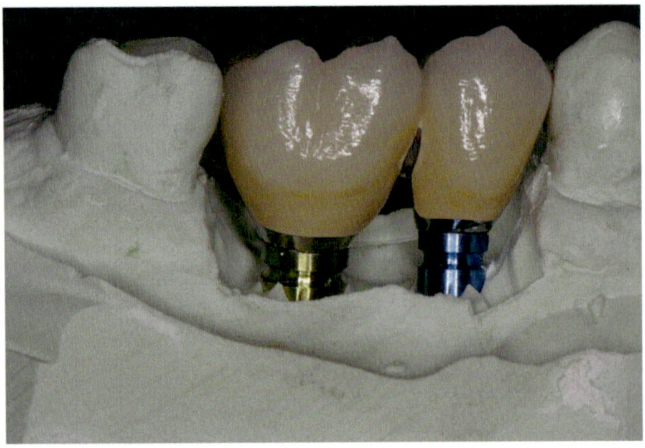

Fig. 12.15 Extra-oral view of the restorations and submucosal contours with soft tissue cast material removed; note the gradual contours from implant platforms to exit profile

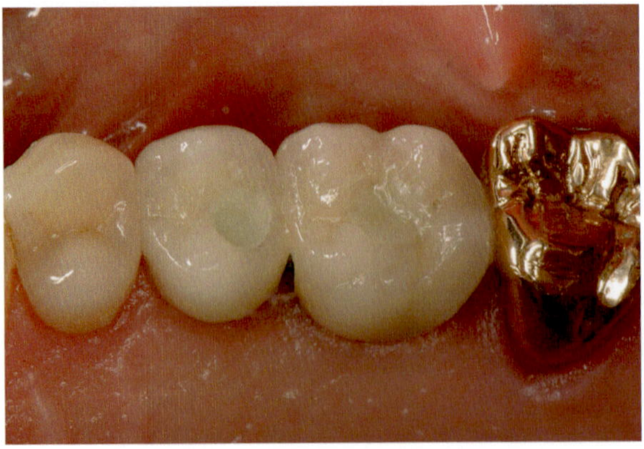

Fig. 12.16 Occlusal view of the implant restorations intra-orally

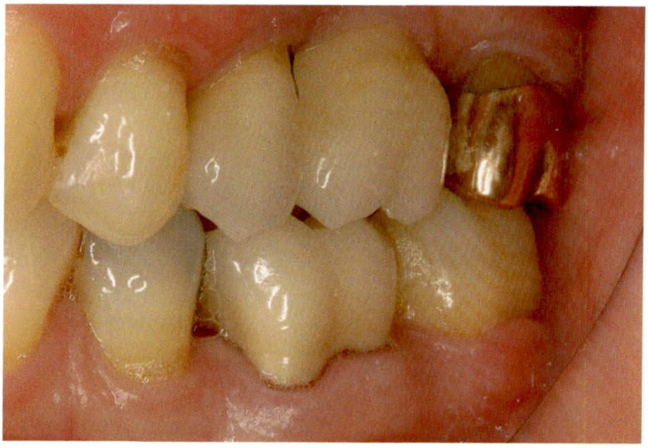

Fig. 12.17 Lateral view of the maxillary restorations with restorations that simulate teeth

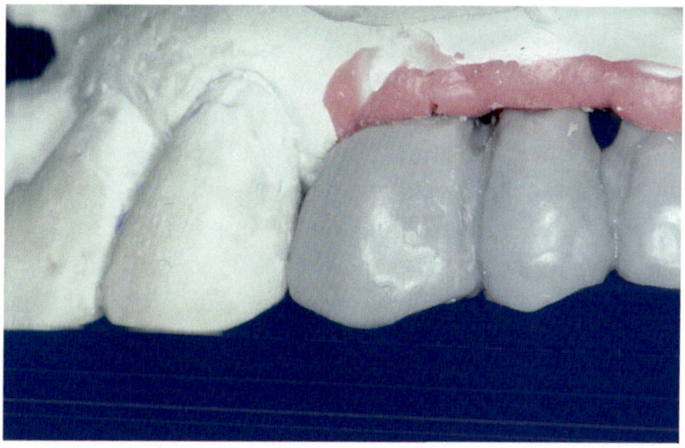

Fig. 12.18 Lateral view of wax-ups on cast when implant is placed too distally to allow proper contours

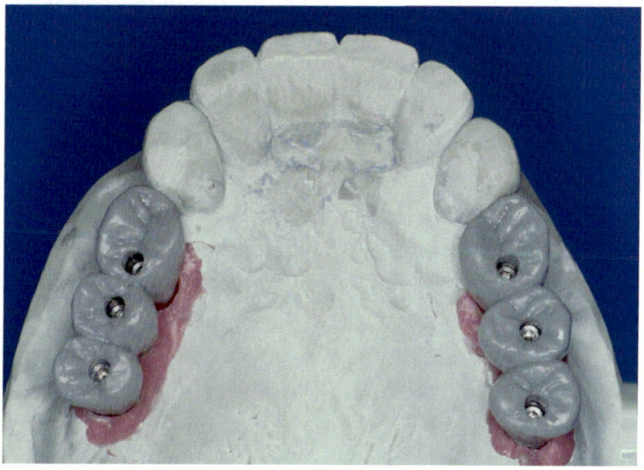

Fig. 12.19 Occlusal view of wax-ups on cast illustration of distally placed implants

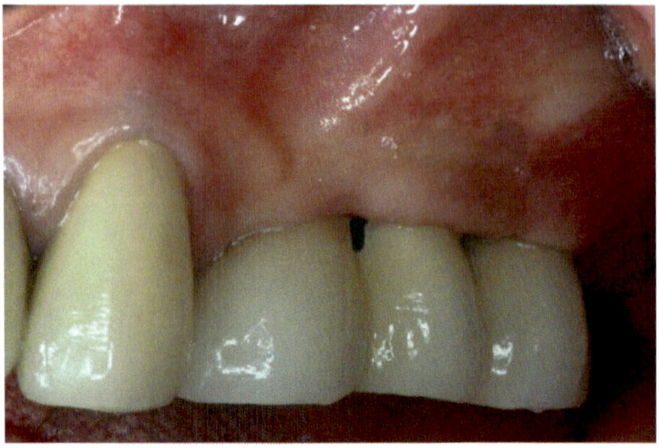

Fig. 12.20 Intra-oral view of restorations with less-than-ideal aesthetics

12.2 Occluso-Gingival

Once teeth are removed, there is a remodelling of the alveolar bone; in the maxilla, the resorptive pattern shifts apically and toward the centre of the arch form, and on the mandible, the shift is apically and away from the centre of the arch.

Replacing premolar and molar teeth requires approximately 10 mm of space between the residual ridge and the opposing occlusion. 7 mm would be considered the bare minimum when aesthetics is an issue. Often, when teeth are missing for prolonged periods of time, opposing teeth over-erupt and compromise the restorative space. If this is minimal, enameloplasty or minimal restorative therapy may create space sufficient to accommodate implant-supported restorations. On occasion, teeth opposing the edentate space can over-erupt; the magnitude of the over-eruption can range from minimal to the extent that they contact the opposing residual ridge.

When occluso-gingival space less than 7 mm or so is present, decisions need to be made whether to resect bone to obtain occluso-gingival space to accommodate restorations to mimic teeth. In case of larger dimensions that may exceed 10 mm of space, a bone graft may be considered to reduce the existing space or a taller prosthesis can be delivered with prosthetic soft tissue analogue [14]. A simple way to aid in decision-making would be to fabricate a removable try-in prostheses that will have simulated tooth forms to emerge from the ridge crest to occlude with the opposing dentition (Figs. 12.21, 12.22, 12.23 and 12.24). This try-in prostheses would allow the patient to visualize the outcome of the display of the restorations; they may accept the presenting anatomy and tooth display or decide on more ideal appearances and accept procedures to alter the current situation. If any procedures to alter the presenting anatomy are required, the extended treatment time, costs and risks need to be explained to patients (Figs. 12.25, 12.26, 12.27, 12.28 and 12.29).

Once decisions are made, the try-in prostheses can be converted to a surgical guide to have the implants placed in accordance with the planned restoration positions. Should a patient present with a removable prosthesis with flanges, they should not use these for a template to fabricate a surgical guide as the flanges will not provide the correct information for implant positions (Figs. 12.21, 12.22 and 12.23).

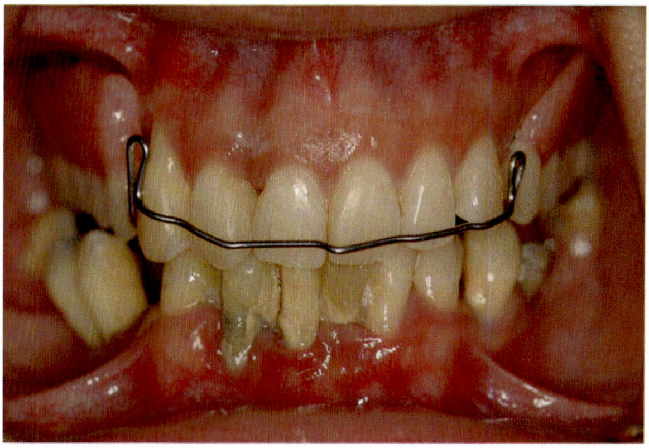

Fig. 12.21 Intra-oral view of a maxillary removable partial denture with posterior teeth emerging from the denture flange (Figs. 12.21, 12.22, 12.23, 12.24, 12.25, 12.26, 12.27, 12.28 and 12.29 courtesy of Dr. Aaron Wu)

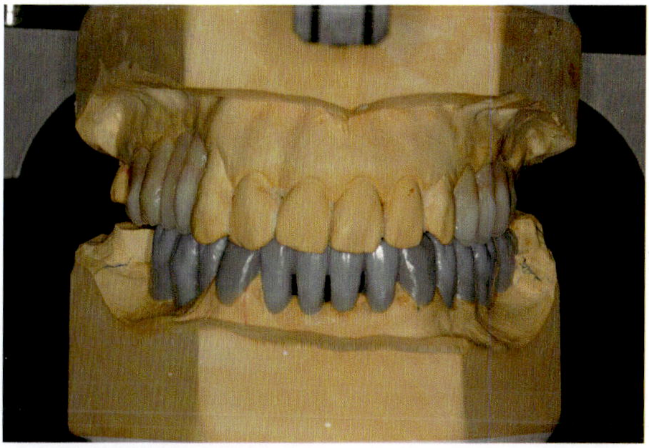

Fig. 12.22 The posterior teeth for the try-in removable prosthesis to emerge from the ridge crest

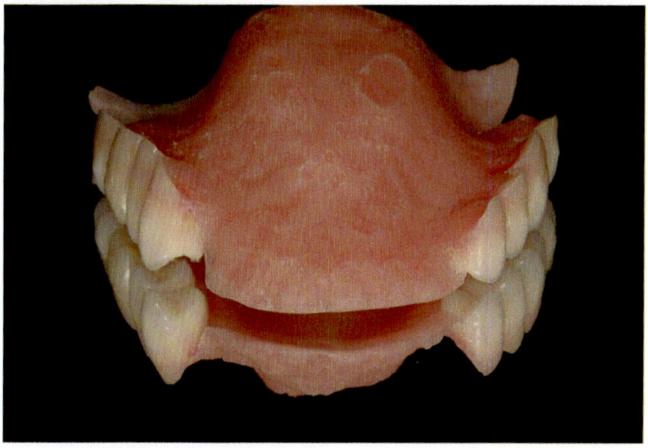

Fig. 12.23 Image of the try-in prosthesis—note that there is no flange on the prosthesis; this try-in prosthesis will also be a template for radiographic guides for CT scans and for surgical guides

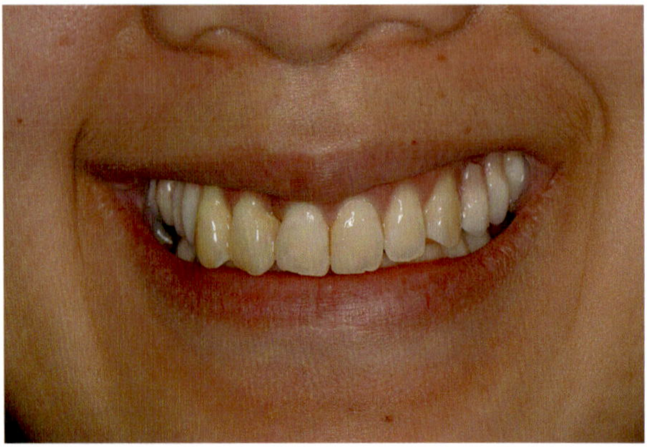

Fig. 12.24 Image of the try-in prostheses to visualize the appearance of the tooth display on the patient's right side; the ridge is more severely resorbed than the left side; the patient may consider grafting on the right side to have similar occluso-gingival dimensions of both sides or resection of the left side to have similar tooth heights

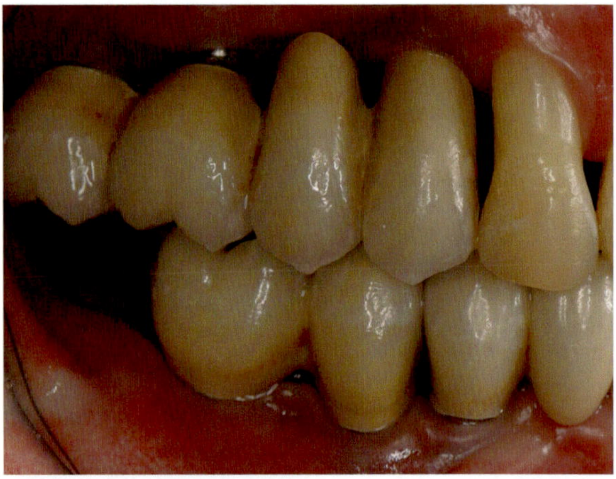

Fig. 12.25 Image of right side of the maxillary posterior sextant

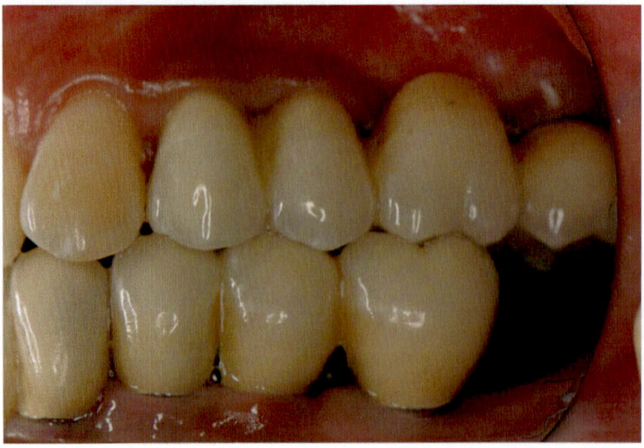

Fig. 12.26 Image of the left side of the maxillary posterior sextant

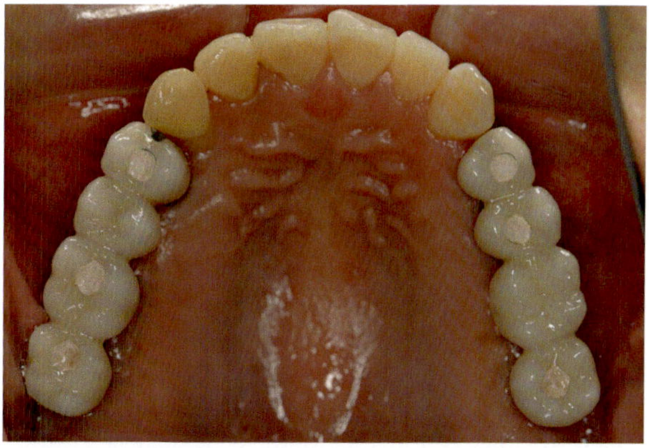

Fig. 12.27 Occlusal view of the arch form intra-orally; mesio-distal dimensions are well distributed with implants placed ideally to have screw channels exit through the occlusal aspects of restorations

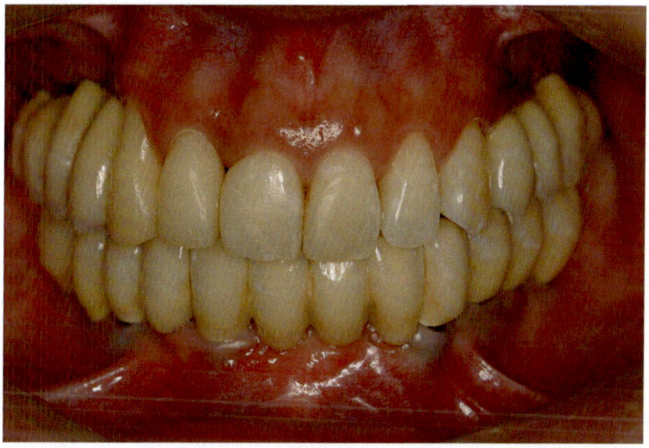

Fig. 12.28 Anterior view of the completed implant-supported restorations on the left and right sextants of the maxilla and the full arch of the mandible

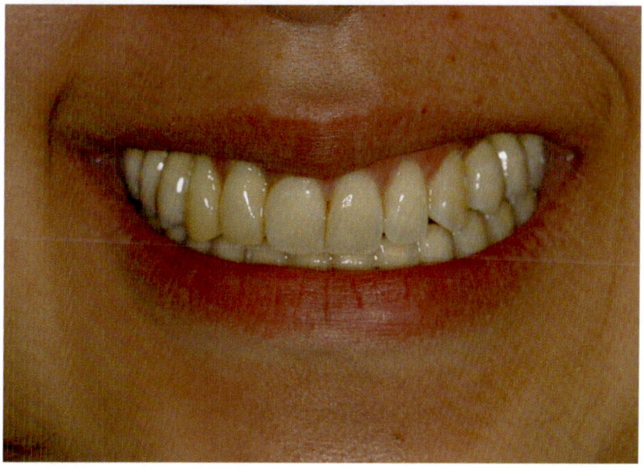

Fig. 12.29 Image of this patient smiling to show similarity of Fig. 12.24, the try-in prosthesis; a comparison of Fig. 12.21 and Fig. 12.24 will demonstrate that the partial denture with flanges should not be used to guide implant placement. In addition, the try-in prosthesis will allow patient and clinician to evaluate tooth display

12.3 Submucosal Contours

When replacing premolars, the transition from the average regular platform (4 mm) of the implant to the exit profile is easily accomplished when the implant is placed 3–5 mm apical to the mucosal margin of the restoration; with a platform-switching design of the implant, the implant would have to be deeper to allow a similar contour to be developed. A wider platform of an implant can allow the implant to be placed less apically and allow a gradual emergence angle. Currently, several authors have reported that when contours are diverging from implant platforms at more than 30°, implants will have exhibited more bleeding on probing and peri-implant bone loss at times. Therefore, more attention should be paid relative to implant depth. It is speculated that the severe divergence of implants from the implant platform can hinder hygiene and plaque removal. However, at present, none of the studies differentiate screw-retained and cemented restorations; the severe divergence of contours may engender cement retention that leads to the symptoms described. In addition, platform-switched dental implant systems can demand deeper implant placement to develop a smooth transition of the submucosal profile [15–19] (Fig. 12.30).

When molars are being replaced, wider implants can be placed when bony anatomy allows; alternatively, when anatomy precludes wider implants, placement of a third premolar can be placed with gradual emergence profiles (Fig. 12.31).

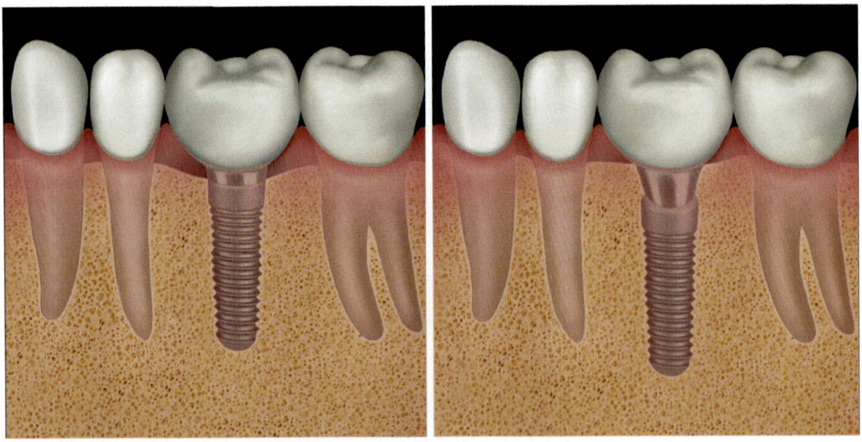

Fig. 12.30 Diagram to show submucosal contours and the difference between having platform-matching implants and platform-switching implants to be placed at different depths

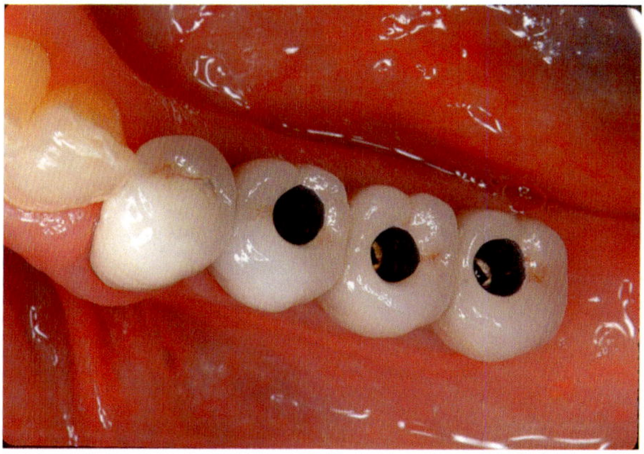

Fig. 12.31 When ridges are narrow from lingual to buccal and limited to depth due to mandibular nerve canal, implants can be placed to accommodate the anatomic limitations; this image shows three premolar-sized implants to be able to have gradual submucosal contours

12.4 Functional Replacement

Functional replacement of implants in the posterior sextants can often be provided if patients are informed of the atypical appearance of the restorations. These restorations may not be similar to teeth but do provide occluding surfaces. Patients do have the option to understand and accept these types of restorations for function and forgo aesthetics, especially when these restorations are not in the aesthetic zone. When patients do not accept restorations that do not appear as teeth, there will be a need to alter the presenting anatomy, restorative space and tooth positions to accommodate implant-supported restorations to mimic tooth forms.

When edentulous posterior sextants are unbounded and not in the aesthetic zones, restorations can be functional and may not have similar appearances to natural teeth; this is often due to implant placement into the most ideal anatomical sites that are receptive to the implants (Fig. 12.32).

Super-eruption of opposing teeth into partially edentulous spaces can be restored with a combination of procedures to develop sufficient occlusal space for implant-supported restorations. In these situations, the restorations are functional and do not resemble teeth (Figs. 12.33, 12.34, 12.35, 12.36 and 12.37). This series of images will illustrate how teeth have erupted into the opposing edentulous space. The erupted teeth are reduced significantly (Fig. 12.34). Crown lengthening is carried out, and endodontic therapy is required as pulp is exposed on reduction of the occlusal tooth structure due to over-eruption. After these ancillary procedures, the teeth are restored with crowns. The combination of these procedures can provide the minimal occluso-gingival restorative space for the restorations as shown in the images, and the restorations are unlike teeth but functional.

When restoring posterior sextants, it also requires an evaluation of the bite forces that are applied to the restorations. Clinicians should evaluate the functional forces that some patients generate. An examination of the remaining teeth can reveal the forces that have been applied, when wear patterns cracked teeth. Likewise, implant-supported restorations can also suffer screw loosening, implant component fractures

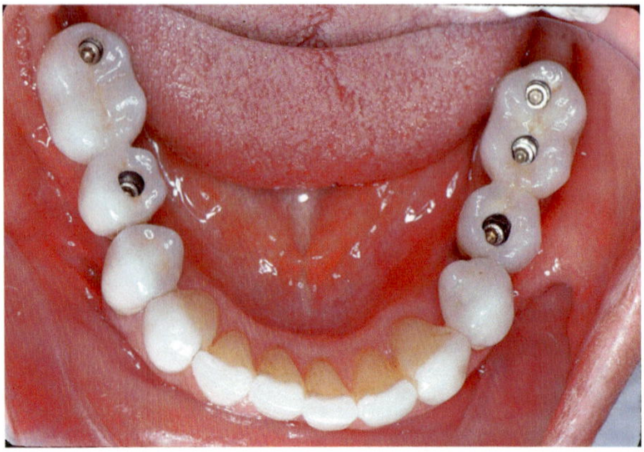

Fig. 12.32 Occlusal view of restorations in posterior that do not mimic the anatomy of teeth; these restorations do provide function

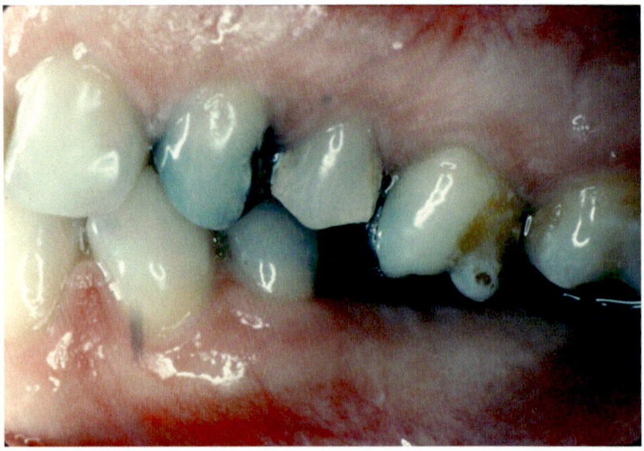

Fig. 12.33 Intra-oral image of supra-erupted teeth and a lack of restorative space

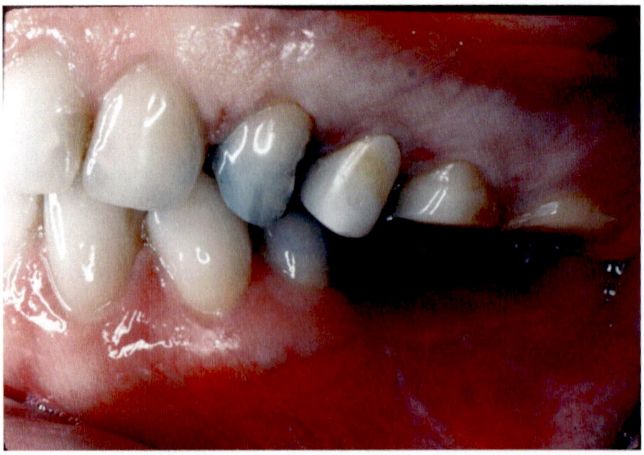

Fig. 12.34 Intra-oral image of supra-erupted teeth that have significant occlusal reduction

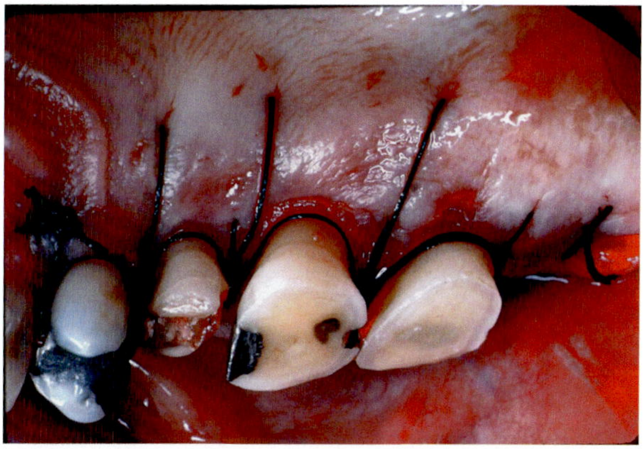

Fig. 12.35 Crown lengthening carried out with caution not to expose root furcations

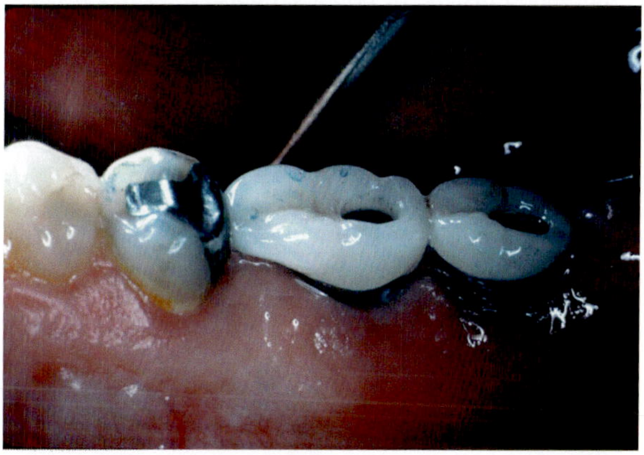

Fig. 12.36 Image of implant-retained restorations that are functional but do not mimic tooth anatomy

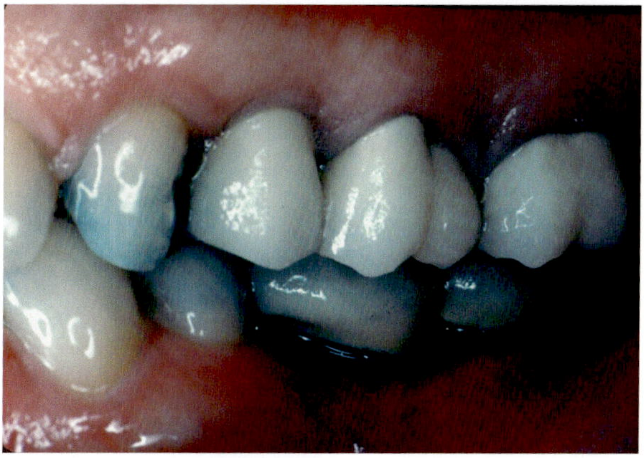

Fig. 12.37 Opposing teeth restored and in occlusion with implant-supported restorations

and chipping implant-supported restorations, especially in posterior sextants where occlusal forces are the strongest. In Chap. 2 discussing biomechanics, this is described in more detail.

A three-implant configuration will eliminate all axes of rotation providing stability of the retaining screws of the restorations; if forces are high in patients, a distribution of implants will reduce screw loosening or fracture significantly. In this example, the implants were also placed to avoid the need for sinus grafting. This allows a reduction of treatment time and placement of the implants into host bone (Figs. 12.38, 12.39 and 12.40).

Another example is where the maxillary sinus is avoided for implant placements due to medical issues with the sinus or the patient's choice of avoiding surgical access to their sinuses. Implants are placed anterior and posterior to the maxillary sinus. If no antagonist teeth are opposed to the implant-supported restorations, then there is no need to have additional tooth units on the restoration, and a connector bar is fabricated instead of pontics. Please refer to Figs. 12.41 and 12.42.

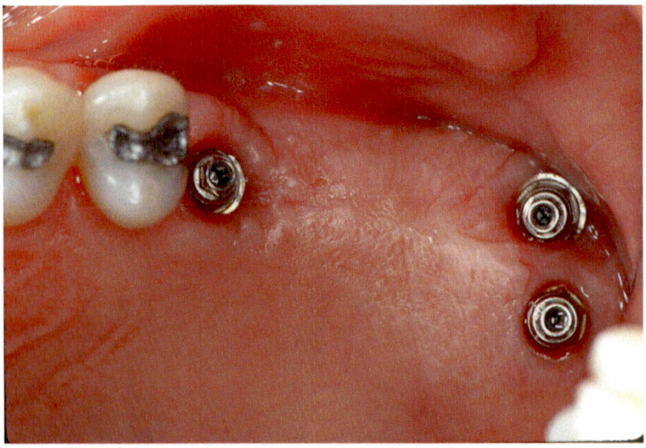

Fig. 12.38 Implants are placed to avoid sinus grafting and placed into host bone; biomechanically, the implant distribution provides stability to the restoration

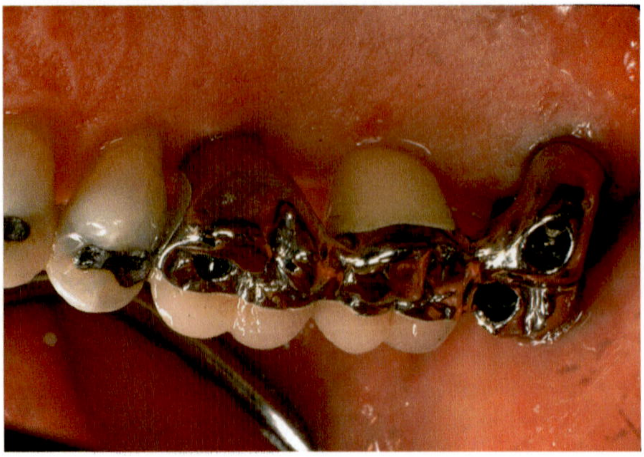

Fig. 12.39 Image of completed restoration; note that the most distal restoration need not have normal tooth morphology

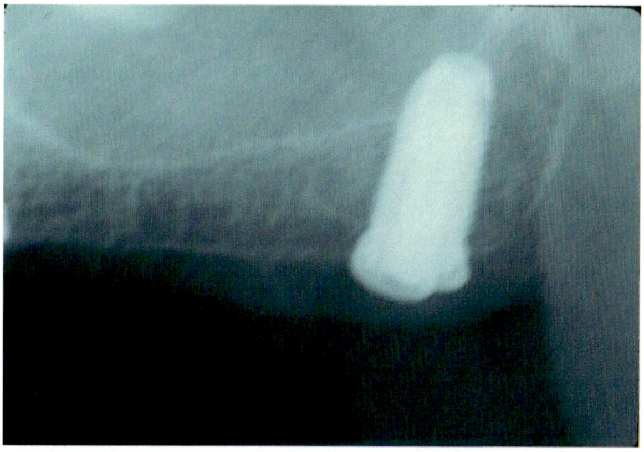

Fig. 12.40 Image of radiograph illustration of implants placed distal to the sinus

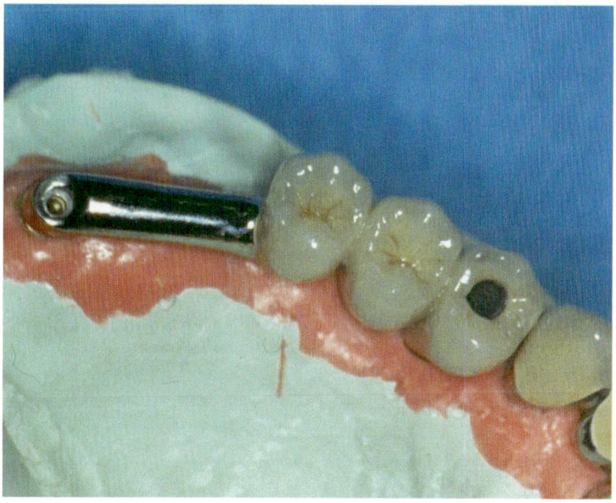

Fig. 12.41 Image of implant connected to restorations with bar; implant is placed to avoid sinus grafting

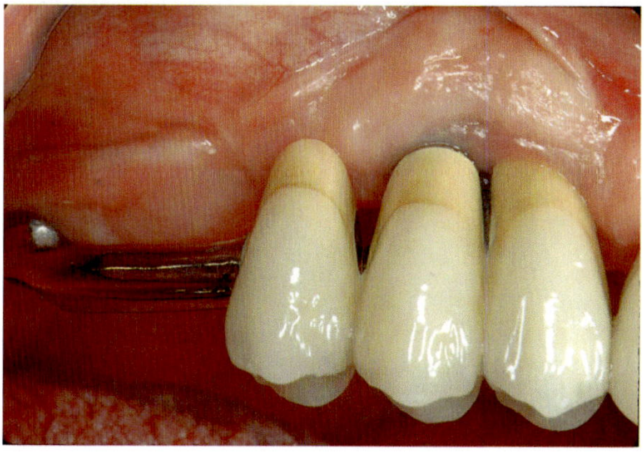

Fig. 12.42 Lateral view of implants intra-orally with implant-supporting restoration distally

12.5 Summary

Function is the dominant factor in posterior sextants whenever function and aesthetics are needed to satisfy both patient and provider. The aesthetic needs in the posterior sextants are more focused on in the maxilla than the mandible because of the tooth display. It is important to evaluate the patient's tooth display, and for more clarity for patient acceptance, a try-in prosthesis will help.

References

1. Åstrand P, Ahlqvist J, Gunne J, Nilson H. Implant treatment of patients with edentulous jaws: a 20-year follow-up. Clin Implant Dent Relat Res. 2008;10:207–17.
2. Lekholm U, Gröndahl K, Jemt T. Outcome of oral implant treatment in partially edentulous jaws followed 20 years in clinical function. Clin Implant Dent Relat Res. 2006;8:178–86.
3. Edelhoff D, Sorensen JA. Tooth structure removal associated with various preparation designs for anterior teeth. J Prosthet Dent. 2002;87(5):503–9.
4. Chee W, Felton DA, Johnson PF, Sullivan DY. Cemented versus screw-retained implant prostheses: which is better? Int J Oral Maxillofac Implants. 1999;14(1):137–41.
5. Dahiya A, Baba NZ, Kattadiyil MT, Goodacre CJ, Mann A. Comparison of the effects of cement removal from zirconia and titanium abutments: an in vitro study. J Prosthet Dent. 2019;121(3):504–9.
6. Korsch M, Walther W. Peri-implantitis associated with type of cement: a retrospective analysis of different types of cement and their clinical correlation to the peri-implant tissue. Clin Implant Dent Relat Res. 2015;17(Suppl 2):e434–43.
7. Wilson TG Jr. The positive relationship between excess cement and peri-implant disease: a prospective clinical endoscopic study. J Periodontol. 2009;80(9):1388–92.
8. Miyazaki T, Nakamura T, Matsumura H, Ban S, Kobayashi T. Current status of zirconia restoration. J Prosthodont Res. 2013;57(4):236–61.
9. Leitão CIMB, Fernandes GVO, Azevedo LPP, Araújo FM, Donato H, Correia ARM. Clinical performance of monolithic CAD/CAM tooth-supported zirconia restorations: systematic review and meta-analysis. J Prosthodont Res. 2022;66(3):374–84.
10. Aloum A, Chee W. Achieving esthetics, function, and retrievability with implant-supported monolithic zirconia restorations while minimizing surgical interventions. Quintessence Dent Technol. 2017;108:256.
11. Goldberg J, Torbati A, Amir A, Chee W. Implant-supported full-arch zirconia fixed dental prostheses for the rehabilitation of a patient with a failing dentition. Quintessence Dent Technol. 2016;39:224.
12. Han HS, Kim PJ, Kim KT, Kim S, Ku Y, Cho YD. Dental implant proximity to adjacent teeth: a retrospective study. Clin Implant Dent Relat Res. 2022;24(6):733–9.
13. Esposito M, Ekestubbe A, Gröndahl K. Radiological evaluation of marginal bone loss at tooth surfaces facing single Brånemark implants. Clin Oral Implants Res. 1993;4(3):151–7.
14. Wicks RA. A systematic approach to definitive planning for osseointegrated implant prostheses. J Prosthodont. 1994;3(4):237–42.
15. Neale D, Chee WW. Development of implant soft tissue emergence profile: a technique. J Prosthet Dent. 1994;71(4):364–8.
16. Katafuchi M, Weinstein BF, Leroux BG, Chen YW, Daubert DM. Restoration contour is a risk indicator for peri-implantitis: a cross-sectional radiographic analysis. J Clin Periodontol. 2018;45(2):225–32.

17. Yi Y, Koo KT, Schwarz F, Ben Amara H, Heo SJ. Association of prosthetic features and peri-implantitis: a cross-sectional study. J Clin Periodontol. 2020;47(3):392–403.
18. Majzoub J, Chen Z, Saleh I, Askar H, Wang HL. Influence of restorative design on the progression of peri-implant bone loss: a retrospective study. J Periodontol. 2021;92(4):536–46.
19. Mattheos N, Janda M, Acharya A, Pekarski S, Larsson C. Impact of design elements of the implant supracrestal complex (ISC) on the risk of peri-implant mucositis and peri-implantitis: a critical review. Clin Oral Implants Res. 2021;32(Suppl 21):181–202.

Treatment Planning of Implants in the Aesthetic Zone

13

Saj Jivraj and Winston Chee

Marketing inquiries have identified aesthetics as one of the major reasons why dentists utilize dental implants within their offices. If we go by that premise, it is reasonable to speculate that the aesthetic results provided with dental implants should be similar to the aesthetics provided with more conventional modes of therapy such as fixed and removable partial dentures. However, achieving aesthetics with implant restorations is significantly more challenging than that with conventional restorations. Diagnosis and appropriate treatment planning are critical in obtaining a successful outcome. Many manufacturers will identify their systems as aesthetic; from an objective perspective, components in of themselves are not aesthetic. There is no single component available from a manufacturer which would deliver an ideal and aesthetic replacement for a maxillary central incisor. Aesthetic outcomes are based on many variables. It is not the specific implant design, surface characteristics or type of abutment that will guarantee an aesthetic result. It is rather the time spent on data collection in reaching a correct diagnosis that pays dividends in terms of function and aesthetics [1].

Root form cylindrical implants placed following surgical techniques described by Branemark et al. have proven to be a predictable method for anchoring replacement teeth to the jawbone [2, 3]. Today, clinicians can prescribe the use of implants with the knowledge and confidence that they will predictably integrate into the jawbone. The successful integration of an implant however is not sufficient to declare success; implants placed in poor restorative positions result in unaesthetic restorations that provide little satisfaction for the clinician or the patient (Figs. 13.1, 13.2, and 13.3). The above illustrations demonstrate the complexity of implant use in aesthetic zones and the importance of proper treatment planning prior to implant placement.

S. Jivraj (✉)
Private Practice, Anacapa Dental Art Institute, Oxnard, CA, USA

W. Chee
Advanced Prosthodontics, Herman Ostrow School of Dentistry, University of Southern California, Los Angeles, CA, USA

W. Chee, S. Jivraj (eds.), *Treatment Planning In Implant Dentistry*, BDJ Clinician's Guides, https://doi.org/10.1007/978-3-031-68726-6_13

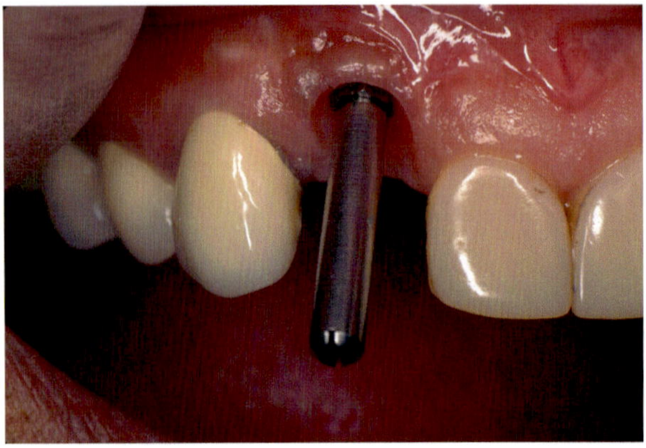

Fig. 13.1 Intra-oral photograph of implant in poor position angled labially and exiting the ridge too apically

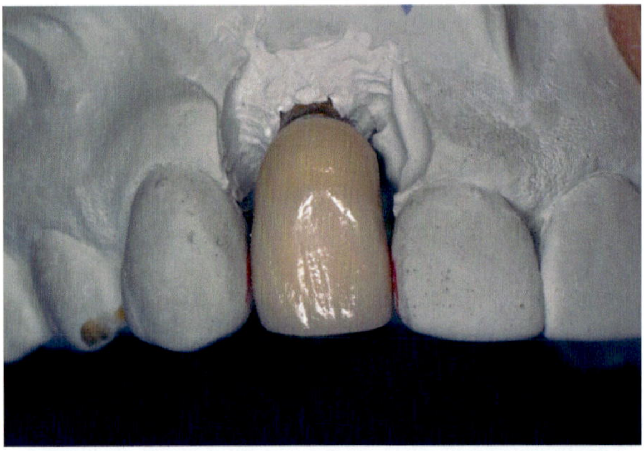

Fig. 13.2 Restoration fabricated for implant in Fig. 13.1; note the length of restoration compared to adjacent teeth

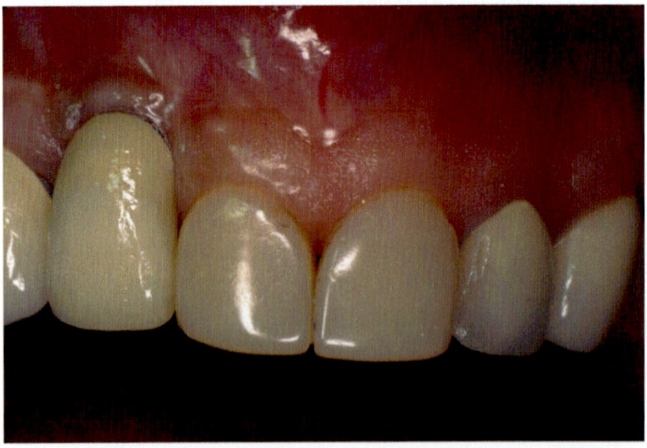

Fig. 13.3 Labial view of restoration for implant on Fig. 13.1; note the poor shape and form of the tooth and a mucosal margin too apical dictated by poor implant position

Providing an aesthetic outcome requires understanding of the objective and subjective criteria related to hard and soft tissue aesthetics [4]. Both dental and gingival aesthetics act together to provide a smile with harmony and balance. The clinician must be aware of parameters related to gingival morphology, form and dimension, characterization, surface texture and colour [5] (Fig. 13.4). Ceramists can often

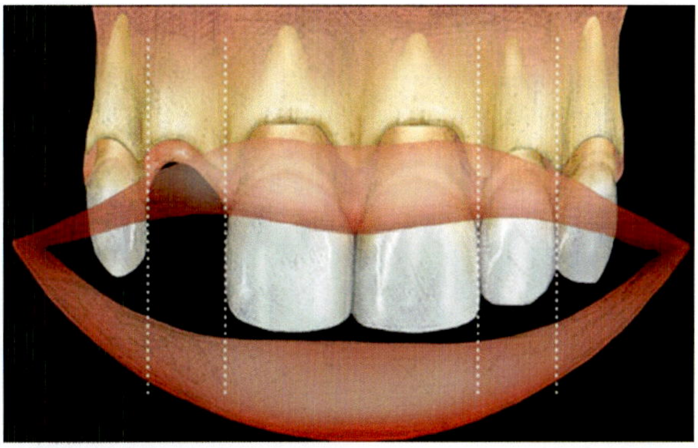

Fig. 13.4 Restoration of implants must satisfy objective and subjective aesthetic criteria. There should be sufficient inter-radicular space for placement of the implant and sufficient inter-tooth distance for fabrication of an aesthetically pleasing restoration

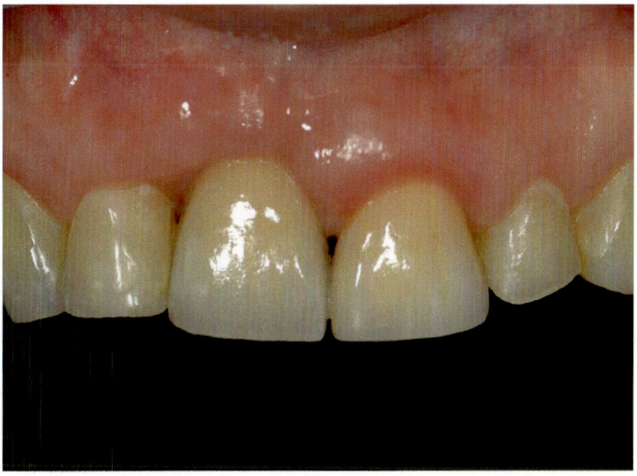

Fig. 13.5 Note that the ceramics of the right central incisor matches that of the left central incisor; however, reconstruction of the deficient hard tissue has not been achieved resulting in a restoration that does not satisfy the objective criteria of aesthetics

produce restorations to match adjacent teeth in terms of colour; however, if the surrounding tissues are not reconstructed, an aesthetic outcome is not likely (Fig. 13.5). The ultimate aim is for the implant restoration to harmonize into the frame of the smile, face and, more importantly, individual.

Treatment planning must address hard and soft tissue deficiencies and combine this with precision in implant placement; only with this approach can implant restorations be indistinguishable from the adjacent teeth (Fig. 13.6).

Recreating what nature provided can be a formidable challenge. The physiology of wound healing after tooth extraction creates an unfavourable soft tissue complex. The remaining mucosa often recedes palatally and apically. Often, this results in a restoration that appears long, and this is compounded by the absence of interdental papilla (Fig. 13.7).

The predictability of the aesthetic outcome of an implant restoration is dependent on many variables including, but not limited to:

1. Patient selection and smile line
2. Tooth position
3. Root position of the adjacent teeth

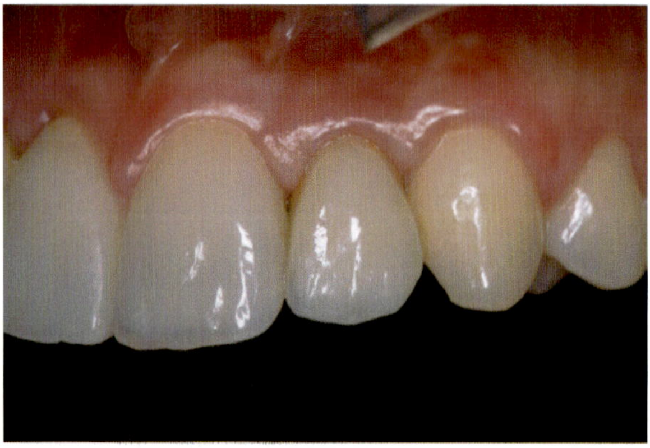

Fig. 13.6 Implant restoration on left lateral incisor in harmony with the existing hard and soft tissue

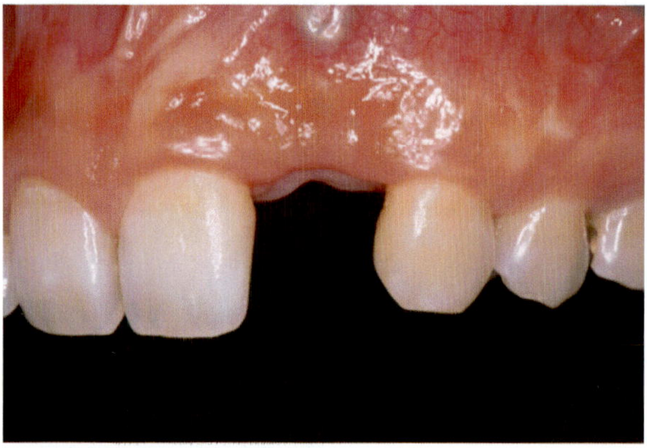

Fig. 13.7 Wound healing following extraction of a tooth can result in apical and palatal migration of the interdental papilla

4. Biotype of the periodontium and tooth shape
5. The bony anatomy of the implant site
6. The position of the implant

13.1 Patient Selection and Smile Line

Patients who are candidates for replacement of an anterior tooth with an implant-supported restoration must understand the benefits of an implant restoration. They must also understand the additional length of time required for treatment and additional costs that will be incurred. The clinician must also understand the patient's desires. In most cases, the patient's primary demand is an aesthetic tooth replacement; with this in mind, it is important to establish sound clinical concepts with clearly defined parameters that lead to successful aesthetics with long-term stability of the peri-implant tissues.

The major indication for a single-tooth implant restoration is preservation (non-preparation) of one or more of the adjacent teeth (Fig. 13.8) and reduction in the rate of alveolar resorption. Additional indications would be restoration of a missing

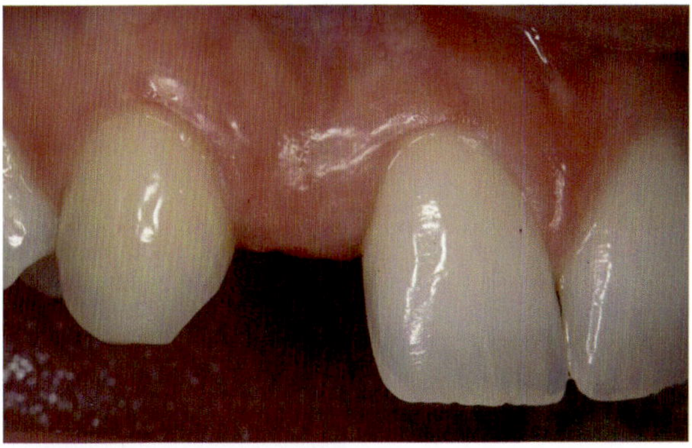

Fig. 13.8 A perfect indication for a dental implant with adequate periodontal attachment levels presented by adjacent teeth

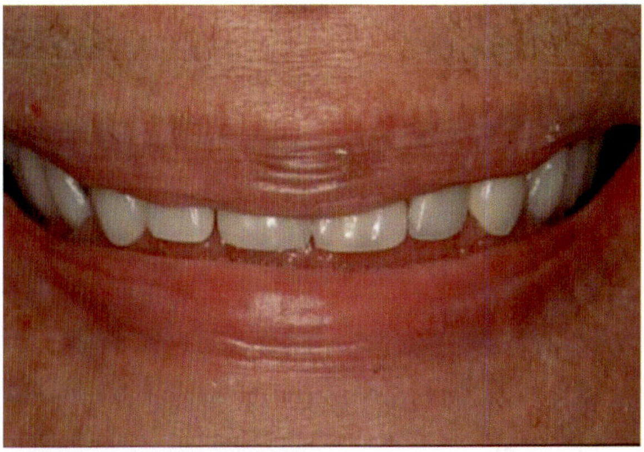

Fig. 13.9 Low smile line

tooth to maintain a diastema, to have teeth that are rotated to appear more natural and preservation of extensive fixed restorations that are intact.

A patient's aesthetic expectations must also be evaluated together with their lip activity and lip length. In an average smile, 75–100% of the maxillary incisors and the interproximal gingiva are displayed. In a high smile line, additional gingival tissue is exposed. Less than 75% of the incisors are exposed in a low smile line (Figs. 13.9, 13.10 and 13.11) [6]. The clinician should be aware that the patient who presents with unacceptable tooth health, shade or position may not give a full smile when asked. Previous photographs may aid in determining the natural position of the patient's lip when smiling.

A high smile line poses considerable challenges when planning for implant-supported restorations in the aesthetic zone because the restoration and gingival tissues are completely displayed. In these types of clinical situations, maximal efforts towards maintaining peri-implant tissue support throughout the planning, provisional, surgical and restorative phases will be required. A book chapter later in the series will discuss soft tissue management with provisional restorations.

The low smile line is a less critical situation because the implant restoration interface will be hidden behind the upper lip. However, this cannot be assumed, and

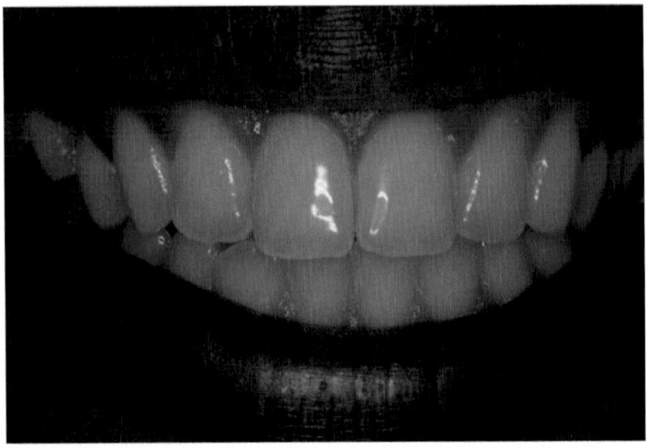

Fig. 13.10 Average smile line

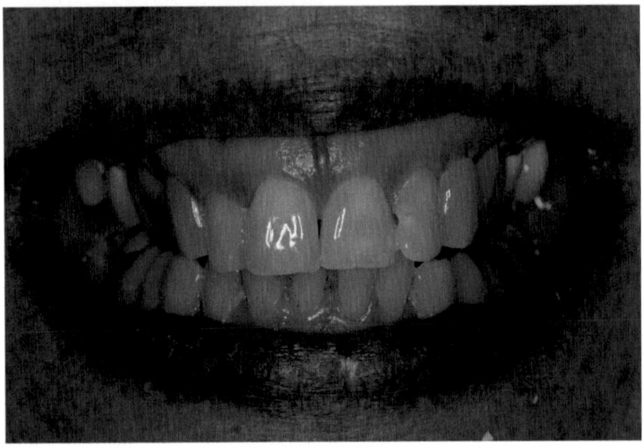

Fig. 13.11 High smile line. The colour and contour of the restorations and associated hard and soft tissues become very visible to the patient and observer

the patient's input must be sought to confirm this. "The aesthetic zone is where the patient thinks it is" (Dr. Jack Preston D.D.S.).

13.2 Tooth Position

The tooth needs to be evaluated in three planes of space: apico-coronal, facio-lingual and mesiodistal. The existing tooth position will significantly influence the presenting gingival architecture. In many instances, teeth with a poor prognosis are thoughtlessly extracted. These teeth can significantly influence both the hard and soft tissue configuration.

13.2.1 Apico-Coronal

On assessment of the apico-coronal position of the tooth, it may be more apical, more coronal or ideal and mimic the level of the adjacent gingival margin (Fig. 13.12). Numerous authors have shown that following extraction and insertion

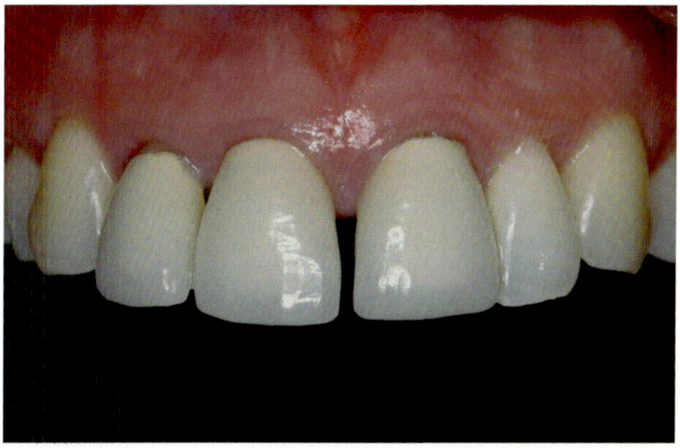

Fig. 13.12 The right lateral incisor has been treatment planned for an implant restoration. The level of the soft tissues mimics that of the contralateral tooth

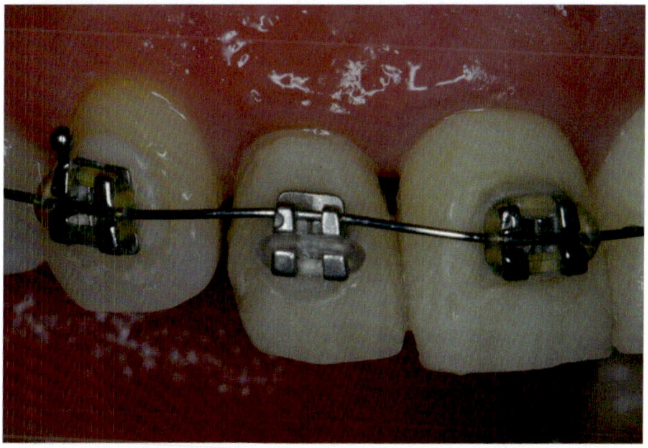

Fig. 13.13 Immediate extraction of the right lateral incisor would result in apical migration of the soft tissue. Orthodontic extrusion will allow the clinician to position the tissue more coronally so that on extraction there is a margin of error

of an ovate pontic, there is likely to be up to 2 mm of gingival recession [6], and on extraction and placement of an implant immediately, the migration of the gingival margin is likely to approximate 0.2 mm [7].

The implication of this is that if there is a hopeless tooth positioned ideally or apically and this is extracted, the gingival margin is likely to migrate apically. Restoratively, long clinical crowns, pink porcelain or visible metal margins will compromise the aesthetic outcome. These teeth can benefit from orthodontic extrusion (Fig. 13.13) prior to extraction, which will serve to position the gingival level at a more harmonious level [8, 9].

It is the author's opinion that a cone beam scan be taken of the area of concern. There must be sufficient bone labial to the tooth for orthodontic extrusion to be effective.

13.2.2 Facio-Lingual

In this dimension, the tooth position may present with different concerns. The tooth may be positioned too far facially; this often results in very thin or non-existent labial bone. These teeth are not good candidates for orthodontic extrusion because of inadequate underlying bone. Extraction of these teeth results in significant vertical bone loss and collapse of the gingival architecture. This type of situation would benefit from bone and soft tissue augmentation procedures prior to implant placement. A tooth positioned more lingually would benefit from the presence of an increased amount of facial bone. This situation is more favourable prior to extraction since the resultant discrepancy in the facial free gingival margin may be minimal [8, 10].

13.2.3 Mesiodistal

The proximity of the adjacent teeth necessary to provide proximal support and volume of interdental papillae should be evaluated. Ideally, the mesiodistal tooth width should be equal to that of the contralateral tooth so that an aesthetic outcome can be achieved (Figs. 13.14 and 13.15). Excess or deficiencies in this dimension should be addressed through the use of orthodontics, enameloplasty or restorations. For patients with diastemas, it is imperative that the decision to maintain or close the space be made prior to implant placement. If the patient refuses the above options to close the space and insists on closing the space with the implant restoration, there is a likelihood that a black triangle (open gingival embrasure) may ensue. This results from inadequate support from the adjacent tooth to maintain the papilla. It is important that the clinician discusses this with the patient ahead of time, so disappointment with the final outcome is avoided (Figs. 13.16 and 13.17).

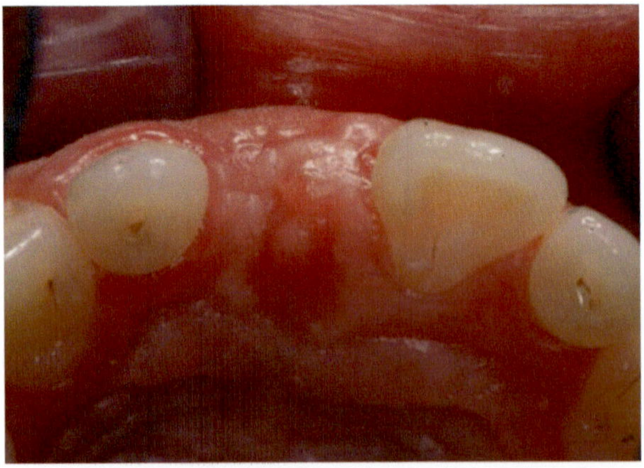

Fig. 13.14 The mesiodistal width of the tooth requiring replacement must equal that of the contralateral tooth

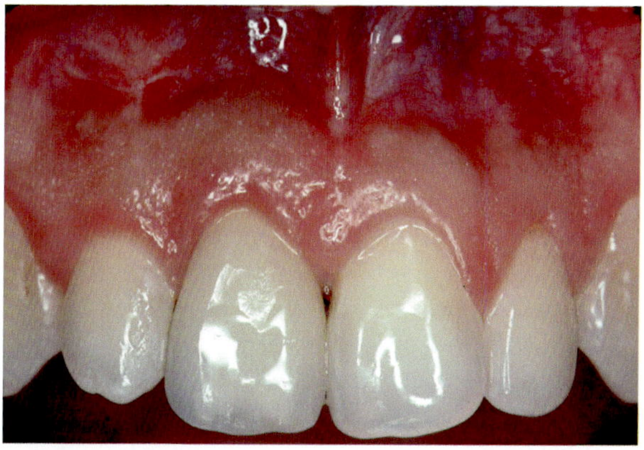

Fig. 13.15 Implant restoration replacing the right central incisor

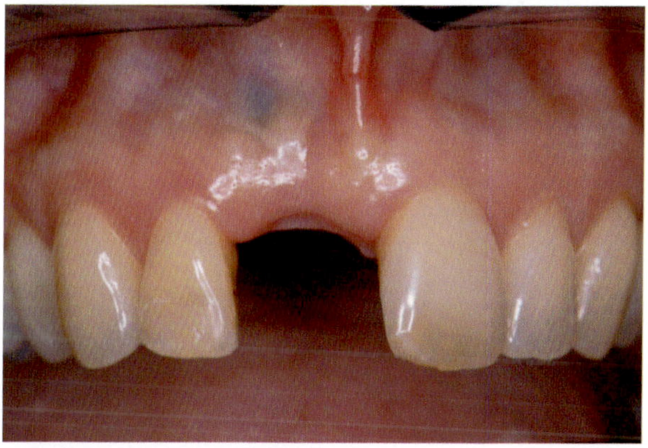

Fig. 13.16 Excessive mesiodistal space in the region of the tooth requiring an implant restoration

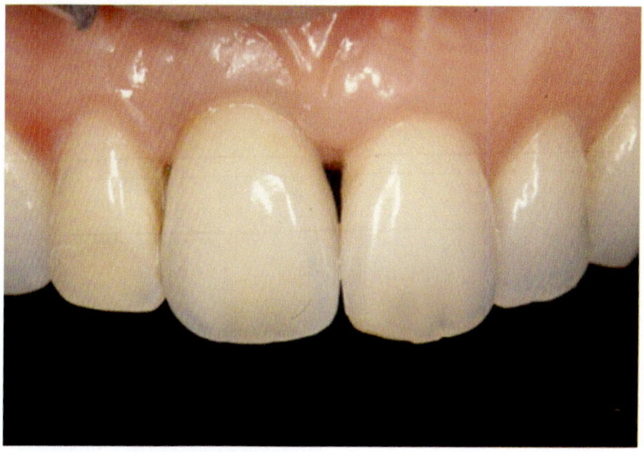

Fig. 13.17 Implant restoration in the region of the right central incisor. Note the absence of interdental papilla as a result of inadequate support of the soft tissue by the restoration

13.3 Root Position of Adjacent Teeth

Part of the diagnostic work for patients who need implants is a periapical radiograph, as often root position will preclude placing of implants. Many of these patients can benefit from orthodontics to reposition malposed teeth.

If the patient illustrated in Figs. 13.18 and 13.19 desired implant restorations to replace congenitally missing lateral incisors, orthodontic therapy would be necessary to move the roots of the cuspid and central incisor to allow room for ideal implant placement.

Teeth with root proximity also possess very little interproximal bone; this thin bone creates a greater risk of lateral resorption, which will decrease the vertical bone height after extraction or implant placement. When teeth are present, the use of orthodontics serves as a valuable adjunct to create space. This can be advantageous for support of proximal gingival architecture [11, 12].

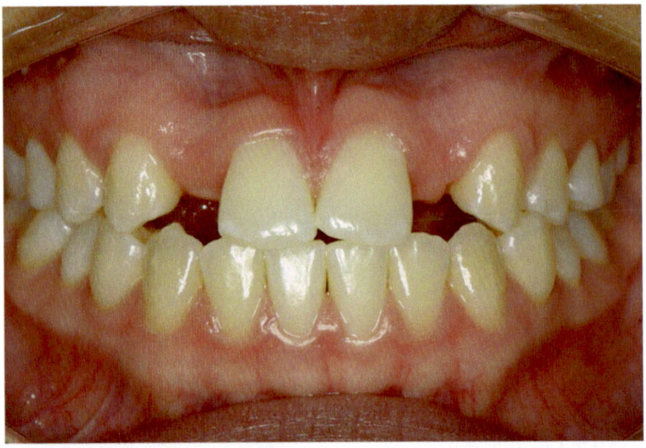

Fig. 13.18 Clinical presentation of patient with congenitally missing maxillary lateral incisors post-orthodontic treatment

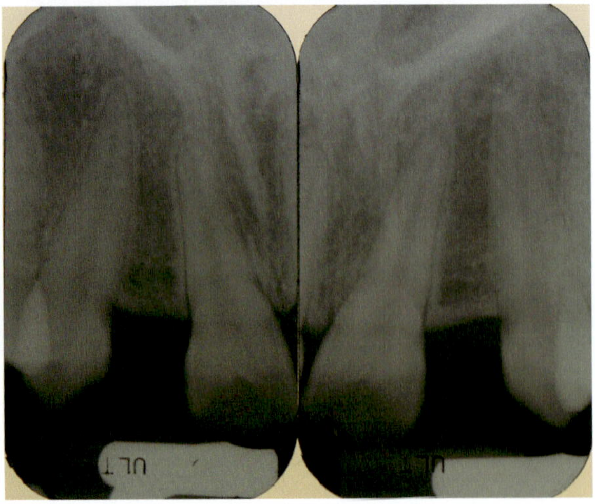

Fig. 13.19 Radiograph of the patient in Fig. 13.18 revealing that there is insufficient inter-radicular space for implants

13.4 Biotype of Periodontium and Tooth Shape

The periodontal status of the adjacent teeth will have a direct impact on the peri-implant tissue and must be evaluated. The maintenance of peri-implant tissues is something patients must be educated on. If the patient lost teeth because of periodontal disease, the patient will likely be susceptible to peri-implantitis.

The position of the gingival tissue around a tooth is determined by the connective tissue attachment and by the bone level. Two different periodontal biotypes have been described in relation to the morphology of the interdental papilla and the osseous architecture—the thin scalloped periodontium and the thick flat periodontium [13].

The thin scalloped periodontium, found in less than 15% of cases, is characterized by a delicate soft tissue curtain and a scalloped underlying osseous form and often has dehiscence and fenestrations present, and a reduced quantity and quality of keratinized mucosa. Generally, interproximal tissue does not completely fill the space between adjacent teeth. This form of gingiva reacts to insults by receding facially and interproximally. As recession occurs and the inter-root bone resorbs, the subsequent soft tissue loss compromises the overall aesthetic result (Fig. 13.20).

The tooth form in this type exhibits a contact point towards the incisal third essentially triangular anatomic crowns and contact areas of teeth that are small facio-lingually and apico-coronally. Due to extreme taper of the roots, the bone interproximally tends to be thicker.

Characteristics of the soft tissue biotype will play a prominent role in the final planning for the position of the implant platform. A thin biotype with highly scalloped tissue will require the implant body and shoulder to be placed more palatal to mask any titanium show through. When implants are placed towards the palate, a slightly deeper placement is required to allow for proper emergence profile.

Combining previous factors in a patient with a high lip line and a thin biotype is extremely difficult to treat. Patients who fit into these treatment categories should be made aware of the challenges involved in obtaining an aesthetic result before

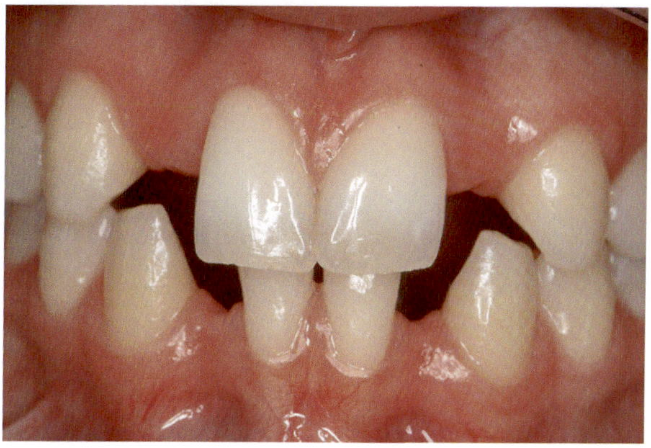

Fig. 13.20 Biotype 1 periodontium; note the thin and scalloped tissue

treatment begins. Often in these types of patients, the use of zirconia or anodized cement abutments when the tissue thickness is less than 2 mm yields a more optimal aesthetic outcome. If screw-retained restorations were used, the ceramic submucosal restorations would help with thin biotypes.

The thick flat periodontal biotype is characterized by a denser, more fibrotic soft tissue curtain, a flat thicker underlying osseous form and an increased quantity and quality of attached keratinized gingiva. This tissue often reacts to insults by pocket formation. Flat gingiva is associated with a tooth form in which more bulbous contact areas are located more towards the middle third of the tooth, primarily square anatomic crowns and contact areas that are wide facio-lingually and apico-coronally (Fig. 13.21).

The tooth morphology appears to be correlated with the soft tissue quality. The triangular tooth shape is associated with the scalloped and thin periodontium. The contact area is located in the coronal third of the crown, underlining a long and thin papilla. The square anatomic crown shape combines with a thick and flat periodontium. The contact area is located at the middle third, supporting a short and wide papilla.

Loss of interproximal tissue in the presence of a triangular tooth form will display a wider black triangle than in a situation when a square tooth is present (Fig. 13.22). In some cases, when the adjacent teeth are to be restored, the crown form can be modified prosthetically to compensate for partial interproximal tooth loss. The contact area of the prosthetic tooth is positioned more apically, reducing the volume of the interdental space.

The presenting tooth shape will also influence the implant restoration shape. The implant restoration should mimic its contralateral natural tooth's free gingival margin. The submucosal contour of the restoration must take into account the existing height of the mucosal margin and its comparison with the contralateral tooth. If the existing mucosal margin is apical, a concave subgingival contour is encouraged to allow the soft tissue to drape more coronally. If the existing mucosal margin is more coronal, a fuller subgingival contour is required to push the soft tissue more apically (Fig. 13.23).

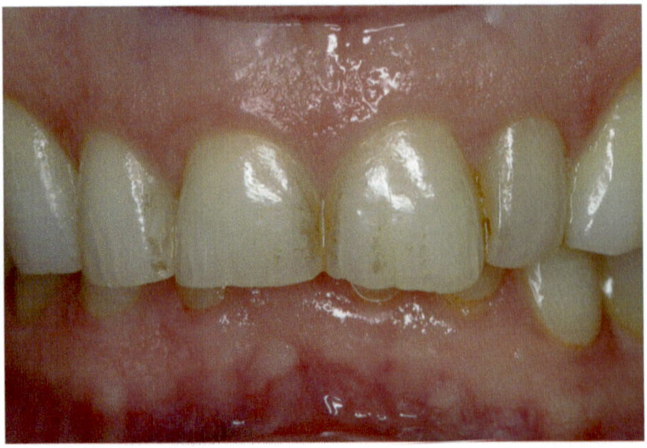

Fig. 13.21 Biotype 2 periodontium; not thick and flat tissues

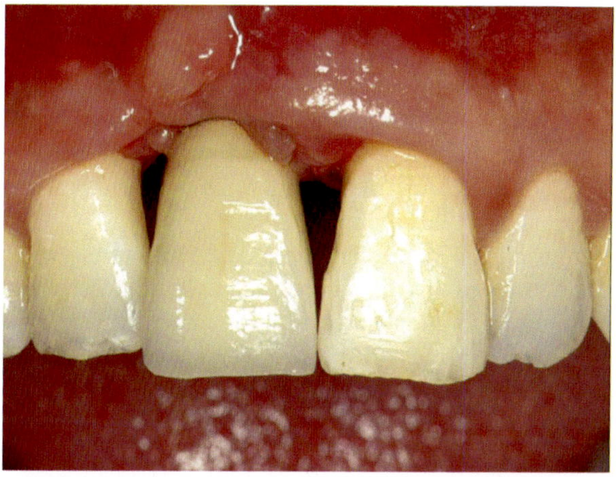

Fig. 13.22 Loss of interproximal soft tissue in the presence of a triangular tooth form can result in unsightly black triangles

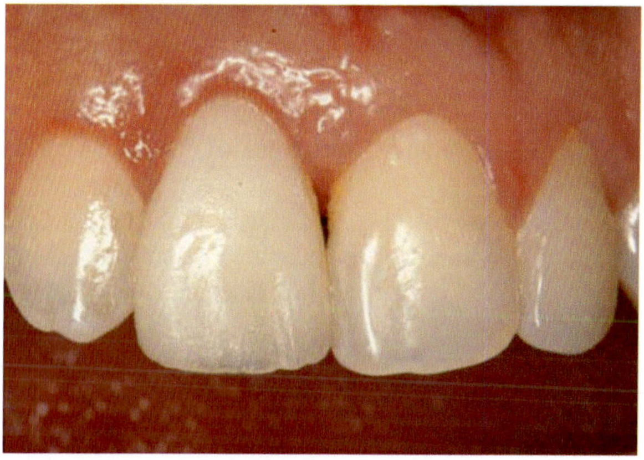

Fig. 13.23 Overcontour of the implant restoration as it emerges from the free gingival margin can result in apical migration of the soft tissues

13.5 Bony Anatomy of the Implant Site

For successful aesthetic restoration of implants, the bony housing must have a three-dimensional configuration that permits placement of an implant in a restoratively ideal position [14]. If the bony anatomy is inadequate, a bone grafting procedure may be required to enhance the site.

When these situations are encountered, the patient must be made to understand that a successful outcome will involve replacing more than just a "missing tooth". The patient must also understand that the missing hard and soft tissue architecture will need to be rebuilt so that optimum aesthetics can be achieved.

The definitive implant restoration needs to be surrounded by a hard and soft tissue environment that is in harmony with the surrounding dentition. It is not only the amount of bone and soft tissue present prior to implant surgery but also the precision of surgical execution that leads to an overall favourable outcome. Several key analyses need to be performed prior to commencing with implant placement. A diagnostic wax-up, which highlights tissue deficiencies and final tooth positioning, can assist in the planning process (Fig. 13.24).

Facio-lingual ridge anatomy should be evaluated to determine if there is sufficient crest width to house the implant. Deficient alveolar crest width will require a bone augmentation procedure to allow the implant to be placed in the ideal position (Figs. 13.25, 13.26, 13.27, and 13.28). A cone beam scan can assist in diagnosing deficiencies in this dimension.

Mesiodistal space should be equal to that of the contralateral tooth; excess or deficiencies in this dimension need to be addressed through orthodontics, enameloplasty or restoration either prior to or after implant placement.

The most critical dimension remains the apico-coronal dimension. Deficiencies in this dimension can result from periodontal disease, trauma, atrophy and infection. Vertical grafting is complex, and the site may require several surgeries to achieve an optimal configuration.

Two anatomic structures are important in determining predictability of soft tissues after implant placement. The first is the height and thickness of the facial bony wall, and the second is the bone height of the alveolar crest in the interproximal areas.

13.5.1 Height and Thickness of Facial Bony Wall

The position of the osseous crest is an important predictor for gingival levels. A survey of 100 patients [15] classified patients as having high, normal or low crests. This was based on the vertical distance of the osseous crest to the free gingival

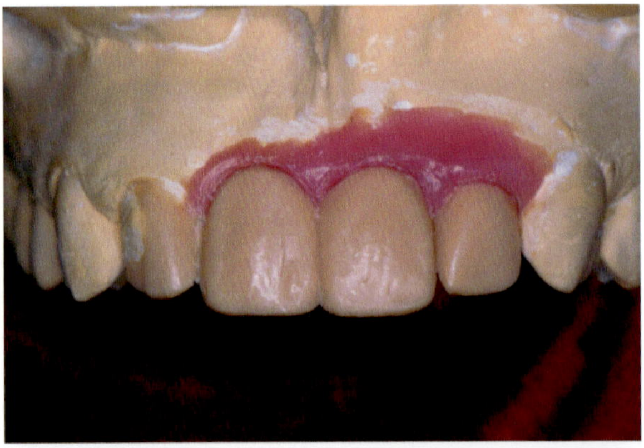

Fig. 13.24 A diagnostic wax-up can highlight the deficiency of the hard and soft tissue and can indicate to the surgeon how much augmentation is required

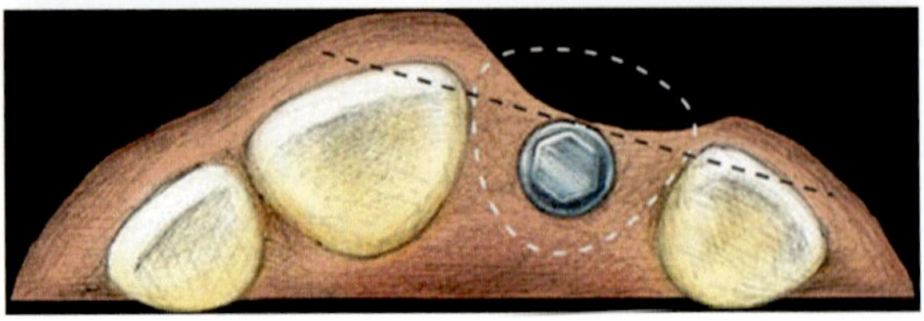

Fig. 13.25 A deficient alveolar crest will not allow the implant to be placed in an ideal position. There will be insufficient bony housing to accommodate the fixture

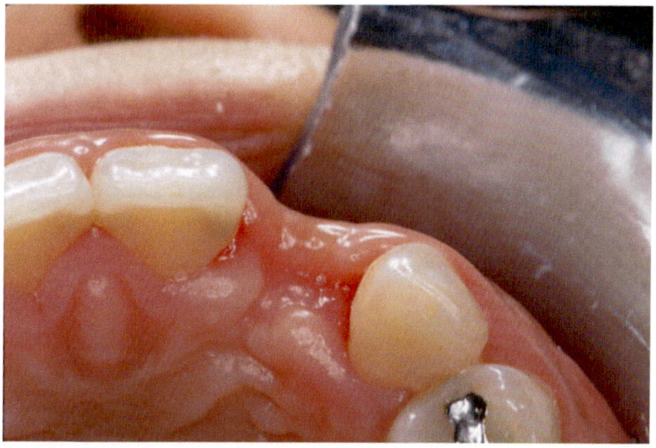

Fig. 13.26 Clinical slide of inadequate buccolingual width for implant placement

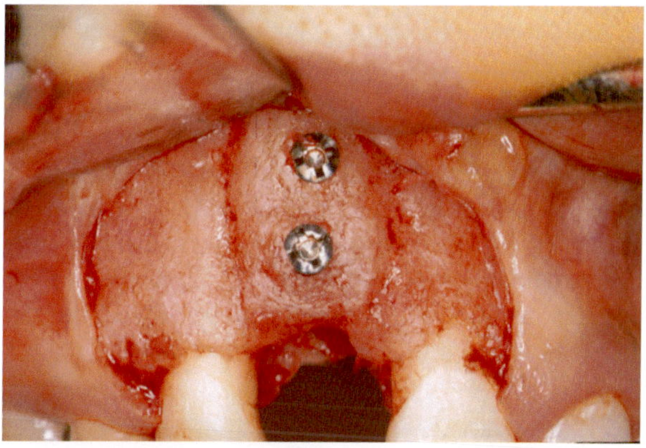

Fig. 13.27 Bone augmentation of the site pictured in Fig. 13.26

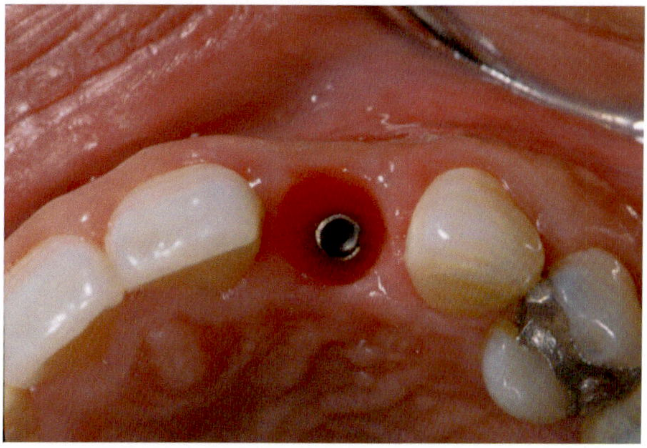

Fig. 13.28 Ideal implant placement; note the adequate ridge contours

margin. The greater the distance from the osseous crest to the free gingival margin, the greater the risk of tissue loss after an invasive procedure. Kois proposed that if the total vertical distance of the total dento-gingival complex on the mid facial aspect is 3 mm, a slight apical loss of tissue up to 1 mm is anticipated after extraction and immediate implant placement. Measuring the distance from the free gingival margin to the osseous crest prior to extraction is an important diagnostic predictor of the anticipated final position of the free gingival margin.

13.5.2 Height of Bony Crest in the Interproximal Area

The interproximal bony crest plays a critical role in the presence or absence of peri-implant papillae. A clinical study around teeth measured the distance from the interproximal contact to the vertical height of bone and observed how frequently the interproximal space would be filled completely by soft tissue [11]. When the contact point to the bone was 3–5 mm, papilla always filled the space. When the distance was 6 mm, papilla was absent 45% of the time, and with a distance of 7 mm, papilla did not fill the space 75% of the time.

A difference of 1–2 mm is significant in obtaining soft tissue aesthetics. This has been confirmed with implant-supported restorations [16]; multiple authors have also shown that the height of peri-implant papillae in single tooth gaps is dependent on the periodontal attachment and proximal bone level of the adjacent teeth. From a diagnostic perspective, sounding from the tip of the papilla to the interproximal bone crest of the adjacent tooth would be an important predictor (Figs. 13.29 and 13.30). If this distance is 5 mm or less, there is an increased likelihood that the interproximal tissues will be predictably maintained following implant placement and restoration. If the distance is greater than 5 mm, the papilla cannot be predictably maintained after surgical intervention.

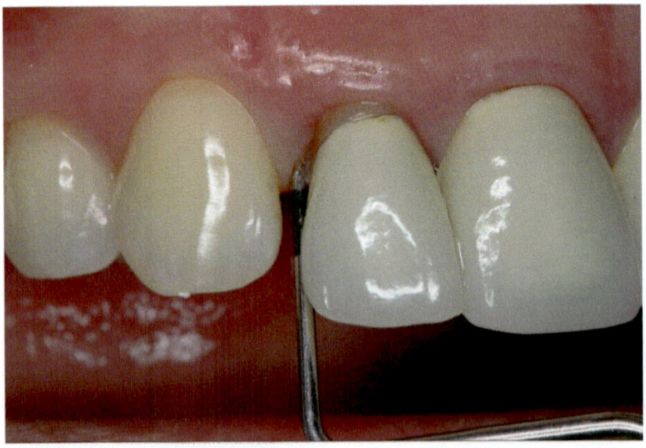

Fig. 13.29 Diagnostic sounding of the bone interproximally is a good clinical indicator in predicting post-treatment papilla levels

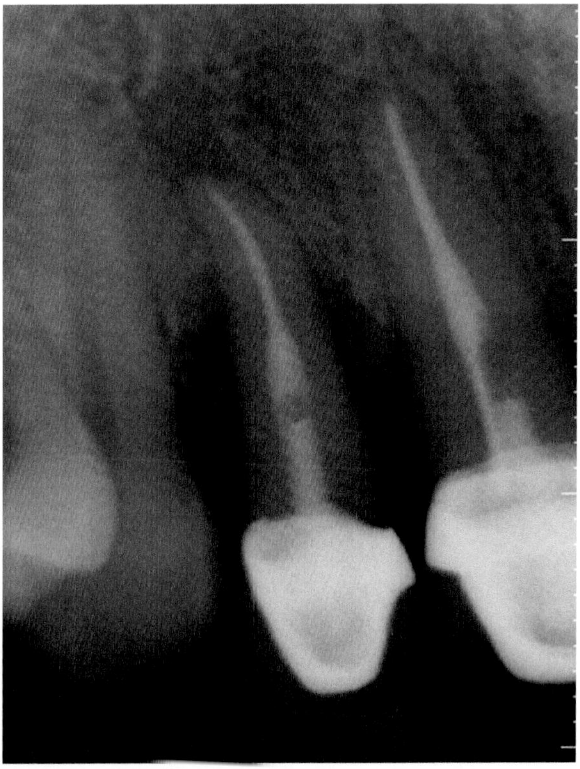

Fig. 13.30 Radiograph of Fig. 13.29; the right lateral incisor has been treatment planned for an implant restoration. Due to attachment loss on the adjacent canine, it is unlikely that the interproximal papilla will be maintained

13.6 Implant Position

Aesthetic implant placement is driven by both a restorative and biological philosophy. Aesthetically, the implant should be placed to satisfy the parameters of contour so that the restoration is pleasing. Biologically, it should be placed to allow maintenance of both hard and soft tissue architecture. If the tooth to be replaced has not yet been removed, several determinations should be made prior to the extraction.

Immediately placing the implant after extraction helps to shorten the treatment time and may reduce the amount of ridge width reduction that accompanies tooth extraction. Studies show that immediate implant placement fails to completely prevent bone resorption but may partially reduce its extent. A major desirable advantage of immediate placement and restoration for patients is the psychological advantage of having a permanent tooth at the time of extraction. A high level of technical competence and experience is required for immediate placement and restoration. Careful patient selection is required to achieve an aesthetic outcome.

Additional strategies, if bone deficiencies are present including orthodontic eruption of the tooth prior to extraction, help increase the amount of hard and soft tissue at the future implant site [17]. More recently, partial extraction therapy has been proposed as a solution for maintaining bone and soft tissue height. The theory is to maintain the facial part of the root and its associated ligament, which in turn maintains bone and soft tissue. Initial results appear promising, but long-term studies are not available to validate this approach.

In most situations involving a single anterior implant restoration, the aesthetic considerations are more important than functional considerations. As such, axial loading is not as critical as it is with posterior implant restorations. Implant position is critical to the final aesthetic outcome and needs to be considered in all three dimensions and in relation to the adjacent teeth. Misalignment of the implant in the prosthetic space can have adverse aesthetic consequences.

13.6.1 Apico-Coronal Placement

Apico-coronal positioning appears to be the most critical aspect. Deficient tissue in this dimension can result from several factors. This type of tissue needs to be addressed during treatment planning. Because of the complexity of vertical hard and soft tissue grafting, these patients are placed in a high-risk group.

Most often tooth loss is followed by bone loss of minor or major importance. It is necessary to evaluate the discrepancy between the bone level at the proposed implant site and the level at the adjacent teeth. Too large a difference represents a risk to both periodontal and peri-implant tissue health. Facing this, the surgeon should consider reconstructing the ridge prior to implant placement.

The apico-coronal positioning of the implant is the vertical discrepancy between the occlusal surface of the implant and the peaks of the bony septa proximal to the adjacent teeth; the most pleasing aesthetic result occurs when this discrepancy is minimal.

To obtain appropriate apico-coronal positioning of the implant, a diagnostic wax-up needs to be completed, and from this, a surgical guide is made. The emergence profile and the shape of the restoration are reproduced on the guide to verify the implant positioning on placement. The modern use of digital technology which includes CBCT, IOS and associated implant planning software allows the clinician to view hard tissue structures in axial coronal and sagittal views enhancing the ability of the clinician to place the implant in the correct three-dimensional position.

A maxillary central incisor measures on average 7–8 mm mesiodistally and 6 mm facio-lingually at the emergence from the soft tissue. A 4.0 mm implant needs to be placed 3–4 mm apical to the gingival margin of the contralateral tooth to allow the restoration to emerge with a natural profile. A vertical distance of 3–4 mm is needed for gradual transition from the 4 mm diameter of the implant platform to the 7–8 mm dimension at the gingival margin. If a lateral incisor is being replaced, the implant would not have to be placed so apically since the average diameter of the crown at the gingival margin is 5 mm and less room is required for transition (Figs. 13.31, 13.32, 13.33, 13.34, 13.35 and 13.36).

Apico-coronal implant placement may also be influenced by the design of implant and abutment complex used. Connections can be platform matched or platform switched (Figs. 13.36 and 13.37). In the platform switching concept,

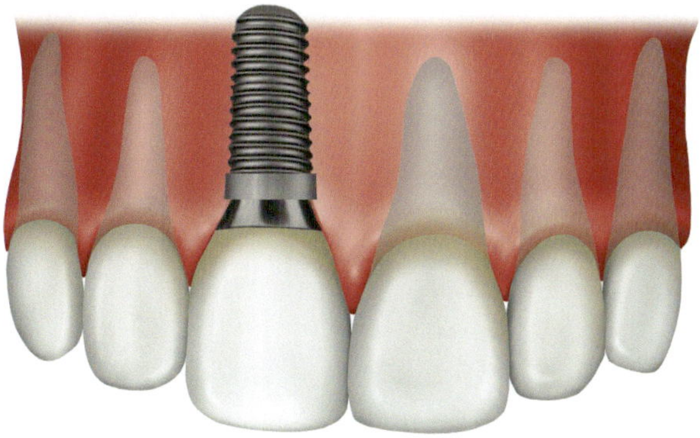

Fig. 13.31 Ideal implant placement for central incisor. Implant should be placed 3–4 mm apical to the existing free gingival margin. Adequate room is required for transition from the head of the implant to the point where the restorations exit the free gingival margin. Note the minimal bone discrepancy between the implant and the adjacent teeth

Fig. 13.32 Laboratory slide depicting ideal implant placement and transition required

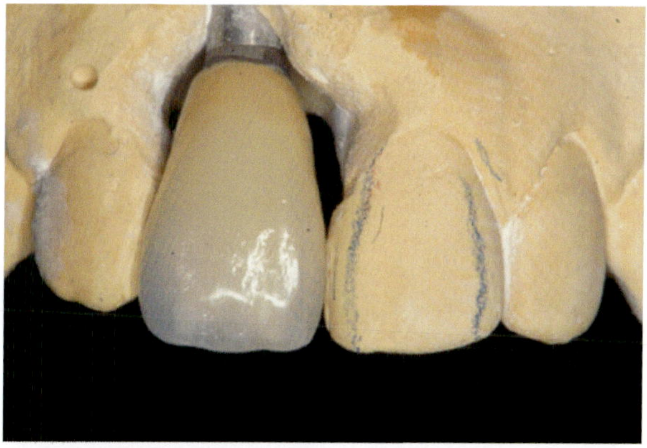

Fig. 13.33 Occlusal view of implant restoration shown in Fig. 13.32

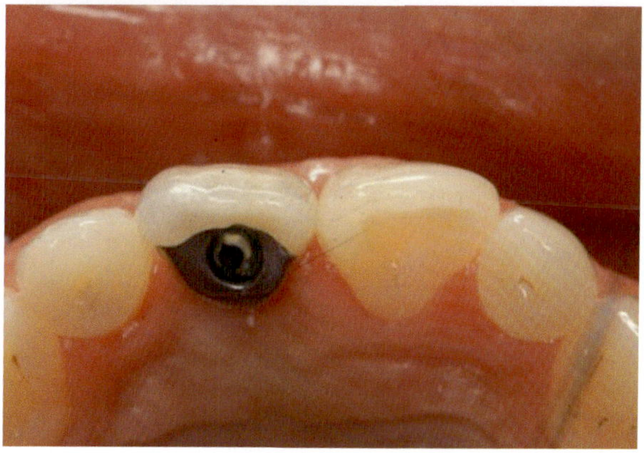

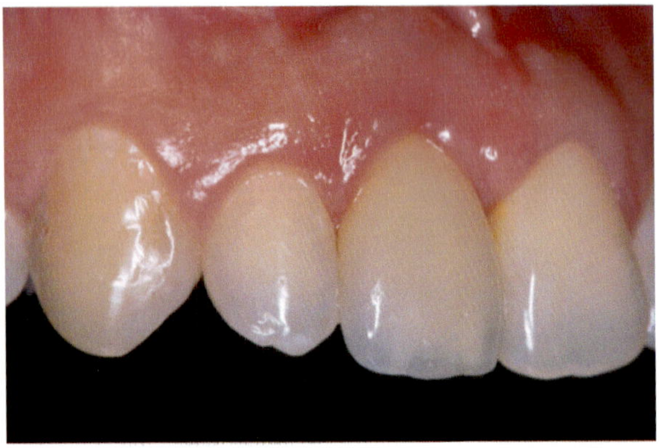

Fig. 13.34 Lateral view of implant restoration in Fig. 13.33 showing the fill of interproximal soft tissue

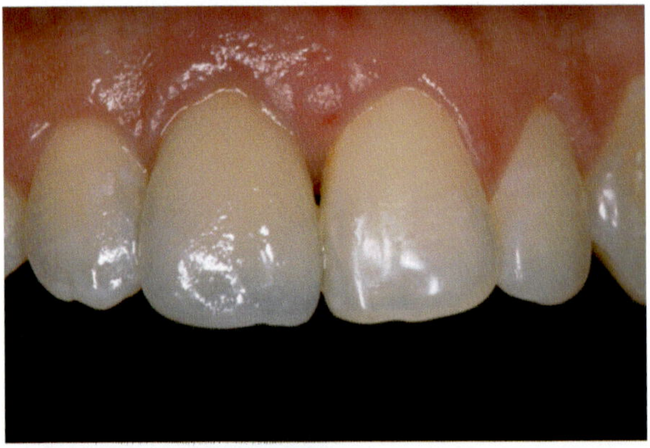

Fig. 13.35 Facial view of implant restoration in Fig. 13.34 showing aesthetic harmony

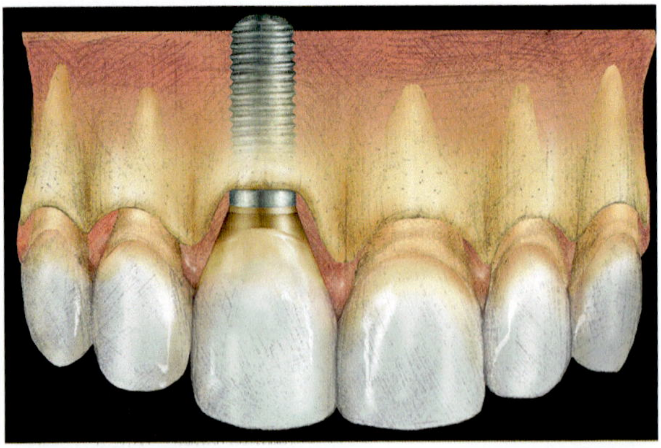

Fig. 13.36 Implant placed without platform switch and an external connection

the implant abutment junction is moved medially away from the bone. The theory is that this will maintain the bone. Most clinicians anecdotally believe that implants with an internal connection yield superior aesthetic outcomes, yet there is no objective data to support this. Most clinicians believe that leakage

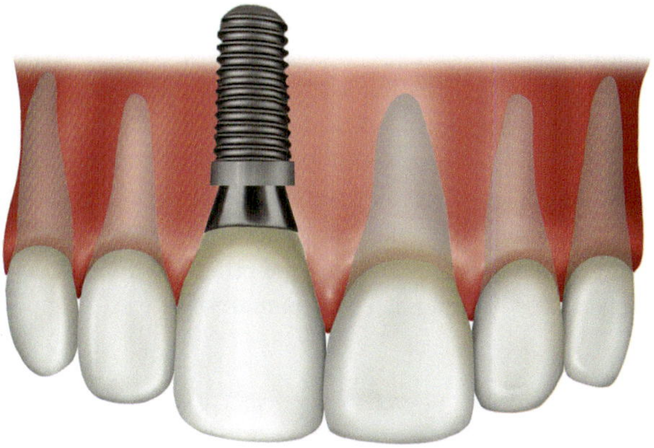

Fig. 13.37 Implant placed with platform switch and internal connection needs to be placed deeper

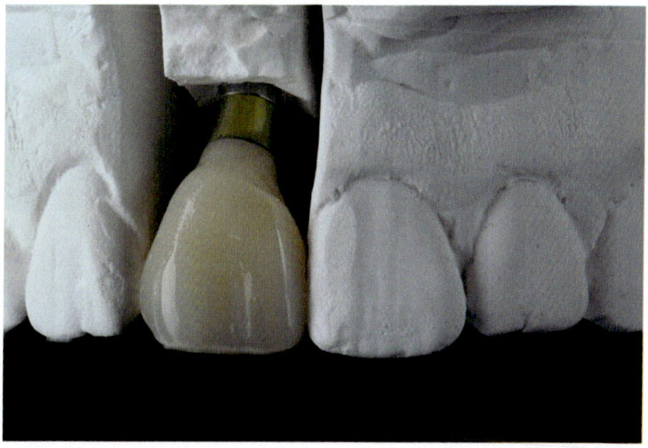

Fig. 13.38 Example of deeper implant placement

at the implant abutment connection in an implant causes bone loss which impacts the aesthetic outcome. This also cannot be validated by objective clinical data.

The design of the implant abutment complex will impact the depth of placement. Implants with a platform switch will need to be placed slightly deeper so the clinician can develop the emergence profile from a narrower base. Implants with a platform match do not need to be placed as deep. From a biological perspective, the implant must be placed no deeper than required to develop an optimal emergence profile (Fig. 13.38).

There are also situations in which there is excess tissue height, and these require attention as well. In these types of patients, a bone scalloping procedure is required to allow placement of the implant shoulder in a subgingival position; once again, the most efficient way to examine this is through a surgical guide highlighting the proposed gingival margin.

Errors in apico-coronal implant placement can have serious aesthetic and biomechanical implications. An implant placed too coronally will not allow adequate transition from the head of the implant to the point where the restoration exits from the free gingival margin. The restoration will look short in comparison to the contralateral tooth. The only prosthetic "bailout" for this type of situation is to provide a ridge-lapped restoration with contours that are pleasing to the observer's eye (Figs. 13.39a, b and 13.40).

Problems can also result when implants are placed too apically. Clinically, if an implant is placed too apically with excessive countersinking procedures, an unnecessary amount of bone loss will occur. Because this bone loss takes place circumferentially, it will affect not only the proximal bone structure but also the height of the facial bone wall and can lead to undesirable soft tissue contours.

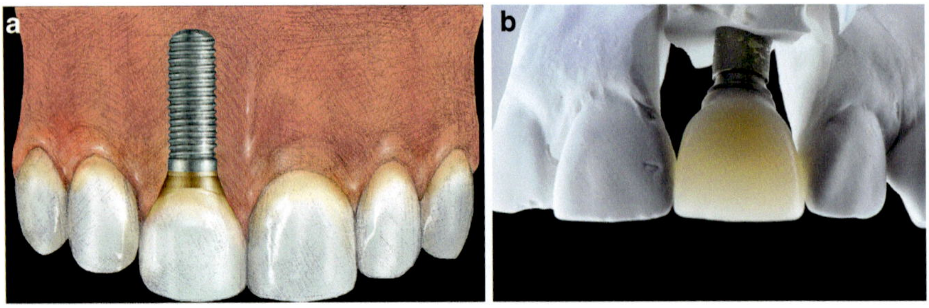

Fig. 13.39 (**a**) Placement of an implant too shallow will result in inadequate space for transition and a short restoration in length. (**b**) Example of implant placed too shallow

Fig. 13.40 A prosthetic bailout for too shallow implant placement is to ridge lap the restoration onto the tissues

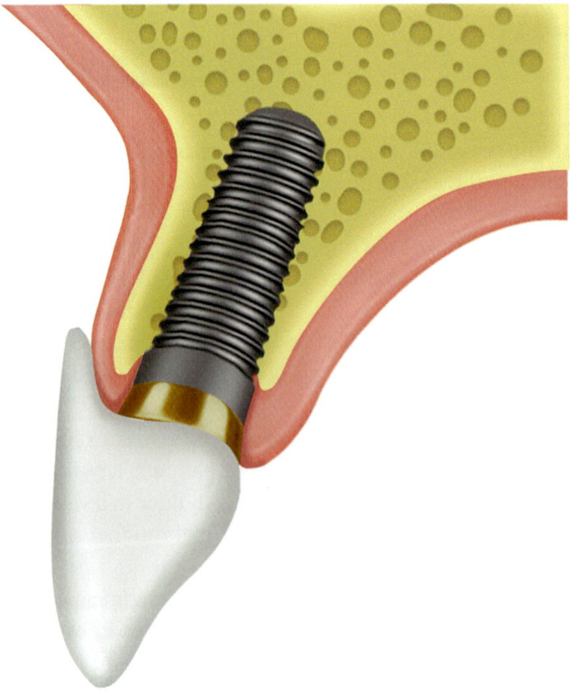

A practical problem in placing an implant too deeply is access for instrumentation. Making an impression of a deeply placed implant can be a difficult experience (Figs. 13.41 and 13.42)—the soft tissue tends to collapse, there is tissue impingement when trying to locate the head of the implant and seating is difficult to evaluate. This is specific to external hex systems.

If an implant is placed too deep, a screw-retained restoration is the treatment of choice. The literature shows that removing all the cement when an implant is placed so deeply can prove to be a difficult endeavour. Agar et al. [18] found that when six experienced investigators were asked to remove cement, there was a surprising amount of cement left behind; this can lead to serious soft tissue complications.

13.6.2 Mesiodistal Placement

Improper mesiodistal positioning of implants can also have a substantial effect on the generation of interproximal papillary support as well as on the osseous crest of the adjacent tooth. An implant should be placed 1.5–2 mm from an adjacent tooth.

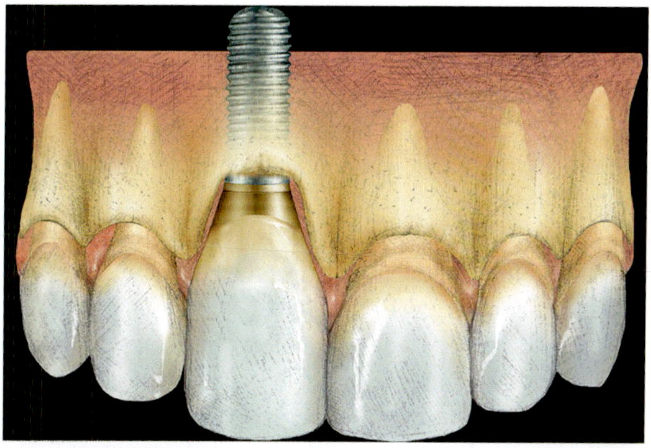

Fig. 13.41 Too deep an implant placement can result in biomechanical and biological problems. Note the level of the bone around implant in relation to the adjacent teeth. This deep placement can result in fistula formation and constant post-operative maintenance problems

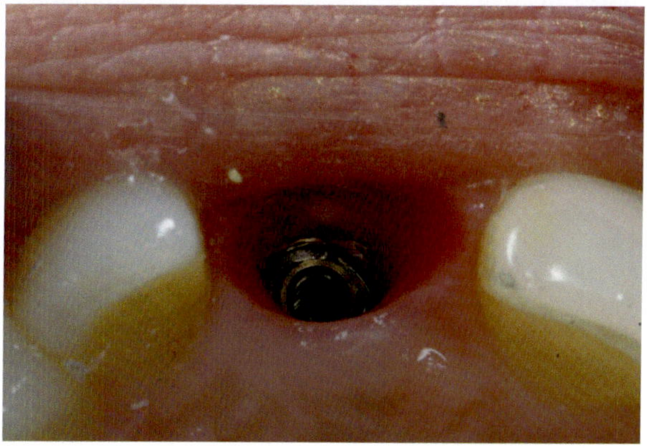

Fig. 13.42 Too deep an implant placement can result in soft tissue collapse and difficulty in instrumentation

Placement too close to the adjacent tooth can cause resorption of the interproximal alveolar crest to the level of that on the implant [19]. With this resorption comes a reduction in papillary height. Restorative problems exist as well. Poor embrasure form and emergence profile will result in a restoration with a long contact zone and compromised clinical outcomes.

The loss of crest height on adjacent teeth is caused by circumferential bone loss routinely found around the implant shoulder in implants. This has two dimensions: horizontal and vertical. Radiographs only demonstrate the horizontal aspect of the bone loss; the proximal bone loss measures 1–1.5 mm from the implant surface. This distance needs to be respected on implant placement to prevent vertical bone loss on adjacent teeth [20].

13.6.3 Facio-Lingual Placement

The crest width needs to be examined to determine the presence or absence of bone atrophy.

Placement will vary depending on the mechanism of retention of the final restoration (screw retained versus cement retained).

Deficient alveolar crest width may require augmentation so that the implant can be positioned in the correct facio-lingual position.

Computerized tomographic scan techniques are useful in assisting to determine width. The amount of bone available should be at least 1 mm greater than the implant diameter on each side. Hence, a 4 mm diameter implant would require 6 mm of bone. This is the minimum amount of bone required to house the implant. The single implant placed in the maxillary anterior region should be situated palatal to an imaginary line that outlines the curve of the arch formed by the facial surfaces of the adjacent teeth (Fig. 13.43).

Implants placed too palatal complicate development of hygienic contours. Biomechanical complications can also arise as a result of cantilever forces on the screw joint of external hex systems (Figs. 13.44, 13.45 and 13.46a–e). Implants are often mistakenly placed too facial. This error results in excessive resorption of the supporting osseous structure resulting in a restoration that will appear long in comparison to the contralateral tooth. Placement of a restoration such as this in the aesthetic zone is certainly unlikely to meet the patient's desires (Figs. 13.47, 13.48 and 13.49a, b).

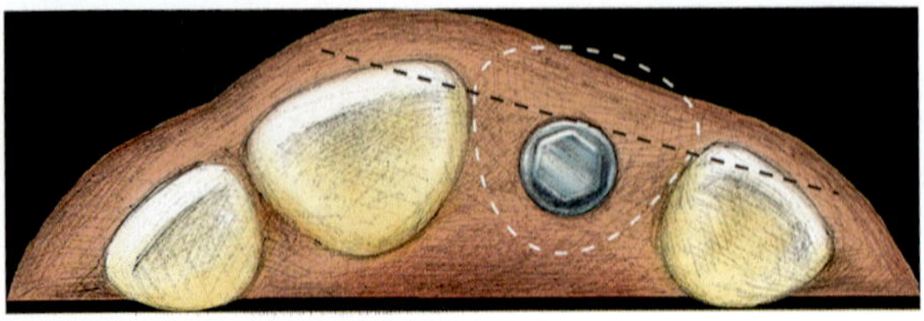

Fig. 13.43 Ideal implant placement should be palatal to an imaginary line that outlines the curvature of the teeth. (Modified from Parel and Sullivan [28])

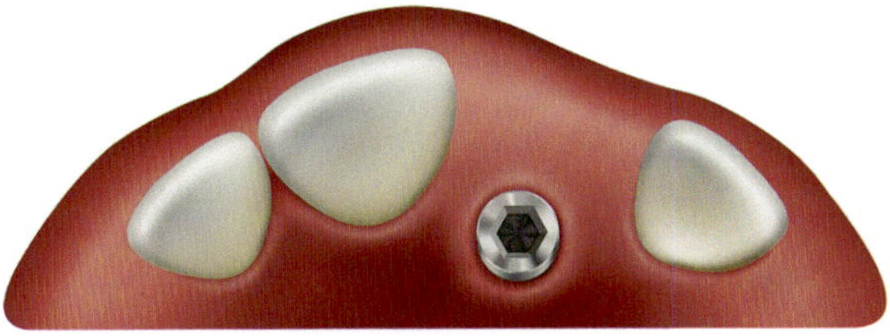

Fig. 13.44 Too palatal an implant placement

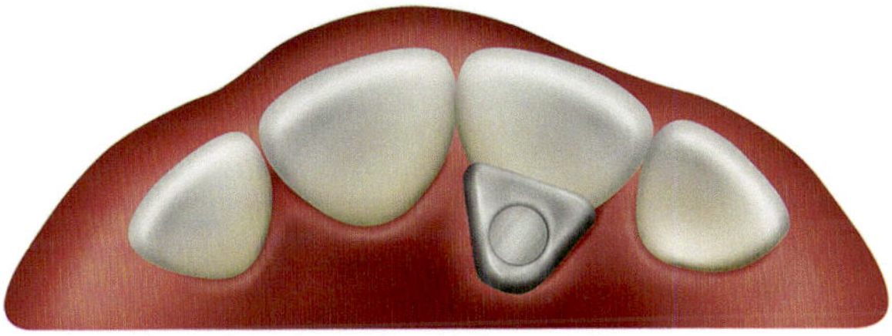

Fig. 13.45 The restoration for the implant placement in Fig. 13.43 would require an excessive facial cantilever

The inclination of the implant may differ depending on the bone trajectory. The clinician's goal is always to have an abundance of bone buccal to the implant to enhance long-term stability. Often in the maxilla, the trajectory of the bone is such that the screw access hole would exit through the incisal edge. In these situations, two options exist for the clinician:

1. To design a customized cement-retained abutment where the cement margin follows the scallop of the gingival contours. From an aesthetic perspective, having the cement margin 1 mm subgingival is preferred. Ideally, the cement margin on implant abutments should always be visible for intra-oral cementation (Figs. 13.50 and 13.51).
2. To fabricate a screw-retained restoration with an angulated screw channel (Fig. 13.52a, b).

13.6.4 Strategies to Reduce Bone Loss Around Implants

Clinicians have often questioned the reasons for small changes in crestal bone height following implant restoration. Clinical techniques have been developed to attempt to mitigate the bone loss.

Several theories exist as to the observed changes in crestal bone height. Amongst them are:

1. Surgical trauma
2. Stress concentration at the coronal region of the implant when implants are placed into function [21]
3. Bacterial leakage due to configuration and position of the implant-abutment microgap [22]. Localized inflammation at the implant-abutment interface [23]

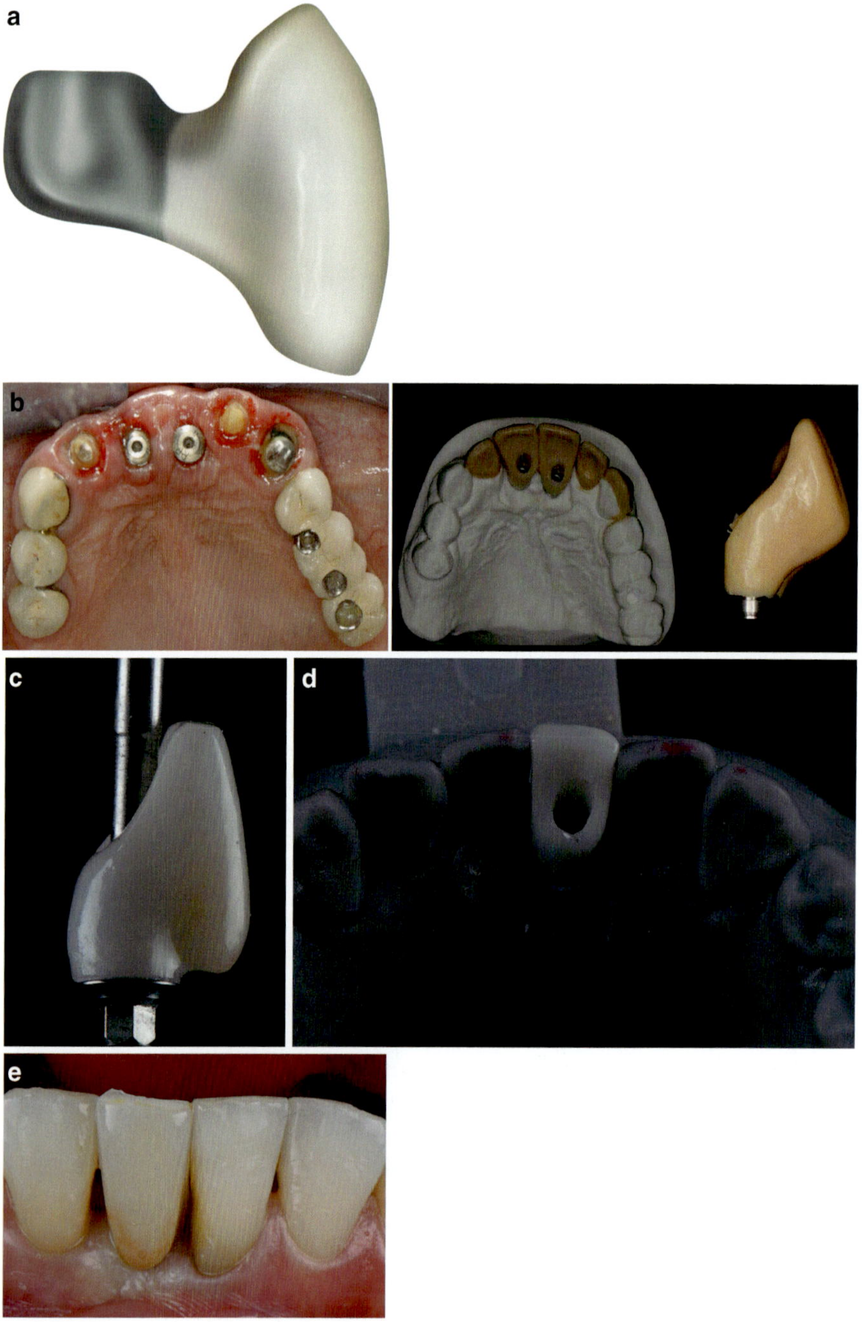

Fig. 13.46 Profile of restoration in Fig. 13.44 illustrating a biomechanical and hygienic compromise

Fig. 13.47 Too facial an implant placement

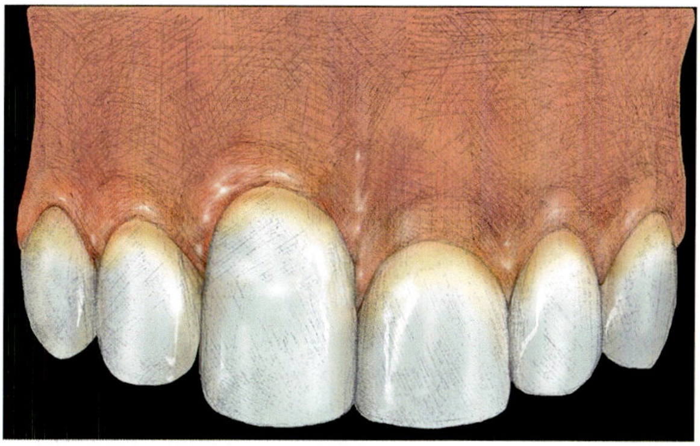

Fig. 13.48 Too facial an implant placement

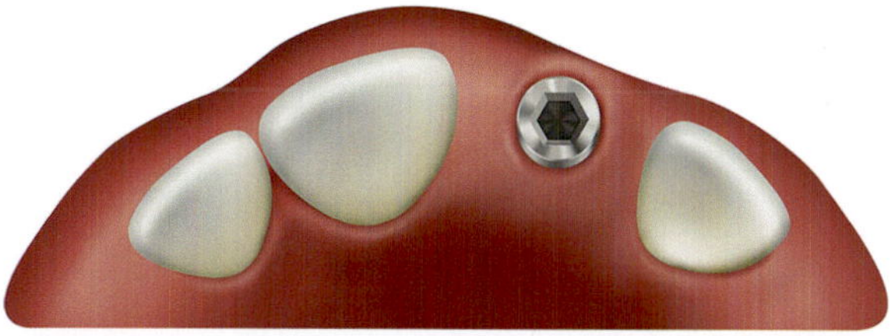

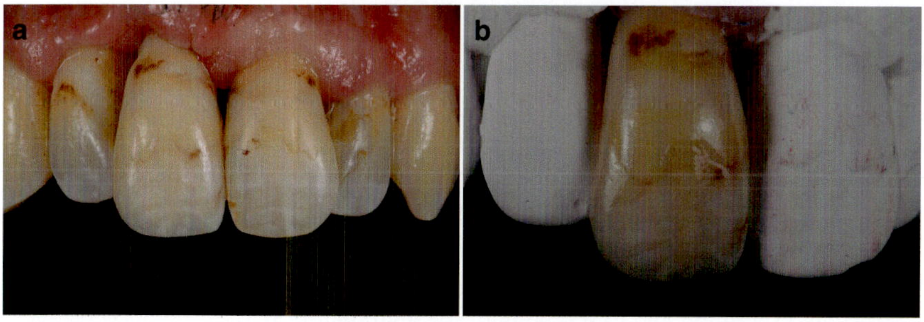

Fig. 13.49 (a, b) Too facial an implant placement; note the soft tissue position

Fig. 13.50 Custom zirconia abutments showing designing of cement line

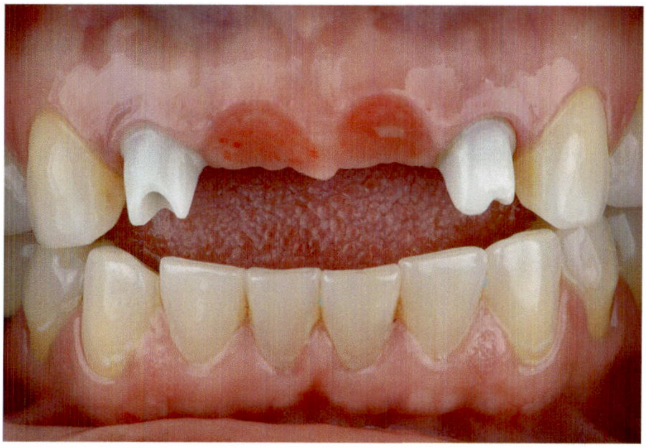

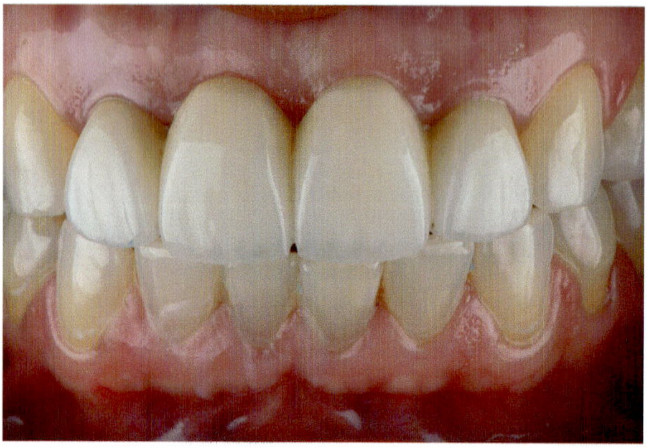

Fig. 13.51 Cemented zirconia implant-supported restoration

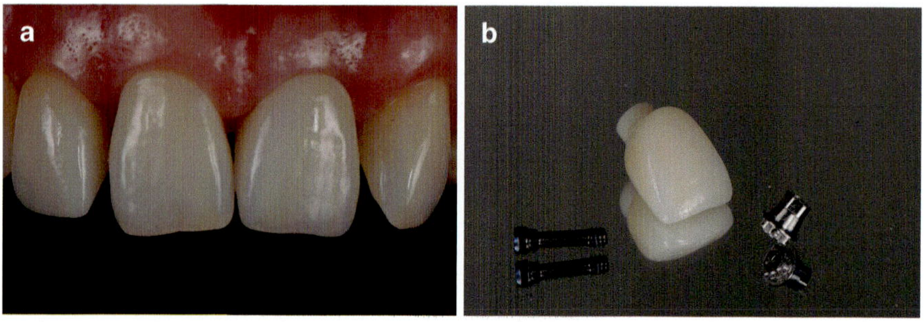

Fig. 13.52 (**a**) Screw-retained anterior implant restoration with angulated screw channel. (**b**) Components of cement-free screw-retained angulated screw channel

4. Biological width theory whereby the soft tissue attempts to establish a mucosal barrier around the coronal aspect of the implant [24]
5. Micromovement of the prosthetic components
6. Repeated screwing and unscrewing of the abutment [25]
7. Implant neck geometry
8. Presence of infection

Implant companies have attempted to address the causes of bone loss and have incorporated design features to attempt to minimize it. Clinicians have also varied implant placement techniques to maximize bone preservation.

Features included to minimize bone loss include:

1. Altering the implant neck design
2. Micro-threads at the coronal aspect of the implant
3. Altering implant surface characteristics
4. Altering the diameter of implant used
5. Use of one-piece implants
6. Placing implants in relation to the alveolar crest

7. Platform switching
8. Partial extraction therapy

13.6.4.1 Altering Implant Neck Design

There is no evidence to show that improved marginal bone preservation is obtained by altering the marginal neck geometry.

Bateli et al. [26] performed a systematic review which included changes in implant neck length and design, implant surface characteristics, implant diameter and/or insertion depth; the addition of micro-threads; the use of one-piece implants; and the concept of platform switching. After subsequent filtering, 20 studies were finally selected and involved the following methods: the use of micro-threads (1 study); modifications in implant surface characteristics (11 studies), implant diameter (4 studies) or insertion depth (2 studies); the use of one-piece implants (3 studies); and platform switching (1 study). Because of the heterogeneity of the studies, it was not possible to analyse the data statistically. No evidence was found regarding the effectiveness of any specific modification in the implant neck area in preserving marginal bone or preventing marginal bone loss. They concluded that current literature provides insufficient evidence about the effectiveness of different implant neck configurations in the preservation of marginal bone. Long-term randomized controlled clinical trials are needed to elucidate the effects of such modifications.

13.6.4.2 Micro-Threads at the Coronal Aspect of the Implant

Micro-threads have been added in the implant neck area by the manufacturer; their purpose is to distribute the forces around an implant when an implant is under functional load and also to increase the bone-to-implant contact. Commercially available implant systems employing this modification present a pitch distance of 0.185 mm between threads. A 5-year prospective study by Palmer [27] looked at Astra-Tech implants with micro-threads. The mean marginal bone loss in the study was 0.39 mm after 5 years, which is much lower than the original machined surface external hex implants. However, the research did not specifically isolate this design feature, so the conclusion cannot be made that the micro-threads were responsible for the bone preservation.

13.6.4.3 Implant Surface Characteristics

There have been many modifications of the implant surface in an attempt to increase bone-to-implant contact. Techniques such as oxidizing, sandblasting and acid etching have been employed to accelerate the process of osseointegration. The rough surface implants do have a better osteoconductive capacity than the machined implants and have improved bone-to-implant contact [28].

Surfaces were compared to determine if a rougher surface resulted in better bone maintenance of bone around dental implants. Wennstrom et al. [29] compared implant groups with the same implant design, but they only differed in their surface characteristics. Their conclusion was that there was no significant difference attributable to the enhanced surface. There is no evidence to support marginal bone preservation for any specific surface modification.

13.6.4.4 Implant Diameter

Wide-diameter implants were designed to be placed in compromised situations where available bone height and quality were limited. Manufacturers suggested that wide-diameter implants may exhibit less horizontal bone resorption than regular diameter implants. It was claimed that increasing the diameter of the implant would decrease the stress and strain on the alveolar crest and lead to less bone loss. Ivanoff [30] showed that 5 mm diameter implants demonstrated the highest failure rates in comparison to 3.75 and 4.00 mm implants. Long-term randomized controlled trails with split-mouth designs are needed to substantiate the claim that wide-diameter implants are effective in the preservation of marginal bone levels.

13.6.4.5 One-Piece Implants

A one-piece implant is defined as an implant in which the bone anchoring portion, the soft tissue traversing portion and the prosthetic abutment are all in one piece [31].

The theory behind one-piece implants is that they are placed in a one-stage surgery and therefore bypass the two-stage procedure, avoiding further manipulation of the soft and hard tissues, and are supposed to eliminate the implant abutment microgap. It was claimed that the elimination of the microgap through the use of one-piece implants resulted in less bone loss [32]. Other studies have shown no difference in bone loss when a two-piece implant system was compared to a one-piece implant system [33]. Currently, the evidence is not clear if one-piece implants serve an advantage over two-piece implants in terms of bone maintenance.

13.6.4.6 Insertion Depths

Clinicians have altered the placement of two-piece implants at varying locations with respect to the gingival margin and marginal bone levels to determine if this has an influence on bone loss. Callan et al. [34] suggested that more bone loss was associated with implants where the implant-abutment interface is placed below the mucosal margin. Hartman [35] found a relationship between the amount of bone remodelling and the location of the rough-smooth border placed at or near the alveolar crest. Although these studies provide us with some information, the possible interference of surface modifications of the studies referring to insertion depth makes it difficult to draw any reliable conclusions about the outcome of the varying locations of the implant-abutment interface in two-piece implants with respect to the mucosal margin or alveolar crest.

13.6.4.7 Platform Switching

This concept refers to the inward horizontal repositioning of the implant abutment junction so that it is positioned away from the outer edge of the implant and adjacent bone. Lazzara et al. [36] introduced the concept by using standard diameter components on wide-platform implants. They found a reduction of the expected post-restoration crestal bone remodelling in comparison to the "standard" implants. There are multiple theories as to why the platform switching concept works.

1. **The biomechanical theory**: Connecting the implant to a smaller diameter abutment may limit bone resorption by shifting the stress concentration zone away from the crestal bone-implant interface and directing the forces of occlusal loading along the axis of the implant.
2. **The biologic width theory**: Shifting the implant-abutment connection may medialize the location of the biologic width and minimize the marginal bone resorption. Placing the IAJ at or below the crestal bone level may cause vertical bone resorption to re-establish the biologic width.
3. **The inflammation at IAJ theory**: This theory postulates that bone resorption is caused by an inflammatory infiltrate at the IAJ. The presence of peri-implant microbiota was suggested to influence the crestal bone resorption by maintaining the inflammatory cell infiltrate at the IAJ. The physical repositioning of the IAJ away from the outer external edge of the implant and neighbouring bone may limit bone resorption by containing the inflammatory cell infiltrate within the angle formed at the interface away from the adjacent crestal bone.

The question becomes does "platform switching" influence bone remodelling. Just as there are many studies to support this concept, there are many studies that refute it.

Canullo et al. [37] placed 22 implants of 5.5 mm diameter immediately in extraction sockets in the maxilla. They were randomly divided where 11 implants were connected with 3.8 mm diameter abutments and 11 implants had 5.5 mm diameter abutments. The follow-up was 25 months. They found lower crestal bone loss in the platform-switched group compared to the non-platform switched. They also found a wider and more resistant zone of connective tissue in the platform-switched group when compared to the platform-matched group.

Hurzeler et al., Atieh et al. and Rodriguez-Ciurana et al. [37–39] found similar results supporting the platform switching concept. The conclusions from these studies were that the biologic width around platform-switched implants is located more coronally and there is a reduction in the vertical and horizontal components of bone loss.

Just as there are many studies supporting the concept, there are many studies refuting the claim that platform switching actually works.

Studies by Baffone et al., Batelli et al., Enkling et al., Van Steenbergh et al. and Jacobs et al. question the platform switching concept [40–44].

Conclusion from their studies were as follows:

1. Geometry of the implant-abutment connection was of limited importance in the preservation of hard and soft tissues.
2. No evidence in a meta-analysis to show that the implant neck configuration contributed to the preservation of marginal bone level and marginal bone loss occurred regardless of all the efforts to eliminate it.
3. Bacterial colonization can occur as a consequence of leakage at the IAJ or as a result of contamination during implant placement.

4. A split-mouth design comparing Astra-Tech and Branemark implants showed that there was no significant difference in probing depths, presence of plaque or change in marginal bone level.
5. Mean radiographic bone loss after the first year was small and was below 0.5 mm for both implant systems up to 15 years after prosthetic loading.

13.6.4.8 Partial Extraction Therapy

Understanding the periodontium and the post-extraction loss of tissues is related to the fundamental procedure of tooth removal, which involves cutting off the highly vascular PDL system that supplies blood and nutrition to the bundle bone [45]. Resorption of the socket after extraction is therefore inevitable.

Several strategies and therapies have been developed to reduce the resorption of alveolar bone. Immediate implant placement, atraumatic extraction, socket preservation procedures and placement of various grafts maintain the dimensions of the alveolar ridge by preventing the collapse of cortical plates. These methods are frequently used to reduce bundle bone loss. Although studies have not shown that these procedures completely preserve the alveolar socket, they do have a considerable impact on keeping the post-extraction alveolar bone.

Partial extraction therapies denote a collective term used to describe the maintenance of a root or a part of the root with the aim of preserving the natural contours of bone and soft tissue around implant-retained restorations.

When a tooth is extracted, the bundle bone-periodontal ligament complex is lost and reduction in alveolar bone is inevitable.

The socket shield techniques maintain part of the buccal root fragment and its associated periodontal ligament with the intention of preserving the buccal plate. The theory is that there will be minimal resorption of the buccal plate in the long term, thus providing long-term aesthetics.

Initial clinical outcomes of partial extraction therapies appear to be promising when executed by highly trained clinicians in a controlled environment. Their exact guidelines are in a process of evolution. The procedures are technique sensitive, and the learning curve is steep. The clinician must be aware that complications may arise that may impact aesthetics in a negative way. These complications include but are not limited to:

1. Shield mobility
2. Shield migration
3. Shield exposure
4. Infection

Although partial extraction therapies may be beneficial in preserving the buccal bony plate, further long-term randomized clinical trials are required which compare these techniques over standard placement procedures. The clinician and patient should both be aware of the risks involved should the technique fail. Additional treatment may be required to correct any soft tissue disfigurement.

There are many causes of bone loss around dental implants, and many clinicians have studied various aspects of implant design in an attempt to reduce the bone loss that is seen.

Manufacturers have attempted to incorporate all the features within their individual systems to aid clinicians in achieving the ultimate in aesthetics and biomechanics.

The clinician's goal is to produce a restoration that mimics nature.

As our quest for the perfect restorations continues, we must realize that there is still a lot that is unknown, and despite our best efforts to maintain bone, the bone loss is multifactorial and cannot be isolated to one aspect of implant design. Operator variables and systemic health of the patient will also influence the bone loss that is seen. As clinicians, we can only utilize all the tools that are available to us in the hope that the bone will be maintained, and this will ultimately result in a lifelike restoration.

13.6.5 Considerations for Multiple Implants

Patients with extended edentulous spaces present greater anatomic and aesthetic challenges, making it even more difficult to obtain an aesthetic result with certainty.

Following extraction and wound healing of two adjacent teeth, the ensuing apical and facio-lingual resorption results in an edentulous segment that is flattened. The same diagnostic considerations need to be addressed when looking at single tooth edentulous sites.

The aim prior to implant placement is to have a three-dimensional configuration of hard and soft tissue, which will allow placement of implants in an ideal position. The placement of two missing central incisors poses an additional challenge. Following surgical placement, an additional peri-implant bone remodelling takes place. In the frontal plane, two processes occur—one between the implant and the adjacent natural tooth and one between the two adjacent implants.

On the tooth implant side, the predictability of the interdental papilla is governed by the height of the interproximal bone crest of the tooth. If this height is favourable, there is a good certainty that the interdental papilla will be maintained following implant placement. The bone crest between the two implants is likely to undergo further resorption in an apical direction. This is accompanied by a loss of interimplant soft tissue that, in the case of multiple edentulous sites, will result in black triangles between the adjacent restorations.

Many clinicians have sought after the ideal implant distance required to maintain the interdental papilla. Tarnow et al. [46] performed a radiographic study to address this clinical problem. Radiographic measurements were taken at a minimum of 1 and 3 years after implant exposure. All radiographs were taken with a paralleling technique.

Radiographs were computer scanned, imaged and magnified for measurement. The following measurements were taken:

1. Lateral distance from the crest of the inter-implant bone to the implants
2. Vertical crestal bone loss
3. Distance between the implants at the implant-abutment interface

When implants were placed too close together, the bone remodelling overlapped to a great degree and consequently resulted in loss of vertical bone height, and this subsequently had soft tissue implications.

When implants were placed 3 mm apart measured from the external diameters and greater, lateral bone loss from the adjacent implants did not overlap with minimal resultant crestal bone loss.

They concluded that it is more difficult to create or maintain papilla between two adjacent implants than it is between an implant and a natural tooth. Their recommendation was that when two implants are placed adjacent to each other in the aesthetic zone, a minimum of 3 mm of bone should be retained between them at the implant-abutment level (Figs. 13.53 and 13.54).

This particular study addressed bone loss between the implants. It should be remembered that bone loss has two dimensions—horizontal and vertical. Radiographs only demonstrate the horizontal aspect of bone loss. Bone loss occurs circumferentially around the implant, and when two implants are placed adjacent to each other, facial bone loss also occurs (Figs. 13.55 and 13.56). This has implications in terms of stability of the facial gingival margin. If the implants are placed too far facially, there will be less facial bone, and this will ultimately result in apical migration of the mucosal margin (Fig. 13.57).

Placement of adjacent implants is also critical for restorative contours; placing implants too close together makes it difficult for the laboratory technician to fabricate restorations with pleasing aesthetic contours (Figs. 13.58 and 13.59).

Tarnow et al. [46] also performed a study to determine the height of the soft tissue to the crest of the bone between two adjacent implants. This was done independent of the location of the contact point.

They looked at 136 inter-implant papillary heights in 33 patients by eight examiners. A standardized periodontal probe was used and placed from the height of the papilla to the crest of the bone.

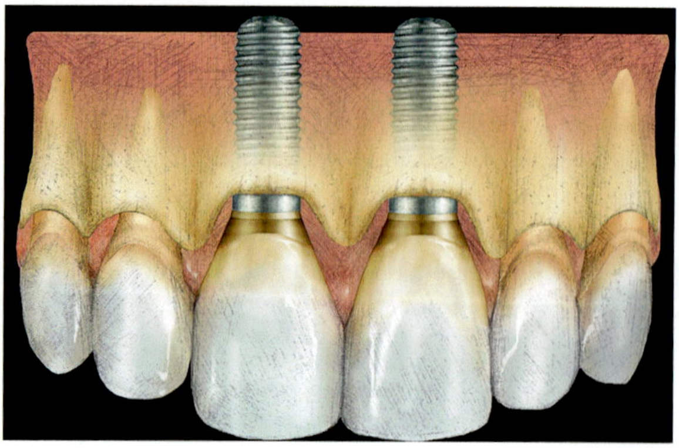

Fig. 13.53 When implants are placed 3 mm and greater apart, the bone loss from the adjacent implants does not overlap resulting in minimal crestal bone loss. (Modified from Tarnow et al. [11])

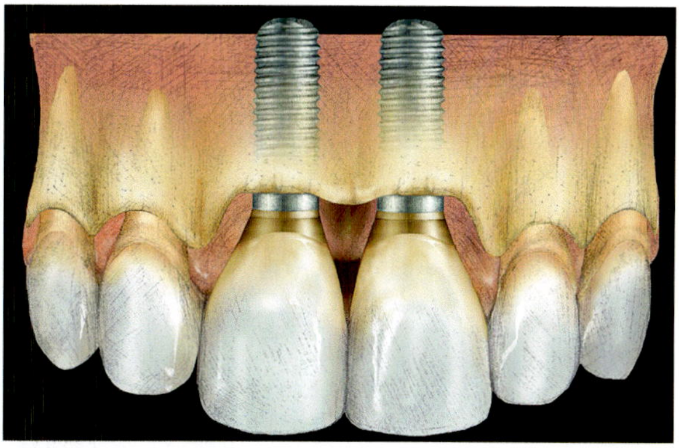

Fig. 13.54 When implants are placed too close together, bone loss from adjacent implants overlaps resulting in additional loss of the crestal bone. (Modified from Tarnow et al. [11])

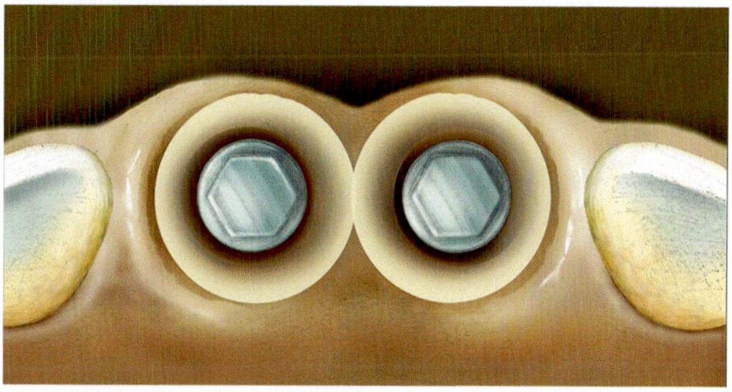

Fig. 13.55 Bone loss is circumferential around the implants. When implants are placed too close together, the vertical and horizontal components of bone loss compromise the peak of the interproximal bone and thus the resulting soft tissues

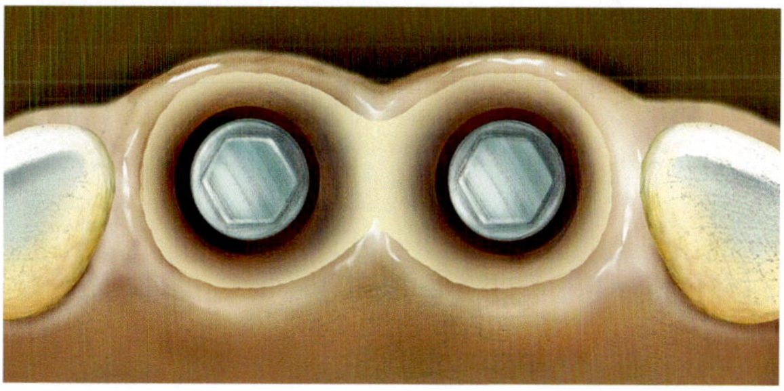

Fig. 13.56 Ideal implant placement theoretically will maintain the interproximal peak of bone; however, there are no long-term studies to support this

They found that the mean height of papilla between two adjacent implants was 3.4 mm with a range of 1–7 mm.

Although this was a retrospective study and there were many variables such as operator, implant type, placement and so forth, it did give us information that soft tissue between two adjacent implants in the aesthetic zone is not a predictable procedure. The patient must be aware of this when treatment planning or alterations must be made in the treatment plan to provide an aesthetic result.

Recreating interdental papilla between two adjacent implants is a formidable task. Restoratively, clinicians alter the position of the contact point to give the illusion of papilla. The thin spicule of bone remaining between the implants may be

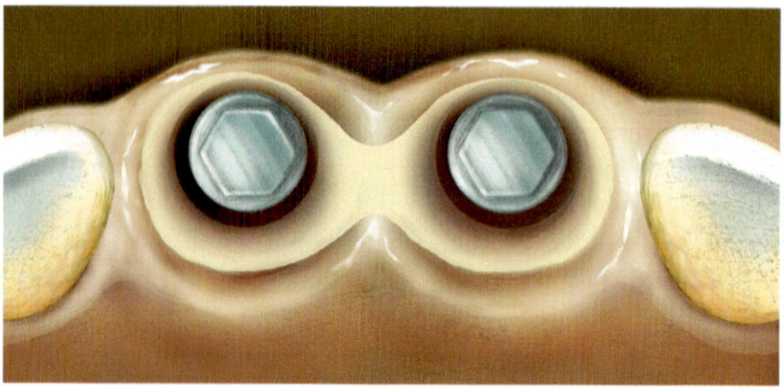

Fig. 13.57 If implants are placed too facial, this will compromise the thickness of the facial bony plate, which can eventually resorb. This will result in apical migration of bone followed by the soft tissue

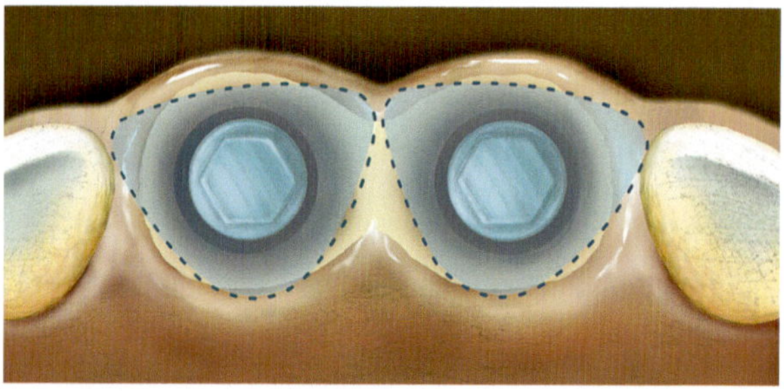

Fig. 13.58 Ideal implant placement will allow fabrication of restorations with ideal contours

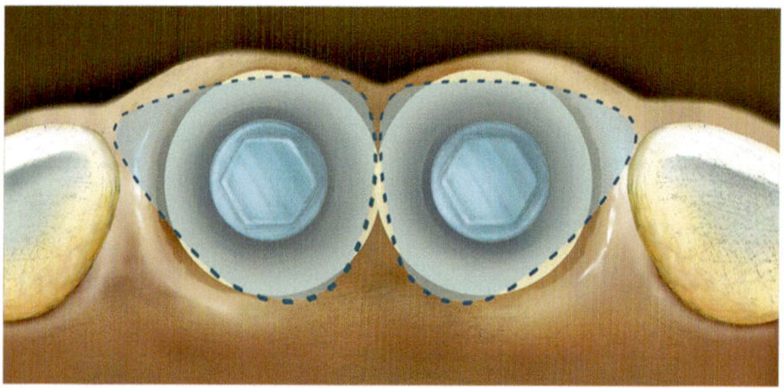

Fig. 13.59 Implants placed too close together will result in compromised restorative contour

sufficient to maintain the papilla during the first few years of the restoration service but may resorb over time resulting in loss of soft tissue.

Another clinically challenging situation is replacement of a maxillary canine and adjacent lateral incisor. This becomes clinically more challenging because the edentulous space is smaller and the inter-implant soft tissue tends to be less voluminous. Consideration in this instance should be given to placement of a single implant in the canine region and cantilevering a lateral incisor from it. Placement of the implant should follow all the principles discussed previously.

Replacement of several missing teeth with implants allows for the use of fixed partial dentures and the opportunity to utilize ovate pontics to help support the soft tissue and give an illusion of papillae. The authors have encountered many situations where one implant per tooth philosophy is espoused to. This can be particularly detrimental in the aesthetic zone. The literature is quite clear that maintaining papillae between implants is not predictable. Even with the advent of more sophisticated implant designs, there are no long-term studies showing papilla maintenance. For an aesthetic outcome, it is more predictable to place implants away from each other so that the intervening soft tissue can be sculpted to give the illusion of papilla. One common error often published in the literature is placement of four implants to replace lateral incisor to lateral incisor. This philosophy of implant placement will not yield an aesthetic outcome (Figs. 13.60 and 13.61).

If the patient is missing maxillary lateral incisor to lateral incisor, there are many combinations of implant placement which can be considered; the clinician must look at the variables that will influence the aesthetic outcome, which include but are not limited to:

1. Ridge width
2. Soft tissue volume
3. Smile line

If there is an adequate volume of bone placement of two implants in both lateral incisor regions and fabrication of a fixed partial denture, sculpting the intervening tissue with ovate pontics is likely to produce an illusion of papilla, which will be more pleasing to the observer's eye [47, 48]. The diameter of implant selected will be relative to the bone width, with the clinician's objective being to have a maximal amount of bone facial to the implant. This placement philosophy can also be reserved for extended edentulous spans where aesthetics is of paramount importance (Figs. 13.62a, b, 13.63a, b, 13.64 and 13.65).

Placement of implants in multiple edentulous spaces must follow the same principles as for single tooth situations; placement must follow appropriate diagnosis and treatment planning, which includes a diagnostic wax-up and fabrication of a surgical guide to facilitate implant placement. If these techniques are not followed, it is all too easy to find implants in the wrong position where prosthetic strategies have to be utilized to satisfy the patient's demand for aesthetics. In situations like these, patient expectations are unlikely to be met (Figs. 13.66, 13.67 and 13.68).

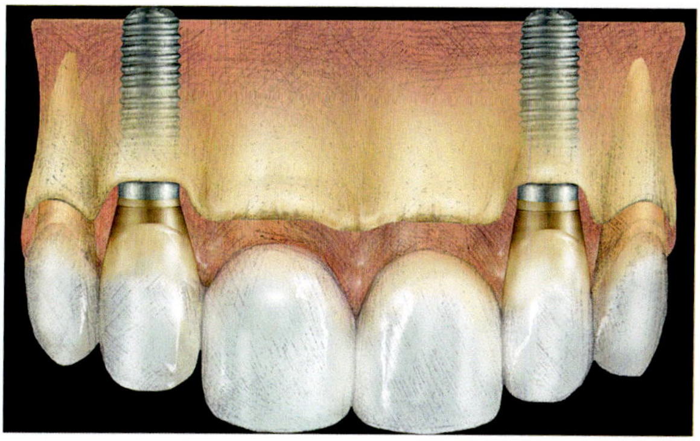

Fig. 13.60 Placement of implant in lateral incisor position so centrals can be moulded with pontic sites

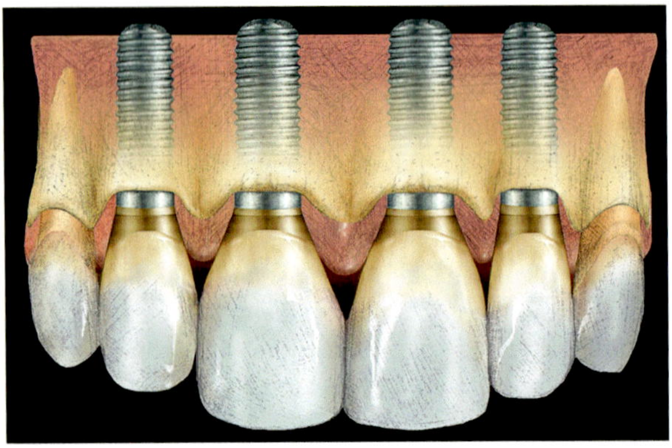

Fig. 13.61 Placement of four implants for four incisors may result in inferior aesthetic results due to proximity of the implants

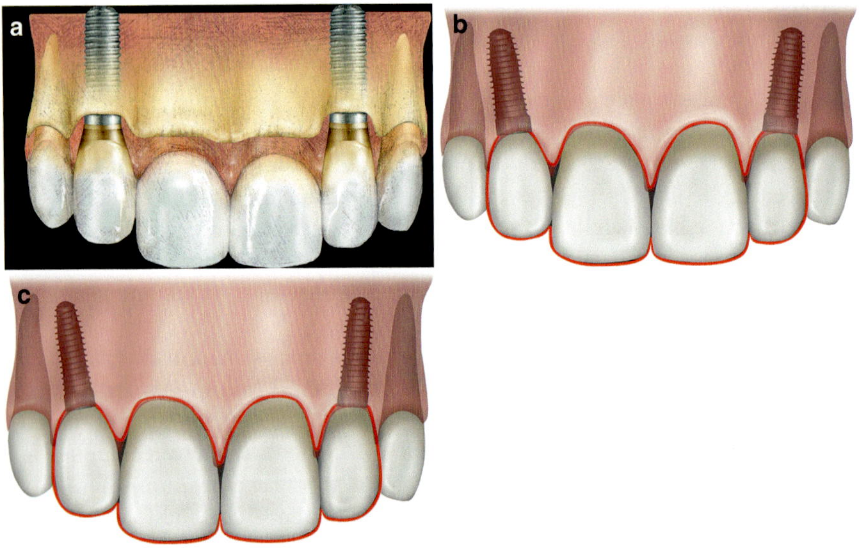

Fig. 13.62 (**a**) Standard platform implants placed in lataral incisor region when bone width allows (**b**) It is easier to develop the illusion of papilla between an implant and an adjacent pontic. Implant placement philosophy should take advantage of such techniques. (**c**) Placement in lateral incisor position may necessitate narrower platform implants because of bone availability

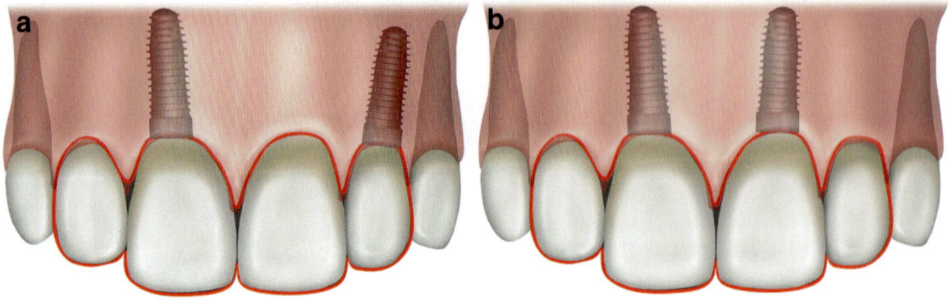

Fig. 13.63 (**a**) Placement of implants in central and lateral regions with pontics in between. (**b**) Placement of implants in the central region. Placement is critical. Laterals can be cantilever from centrals

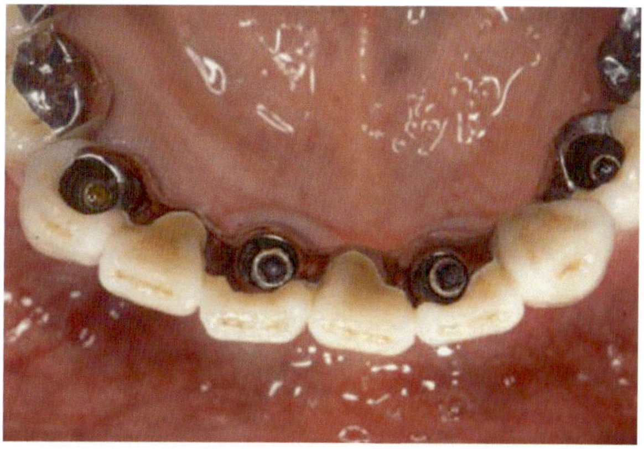

Fig. 13.64 Clinical slide showing implant placement so that illusion of papilla can be developed

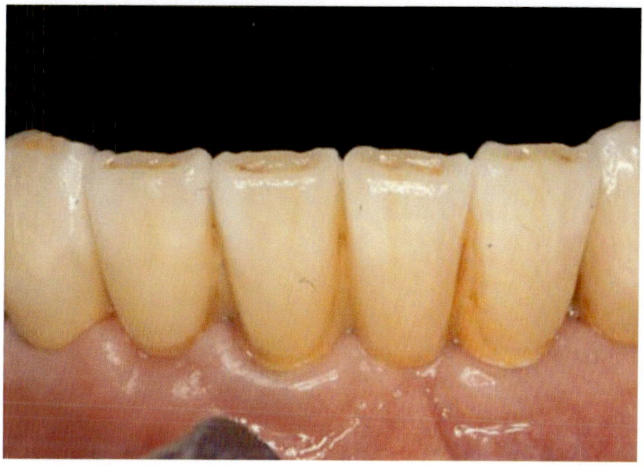

Fig. 13.65 Facial view of image in Fig. 13.64

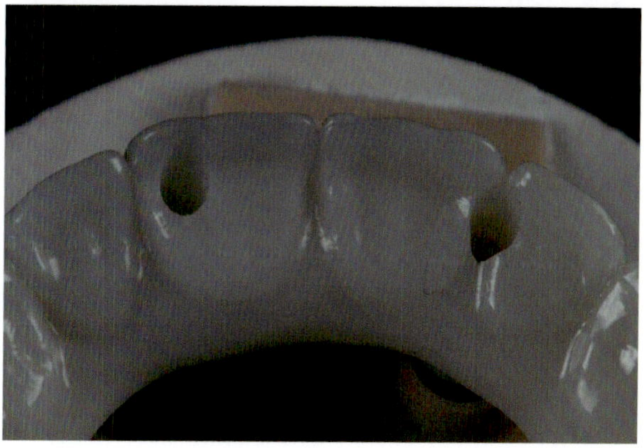

Fig. 13.66 Implants placed in interproximal region, compromising restoration

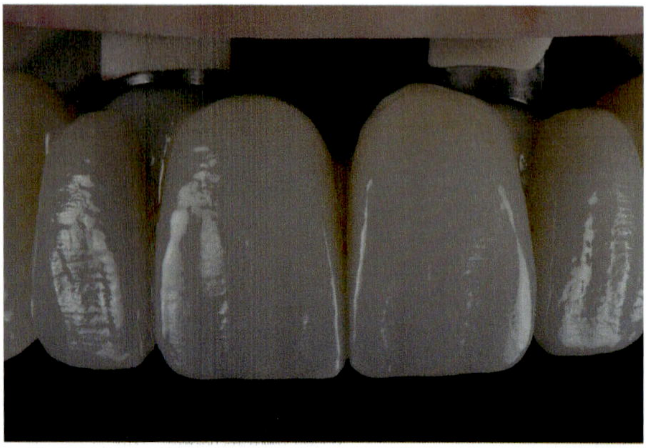

Fig. 13.67 Facial view compromising aesthetics

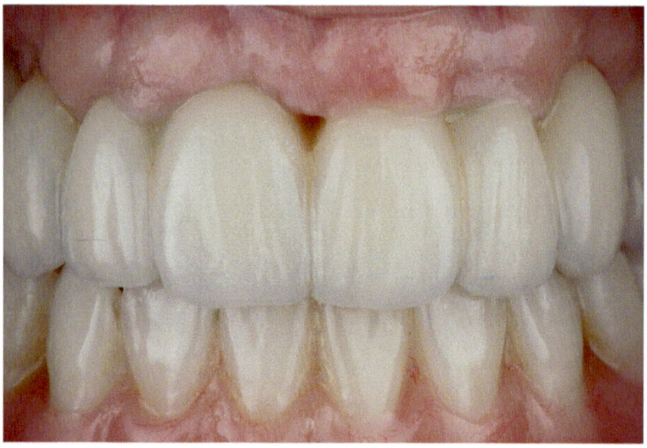

Fig. 13.68 Clinical view of case in Fig. 13.63

13.7 Clinical Cases

Case 1: Retreatment of a Failed Implant
This patient presented with a failing implant in the upper right central incisor region.

The following clinical observations were made:

1. Patient selection and smile line: The patient presented with a high smile line and even gingival levels. Inflammation was present due to the failing implant. The patient's request was not to be in removable provisional at any time during the treatment process (Fig. 13.69).
2. Tooth position: There was adequate three-dimensional space to be able to provide the patient with an aesthetic restoration. Caution would need to be exercised during the surgical phase to minimize tissue recession.
3. Root position of the adjacent teeth: Sufficient inter-radicular space; the roots were tapering.

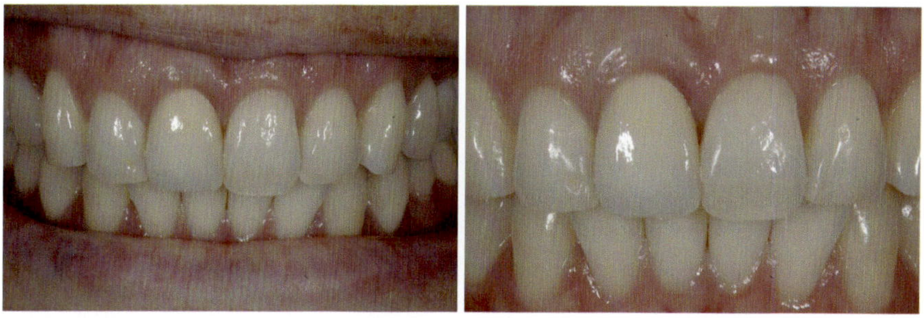

Fig. 13.69 Facial view of failing implant restoration for upper right central incisor

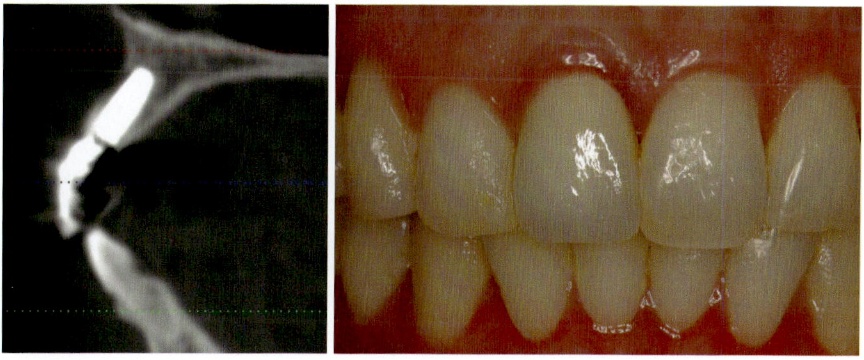

Fig. 13.70 Lateral CT view showing fenestration

4. Biotype of the periodontium and tooth shape: The patient presented with a thick biotype. On removal of the implant, tissue would be deficient over the socket.
5. The bony anatomy of the implant site: This area would be deficient once the implant is removed. There was a fenestration buccal to the existing implants (Fig. 13.70).
6. The position of the implant: The implant was inclined buccally due to the trajectory of the premaxilla.

Treatment Plan

1. Preoperative diagnostics and hygiene.
2. Pre-surgical fabrication of metal-based resin-bonded provisional to serve as a provisional during grafting and implant placement (Fig. 13.71).
3. Removal of the implants, curettage of the socket, irrigation and placement of allograft with resorbable membrane (Fig. 13.72).
4. Grafting of the socket to increase the amount of keratinized mucosa simultaneously with the bone grafting procedure (Fig. 13.73).
5. Bonding of the provisional restoration (Fig. 13.74).
6. Implant placement post-graft healing; rebonding of the metal-based provisional (Figs. 13.75, 13.76 and 13.77).

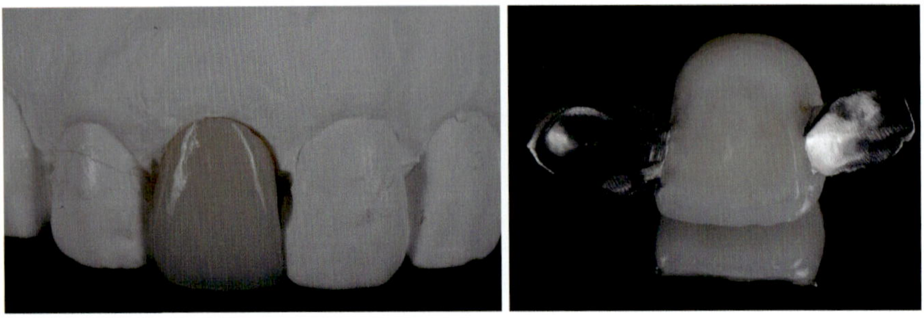

Fig. 13.71 Base metal resin-bonded bridge

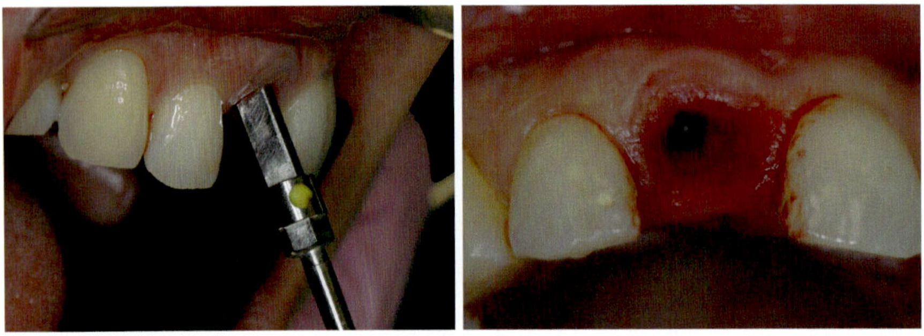

Fig. 13.72 Implant explanted and allograft placed

Fig. 13.73 Soft tissue graft placed over socket

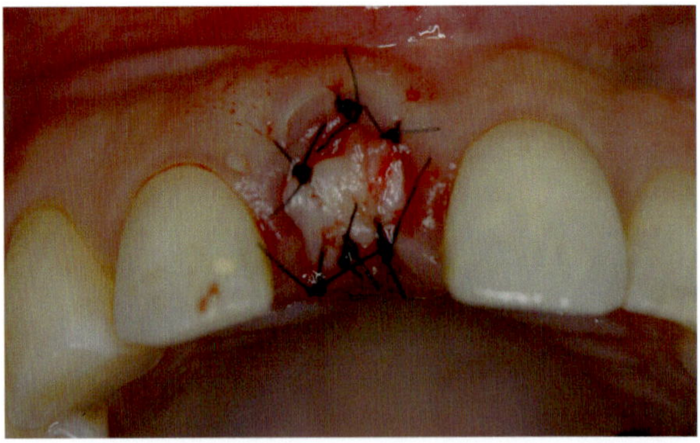

7. Fabrication of an implant-supported provisional to sculpt tissue (Figs. 13.78 and 13.79).
8. Maturation of tissue and implant impression using customized impression coping (Fig. 13.80).
9. Layered zirconia restoration with angulated screw channel used as definitive restoration; highly polished zirconia to be in contact with tissue sub-gingivally (Figs. 13.81, 13.82 and 13.83).

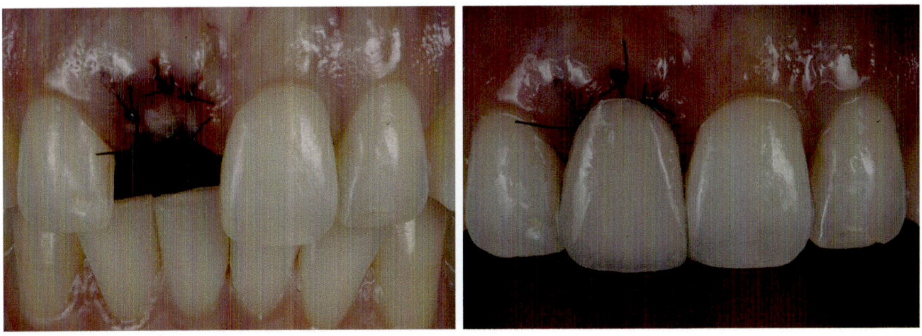

Fig. 13.74 Bonding of resin-bonded FPD (bridge)

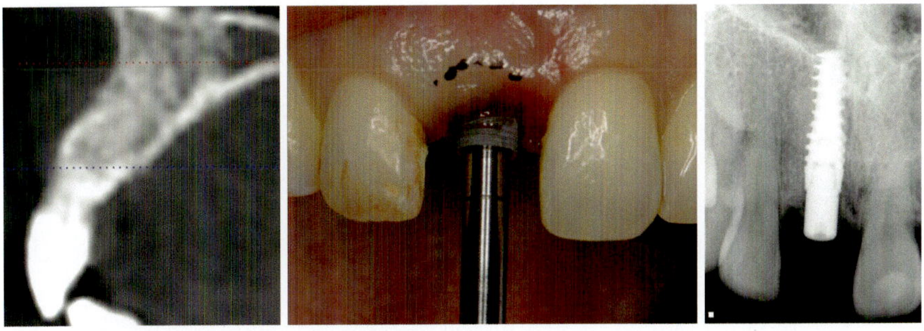

Fig. 13.75 Implant placement in adequate dimension of bone

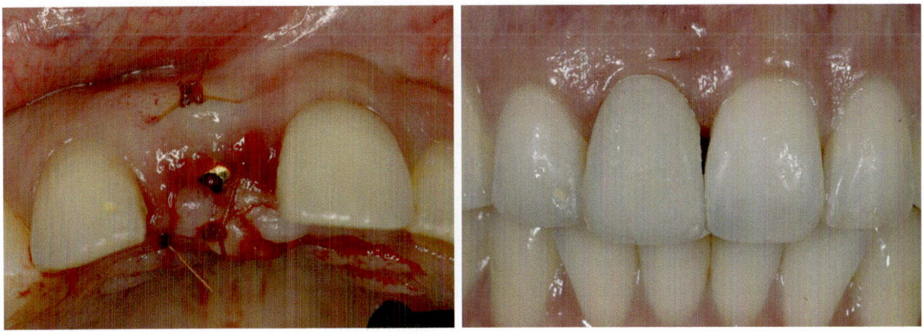

Fig. 13.76 Rebonding of same resin-bonded bridge

Case 2: Single Tooth Implant-Deficient Bone and Soft Tissue
Patient presented with a failing upper right central incisor which had previously been endodontically treated. Adjacent teeth had been treated with ceramic veneers. The patient's request was to have a fixed provisional throughout the entire treatment process.

1. Patient selection and smile line: Patient presented with a medium smile line (Fig. 13.84).
2. Tooth position: The three-dimensional space was ideal; mesiodistally, the tooth was slightly wider than the contralateral central incisor. The patient was made

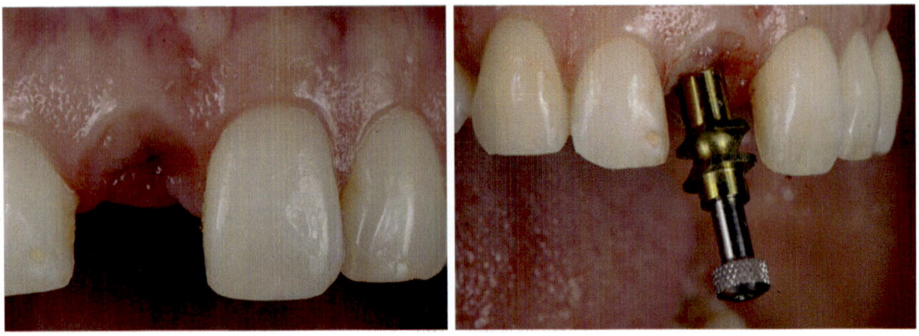

Fig. 13.77 Impression of implant. Look at the abundance of soft tissue

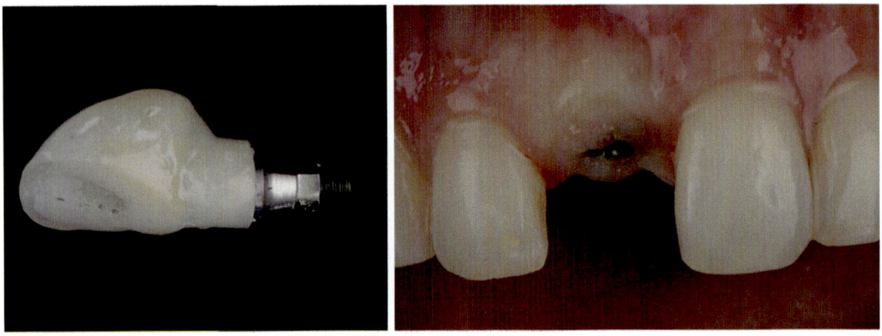

Fig. 13.78 Acrylic provisional fabricated

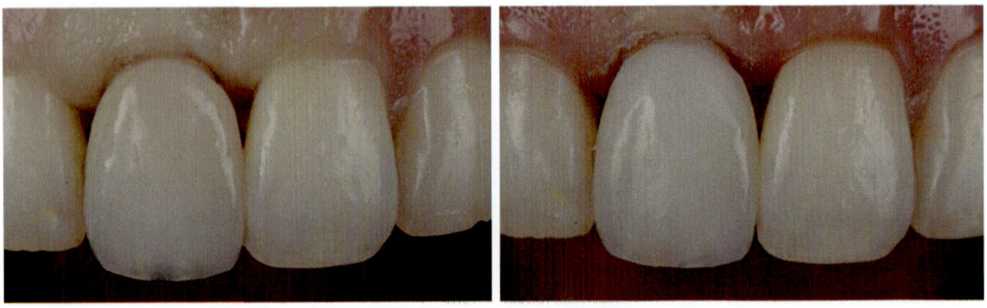

Fig. 13.79 Tissue maturation around provisional restoration

aware of this, and replacement of the adjacent ceramic veneer was discussed. The patient declined this (Figs. 13.85 and 13.86).

3. Root position of the adjacent teeth: There was sufficient inter-radicular space, and roots were tapering (Fig. 13.87).
4. Biotype of the periodontium and tooth shape: Biotype was thin, and tooth shape was triangular. This bears significance. If there is recession during the surgical procedure, a black triangle may develop.
5. The bony anatomy of the implant site: The site was deficient due to the per-apical infection and bone loss.

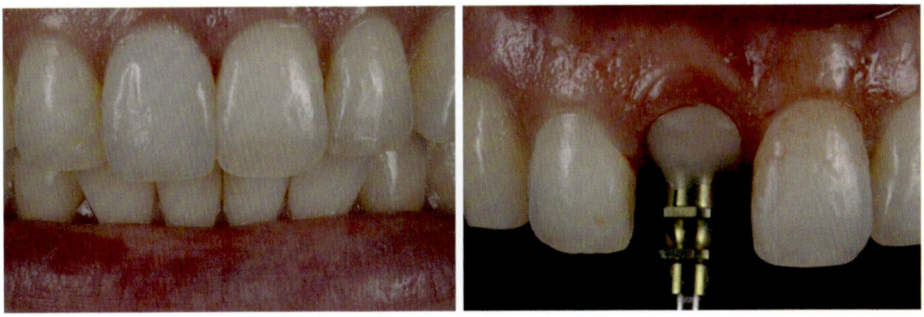

Fig. 13.80 Customized impression coping to transfer to laboratory

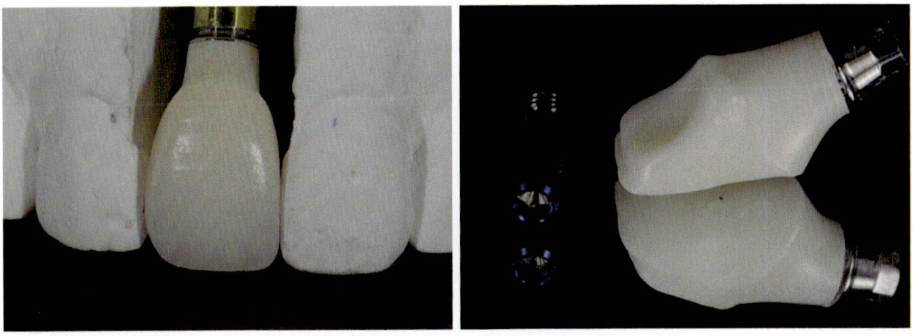

Fig. 13.81 Layered zirconia restoration with angled screw channel

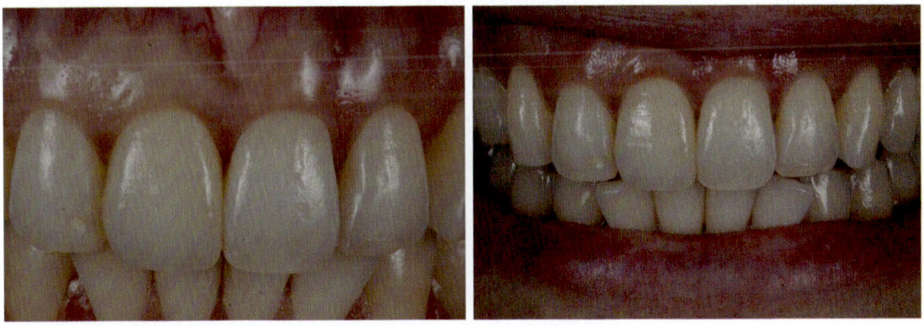

Fig. 13.82 Definitive restoration in place

6. The position of the implant: The site would need to be developed for ideal three-dimensional positioning of the implant.

Treatment Plan

1. Preoperative diagnostic and hygiene.
2. A resin-bonded fixed provisional was fabricated prior to the surgical procedure (Fig. 13.88).

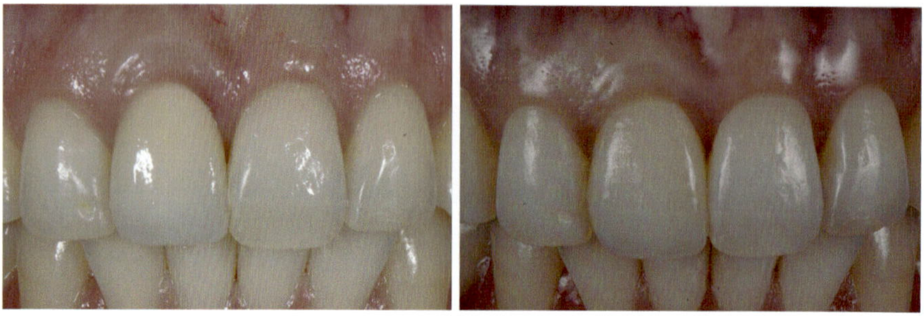

Fig. 13.83 Before and after. Not the position of soft tissue despite multiple surgical procedures

Fig. 13.84 Patient presented with failing maxillary right central incisor. All other maxillary anterior teeth had been restored with porcelain veneers

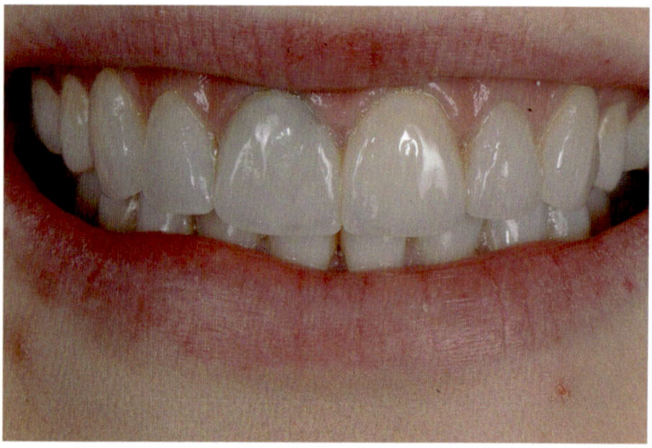

Fig. 13.85 Close-up intra-oral view

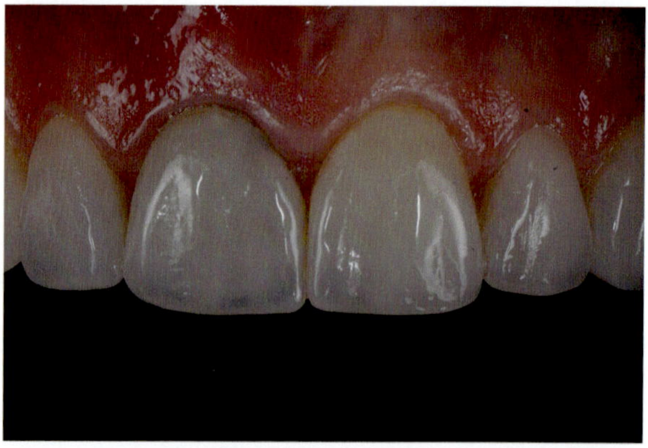

3. The tooth was extracted, socket grafted and resin-bonded provisional placed (Figs. 13.89 and 13.90).
4. A connective tissue graft was performed to improve the biotype. The resin-bonded provisional was rebonded (Figs. 13.91, 13.92, 13.93, 13.94 and 13.95).
5. Implant was placed using a surgical guide to ensure correct three-dimensional positioning (Figs. 13.96, 13.97 and 13.98).

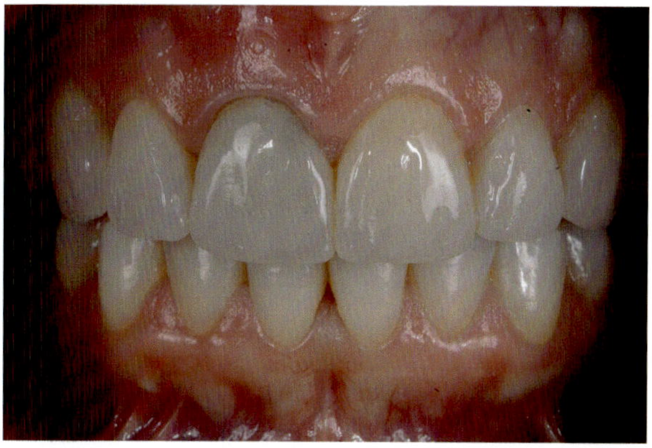

Fig. 13.86 Look at symmetry of tissue and thin biotype

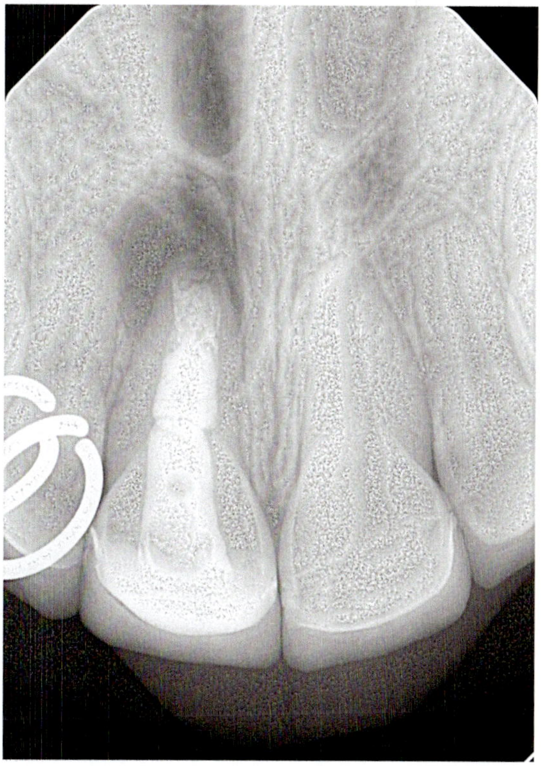

Fig. 13.87 Periapical showing pathology at the apex of root

6. Post-integration impressions were taken, and a fixed implant-supported provisional was fabricated to sculpt the tissue (Figs. 13.99, 13.100, 13.101 and 13.102).
7. The definitive restoration was a layered lithium disilicate restoration (Figs. 13.103, 13.104, 13.105 and 13.106).

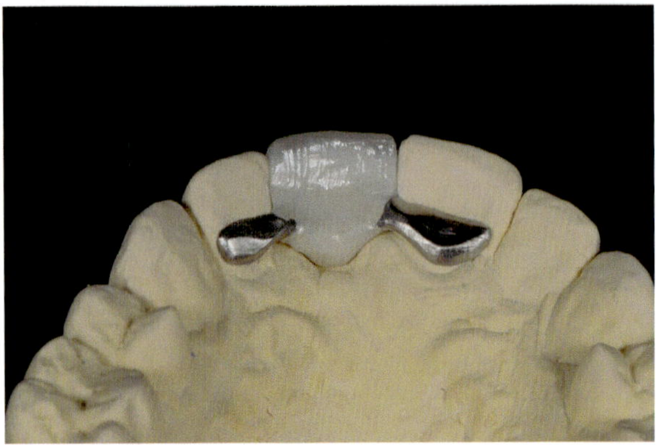

Fig. 13.88 Resin-bonded fixed partial denture made to be delivered at the time of surgery

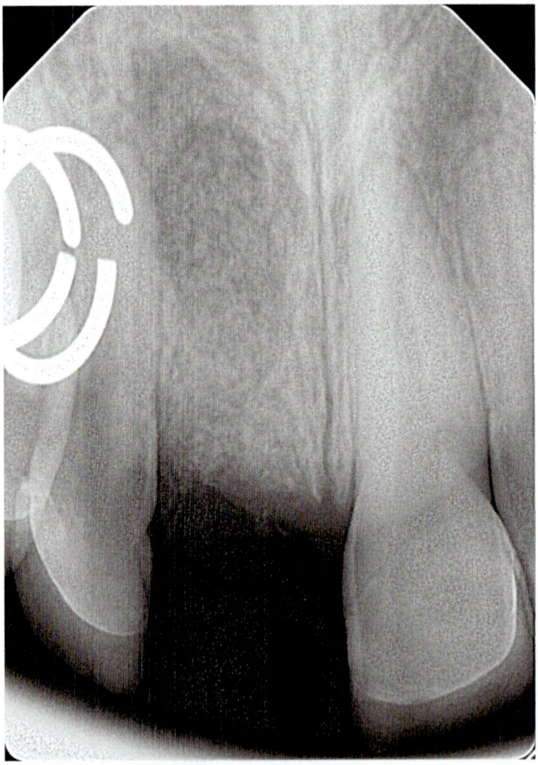

Fig. 13.89 Tooth extracted allograft and membrane place

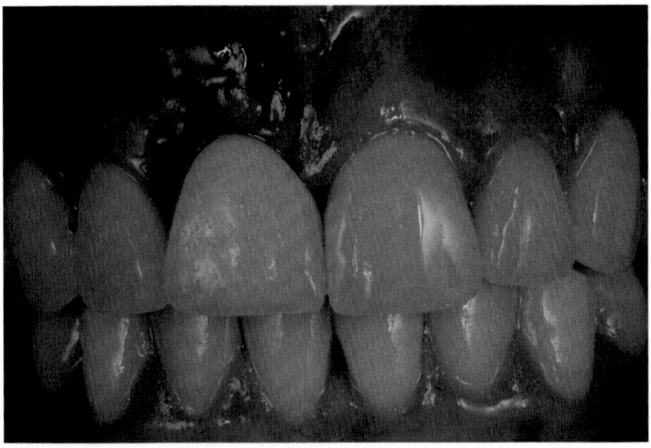

Fig. 13.90 Resin-bonded bridge delivered as a provisional

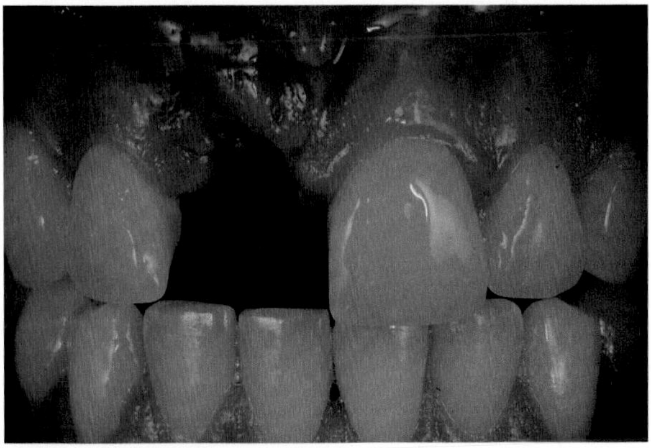

Fig. 13.91 Soft tissue healing

Case 3: Restorations of Implants That Were UnAesthetic

This patient presented having recently undergone implant therapy for her two central incisors and conventional crowns for the lateral incisors. She was unhappy with the aesthetics of the final outcome and wanted to explore options to improve them.

1. Patient selection and smile line: The patient was a dentist, and her smile line was low (Figs. 13.107, 13.108 and 13.109).
2. Tooth position: There was sufficient mesiodistal space to re-restore the teeth. The implants in the central incisor region were a little shallow.
3. Root position of the adjacent teeth: The root position did not interfere with any proposed restorative therapy.
4. Biotype of the periodontium and tooth shape: Biotype was thick. Tooth shape was short and square, and the gingival margins of the lateral incisors were low.
5. The bony anatomy of the implant site: No surgery was to be undertaken except crown lengthening for the lateral incisors.

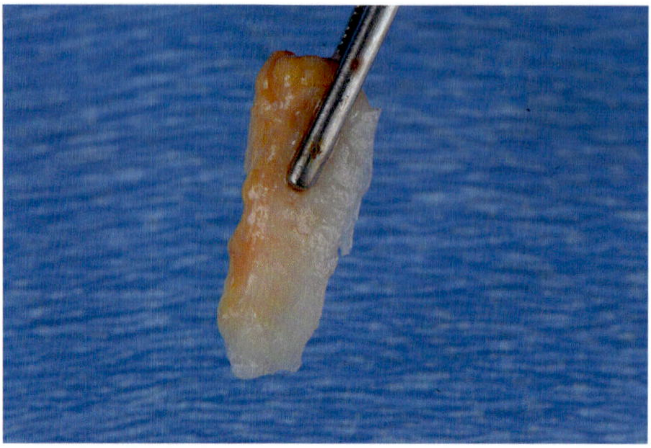

Fig. 13.92 Connective tissue graft harvested from palate

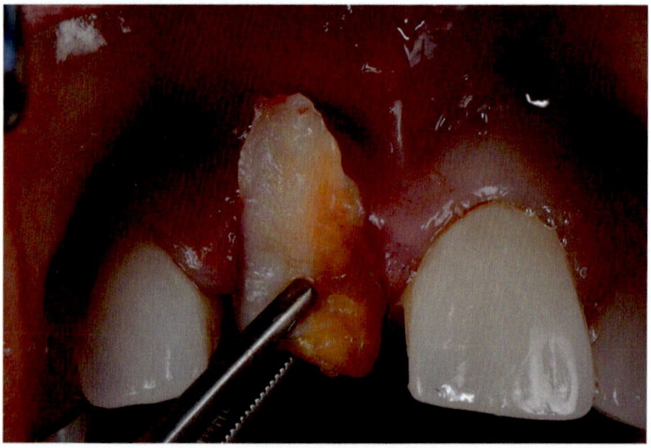

Fig. 13.93 Placement of connective tissue graft to improve biotype

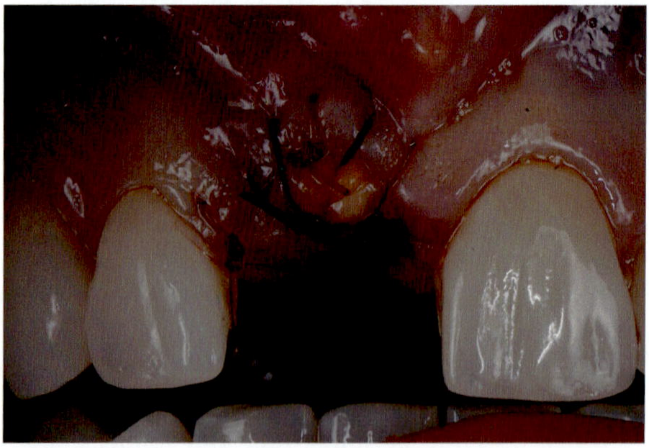

Fig. 13.94 Healing of graft

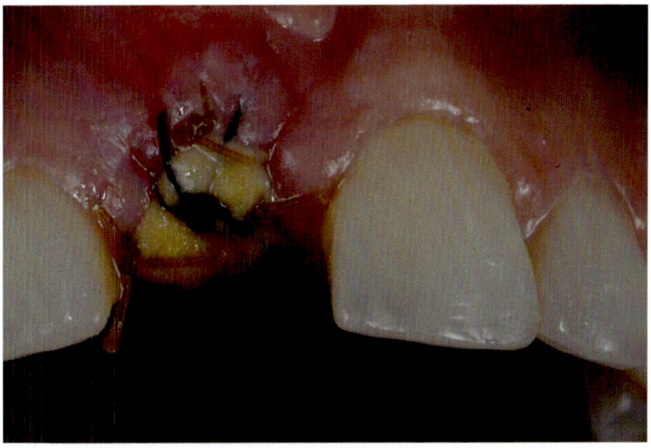

Fig. 13.95 Healing of graft at 1 week

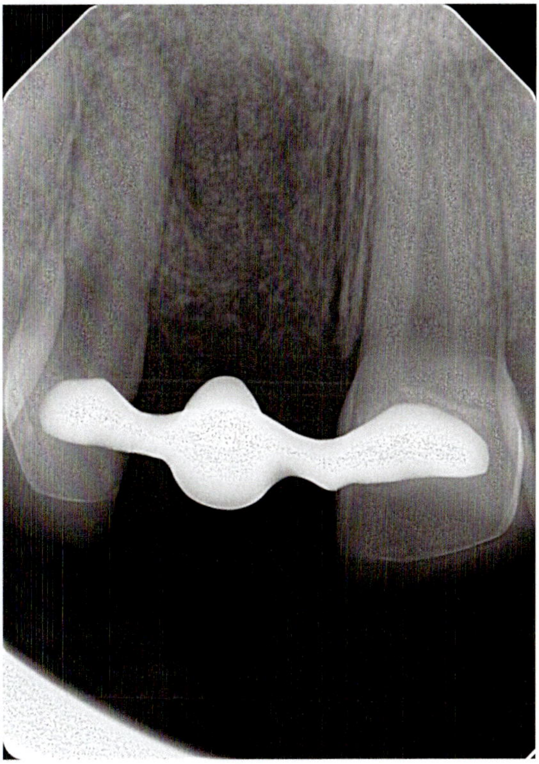

Fig. 13.96 Resin-bonded bridge replaced

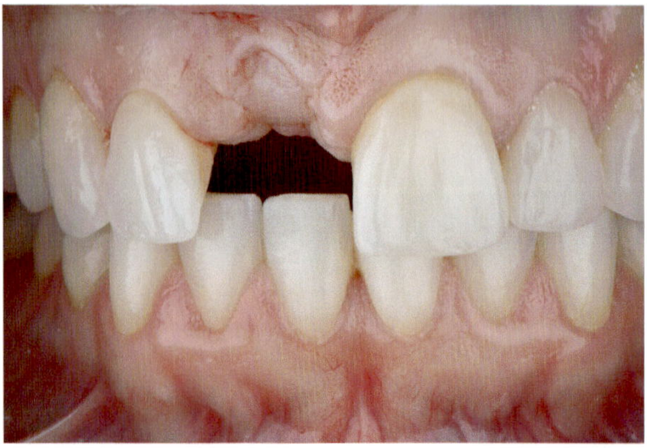

Fig. 13.97 Soft tissue healing

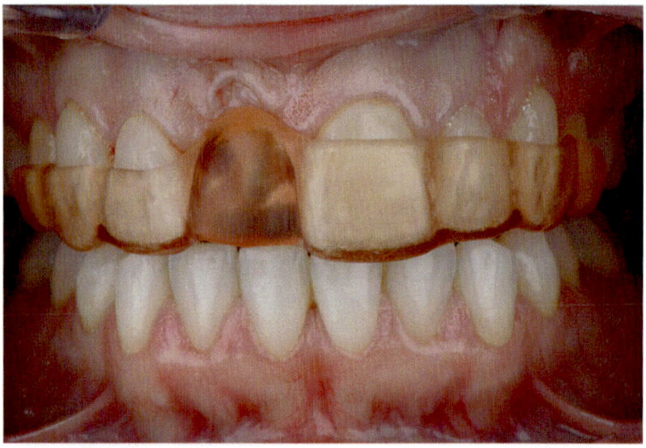

Fig. 13.98 Surgical guide for implant placement

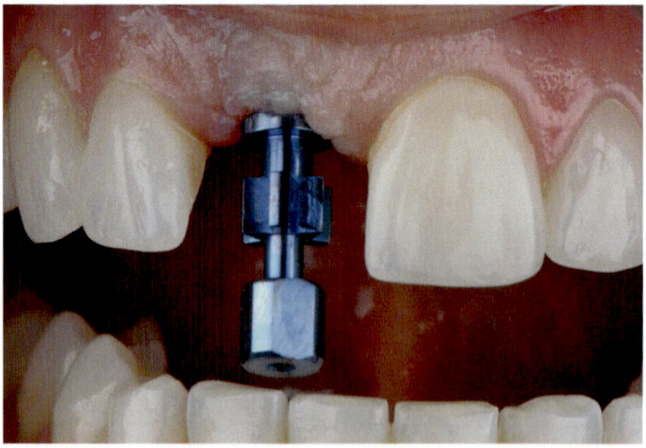

Fig. 13.99 Implant impressions

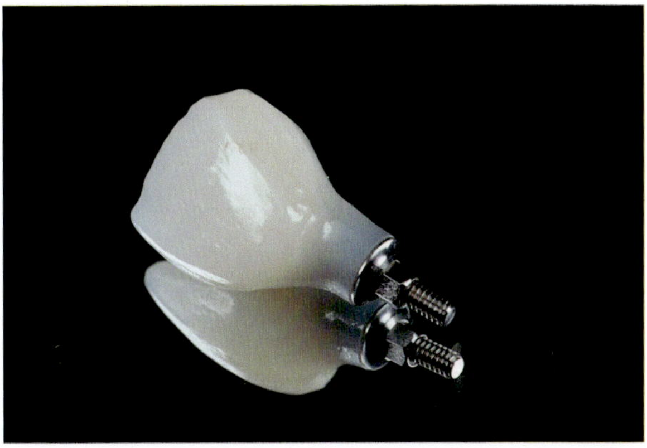

Fig. 13.100 Laboratory-fabricated provisional restoration

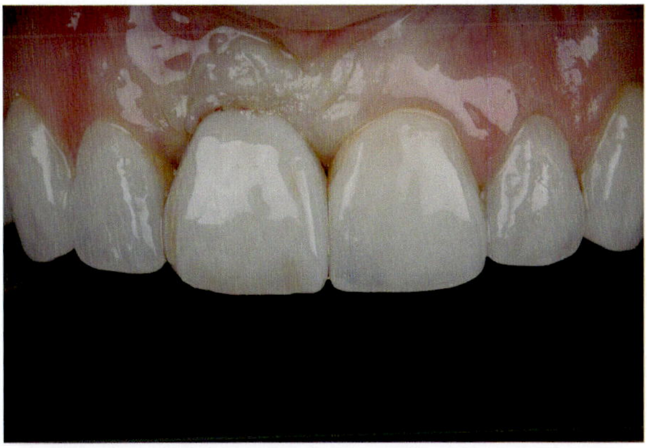

Fig. 13.101 Provisional restoration in situ

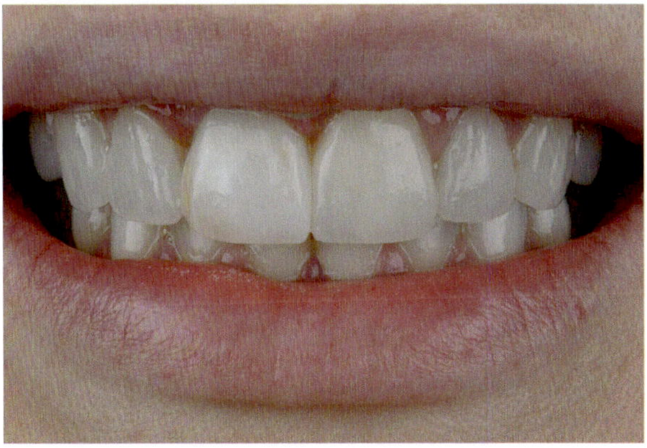

Fig. 13.102 Smile view of provisional restoration

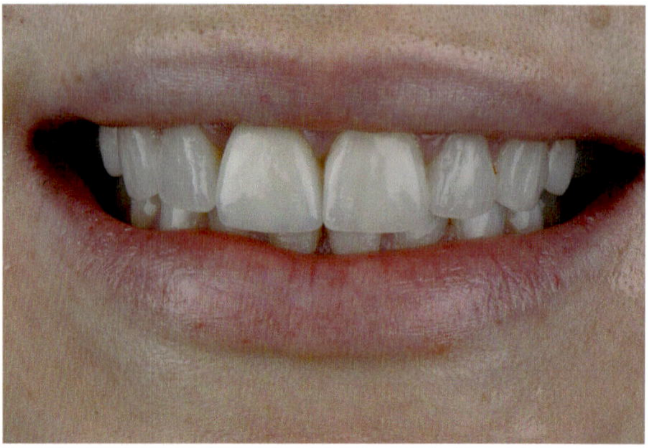

Fig. 13.103 Smile view of definitive restoration

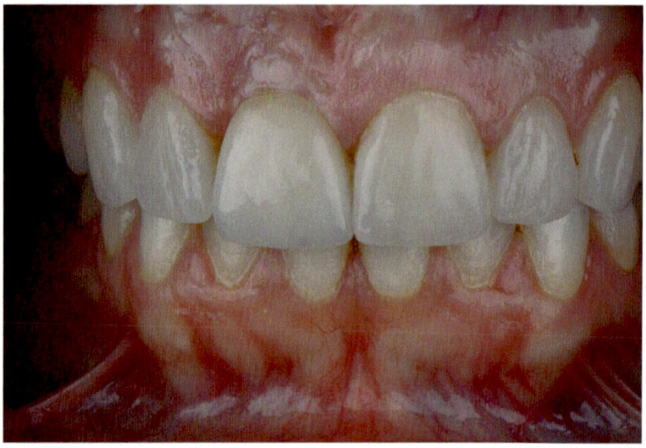

Fig. 13.104 Intra-oral view of definitive restoration

6. The position of the implant: The position was shallow but within an acceptable range to provide aesthetic restorations.

Treatment Plan

1. An ideal treatment plan to restore aesthetics and function as creative. The objective of this treatment plan was to improve the shape and proportions of the teeth. The gingival levels would also be addressed.
2. An impression was made of the implants and teeth. A diagnostic wax-up to visualize the end result was undertaken. Acrylic provisional restorations were fabricated (Fig. 13.110).
3. Crown lengthening was performed on the lateral incisors, and the patient was provisionalized (Fig. 13.111).
4. Post-gingival healing and additional set of provisional restorations were fabricated to finalize the tissue position and seek approval from the patient in regard to aesthetics (Fig. 13.112).
5. Definitive restorations were made from zirconia with a layered feldspathic ceramic (Figs. 13.113, 13.114, 13.115 and 13.116).

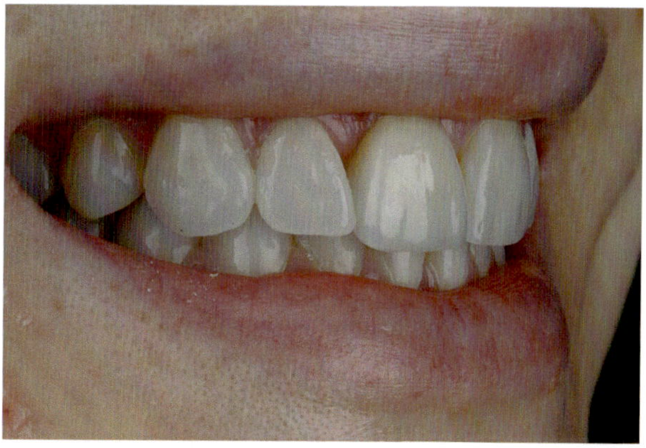

Fig. 13.105 Side view of definitive restoration

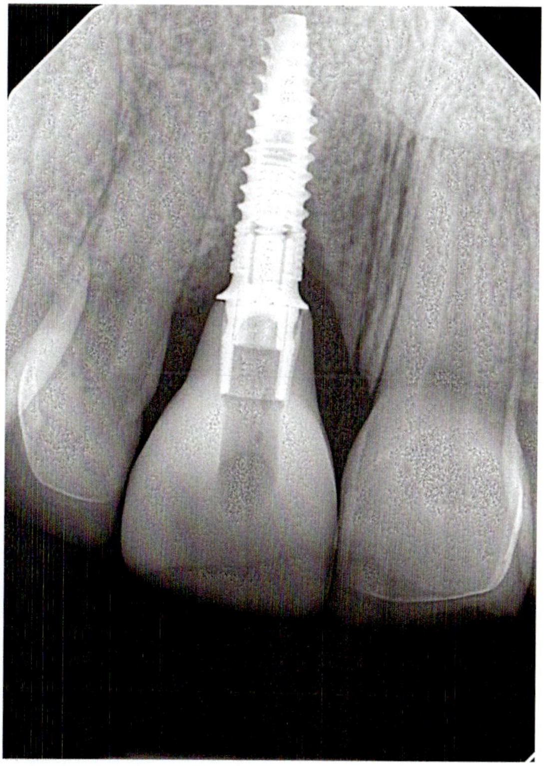

Fig. 13.106 Periapical radiograph of definitive restoration

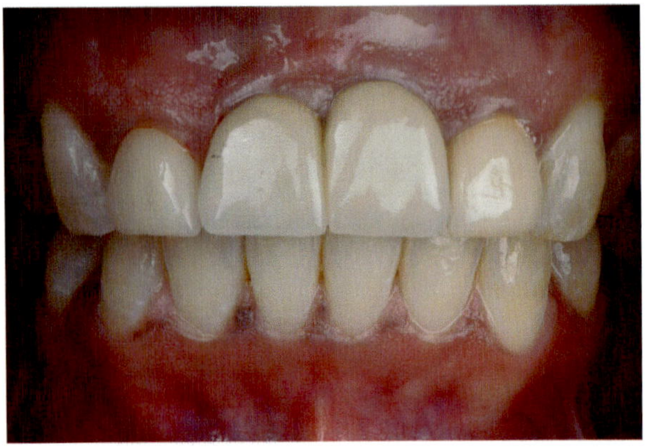

Fig. 13.107 View on presentation showing asymmetric gingival levels

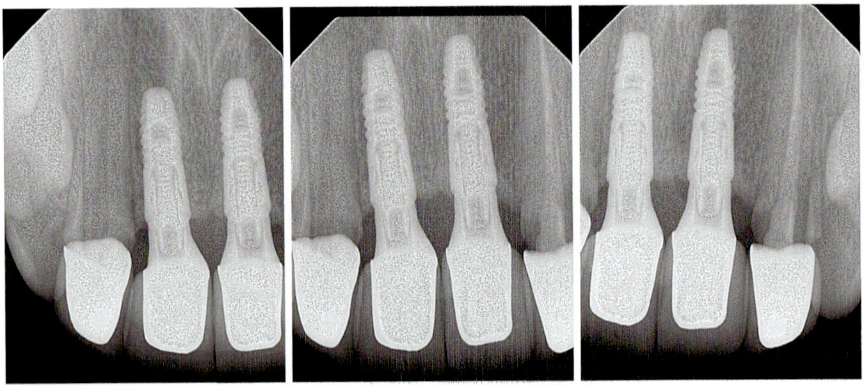

Fig. 13.108 Presenting radiograph

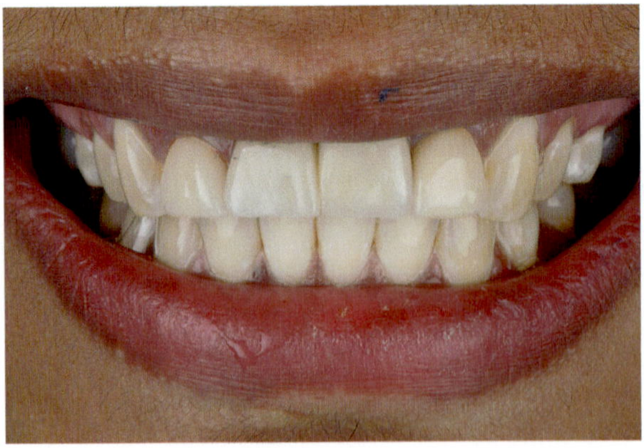

Fig. 13.109 Smile view

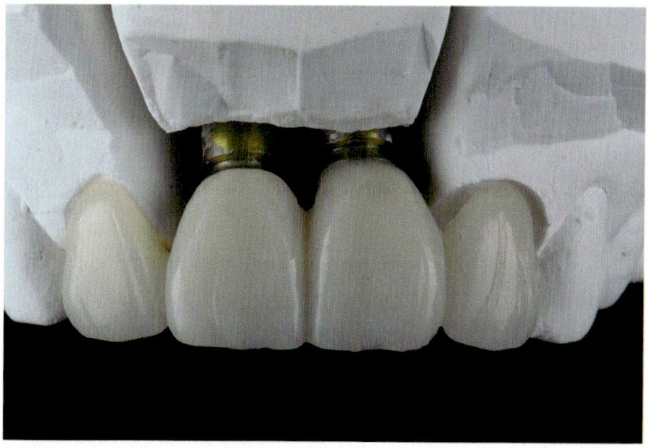

Fig. 13.110 Lab-fabricated provisional restorations

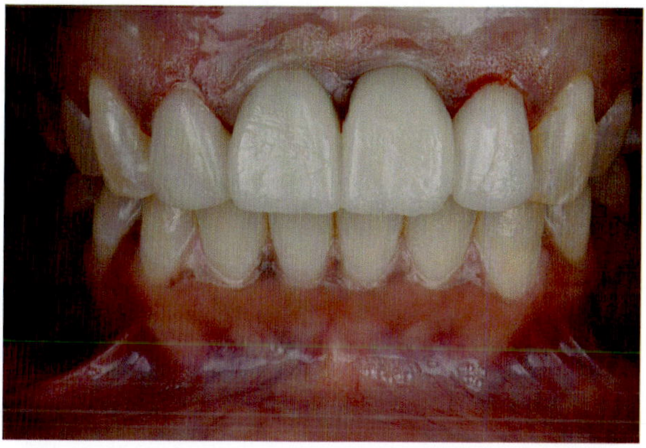

Fig. 13.111 Provisional restorations in situ post-crown lengthening

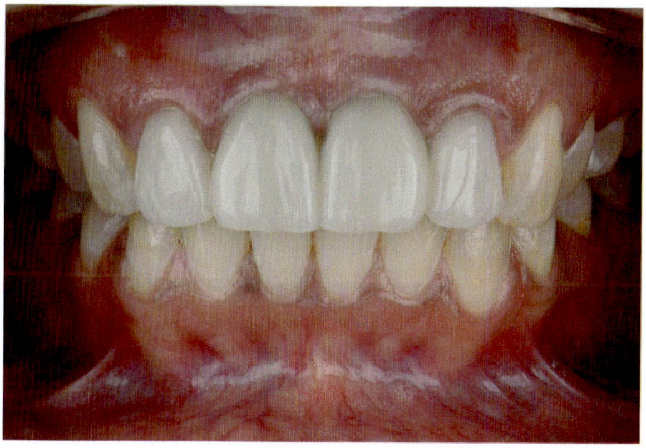

Fig. 13.112 New provisional restorations fabricated following tissue maturation

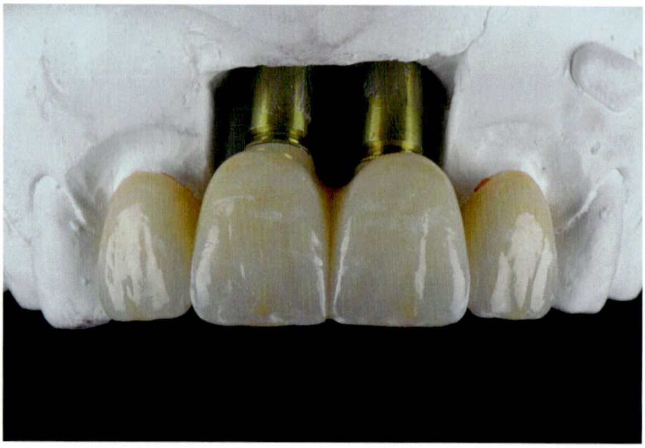

Fig. 13.113 Definitive zirconia-based restorations

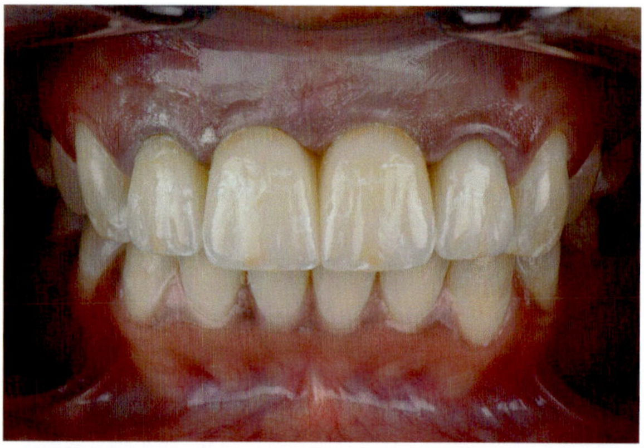

Fig. 13.114 Definitive restorations in situ. Note the gingival symmetry and tooth proportions

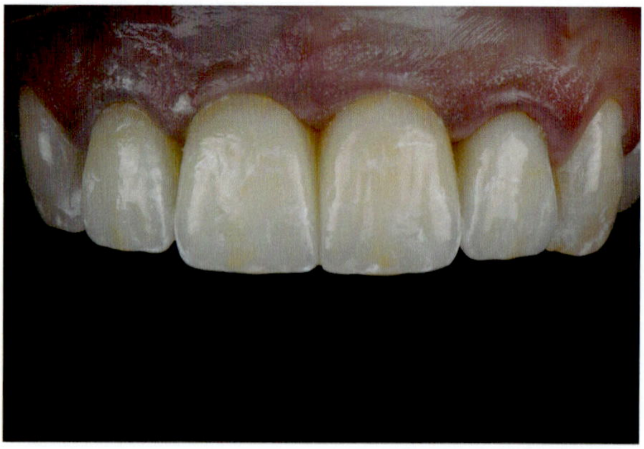

Fig. 13.115 Close-up view of definitive restorations

Fig. 13.116 Smile view

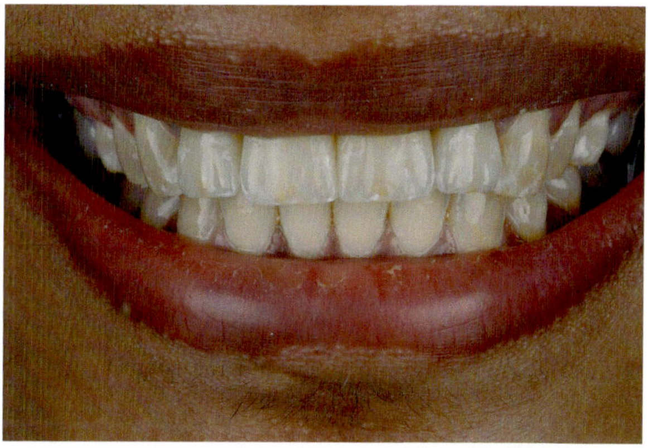

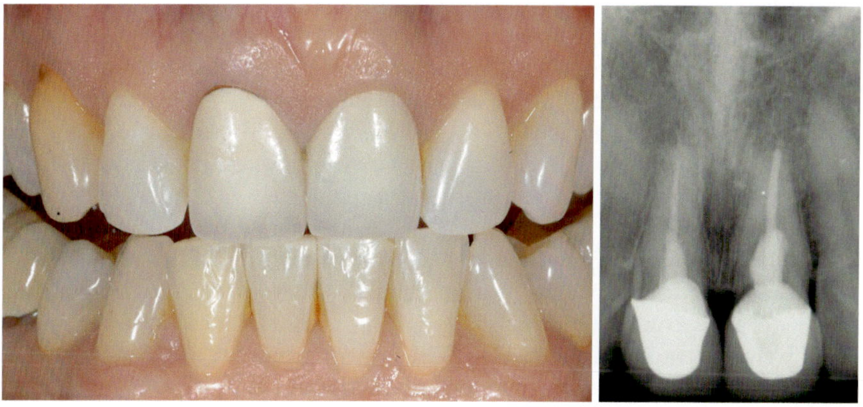

Fig. 13.117 Initial presentation, maxillary central incisors failing endodontically

Case 4: Treatment of Two Failing Central Incisors

This patient presented with two endodontically failing central incisors. They were deemed to be of poor prognosis, and dental implant therapy was planned.

On clinical examination, the following observations were made.

1. Patient selection and smile line: Patient had a low smile line (Fig. 13.117).
2. Tooth position: The patient presented with a deep vertical overlap.
3. Root position of the adjacent teeth: The adjacent root shape was tapering, and there was sufficient inter-radicular place for implant placement.
4. Biotype of the periodontium and tooth shape: Biotype was thick.
5. The bony anatomy of the implant site: There appeared to be an abundance of bone around the teeth. The trajectory of the bone was facially inclined.
6. The position of the implant: Two dental implants were planned, and there was sufficient space mesiodistally and sufficient bone apico-coronally to put them in an ideal position.

The patient requested that at no time during the treatment process would she accept a removable provisional restoration. Implant placement and immediate loading were planned. The patient was informed of the risk of the procedure and made aware that implant loading and lasting provisional restorations would only be delivered should the primary stability of the implants be adequate.

Treatment Plan

1. Diagnostics and hygiene.
2. Impressions and fabrication of tooth-supported surgical guides.
3. Extraction of the teeth and placement of two implants with an aggressive thread design (Figs. 13.118 and 13.119).
4. Fabrication of splinted implant provisionals. These provisionals were out of occlusal contact. Interproximal contacts were also relived. The patient was advised to have a soft diet. A soft night guard was fabricated for the opposing dentition (Figs. 13.120, 13.121 and 13.122).
5. Due to the trajectory of the bone in the premaxilla, the implants were placed with the access holes exiting from the incisal edge. An angulated screw channel option was utilized to ensure that the patient was provided with a screw-retained definitive zirconia restoration (Figs. 13.123, 13.124, 13.125 and 13.126). The clinician should be aware that angulated screw options are not similar from all companies and certain ones are prone to fracture.

Case 5: Failing Maxillary Lateral and Central Incisors

This patient presented with ill-fitting crowns and recurrent caries beneath existing crowns from lateral incisor to lateral incisor. Root length was short. Teeth were all tender to percussion. The patient's request was not to wear a removable provisional at any time during the treatment process.

The following clinical observations were made:

1. Patient selection and smile line: The patient had a low smile line. Considerations for treatment would be the restorability of the teeth following crown removal. Other factors include root length, opposing occlusion and medical history.

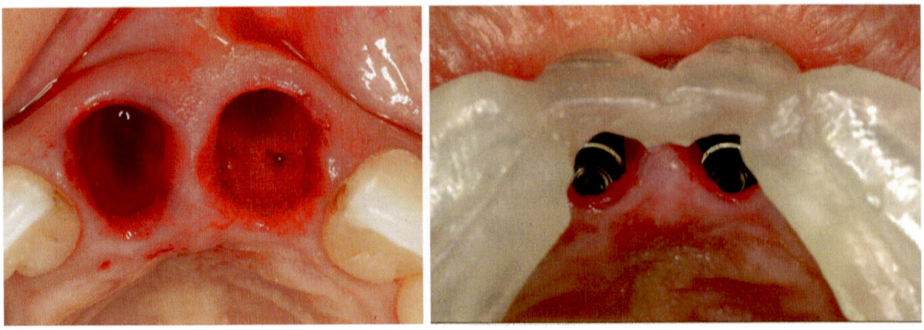

Fig. 13.118 Extraction and implant placement utilizing a tooth-supported surgical guide

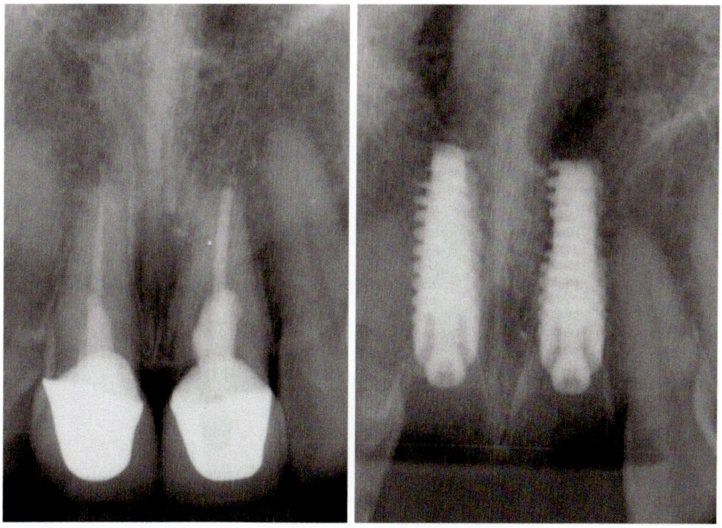

Fig. 13.119 Radiographs pre- and post-implant placement

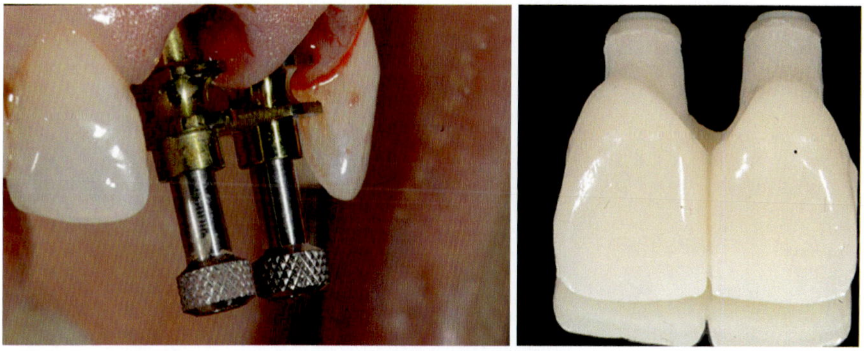

Fig. 13.120 Implant positioning and fabrication of splinted provisional restorations

2. Tooth position: There was sufficient mesiodistal space to restore the patient with a combination of tooth- and implant-supported restorations. The goal was to provide individual units.
3. Root position of the adjacent teeth: Roots were tapering and would not interfere with implant placement.
4. Biotype of the periodontium and tooth shape: Biotype was thick.
5. The bony anatomy of the implant site: The CBCT scan revealed adequate bone dimensions apico-coronally and buccolingually for regular platform implants in all sites if needed.
6. The position of the implant: This would depend on sites chosen.

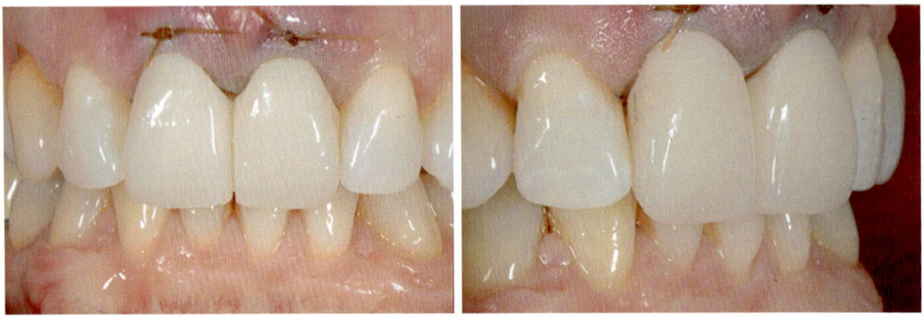

Fig. 13.121 Provisional restorations in situ

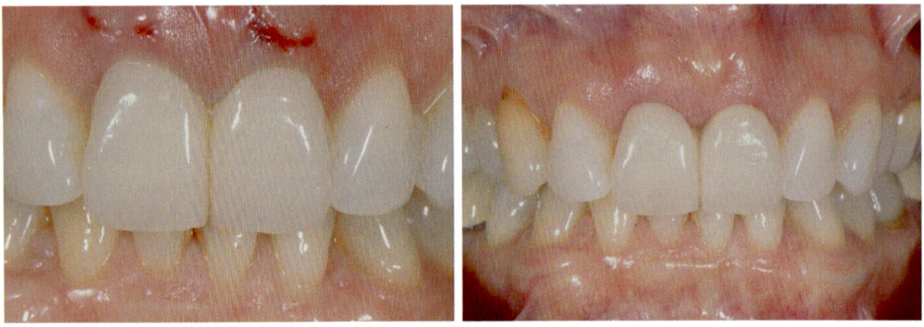

Fig. 13.122 Tissue maturation

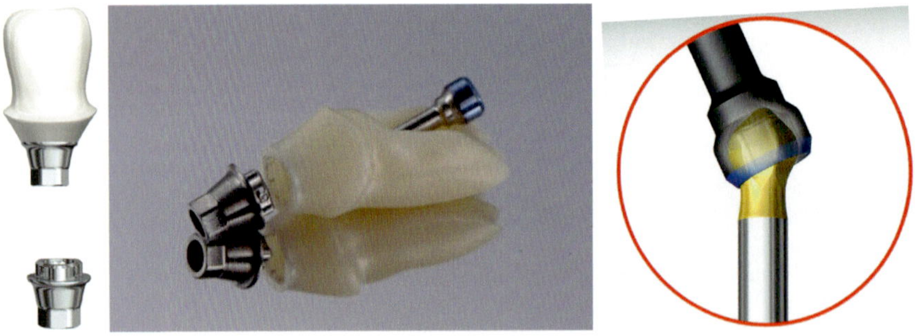

Fig. 13.123 Restorations fabricated utilizing an angled screw channel concept

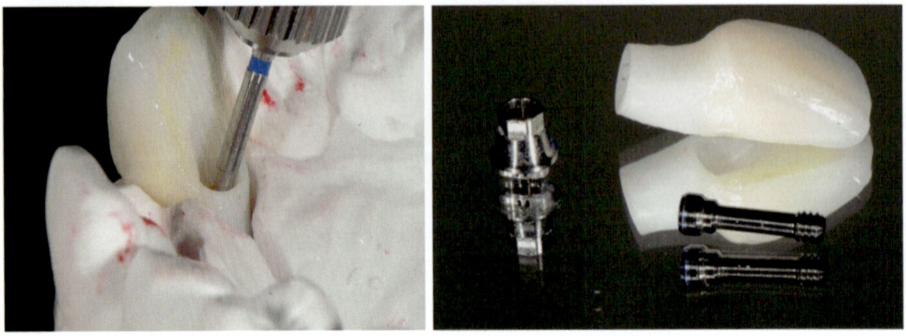

Fig. 13.124 Definitive zirconia-based restorations

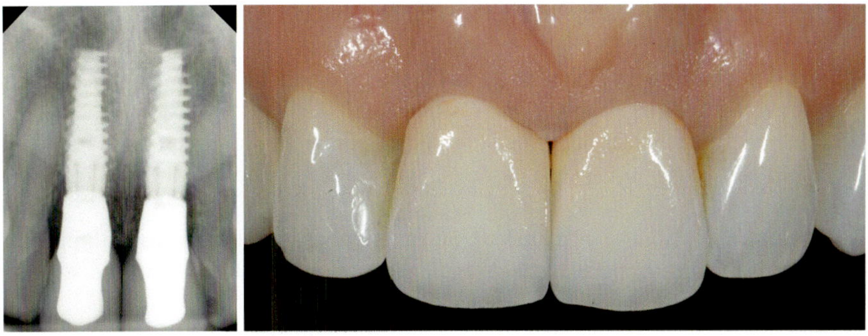

Fig. 13.125 Restorations in situ

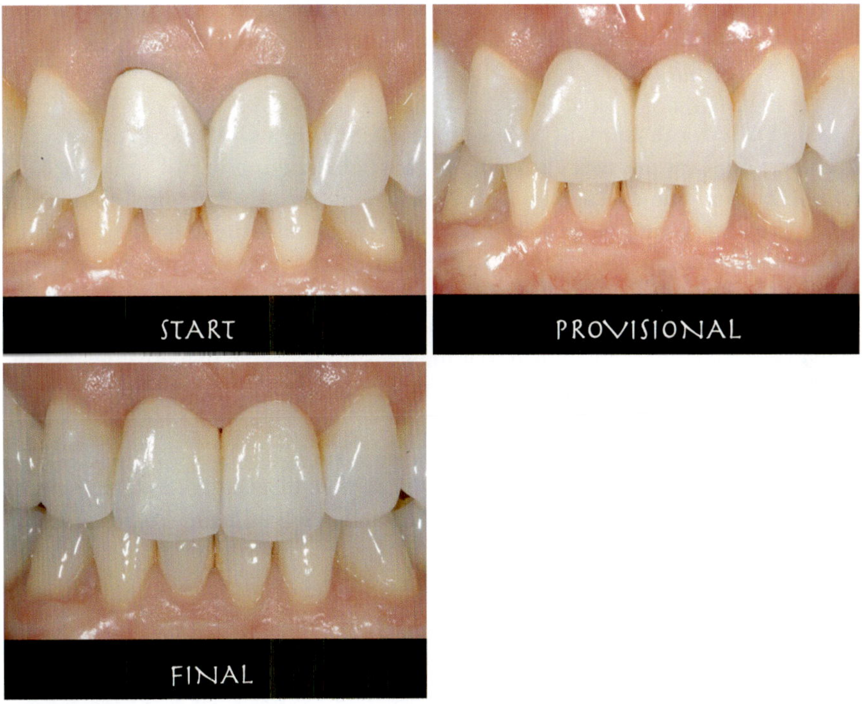

Fig. 13.126 Before provisional and definitive restorations

Treatment Plan

This would depend to a major degree on tooth structure and restorability of the teeth

1. Diagnostics and hygiene.
2. Fabrication of splinted shell provisional for the four incisors.
3. Removal of existing crowns and evaluation of tooth structure. Extensive recurrent caries was present in all four teeth. Due to the tapering and short root length, a decision was made that ultimately all four incisors would be extracted and two implants would be placed to provide a four-unit implant-supported restoration.

4. The central incisors were temporarily kept supporting a fixed tooth-supported provisional.
5. Dental implants were placed in the lateral incisor region. The patient was transitioning in a fixed tooth-supported restoration.
6. Once the implants had integrated, an impression was made and a fixed implant-supported provisional was fabricated with ovate pontics in the central incisor region.
7. The central incisors were extracted, and a mix of allograft and xenograft placed. A fixed implant-supported provisional restoration was placed until the sockets had healed.
8. Impressions were made, and zirconia custom abutments were fabricated for a cement-retained restoration. The cement margin followed the scallop of the tissue to ensure that cement could be cleaned.
9. The definitive restoration was a four-unit minimally layered zirconia restoration compressing the pontic sites in the central incisor region (Figs. 13.127, 13.128, 13.129, 13.130, 13.131, 13.132, 13.133, 13.134, and 13.135).

Case 6: Full-Mouth Implant Rehabilitation Utilizing a Graftless Protocol

Aesthetic implant dentistry can be the most challenging in full-arch implant rehabilitation. The extraction of the teeth between the implants causes the tissue to collapse, and ultimately a flat gingival architecture results. The clinician must take further steps in sculpting the tissue with provisional restorations.

Often patients refuse additional grafting procedures, and there is insufficient bone to be able to place more than four implants in each arch. In these clinical situations, the patient must be made aware of the advantages and disadvantages of such treatment protocols and must be fully aware of the clinical and financial consequences of implant failure.

The following patient presentation illustrates the philosophy of minimally invasive implant therapy for full-arch implant rehabilitation utilizing four implants in each arch and digital technologies.

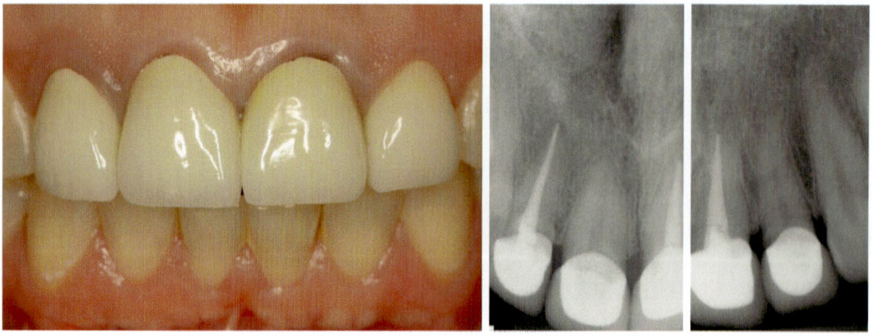

Fig. 13.127 Initial presentation. Four failing incisors

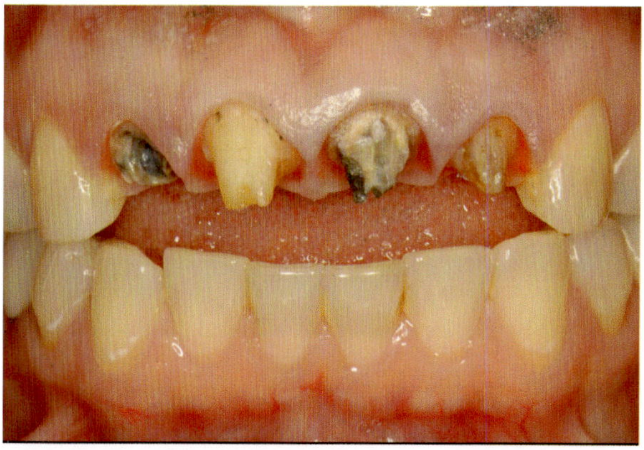

Fig. 13.128 Crowns removed, teeth deemed unrestorable

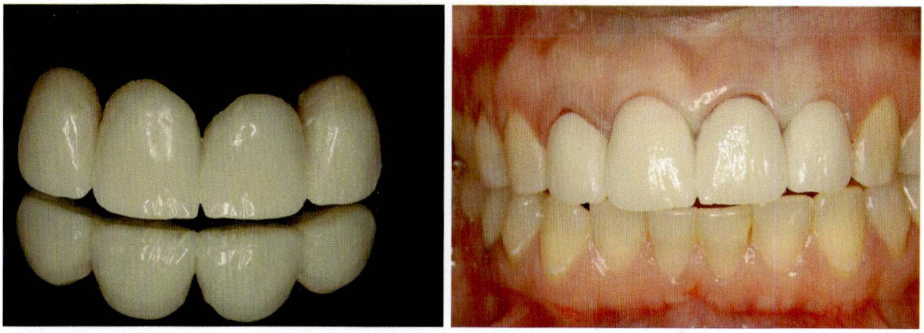

Fig. 13.129 Shell provisionals had been fabricated ahead of time. Two teeth chosen to support the provisional restoration

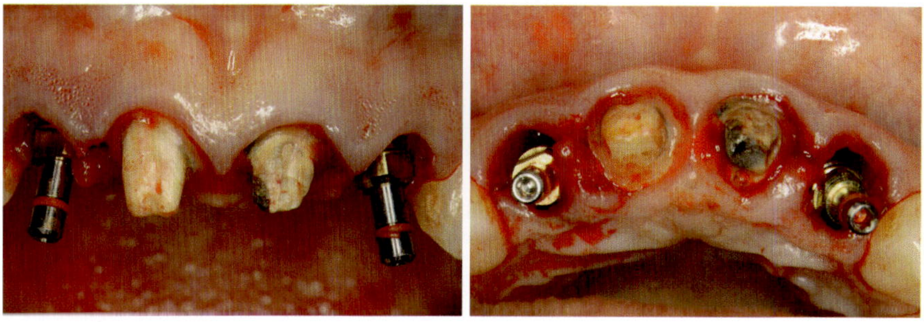

Fig. 13.130 Dental implants placed in lateral incisor region

A 62-year-old female presented seeking a solution to her failing maxillary and mandibular dentition. A detail medical and dental evaluation was performed. Specific concerns in treatment planning were multiple medications that resulted in the patient being xerostomic. The patient's teeth had been compromised due to caries and periodontal disease (Figs. 13.136 and 13.137).

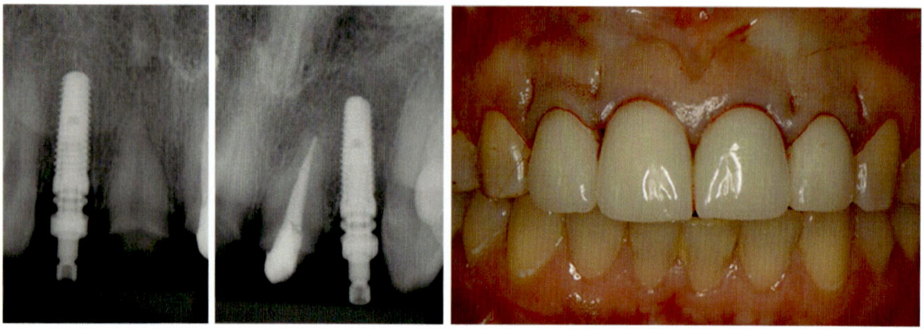

Fig. 13.131 Provisionals replaced on central incisors

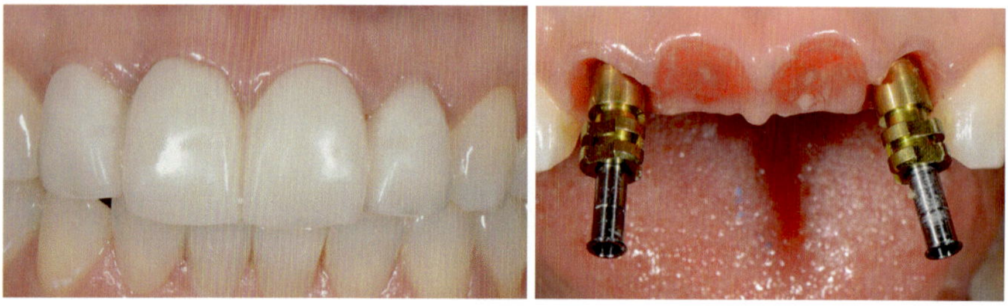

Fig. 13.132 Implant-supported provisionals fabricated

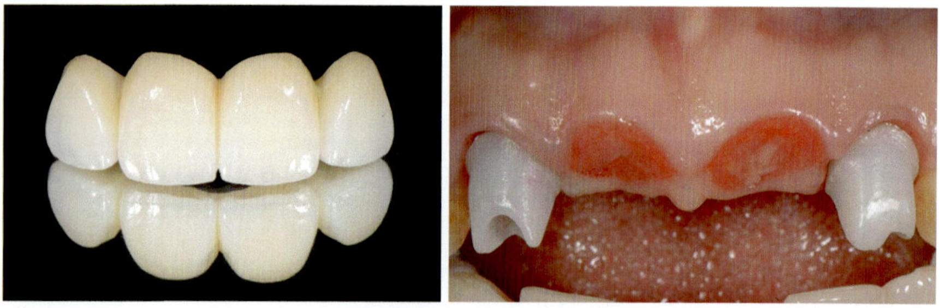

Fig. 13.133 Cementable abutments and definitive zirconia restoration

The following diagnosis was made:

1. Caries
2. Periodontal disease
3. Lack of posterior support

On clinical and radiographic examination, her maxillary and mandibular dentition was deemed to be of poor prognosis. Alternative treatment plans were discussed which included grafting. The patient declined.

The following clinical issues required attention:

1. Lack of bone in the posterior maxilla
2. Over-eruption of teeth compromising restorative space

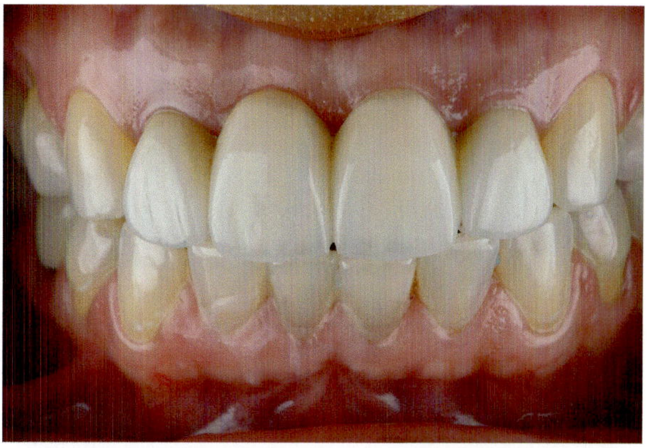

Fig. 13.134 Intra-oral view of definitive zirconia restorations

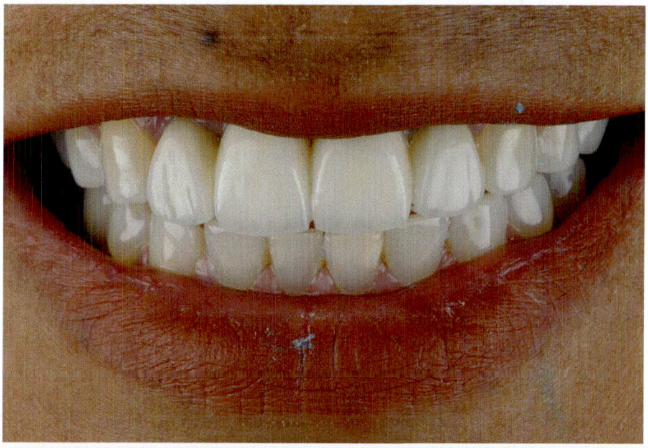

Fig. 13.135 Smile view

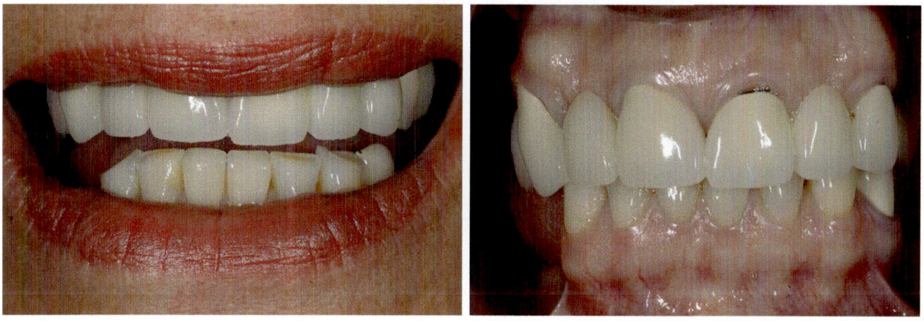

Fig. 13.136 Initial presentation of terminal dentition

3. Short square teeth
4. Posterior bone resorption in the mandible

The patient's concerns were the following:

1. The patient did not want to wear a removable appliance at any point during the treatment process.
2. The patient did not want to go through bone grafting procedures.

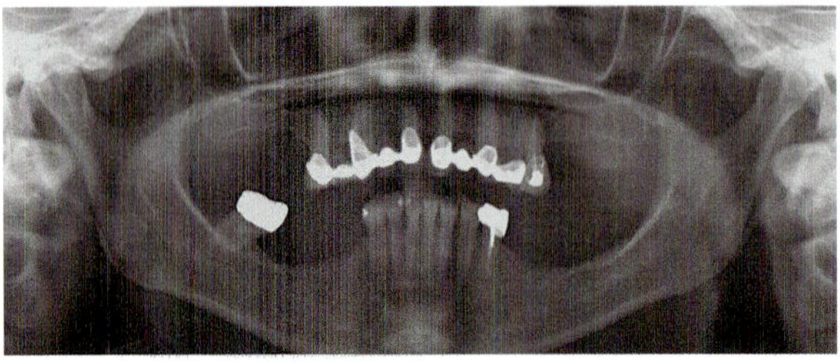

Fig. 13.137 Panoramic radiograph showing pneumatized sinuses and posterior mandibular resorption

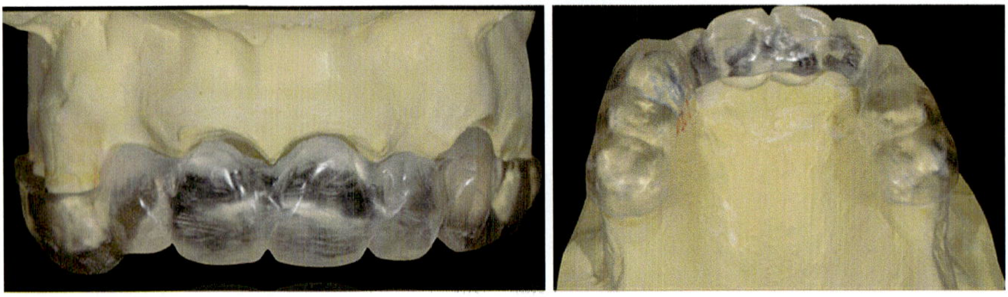

Fig. 13.138 Tooth-supported surgical guide fabricated

Considerations in implementing care were the following:

1. Multiple medications causing the patient to be xerostomic.
2. The patient's smile line was low. The patient had a short lip. It is the author's opinion that bone reduction and use of pink prosthetics in these types of clinical situations are contraindicated.
3. Preservation of bone.
4. Providing an FP1 prosthesis and maintaining bone.
5. Providing an anteroposterior spread that is optimal. Placement of implants that do not compromise connector size for the definitive restorations.
6. Minimal alveolar bone recontouring to lift the maxillary occlusal plane up and to lower the mandibular occlusal plane.
7. Transitioning the patient with fixed restoration during the entire treatment process.

The above considerations required a more cautious approach in treatment planning and execution.

Treatment Plan and Sequence

1. Intra-oral scans were completed (Trios 3 Shape Technologies), and shell provisionals were milled (Pro Art CAD Ivoclar Vivadent) (Figs. 13.138 and 13.139).
2. The patient was treated surgically and prosthetically in 1 day, utilizing laboratory-fabricated static surgical guides. No guided surgery was performed per se. The surgical guides were stabilized on retained teeth, and osteotomies of the anterior implants were performed. Four implants were placed in the maxilla and four in the mandible. Multi-unit abutments were secured, and soft tissue closure was achieved. Deep sedation with profound local anaesthesia was used to remove

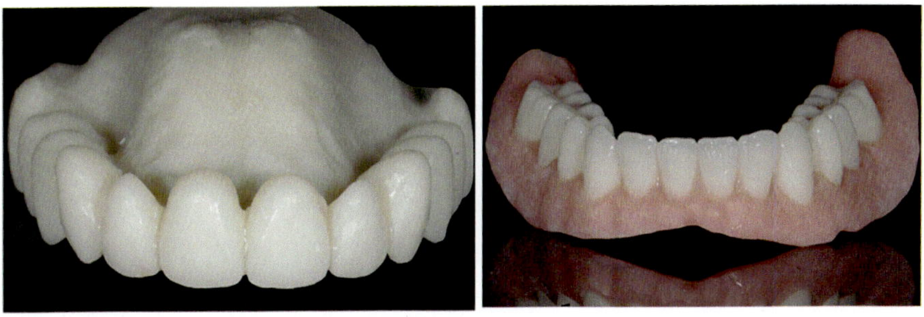

Fig. 13.139 Milled provisional fabricated

all teeth except the ones needed for stability of bone reduction and surgical stent. A tooth-supported surgical guide was provided to ensure accurate three-dimensional placement of implants in the maxilla. This required careful depth placement so that a pre-angled multi-unit abutment could be selected with a minimum collar height. This would allow correction of the flaring of the teeth as well as an optimal emergence profile. Alveolectomy was completed in the mandible to provide appropriate restorative space and correct the mandibular incisal edge position. The mandibular bone was reduced minimally to create a platform for implant placement. The patient was informed that the mandible may require pink prosthetics. The patient's provisional immediate load prosthesis was fabricated on the same day as implant placement. The patient tolerated the procedure well and healed uneventfully.

3. A direct technique for immediate loading was employed. Vertical dimension, centric relation and occlusal plane were verified. After protection of the surgical sites with rubber dam, temporary cylinders were first picked up in the maxillary prosthesis. Patient was guided into centric relation, and a similar pickup of temporary cylinders was performed in the mandibular provisional restoration. The prostheses were removed and transferred to the dental laboratory where the prostheses were processed and finished. The prostheses were adjusted to compress the tissue by 2 mm and to develop the pontic sites from the outset. Twelve teeth were provided in the maxilla and ten teeth in the mandible. Occlusion was adjusted for shimstock hold on the anterior teeth and shimstock drag on the posterior teeth. Vertical dimension was verified on the delivery of the restoration. Extraction of remaining teeth and grafting of extraction sites with a bone xenograft were performed to maintain ridge height and width. Delivery of splinted provisionals was done (Figs. 13.140, 13.141, and 13.142).
4. Tissue maturation and stabilization (Fig. 13.143).
5. Post-integration, an additional provisional restoration was fabricated to ensure verification of aesthetics, phonetics and tissue compression (Figs. 13.144 and 13.145).
6. Splinted open-tray impressions, jaw relation records and tooth try-ins were performed. Aesthetics, phonetics and soft tissue contours were further developed in the provisional restoration. The soft tissue information was communicated to the

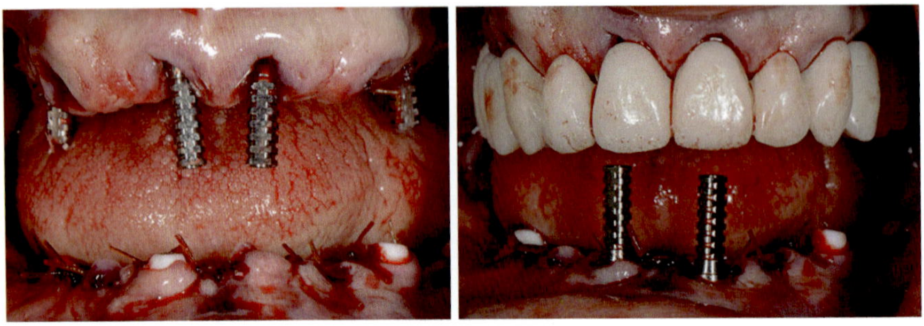

Fig. 13.140 Maxillary implants placed and immediately loaded with provisional

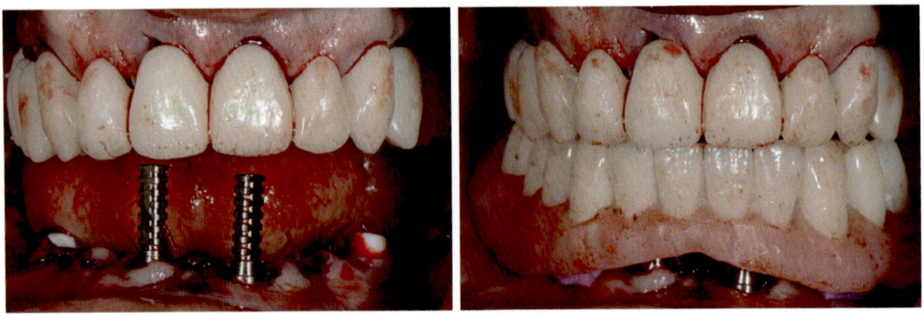

Fig. 13.141 Mandibular implants placed and immediately loaded with provisional

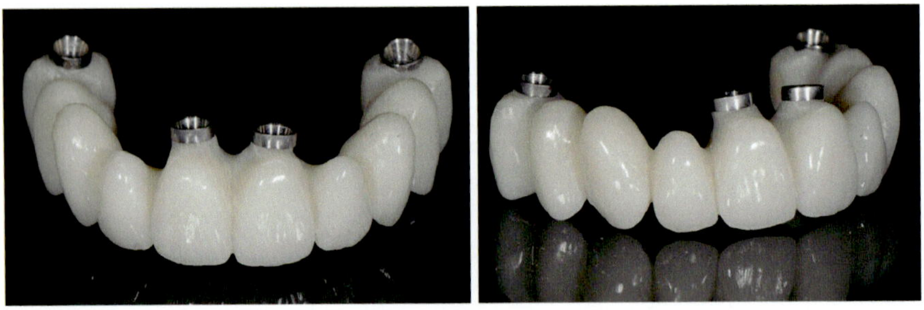

Fig. 13.142 Provisional with ovate pontics

laboratory for adequate tissue compression in the definitive restorations (Fig. 13.146).

7. Minimally layered zirconia restorations were fabricated for the maxillary arch and acrylic titanium prosthesis in the mandibular arch and mandible (Figs. 13.147 and 13.148).
8. The prosthesis was delivered adjusting the undersurface to ensure positive pressure. Dynamic occlusion was adjusted for canine guidance. Static occlusion was adjusted to ensure shimstock hold on canines and premolars. Shimstock drag on anterior teeth and no contact on the cantilevers.

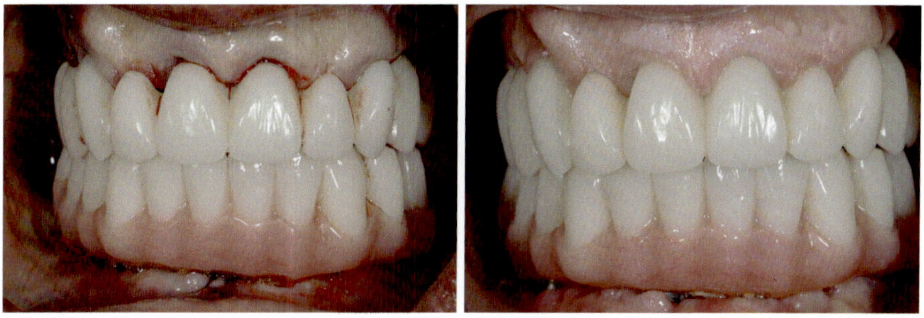

Fig. 13.143 Day of delivery of provisionals and 1 week post-op

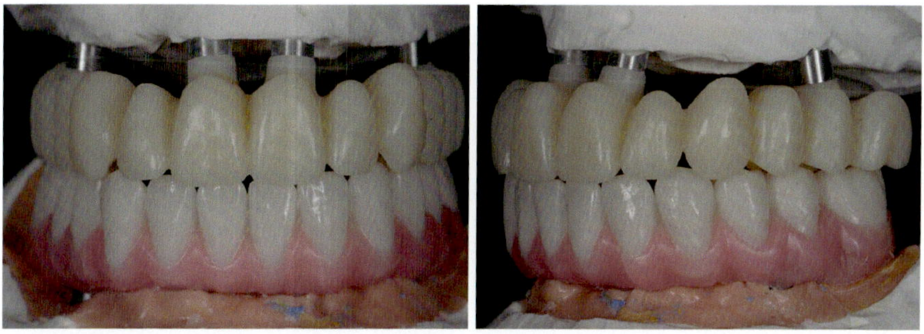

Fig. 13.144 Prototype fabricated to ensure tissue adaptation and compression

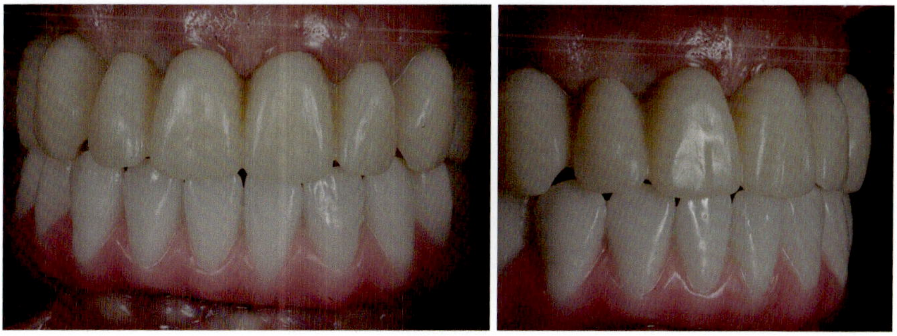

Fig. 13.145 Prototypes in situ, to shape tissue and transfer information to laboratory

9. Screws were torqued according to the manufacturer's instructions, and access holes were sealed using Teflon and composite resin.

By completing the above sequence, the following objectives were met:

1. Transitioning the patient through fixed provisional restorations at all times.
2. Preservation of bone and fabrication of an FP1 prosthesis in the maxilla.
3. Restoration of posterior support.

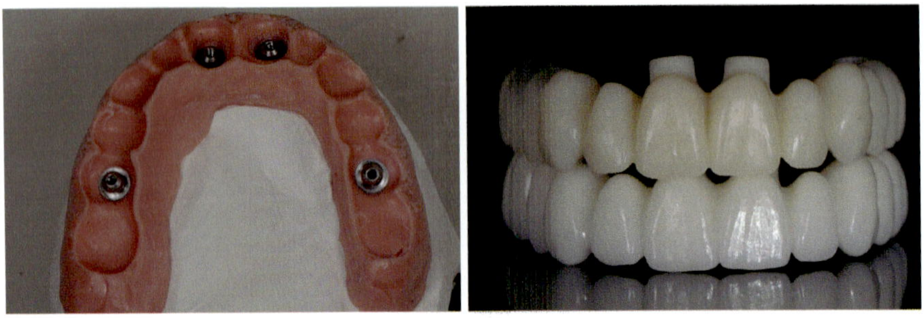

Fig. 13.146 Shaping of tissue on implant model. Definitive zirconia restoration is a copy of the prototype

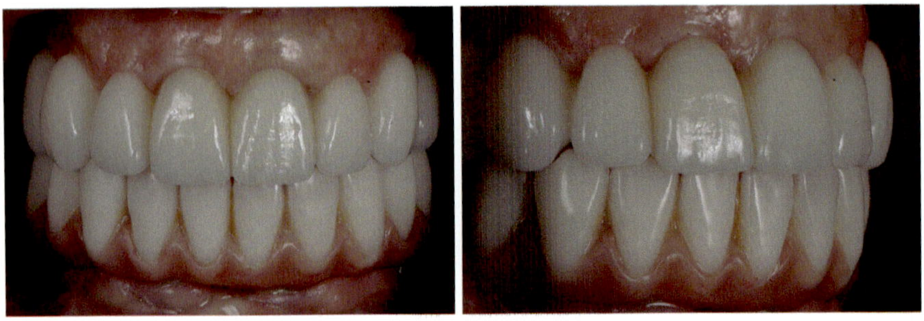

Fig. 13.147 Definitive zirconia maxillary restoration. Mandibular acrylic titanium restoration

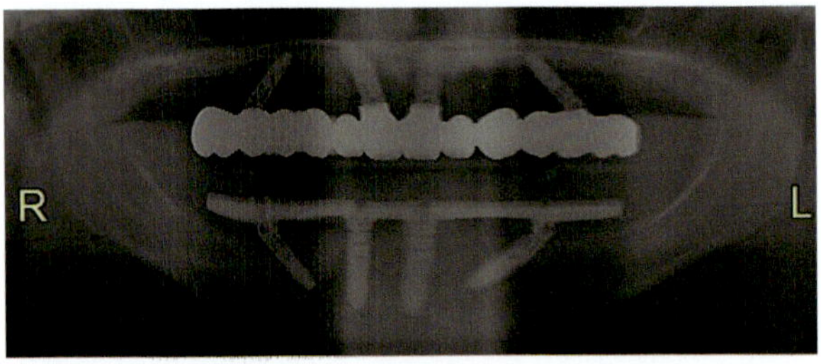

Fig. 13.148 Final panoramic radiograph

4. Satisfying the patient's aesthetic concerns.
5. Utilization of technology to make treatment more efficient prosthetically.

13.8 Summary

When a patient has a missing anterior tooth and desires replacement, a decision must be made by the clinician and patient as to the method of replacement. Common choices would include a conventional fixed partial denture, a resin-bonded fixed partial denture or an implant-borne restoration. Each has its advantages and disadvantages.

The conventional fixed partial denture has the advantages of being an established treatment procedure, having predictable aesthetics and being expedient. It has the disadvantage of requiring preparation of adjacent teeth and potential risk for periodontal and pulpal tissue.

The resin-bonded partial denture has the advantages of preserving tooth structure, having predictable aesthetics and reduced cost. It has the disadvantages of being technique sensitive for the dentist and technician and often losing retention, which may lead to decay.

Implants used to replace missing teeth in the aesthetic zone have many advantages like preservation of unrestored adjacent teeth, halting the resorption of edentulous spaces and providing support. However, at present, it has the disadvantages of long treatment time, requiring a provisional restoration during implant integration, surgical placement of the implant, surgical uncovering of the implant, a provisional after the implant is uncovered and having higher cost.

Much effort is being directed at shortening the treatment time and making delivery of the service more time efficient. Immediately loading implants is one direction that many researchers and clinicians are taking when indicated.

Even with all the disadvantages listed, the implant-supported single-tooth restoration can be successfully executed when all the factors discussed in this series of articles are addressed. When one or more of the adjacent teeth are unrestored or in need of only a minor restoration, the single-tooth implant should be considered the restoration of choice.

References

1. Mankoo T. Maintenance of interdental papillae in the esthetic zone using multiple immediate adjacent implants to restore failing teeth-a report of ten cases at 2 to 7 years follow-up. Eur J Esthet Dent. 2008;3(4):304–22.
2. Sullivan RM. Perspective on esthetics in implant dentistry. Compendium. 2001;22(8):685–92.
3. Belser UC. Esthetic checklist for the fixed prosthesis. Part II: Biscuit bake try in. In: Scharer P, Rinn LA, Kopp FR, editors. Esthetic guidelines for restorative dentistry. Chicago: Quintessence; 1982. p. 188–92.
4. Magne P, Belser U. Natural oral esthetics. In: Bonded porcelain restorations in the anterior dentition. A biomimetic approach. Chicago: Quintessence; 2002. p. 57–99.
5. Tjan AH, Miller GD, The JG. Some esthetic factors in a smile. J Prosthet Dent. 1984;51(1):24–8.
6. Kois JC. Esthetic extraction site development: the biological variables. Contemp Esthet Restor Pract. 1998;2:10–8.
7. Khzam N, Mattheos N, Roberts D, Bruce WL, Ivanovski S. Immediate placement and restoration of dental implants in the esthetic region: clinical case series. J Esthet Restor Dent. 2014;26(5):332–44.
8. Kois JC. Predictable single tooth peri-implant esthetics: five diagnostic keys. Compendium. 2004;25(11):895–905.
9. Salama H, Salama M, Kelly J. The orthodontic-periodontal connection in implant site development. Pract Periodontics Aesthet Dent. 1996;8(9):923–32.
10. Urban IA, Nagursky H, Lozada JL, Nagy K. Int J Periodontics Restor Dent. 2013;33(3):299–307.
11. Tarnow DP, Cho SC, Wallace SS. The effect of inter-implant distance on the height of inter-implant bone crest. J Periodontol. 2000;71(4):546–9.

12. Tarnow DP, Magner AW, Fletcher P. The effect of distance from the contact point to the crest of bone on the presence or absence of the interproximal dental papilla. J Periodontol. 1992;63:995–886.
13. Becker W, Ochsenbein C, Tibbetts L, et al. Alveolar bone anatomic profiles as measured from dry skulls. Clinical ramifications. J Clin Periodontol. 1997;24(10):727–31.
14. Martin WC, Pollini A, Morton D. The influence of restorative procedures on esthetic outcomes in implant dentistry: a systematic review. Int J Oral Maxillofac Implants. 2014;29(Suppl):142–54.
15. Kois JC, Kan JY. Predictable per-implant gingival esthetics. Surgical and prosthodontic rationales. Pract Periodontics Aesthet Dent. 2001;13:691–8.
16. Nisapakultorn K, Suphanantachat S, Silkosessak O, Rattanamongkolgul S. Factors affecting soft tissue level around anterior maxillary single-tooth implants. Clin Oral Implants Res. 2010;21(6):662–70.
17. Chen ST, Buser D. Esthetic outcomes following immediate and early implant placement in the anterior maxilla—a systematic review. Int J Oral Maxillofac Implants. 2014;29(Suppl):186–215.
18. Agar J, Cameron SM, Hughbanks JC, Parker MH. Cement removal from restorations luted to titanium abutment with simulated subgingival margins. J Prosthet Dent. 1997;78(1):43–7.
19. Thilander B, Odman J, Jemt T. Single implants in the upper incisor region and their relationship to the adjacent teeth. An 8 year follow up study. Clin Oral Implants Res. 1999;10:346–55.
20. Esposito M, Ekestubbe A, Grondahl K. Radiological evaluation of marginal bone loss at tooth surfaces facing single Branemark implants. Clin Oral Implants Res. 1993;4(3):151–7.
21. Albrektsson T, Zarb G, Worthington P, Eriksson AR. The long term efficacy of currently used dental implants. A review and proposed criteria for success. Int J Oral Maxillofac Implants. 1986;1:11–25.
22. Pillar RM, Deporter DA, Watson PA, Valiquette N. Dental implant design. Effect on bone remodeling. J Biomed Mater Res. 1991;25:467483.
23. Cappiello M, Luongo R, Di Iorio D, Bugea C, Cocchetto R, Celletti R. Evaluation of peri-implant bone loss around platform-switched implants. Int J Periodontics Restor Dent. 2008;28:347–55.
24. Canullo L, Pellegrini G, Allievi C, Trombelli L, Annibali S, Dellavia C. Soft tissues around long-term platform switching implant restorations: a histological human evaluation. Preliminary results. J Clin Periodontol. 2011;38:86–94.
25. Abrahammson I, Berglundh T, Lindhe J. The mucosal barrier following abutment dis/reconnection: an experimental study in dogs. J Clin Periodontol. 1997;24(8):568–72.
26. Bateli M, et al. Implant neck configurations, for preservation of marginal bone level: a systematic review. Int J Oral Maxillofac Implants. 2011;26(2):290–303.
27. Palmer RM, Palmer PJ, Smith BJ. A 5 year prospective study of Astra single tooth implants. Clin Oral Implants Res. 2000;11:179–82.
28. Albrektsson T, wennerberg A. Oral implant surfaces: Part 1. Review focusing on topographic and chemical properties of different surfaces and in vivo responses to them. J Dent Res. 2006;85:496–500.
29. Wennstrom JL, Ekkestubbe A, Grondahl K, Karlsson S, Lindhe J. Oral rehabilitation with implant supported fixed partial dentures in periodontitis susceptible subjects. A 5 year prospective study. J Clin periodontol. 2004;31:713–24.
30. Ivanoff CJ, Grondahl K, Sennerby L, Bergstrom C, Lekholm U. Influence of variations in implant diameters: a 3 to 5 year retrospective clinical report. Int J Oral Maxillofac Implants. 1999;14:173–80.
31. Ding X, Zhu SH, Zhang XH, Zhang L. Effect of diameter and length on stress distribution of the alveolar crest around immediately loaded implants. Clin Implant Dent Relat Res. 2009;11:279–87.
32. Jones AA, Cochran DL. Consequences of implant design. Dent Clin North Am. 2006;50:339–60.

33. Heijdenrijk K, Raghoebar GM, Meijer HJ, Stegenga B, Van de Reiiden WA. Feasibility and influence of the microgap of two implants placed in a non-submerged procedure: a five year follow up clinical trial. J Periodontol. 2006;77:1051–60.
34. Callan DP, O'Mahoney A, Cobb CM. Loss of crestal bone around dental implants: a retrospective study. Implant Dent. 1998;7:258–66.
35. Hartman GA, Cochran DL. Initial implant position determines the magnitude of crestal bone remodeling. J Periodontol. 2004;75:572–7.
36. Lazzara RJ, Porter SS. Platform switching: a new concept in implant dentistry for controlling post-restorative crestal bone levels. Int J Periodontics Restor Dent. 2006;26(1):9–17.
37. Canullo L, Iurlaro G, Ianello G. Double blind randomized controlled trial study on post extraction immediately restored implants using the switching platform concept. Soft tissue response. Preliminary report. Clin Oral Implants Res. 2009;20(2):141–51.
38. Hurzeler M, Fickl S, Zuhr O, Wachtel H. Peri-implant bone level around implants with platform switched abutments: preliminary data from a prospective study. J Oral Maxillofac Surg. 2007;65(7):33–9.
39. Atieh MA, Ibrahim HM, Atieh AH. Platform switching for marginal bone preservation around dental implants. A systematic review and meta analysis. J Periodontol. 2010;81(10):1350–66.
40. Rodriguez-Ciurana X, Tarnow DP. The effect of interimplant distance on height of the interimplant bone crest when using platform switched implants. Int J Periodontics Restorative Dent. 2009;29(2):141–51.
41. Baffone GM, et al. Influence of various platform configurations on peri-implant tissue dimensions: an experimental study in dog. Clin Oral Implants Res. 2011;22(4):438–44.
42. Enkling N, et al. Effect of platform switching on peri-implant bone levels: a randomized clinical trial. Clin Oral Implants Res. 2011;22(10):1185–92.
43. Van Steenberghe D, et al. A prospective split mouth comparative study of two screw shaped self tapping pure titanium implant systems. Clin Oral Implants Res. 2000;11(3):202–9.
44. Jacobs R, et al. A split mouth comparative study upto 16 years of two screw shaped titanium implant systems. J Clin Periodontol. 2010;37(12):1119–27.
45. Wu DT, Raoof S, Latimer JM, Nguyen TT. Partial extraction therapy: a review of human clinical studies. J Oral Implantol. 2022;48(5):436–54.
46. Tarnow D, Elian N, Fletcher P, Froum S, Magner A, Cho SC, Salama M, Salama H, Garber DA. Vertical distance from the crest of bone to the height of the interproximal papilla between adjacent implants. J Periodontol. 2003;74(12):1785–8.
47. Salama MA, Salama H, Garber DA. Guidelines for aesthetic restorative options and implant site enhancement. Pract Proced Aesthet Dent. 2002;14:125–30.
48. Cascione D, Reshad M, Kim T. A novel approach for non-invasive pontic site development. In: Quintessence of dental technology; 2010. p. 218–23.

The Immediate Placement of Single Implants in the Aesthetic Zone

14

Gian Pietro Schincaglia

Implant-supported restorations have significantly advanced the field of dentistry, providing predictable and durable treatment options for patients from edentulous jaws to single-tooth deficiencies. In the case of single-tooth implant restorations, treatment planning in aesthetic areas requires meticulous attention to detail to achieve optimal outcomes. While successful osseointegration remains a primary objective, modern implant therapy places equal emphasis on integrating the implant-supported restoration seamlessly into the surrounding soft and hard tissues, ensuring a harmonious and natural appearance.

This chapter aims to explore the intricate aspects of surgical treatment planning for immediate single-tooth implant restorations in aesthetic areas. By considering a range of factors, including pre-surgical determinants, surgical procedures, and treatment sequencing, clinicians can optimize the aesthetic results and obtain patient satisfaction. Additionally, we will introduce a comprehensive surgical protocol designed to assist practitioners in navigating the complexities associated with achieving predictable and aesthetically pleasing outcomes in single-tooth implant restorations.

By delving into the nuances of treatment planning and surgical techniques, this chapter presents a goal to equip clinicians with the knowledge and tools necessary to overcome the challenges inherent in immediate single-tooth implant restorations in aesthetic areas. By adhering to a systematic approach and understanding the interplay between many variables, an outcome both functional and aesthetic will please both the recipient and provider of the implant-supported restoration.

G. P. Schincaglia (✉)
Dept. of Periodontics, School of Dental Medicine, Case Western Reserve University, Cleveland, OH, USA

W. Chee, S. Jivraj (eds.), *Treatment Planning In Implant Dentistry*, BDJ Clinician's Guides, https://doi.org/10.1007/978-3-031-68726-6_14

14.1 Pre-surgical Evaluation of the Implant Site

Implant-site evaluation in aesthetic areas requires careful consideration of several determinants, to include the following:

14.1.1 The Smile Line

The position of the smile line is an important consideration in the aesthetic zone; the exposure of amount of tooth surface and gingival tissue that is visible during speech and full smiling is influenced by the tonus of the orofacial muscles that control the movement of the upper lip and the lip length [1, 2]. On average, a smile reveals approximately 75–100% of the maxillary incisors and interproximal gingiva [1]. However, the smile line can vary. A high smile line refers to a smile where gingival tissue apical to the tooth is exposed. In this situation, implant-supported single-tooth restorations in the aesthetic area can pose significant challenges. The restoration and surrounding gingival tissue will be prominently displayed, making it crucial to flawlessly reconstruct the soft tissue contour, colour and shape of the restoration to achieve pleasing aesthetics. The high smile line requires meticulous attention to detail to create a natural-appearing outcome.

Conversely, a low smile line is characterized by the display of less than 75% of the maxillary teeth. In this situation, the implant-restoration interface will be concealed behind the upper lip. While still important, the low smile line poses a less critical challenge for the implant-restoration interface in terms of aesthetics, as it remains largely hidden from direct view.

Determining the position of the lip during a full smile is essential when planning implant-supported single-tooth restorations in the aesthetic area. It guides the decision-making process regarding the design and reconstruction of the restoration, particularly in cases where the smile line is high and demands meticulous attention to achieve optimal aesthetic outcomes. Despite the display of hard and soft tissue that is discussed above where exposure of the "aesthetic" zone is important, there will be a number of patients who might manually lift their lips to expose the entire area of the hard and soft tissues, and clinicians should be aware of the patients' expectations and proceed accordingly.

14.1.2 Soft Tissue Morphology

The position of the gingival tissue around a tooth is determined by the connective tissue attachment levels and by the bone levels. The zenith of the gingival margin of the central incisor and canines should be at the same levels, whereas the gingival margin of the lateral incisors should be 0.5 mm more coronal. Three different periodontal phenotypes have been described in relation to the morphology of the tooth and the thickness of the buccal soft tissue [3]: slender teeth with thin gingival tissue

(A1 phenotype), slender teeth with thick gingival tissue (A2 phenotype) and squared teeth with thick tissue (B phenotype).

The A1 and A2 phenotypes are characterized by scalloped gingival tissue and long interdental papillae. The B phenotype is characterized by a flat morphology and short and wide papillae [3].

In health, the interdental papilla fills the embrasure space to the apical extent of the contact area. Periodontal disease or surgical trauma may lead to attachment loss or bone loss. The thin and scalloped periodontium has the tendency to develop recession following periodontal inflammation. The thick periodontal phenotype is relatively resistant to surgical trauma and recession, and the presence of periodontal infection leads most likely to pocket formation [4, 5].

The recession of the interproximal soft tissue creates an empty space in the interdental area which is referred to as the "black triangle". The loss of the interproximal soft tissue on teeth appears to correlate with the distance between the contact area of the adjacent teeth and the bony crest in the interproximal area [6]. For a distance equal to or less than 5 mm, the interdental papilla is always present. For 6 mm and 7 mm or more, the interdental papilla fills the interproximal space 56% and 27% of the time, respectively [6].

The biological parameters determining the soft tissue position at the proximal site between a tooth and an implant have been investigated [7, 8] indicating a similar response as observed on teeth. Hence, the level of papilla adjacent to a single implant is influenced by the periodontal attachment on the adjacent tooth [7].

The buccal soft tissue contour is an important factor toward the natural appearance of the restoration. The presence of buccal gingival recession on the tooth that needs to be immediately replaced by the implant will prevent optimal soft tissue contour after healing.

14.1.3 Tooth Morphology

As previously mentioned, tooth morphology is closely associated with the periodontal phenotype. Three tooth shapes have been described [9]: slender teeth with rectangular shapes, slender teeth with triangular shapes and squared teeth. The triangular tooth shape represents the most challenging condition since the contact area is in the coronal third of the interproximal space. When interproximal soft tissue loss occurs following surgical manipulation, triangle-shaped teeth tend to exhibit wider black triangles compared to situations where squared teeth are present. The tooth morphology can be modified in the restoration design, to compensate for partial interproximal tissue loss. This is obtained by displacing the contact area in a more apical location. However, in the case of single-tooth restorations, these modifications with triangular teeth often require altering the shape of the teeth adjacent to the restored site [10].

Conversely, squared/rectangular tooth shapes are commonly associated with the contact area positioned at the middle third of the crown presenting a shorter papilla occupying a smaller volume, making it easier to compensate for the loss of interdental tissue by modifying the position of the interproximal contact area [10].

The maxillary central incisor typically measures around 7–8 mm mesiodistally and 6 mm bucco-palatally at its emergence from the soft tissue [11]. For a natural profile, a standard 3.75/4-mm-diameter implant should be placed approximately 3–4 mm apical to the buccal soft tissue level of the adjacent teeth [12, 13]. This positioning allows for a smooth transition from the 4 mm diameter of the implant platform to the 7–8 mm dimension of the crown at the gingival margin. If a platform-switching implant design is used, it would require more space for the transition and a more apical placement of the platform. In the case of a maxillary lateral incisor replacement, less apical positioning is needed since the average crown diameter at the gingival level is 5 mm, necessitating less space for the transition.

A surgical guide, created based on the diagnostic wax-up, is utilized to verify the implant position during placement. The guide replicates the emergence profile and shape of the restoration, aiding in accurate implant placement.

14.1.4 The Bone Morphology

The housing of a 3.5–4-mm-diameter implant requires about 7–8 mm of bone in a buccolingual dimension and 7 mm in a mesiodistal dimension [14–16].

The bony architecture of the alveolar bone has been described by Becker et al. [17]. Three types of alveolar configurations were identified: flat, scalloped and pronounced scalloped based on the vertical distance from the interproximal septum and the buccal contour of the alveolar crest of the socket. This distance ranged from 2.1 mm for the flat configuration to 4.1 mm observed in the pronounced scalloped anatomy [17]. In addition, a higher prevalence of fenestration and dehiscence was observed in the pronounced scalloped anatomic profile. A correlation between alveolar bone thickness and soft tissue thickness in the maxillary anterior teeth was reported by Cook et al. [18]. The presence of a thick tissue phenotype and width of keratinized gingiva seemed to be directly correlated with thicker underlying alveolar bone [19].

Periodontal disease, endodontic infection and bone modelling processes after tooth extraction may reduce the bone volume available for implant placement.

Limitations in bone quantity in the mesiodistal dimension may be due to the root position of the adjacent teeth. Orthodontic movement should be used to alter the root position to provide the space for implant insertion. A reduced horizontal distance between the tooth and the neighbouring implant may adversely affect the bone level at the tooth surface [16]. A minimum of 1.5 mm of bone between the implant surface and the root surface should be present [16]. The bone volume at the implant site is measured on cone beam computed tomography (CBCT) scans taken with a radiographic template or merged with a virtual wax-up on planning software representing the position and shape of the final restoration.

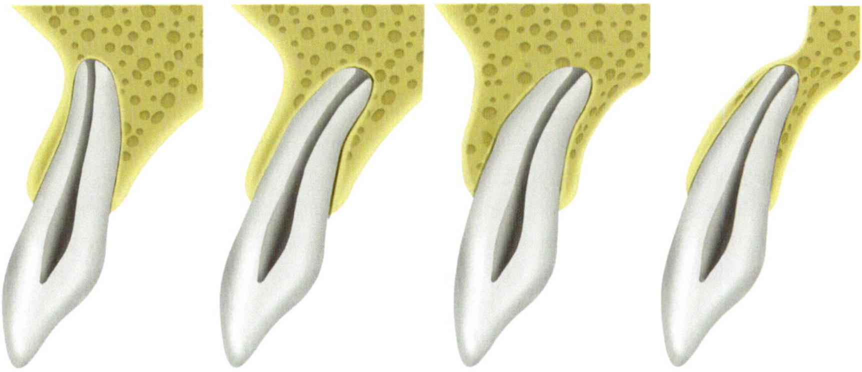

Fig. 14.1 Classification of sagittal root position [20]. Class I is present in 80% of the cases and represents the most favourable anatomical condition for immediate implant placement

14.1.5 Sagittal Root Position

The anatomy of the socket is a critical factor in the immediate implant placement endeavour. A recent classification of the sagittal root position has been proposed for the maxillary anterior teeth (Fig. 14.1) [20]. The class I position refers to the most frequent configuration (81% of the cases), and it is characterized by a buccal orientation of the root and the presence of bone within the palatal wall of the socket. In this condition, the palatal bone volume allows for the housing of the implant. The class II position is described by a centred position of the root in the alveolar housing with even distribution of bone thickness buccally and palatally. This condition is represented in about 6% of the cases and allows for immediate implant placement along the socket orientation only if at least 5 mm of bone is present apically to the socket. In class III, the root housing is oriented toward the palatal aspect of the ridge; this condition is represented by <1% of the cases and allows for immediate implant placement if 5 mm of bone is available apical to the socket. Class IV is described with a centred position of the root in the alveolar ridge with a minimal amount of bone lining the socket. This is considered the least favourable socket anatomy for immediate implant placement, and it has been described in 12% of the sites.

14.2 Immediate Implant Placement

14.2.1 Rationale and Treatment Considerations

Traditionally, a waiting period of 3–6 months between tooth extraction and implant placement has been recommended as the standard protocol [21]. However, delaying implant placement after the healing of the socket can result in advanced resorption of the alveolar crest, leading to a tapering defect that lacks adequate volume for the housing of the implant. Prolonged functional stimulation interruption following tooth extraction may further contribute to a reduction in osseous trabecular pattern and capillary density [22, 23]. The most significant amount of resorption occurs within the first year post-extraction, with 50% of the lost volume observed in the initial 3 months, particularly in the mandible's sagittal plane and more in the buccal and horizontal direction in the maxilla [23, 24].

To counteract the impact of bone modelling at the extraction site, the concept of immediate implant placement into fresh extraction sockets has been introduced [25]. Although the latest studies have shown that immediate placement of implants does not prevent socket bone modelling [26–28], numerous clinical studies and systematic reviews have confirmed survival rates of immediately placed implants comparable to the success rates of implants placed in healed sites [29].

14.2.1.1 Advantages of Immediate Implant Placement

- Reduced treatment time: The restorative procedures can start as early as immediately at the time of placement to 2 months after tooth extraction.
- Improved soft tissue support: Immediate placement in combination with immediate provisional or customized healing abutments has shown improved soft tissue healing in the case of thick phenotype.

14.2.1.2 Indications

Indications include a failing tooth due to trauma without bone loss, endodontic lesion, root fracture, and extensive caries; adequate bone support for implant stabilization; and intact soft tissue morphology for aesthetics.

14.2.1.3 Contraindications

Contraindications include:

- Active infection fistulous track and suppuration
- Extensive osseous defects or unfavourable socket anatomy preventing the insertion of the implant in an optimal position or the achievement of implant stability
- Extensive soft tissue defect so that an aesthetic outcome cannot be anticipated

14.2.2 The Immediate Implant Site in the Aesthetic Zone

Not all sites that require tooth extraction in the aesthetic zone are suitable for immediate implant placement, and various clinical classifications have been proposed to aid in site selection [12, 30–32]. A previously published clinical classification from our group includes the treatment algorithm that should be implemented in different conditions [12, 32].

When planning for surgical treatment of an implant placed into an extraction site in aesthetic areas, the previously discussed pre-surgical parameters need to be carefully considered:

14.2.3 Immediate Implant-Site Classification and Treatment Algorithms

14.2.3.1 Type I Immediate Implant Site

The only clinical condition that allows for immediate placement in the aesthetic zone is represented by the site described as type I.

The type I immediate implant site is characterized by ideal soft tissue morphology, with intact interproximal papillae, and an ideal position of the mid-buccal gingival margin (Fig. 14.2a). The bone configuration displays intact bone support in the coronal aspect of the root. Upon CBCT scan evaluation, the palatal thickness of the socket wall is ≥3 mm when evaluated 3–5 mm apical to the buccal gingival zenith (Fig. 14.2b). This condition is consistent with a class I sagittal root position according to Kan et al. [20]. Class II and III sagittal positions can also be included, provided that a 5 mm of bone apical to the socket is available for implant housing. Another important element that defines the type I immediate implant site is the presence of the buccal wall of the socket. The average thickness of the buccal wall of the socket in the maxillary anterior teeth is reported to range between 0.6 and 0.8 mm [33]. However, there are limitations on the accuracy of the CBCT scan image in detecting the presence of the buccal wall if the thickness is less than 0.4 mm [27]. Hence, in the presence of a buccal wall thickness <0.5 mm, the final decision to perform an immediate implant placement may occur at the time of extraction. A thin buccal bony wall is usually associated with a thin and scalloped bone morphology [17]. Immediate placement of implants in extraction sockets of thin phenotype has been related to a higher risk of mid-buccal gingival recessions [34, 35].

14.2.4 Treatment Sequence for Immediate Implant Placement in the Aesthetic Zone

Restorative Planning The very first step in the planning process is to develop a diagnostic wax-up of the tooth to be replaced. If the natural crown of the tooth is still present, it can be used to design the final crown. If tooth shape modifications are needed, they should be incorporated at this stage.

A surgical guide is developed based on the diagnostic wax-up. The surgical guide can be analogic or computer generated depending on whether a free hand or a navigation approach is used.

Minimally Traumatic Extraction The minimally traumatic removal of the tooth is critical to prevent damage to the socket walls. Several approaches have been described in the literature. The use of a small sharp periotome is recommended. In the presence of difficult root anatomies, root separation with a thin fissure bur should be performed. Luxation of the tooth with bucco-palatal movements using forceps should be avoided.

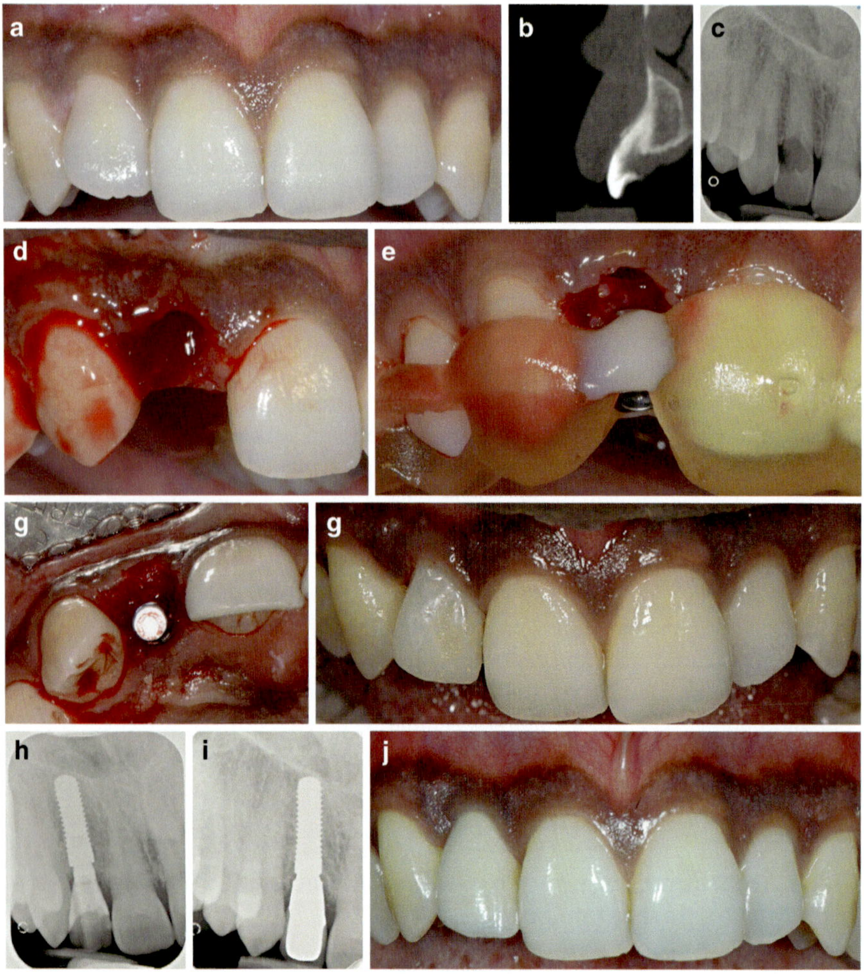

Fig. 14.2 Type I immediate implant site. Tooth #7 presents internal/external root resorption and requires extraction (**b**, **c**). Soft and hard tissue conditions present an ideal configuration for immediate placement (**a**, **b**). Flapless extraction is performed (**d**), and the implant is placed using a computer-generated guide (**e**, **f**), followed by immediate provisional (**g**, **h**). The final restoration shows adequate soft tissue and hard tissue morphology surrounding the implant (**i**, **j**). (Surgery by Dr. Simpson—Resident in Periodontics WVU-School of Dentistry, Restoration by Dr. Chertok Resident in Prosthodontics WVU-School of Dentistry)

Once the root is removed, the socket is inspected for the integrity of the buccal wall (Fig. 14.2d). Partial extraction technique, also known as the "socket shield" technique, has been proposed in the literature [36]. The rationale for the partial extraction is to retain the buccal fragment of the root together with the PDL to reduce post-extraction bone modelling [37, 38]. Recent systematic reviews and meta-analyses indicated improved clinical parameters in the short term when implants were placed with socket shields compared to full extraction sockets [39].

However limited information is available for long-term results [39]. It is the opinion of the authors that this approach should be used with caution since the clinical predictability and long-term results are still warranted.

Osteotomy Preparation and Implant Position The position of the implant in the extraction socket is critical for the short- and long-term success of the immediate placement approach. The osteotomy direction should satisfy vertical, mesiodistal and buccolingual positioning criteria.

The vertical position of the implant platform should be 3–5 mm apical from the gingival zenith of the adjacent or contralateral tooth. The deepest vertical position should be reserved for a more palatal location of the buccal rim of the implant platform. The vertical position of the platform directly influences the angle of emergence of the crown. Recent data recommend an emergence angle of the crown less than 30° to reduce the risk of peri-implantitis [40]. Hence, the vertical placement of the implant platform should be based on the buccal emergence profile of the crown. The platform position should also consider the buccal crestal margin of the socket. Clinical studies [28, 41] indicated that the optimal vertical placement of the platform should be 1 mm apical to the buccal bony crest and 2 mm horizontal from the buccal wall of the socket.

The mesiodistal position of the platform should be >1.5 mm from the adjacent teeth. A closer position of the implant shoulder to the adjacent teeth can induce bone resorption on the tooth and affect the final height of the interdental papilla between the implant crown and tooth [16].

The buccolingual angulation is determined by the buccolingual anatomy of the socket and the position of the crown. Ideally, the long axis of the implant should fall inside the projection of the crown's cingulum if a screw-retained restoration is planned (Fig. 14.3a). This is not always possible in the case of a proclined premaxillary ridge profile [42]. In these conditions, it has been suggested to aim at the incisal edge of the crown instead of the cingulum; this will increase the distance of the implant apex from the buccal wall of the socket and allow engaging more apical bone and improving the emergence angle of the crown (Fig. 14.3b). If immediate loading is attempted, the apical extension of the osteotomy should engage 5 mm of native bone for good primary stability. The implant-screw access located on the incisal edge of the crown does not preclude the fabrication of a screw-retained restoration. Angled screw-channel components permit the creation of screw-retained restorations with up to 25° of angle between the crown and the implant axis [42, 43]. In addition, recent studies from our group showed similar mechanical performance of angled screws when compared to straight abutment screws [44].

Flapless vs. Flap Choosing between a flapless approach and raising a flap during implant surgery may be based on the clinical condition and bone quality. Flapless surgery is less invasive but requires precise planning while raising a flap might allow for better visualization and access (Fig. 14.2f, g). Although the use of flapless implant placement should reduce the amount of bone modelling since it prevents

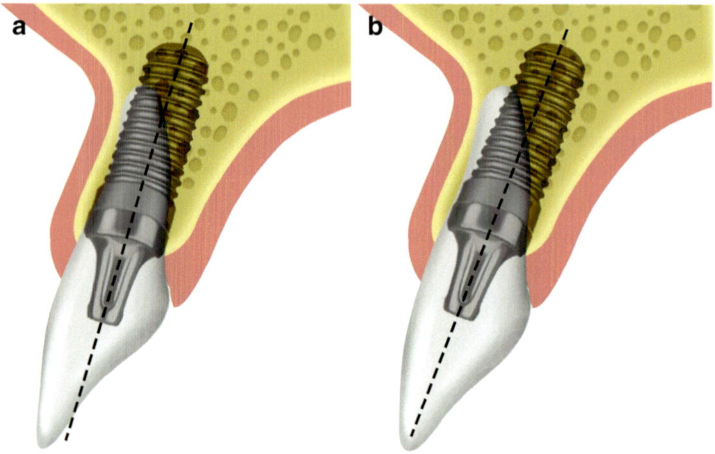

Fig. 14.3 Sagittal implant angulation within the projection of the cingulum of the tooth (**a**) for a screw-retained crown. With this position, the restoration presents a wider angle of emergence, and the apical section of the implant is close to the buccal plate. If an angled screw channel abutment is used, the implant can be oriented toward the incisal edge of the crown (**b**). This position improves the implant bone anchorage and allows for a reduced angle of emergence of the restoration

disruption of the blood supply, clinical research data were unable to show clinically significant advantages of flapless versus flap procedures [45].

Grafting the Gap vs. No Grafting Deciding whether to graft the gap between the implant and the socket wall is often based on the size of the gap and the thickness of the buccal bone. Recent systematic reviews suggested a moderate improvement of soft and hard tissue volume when the graft is used [46].

Clinical studies indicate a higher amount of vertical loss of crestal bone observed in the presence of a thin buccal crest and narrow (<1 mm) gap [28]. However, the least amount of vertical resorption of the crest and greater filling of the gap were observed with a larger gap (>1 mm) and thick buccal socket wall [28]. Grafting the gap may be recommended in case of a thin buccal bony wall despite the dimension of the gap. In the presence of a thick buccal wall of the socket (>1 mm), grafting the gap may not be necessary [28].

Connective Tissue Graft The use of an autogenous connective tissue graft at the time of immediate implant placement has been proposed to improve aesthetic results. Systematic reviews and meta-analysis data indicate that this may be a consideration in cases with thin phenotype to improve soft tissue volume and quality [47]. In addition, increasing the peri-implant connective tissue thickness using connective tissue grafting may be indicated to mitigate gingival discoloration due to the transparency of the restorative material [48].

Immediate Provisional vs. Delayed Restoration Deciding between placing a provisional crown immediately and delaying the restoration can be based on factors such as the primary stability of the implant, the patient's occlusion and aesthetic demands. The clinical data indicates a 3.2 times higher risk of complications when immediate placement and loading are used on a single-tooth replacement in comparison to a one-stage approach [49].

However, the use of an immediate provisional has shown a better restorative outcome with 2.5 times less mid-facial recession when compared to a delayed loading [50] (Fig. 14.2g, i).

14.2.4.1 Type II Immediate Implant Site

A type II immediate implant site entails a soft tissue dehiscence or partial collapse of the interproximal soft tissue. The buccal wall is partially or totally resorbed. The palatal wall of the socket measures >3 mm in the buccolingual dimension at a depth of >5 mm from the soft tissue level [12, 32]. These features can also be combined with active infection due to root/tooth damage. This type of condition prevents the immediate insertion of the implant in the correct restorative position (Fig. 14.4a, b).

The treatment options available to address these cases are (1) orthodontic implant site development (OISD) [51] followed by immediate placement or (2) immediate delayed (early) approach [52] in combination with GBR and soft tissue grafting.

The orthodontic forced eruption has been largely discussed in the literature for the treatment of intra-bony defects, crown lengthening and implant-site development [53–55]. With this procedure, a tooth is deliberately moved in the coronal direction, using orthodontic appliances. This movement stretches the gingival fibre apparatus, creating tension across the osseous housing of the tooth. Such tension stimulates bone formation at the alveolar crest, as well as coronal migration of soft tissue expanding the zone of the gingiva. Amato et al. [51] reported an average gain of vertical bone and gingival height of 4 mm and 3.8 mm, respectively, in combination with a coronal tooth displacement of 6 mm. It is noteworthy that this technique is contraindicated in cases where active infection is present. Hence, the future implant site can be corrected using OISD from a type II to a type I site, using tooth movement.

Once the osseous crest has been satisfactorily repositioned and the soft tissue profile has been restored, the tooth extraction is performed. Subsequently, the dental implant is placed following the criteria described for type I immediate implant sites.

In the situation of a type II site with active infection, OISD cannot be applied. These cases can be treated using a delayed-immediate or early implant placement (Fig. 14.4). This approach was originally proposed by Grunder et al. [56] and consists of extraction of the damaged tooth; after 4–8 weeks of healing, the implant is placed in conjunction with GBR with grafting to correct the hard and soft tissue deficiencies. The 4–8-week healing period allows for the clearance of the infection, and the tissue obtained from the healing of the socket can be used for protecting the barrier/graft during GBR, thus reducing the risk of membrane exposure and graft exfoliation [52, 56]. This approach has limitations if vertical tissue augmentation is

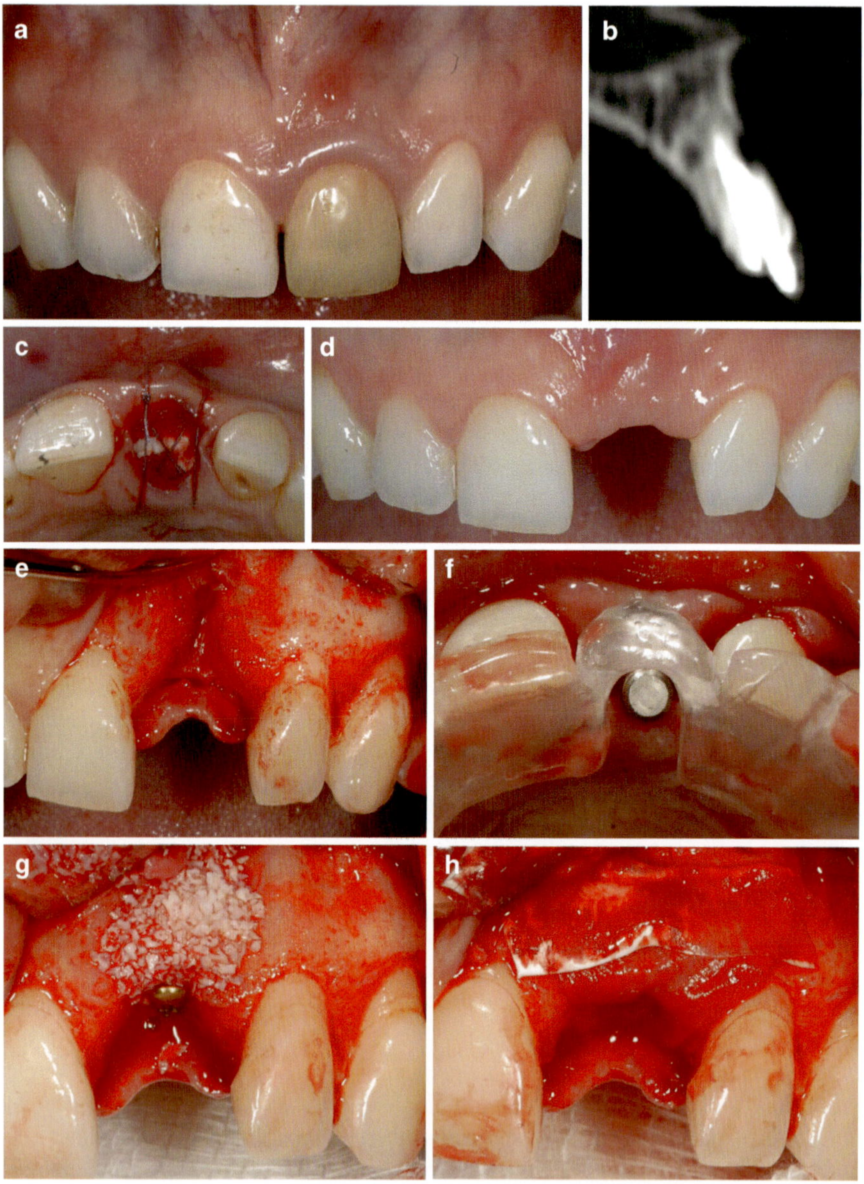

Fig. 14.4 Type II immediate implant site. Tooth #9 presents a root perforation with sinus track and resorption of the buccal plate (**a**, **b**). An early (delayed immediate) implant placement approach is planned. The tooth is extracted, and the socket is dressed with a collagen sponge (**c**). Four weeks later, the implant is placed in combination with guided bone regeneration (GBR) using a resorbable membrane and deproteinized bovine bone allograft (**d**–**h**). The implant uncovering is performed after 4 months of submerged healing. A subepithelial connective tissue graft is placed on the buccal aspect of the implant, and a provisional crown is inserted at the time of uncovering (**i**, **j**). The provisional crown is used to shape the soft tissue contour (**k**), and the permanent restoration can be finalized (**l**). (Restoration by Dr. G. Franceschetti)

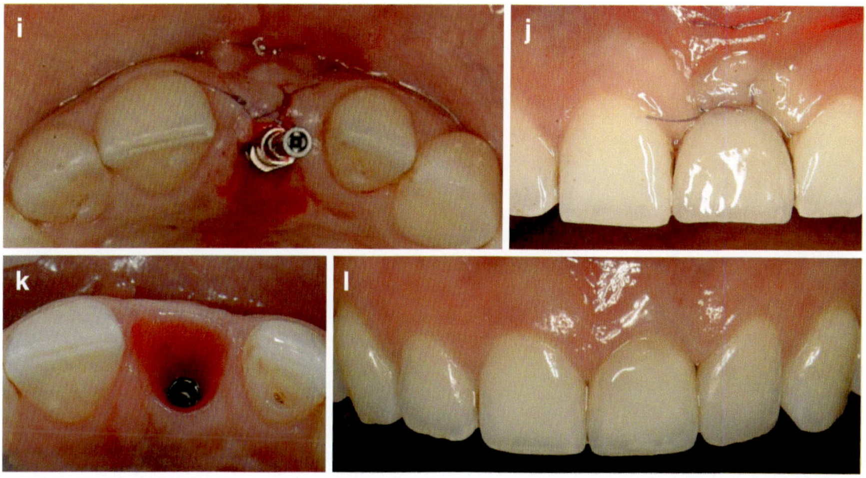

Fig. 14.4 (continued)

needed. The final vertical position of the soft and hard tissue is strictly dependent on the coronal position of the soft tissue after the extraction. If the amount of bone after the extraction is considered not sufficient for a correct vertical position of the implant, the site should be considered as type III (see below).

Practitioners must exercise caution utilizing GBR at the time of extraction and immediate implant placement due to the higher chance of complications [52]. These complications may include membrane exposure, dehiscence of soft and hard tissues or even loss of the implant. It is crucial for clinicians to weigh the potential risks and benefits before deciding on the appropriate approach to address the complexities of a type II immediate implant site.

14.2.4.2 Type III Immediate Implant Site

A type III immediate implant site entails deep soft tissue collapse (>4 mm) either buccal or interproximal, absence of the buccal wall of the socket or presence of extended periapical or periodontal lesions. OISD cannot be performed predictably. The palatal wall measures <3 mm in thickness (Class IV Kan), and the residual bone is insufficient to insert the implant with simultaneous GBR (Fig. 14.5a–c).

In this clinical situation, implant placement requires a staged approach. The treatment sequence requires extraction of the tooth followed by bone grafting procedures as well as soft tissue augmentation procedures. Hard and soft tissue grafting procedures should be performed before implant placement (Fig. 14.5d–g). Optimal aesthetic results cannot be anticipated (Fig. 14.6).

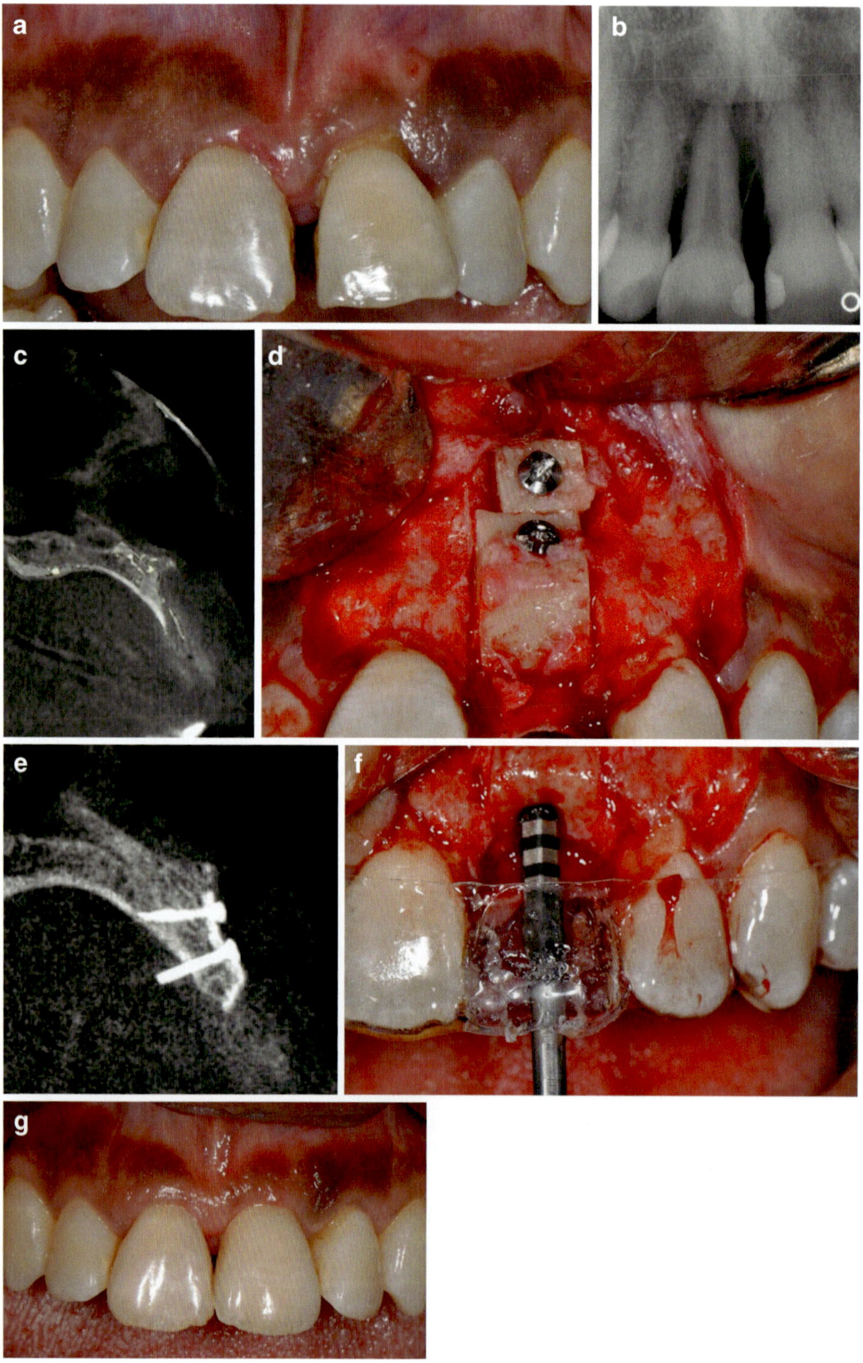

Fig. 14.5 Type III immediate implant site. Tooth #9 is exfoliating with class III mobility and circumferential PD ranging from 8 to 11 mm (**a**, **b**). The residual defect shows vertical and horizontal bone deficiency, and a staged approach is indicated (**c**). A block graft from the mandible is used to rebuild the alveolar ridge (**d**–**e**). After 3–4 months of graft healing, the implant is placed in a submerged fashion (**f**). The final crown is delivered after 12 weeks of healing (**g**). (Restoration by Dr. A. Dingra)

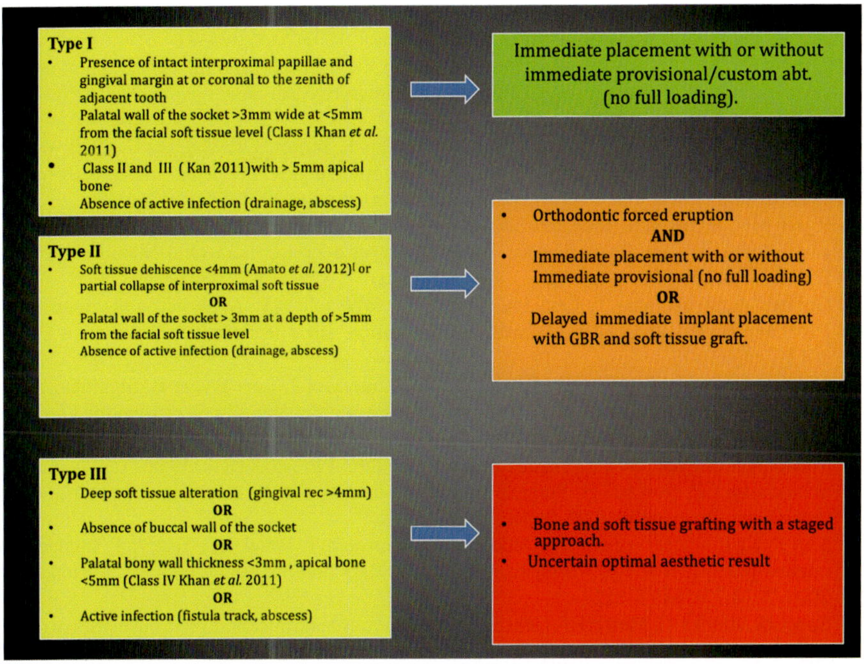

Fig. 14.6 Treatment algorithms for immediate implant sites in the aesthetic zone

14.3 Conclusion

Prosthodontic and surgical treatment planning is essential in the decision-making process about the immediate placement of a dental implant in the aesthetic zone. Proper positioning of the implant and creation of an ideal soft tissue environment surrounding the restoration are critical for achieving long-term success.

Pre-surgical factors have been discussed to address the planning, based on the implant site condition and the morphology of the soft and hard tissues, hence to guide the treatment pathway toward a predictable aesthetic result.

To summarize, achieving aesthetic outcomes in the immediate replacement of an anterior tooth requires thorough prosthodontic and surgical treatment planning. By considering patient expectations and morphology of the surrounding tissues, satisfactory aesthetic results can be achieved.

References

1. Tjan AH, Miller GD, The JG. Some esthetic factors in a smile. J Prosthet Dent. 1984;51(1):24–8.
2. Vig RG, Brundo GC. The kinetics of anterior tooth display. J Prosthet Dent. 1978;39(5):502–4.
3. De Rouck T, Eghbali R, Collys K, De Bruyn H, Cosyn J. The gingival biotype revisited: transparency of the periodontal probe through the gingival margin as a method to discriminate thin from thick gingiva. J Clin Periodontol. 2009;36(5):428–33.
4. Olsson M, Lindhe J. Periodontal characteristics in individuals with varying form of the upper central incisors. J Clin Periodontol. 1991;18(1):78–82.

5. Olsson M, Lindhe J, Marinello CP. On the relationship between crown form and clinical features of the gingiva in adolescents. J Clin Periodontol. 1993;20(8):570–7.
6. Tarnow DP, Magner AW, Fletcher P. The effect of the distance from the contact point to the crest of bone on the presence or absence of the interproximal dental papilla. J Periodontol. 1992;63(12):995–6.
7. Choquet V, Hermans M, Adriaenssens P, Daelemans P, Tarnow DP, Malevez C. Clinical and radiographic evaluation of the papilla level adjacent to single-tooth dental implants. A retrospective study in the maxillary anterior region. J Periodontol. 2001;72(10):1364–71.
8. Ryser MR, Block MS, Mercante DE. Correlation of papilla to crestal bone levels around single tooth implants in immediate or delayed crown protocols. J Oral Maxillofac Surg. 2005;63(8):1184–95.
9. Gobbato L, Tsukiyama T, Levi PA, Griffin TJ, Weisgold AS. Analysis of the shapes of maxillary central incisors in a Caucasian population. Int J Periodontics Restorative Dent. 2012;32(1):69–78.
10. Gobbato L, Paniz G, Mazzocco F, Chierico A, Tsukiyama T, Levi PA, et al. Significance of crown shape in the replacement of a central incisor with a single implant-supported crown. Quintessence Int. 2013;44(5):407–13.
11. Weeler R. Complete crown form and the periodontium. J Prosthet Dent. 1958;11:722–34.
12. Schincaglia GP, Nowzari H. Surgical treatment planning for the single-unit implant in aesthetic areas. Periodontol 2000. 2001;27:162–82.
13. Kan JYK, Rungcharassaeng K, Deflorian M, Weinstein T, Wang HL, Testori T. Immediate implant placement and provisionalization of maxillary anterior single implants. Periodontol 2000. 2018;77(1):197–212.
14. Spray JR, Black CG, Morris HF, Ochi S. The influence of bone thickness on facial marginal bone response: stage 1 placement through stage 2 uncovering. Ann Periodontol. 2000;5(1):119–28.
15. Grunder U, Gracis S, Capelli M. Influence of the 3-D bone-to-implant relationship on esthetics. Int J Periodontics Restorative Dent. 2005;25(2):113–9.
16. Esposito M, Ekestubbe A, Gröndahl K. Radiological evaluation of marginal bone loss at tooth surfaces facing single Brånemark implants. Clin Oral Implants Res. 1993;4(3):151–7.
17. Becker W, Ochsenbein C, Tibbetts L, Becker BE. Alveolar bone anatomic profiles as measured from dry skulls. Clinical ramifications. J Clin Periodontol. 1997;24(10):727–31.
18. Cook DR, Mealey BL, Verrett RG, Mills MP, Noujeim ME, Lasho DJ, et al. Relationship between clinical periodontal biotype and labial plate thickness: an in vivo study. Int J Periodontics Restorative Dent. 2011;31(4):345–54.
19. Zweers J, Thomas RZ, Slot DE, Weisgold AS, Van der Weijden FG. Characteristics of periodontal biotype, its dimensions, associations and prevalence: a systematic review. J Clin Periodontol. 2014;41(10):958–71.
20. Kan JY, Roe P, Rungcharassaeng K, Patel RD, Waki T, Lozada JL, et al. Classification of sagittal root position in relation to the anterior maxillary osseous housing for immediate implant placement: a cone beam computed tomography study. Int J Oral Maxillofac Implants. 2011;26(4):873–6.
21. Branemark PI, Adell R, Albrektsson T, Lekholm U, Lundkvist S, Rockler B. Osseointegrated titanium fixtures in the treatment of edentulousness. Biomaterials. 1983;4(1):25–8.
22. Carlsson GE, Thilander H, Hedegård B. Histologic changes in the upper alveolar process after extractions with or without insertion of an immediate full denture. Acta Odontol Scand. 1967;25(1):21–43.
23. Schropp L, Wenzel A, Kostopoulos L, Karring T. Bone healing and soft tissue contour changes following single-tooth extraction: a clinical and radiographic 12-month prospective study. Int J Periodontics Restorative Dent. 2003;23(4):313–23.
24. Tallgren A. The continuing reduction of the residual alveolar ridges in complete denture wearers: a mixed-longitudinal study covering 25 years. 1972. J Prosthet Dent. 2003;89(5):427–35.
25. Lazzara RJ. Immediate implant placement into extraction sites: surgical and restorative advantages. Int J Periodontics Restorative Dent. 1989;9(5):332–43.

26. Araújo MG, Sukekava F, Wennström JL, Lindhe J. Tissue modeling following implant placement in fresh extraction sockets. Clin Oral Implants Res. 2006;17(6):615–24.
27. Sanz M, Cecchinato D, Ferrus J, Pjetursson EB, Lang NP, Lindhe J. A prospective, randomized-controlled clinical trial to evaluate bone preservation using implants with different geometry placed into extraction sockets in the maxilla. Clin Oral Implants Res. 2010;21(1):13–21.
28. Tomasi C, Sanz M, Cecchinato D, Pjetursson B, Ferrus J, Lang NP, et al. Bone dimensional variations at implants placed in fresh extraction sockets: a multilevel multivariate analysis. Clin Oral Implants Res. 2010;21(1):30–6.
29. Esposito M, Grusovin MG, Polyzos IP, Felice P, Worthington HV. Timing of implant placement after tooth extraction: immediate, immediate-delayed or delayed implants? A Cochrane systematic review. Eur J Oral Implantol. 2010;3(3):189–205.
30. Hämmerle CH, Chen ST, Wilson TG. Consensus statements and recommended clinical procedures regarding the placement of implants in extraction sockets. Int J Oral Maxillofac Implants. 2004;19(Suppl):26–8.
31. Juodzbalys G, Sakavicius D, Wang HL. Classification of extraction sockets based upon soft and hard tissue components. J Periodontol. 2008;79(3):413–24.
32. Furtado Araújo MV, Sommerville D, Dhingra A, Schincaglia GP. Immediate placement and restoration of an implant in an infected socket in the esthetic zone. Clin Adv Periodontics. 2015;5(2):83–9.
33. Huynh-Ba G, Pjetursson BE, Sanz M, Cecchinato D, Ferrus J, Lindhe J, et al. Analysis of the socket bone wall dimensions in the upper maxilla in relation to immediate implant placement. Clin Oral Implants Res. 2010;21(1):37–42.
34. Evans CD, Chen ST. Esthetic outcomes of immediate implant placements. Clin Oral Implants Res. 2008;19(1):73–80.
35. Chen ST, Wilson TG, Hämmerle CH. Immediate or early placement of implants following tooth extraction: review of biologic basis, clinical procedures, and outcomes. Int J Oral Maxillofac Implants. 2004;19(Suppl):12–25.
36. Hürzeler MB, Zuhr O, Schupbach P, Rebele SF, Emmanouilidis N, Fickl S. The socket-shield technique: a proof-of-principle report. J Clin Periodontol. 2010;37(9):855–62.
37. Bäumer D, Zuhr O, Rebele S, Schneider D, Schupbach P, Hürzeler M. The socket-shield technique: first histological, clinical, and volumetrical observations after separation of the buccal tooth segment—a pilot study. Clin Implant Dent Relat Res. 2015;17(1):71–82.
38. Bäumer D, Zuhr O, Rebele S, Hürzeler M. Socket shield technique for immediate implant placement—clinical, radiographic and volumetric data after 5 years. Clin Oral Implants Res. 2017;28(11):1450–8.
39. Atieh MA, Shah M, Abdulkareem M, AlQahtani HA, Alsabeeha NHM. The socket shield technique for immediate implant placement: a systematic review and meta-analysis. J Esthet Restor Dent. 2021;33(8):1186–200.
40. Soulami S, Slot DE, van der Weijden F. Implant-abutment emergence angle and profile in relation to peri-implantitis: a systematic review. Clin Exp Dent Res. 2022;8(4):795–806.
41. Ferrus J, Cecchinato D, Pjetursson EB, Lang NP, Sanz M, Lindhe J. Factors influencing ridge alterations following immediate implant placement into extraction sockets. Clin Oral Implants Res. 2010;21(1):22–9.
42. Kan JYK, Rungcharassaeng K, Kamolroongwarakul P, Lin GH, Matsuda H, Yin S, et al. Frequency of screw-retained angulated screw channel single crown following immediate implant placement and provisionalization in the esthetic zone: a cone beam computed tomography study. Clin Implant Dent Relat Res. 2023;25:789.
43. Berroeta E, Zabalegui I, Donovan T, Chee W. Dynamic abutment: a method of redirecting screw access for implant-supported restorations: technical details and a clinical report. J Prosthet Dent. 2015;113(6):516–9.
44. Goldberg J, Lee T, Phark JH, Chee W. Removal torque and force to failure of non-axially tightened implant abutment screws. J Prosthet Dent. 2019;121(2):322–6.

45. Esposito M, Maghaireh H, Grusovin MG, Ziounas I, Worthington HV. Interventions for replacing missing teeth: management of soft tissues for dental implants. Cochrane Database Syst Rev. 2012;2012(2):CD006697.
46. Seyssens L, Eeckhout C, Cosyn J. Immediate implant placement with or without socket grafting: a systematic review and meta-analysis. Clin Implant Dent Relat Res. 2022;24(3):339–51.
47. Seyssens L, De Lat L, Cosyn J. Immediate implant placement with or without connective tissue graft: a systematic review and meta-analysis. J Clin Periodontol. 2021;48(2):284–301.
48. Jung RE, Holderegger C, Sailer I, Khraisat A, Suter A, Hämmerle CH. The effect of all-ceramic and porcelain-fused-to-metal restorations on marginal peri-implant soft tissue color: a randomized controlled clinical trial. Int J Periodontics Restorative Dent. 2008;28(4):357–65.
49. Atieh MA, Payne AG, Duncan WJ, Cullinan MP. Immediate restoration/loading of immediately placed single implants: is it an effective bimodal approach? Clin Oral Implants Res. 2009;20(7):645–59.
50. De Rouck T, Collys K, Wyn I, Cosyn J. Instant provisionalization of immediate single-tooth implants is essential to optimize esthetic treatment outcome. Clin Oral Implants Res. 2009;20(6):566–70.
51. Amato F, Mirabella AD, Macca U, Tarnow DP. Implant site development by orthodontic forced extraction: a preliminary study. Int J Oral Maxillofac Implants. 2012;27(2):411–20.
52. Buser D, Chen ST, Weber HP, Belser UC. Early implant placement following single-tooth extraction in the esthetic zone: biologic rationale and surgical procedures. Int J Periodontics Restorative Dent. 2008;28(5):441–51.
53. Ingber JS. Forced eruption. I. A method of treating isolated one and two wall infrabony osseous defects-rationale and case report. J Periodontol. 1974;45(4):199–206.
54. Ingber JS. Forced eruption: Part II. A method of treating nonrestorable teeth—periodontal and restorative considerations. J Periodontol. 1976;47(4):203–16.
55. Salama H, Salama M. The role of orthodontic extrusive remodeling in the enhancement of soft and hard tissue profiles prior to implant placement: a systematic approach to the management of extraction site defects. Int J Periodontics Restorative Dent. 1993;13(4):312–33.
56. Grunder U, Polizzi G, Goené R, Hatano N, Henry P, Jackson WJ, et al. A 3-year prospective multicenter follow-up report on the immediate and delayed-immediate placement of implants. Int J Oral Maxillofac Implants. 1999;14(2):210–6.

Treatment Planning of the Edentulous Maxilla 15

Saj Jivraj and Winston Chee

As in all phases of dentistry, diagnosis is critical in obtaining a predictable outcome. An incomplete or erroneous diagnosis can yield unsatisfactory results for both the patient and treating clinician.

Historically, most of the research for implant rehabilitation of edentulous patients was conducted in the mandible. Due to the reduced denture-bearing surface of the mandible and the mobility of the tongue, patients often complained of instability of the denture and an inability to adapt to a removable prosthesis. Many prosthesis designs were evaluated ranging from subperiosteal implants to implant-supported complete dentures.

Patients are more likely to wear and accommodate a maxillary denture compared to its mandibular counterpart. Aesthetics are satisfactory, and the greater retention, support, and stability compared to a mandibular complete denture are also well documented. Patients are also more likely to wear a maxillary prosthesis for longer periods of time before complications arise. When implant rehabilitation of the edentulous maxilla was required, the principles were similar to those of the edentulous mandible. Screw-retained prostheses were fabricated with distal cantilevered pontics. When there was excessive resorption, tall standard abutments were installed which projected above the oral mucosa after which the prostheses were constructed on the abutments. The prostheses fabricated had open spaces under the mandibular prostheses. These procedures were acceptable for mandibular prostheses; however, the open interproximal spaces in the maxilla would compromise both the aesthetics phonetics and function.

S. Jivraj (✉)
Private Practice, Anacapa Dental Art Institute, Oxnard, CA, USA

W. Chee
Advanced Prosthodontics, Herman Ostrow School of Dentistry, University of Southern California, Los Angeles, CA, USA

W. Chee, S. Jivraj (eds.), *Treatment Planning In Implant Dentistry*, BDJ Clinician's Guides, https://doi.org/10.1007/978-3-031-68726-6_15

Following the same prosthetic concepts for the maxilla as in the mandible is not feasible. The long-term prognosis for implants in the maxilla is less secure than that of the edentulous mandible [1]. Following tooth extraction in the anterior part of the maxilla, horizontal bone resorption is almost twice as pronounced as vertical resorption [2]. The vertical distance between the alveolar crest and the base of the nasal sinuses provides a limiting factor for the placement of implants. In the posterior maxilla, vertical and horizontal atrophy occur at about the same rate; in addition, there can be pneumatization of the maxillary sinuses. The width of the ridge is usually sufficient; however, the limiting factor is the vertical distance between the crest and the base of the sinuses. Toda, protocols have been developed which include tilted implant placement. This allows the clinician to bypass extensive grafting procedures and be able to place dental implants in the patient's native bone. This brings significant advantages in terms of cost and time to completion of the maxillary prosthesis for the patient.

The reduced quantity and quality of bone in the maxilla together with increased aesthetic demands make treatment planning more complex. A different approach based on the ultimate aesthetic outcome is required compared to that of the edentulous mandible where function is the more dominant factor.

Restoration of the edentulous patients with dental implants is costly whichever method is used to restore the patient. Fixed reconstructions require more laboratory assistance and implant parts and, thus, are a lot more costly.

Due to economic factors, many patients have been provided with implant- and mucosa-supported overdentures.

However, cost needs to be considered not only during fabrication of the prosthesis but also during maintenance. Overdentures seem to have more post-insertion maintenance than their fixed counterparts. If this is consistent, it could be questioned whether an economic indication for choosing an overdenture could be justified when there is sufficient bone to support implants for a fixed prosthesis. The patient must be made aware that maintenance costs for removable prostheses on implants will be higher than those of a fixed prosthesis. These costs for maintenance are due to wear of the retentive elements that retain the prosthesis to the implants and breakage of the overdenture as the areas that accommodate the retentive attachments have reduced volume of acrylic and lead to fracture. In addition, when wearing a complete denture, some patients complain and feel pain when biting. This is due to pinching the mucosa between the denture base and underlying bone; when implant support is added, bite forces increase as the mucosa is not compressed; unfortunately, this increased occlusal force escalates the frequency of breakage of the overdenture. Today, clinicians are seeing an increasing number of dentate patients where the dentition is terminal. These patients would have been edentulous a long time ago if it had not been for the efforts of skilled restorative dentists. Clinical treatments have involved maintaining non-restorable teeth for as long as possible to avoid a removable appliance. Patients understand that maintaining a terminal dentition has consequences on the bone. However, the fear of edentulism forces them to ignore failing oral conditions.

Despite the increasing numbers of edentulous or soon-to-be edentulous patients, there still appears to be many reasons why patients avoid treatment with dental implants.

These reasons could include:

- The fear of wearing a removable appliance in the transitional phase
- The notion that the proposed treatment is time consuming and unpredictable
- The number of visits involved and the fear of pain
- Cost

Most patients will look toward an implant rehabilitation hoping to acquire a fixed prosthesis. Treatment planning of edentulous patients with fixed restorations on dental implants has undergone a paradigm shift since the introduction of graft-less solutions, in particular, the All on 4 method™.

Today, patients have options whereby with the right indication, complete rehabilitation can be accomplished using four implants per arch. The major advantages of this procedure are reduced number of implants and the ability to bypass extensive grafting procedures. This rehabilitation not only satisfies aesthetics and function but also considerably reduces costs for the patient. This ultimately results in increased patient acceptance and an increased number of patients treated. Very few patients today are able to afford extensive implant rehabilitations on six to eight implants. Thus, the All on 4™ or graft-less protocol is gaining popularity as being the treatment of choice for the edentulous patient [3].

The principles of the All on 4™ concept include but are not limited to the following:

1. Placement of four implants: Posterior implants are tilted. Anterior implants are placed vertically. The posterior implants can include zygomatic implants.
2. Bi-cortical fixation when feasible.
3. Bone reduction to allow for prosthetic gingiva.
4. Procedure is a graft-less solution.
5. Fixed provisional the same day of surgery that is immediately loaded.

Clinicians must be cognizant that the All on 4 concept™ is indicated for specific clinical situations, namely:

1. There is minimal bone, with pneumatized sinuses and posterior mandibular resorption. In this circumstance, the clinician can only place four implants due to anatomical limitations. To avoid grafting, tilted implant concepts are employed.
2. Adequate lip support.
3. Where the patient has lost a significant amount of bone, a strategic implant placement is required to obtain bi-cortical anchorage.
4. Patient refuses grafting procedures and desires a fixed restoration.

There is always going to be a debate over how many implants should be placed in an edentulous arch. The answer to that question is "It Depends". It depends on the patient's medical history, quality of bone, anticipated occlusal force on the restoration and operator's skill. It is a specific surgical, prosthetic and maintenance protocol which has been misinterpreted as a solution for all edentulous or soon-to-be edentulous patients.

It is the author's opinion that more than four implants are required when:

1. There is an abundance of bone and biomechanically cantilevers can be avoided.
2. The patient presents with a dentition that exhibits signs and symptoms of excessive force.
3. The patient has uncontrolled metabolic disease which compromises healing.
4. There is poor-quality bone.

The advantages and considerations of placing more implants and preserving bone include the following:

1. There is the ability to segment the prosthesis, and complication management becomes easier for the clinician.
2. If in the future an implant were to fail, there are enough implants where the patient may not have to undergo surgery again.
3. The thought process that making an impression on four implants is easier than making an impression on five or six does not hold merit. Today, with advancements in digital technologies, analogue impression taking may soon become obsolete at multi-unit abutment level.
4. When placing implants, the clinician must begin with the end in mind visualizing the definitive restoration. Zirconia requires specific connector dimensions and requires appropriate distance between implants. Zirconia also requires specific thickness for biomechanical integrity. The implants together with the multi-unit abutments must be positioned three dimensionally to allow for this.
5. Maintenance of bone in between the implants can be obtained by banking roots.
6. If a catastrophic failure were to occur and all the implants were lost, then the clinician still has the ability to retreat the patient.

Treatment planning should be based on a thorough diagnosis to culminate in an appropriate treatment plan for the patients presenting clinical situation. Unfortunately, the All on 4™ concept has been used as a panacea for full-arch implant reconstruction, and often patients are treated dogmatically with this treatment protocol. Often, bone is removed needlessly to satisfy a certain treatment philosophy. The preservation of bone provides an obvious advantage in providing the patient with restorations that may mimic the natural dentoalveolar complex.

Minimally invasive full-arch implant dentistry adheres to the concept of preserving and maintaining bone. Bone reduction is virtually eliminated, and the patient maintains their own mucosa. Although four implants are considered standard, the placement of additional implants is considered advantageous. As a practicing clinician, implant failure is always a concern, and should one of the four implants fail, the definitive restoration needs to be remade at the restorative dentist's cost. If more than four implants have been placed, then there are reserve implants to work with.

15.1 Diagnosis

George Bernard Shaw once said, "One of the most dangerous diseases is diagnosis". The decision-making parameters when rehabilitating patients require the clinician to make a decision as to whether a fixed or a removable prosthesis would be more suitable. Patients presenting with a satisfactory complete denture requesting transition to an implant-supported restoration may be difficult to satisfy. Patients must be told about the risks and potential pitfalls of treatment. Informed consent must include surgical risks of treatment as well as a realistic assessment of whether the patient's chief complaint can be addressed, and their expectations satisfied.

When restoring the edentulous maxilla with implants, one of the major decisions to make is often whether the patient should be restored with a fixed or removable prosthesis. Several designs can be used to restore patients. With overdenture-type designs, we can obtain support from both the implants and the mucosa; when there are enough implants that are well distributed, the restoration can be entirely implant supported.

Zitzmann and Marinello [4] described in detail parameters that need to be evaluated. A fixed restoration should not be promised to a patient until all diagnostic criteria are evaluated. These criteria must include quality and quantity of bone available to support implants, lip line, lip support and aesthetic demands. Implants should not be placed till a definitive treatment plan has been established as implant positions may vary depending on the type of prostheses to be delivered (Fig. 15.1).

15.2 Extraoral Examination

15.2.1 Facial and Lip Support

The delivery of tooth- and implant-borne prosthetics has been significantly advanced by the rapid introduction of innovative digital technologies into clinical practice. These technologies allow for greater ease, cost efficiencies and improved workflows.

Preliminary digital data acquisition is the entry point into an entire ecosystem of digital workflows that result in precision, predictability and cost and time savings, which in turn create more comprehensive affordable solutions for patients. This phase consists of:

1. Obtaining intraoral scan (IOS) data
2. Cone beam computed tomography (CBCT) imaging
3. Facial scans
4. Adjunctive photography or videography if needed

Despite the introduction of these technologies, the clinician should have a full understanding of the analogue workflow and what factors need to be considered in diagnosis to yield an optimal outcome.

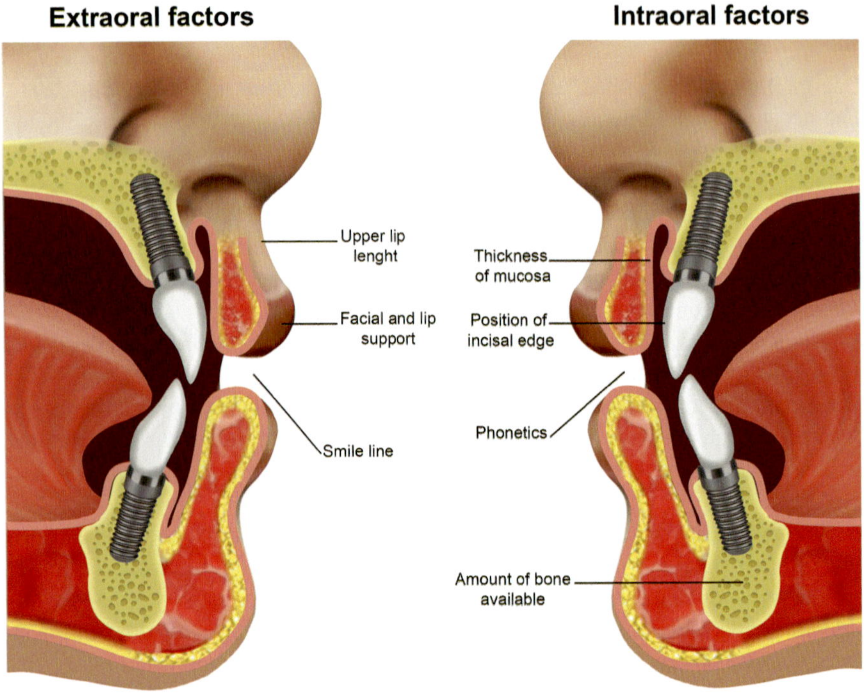

Fig. 15.1 Extraoral and intraoral factors that need to be evaluated. (Modified from Zitzmann and Marinello [3])

One of the best diagnostic tools is the patient's existing maxillary denture. The clinician can evaluate the patient's denture to determine what the likes and dislikes are regarding aesthetics, speech and function. Each point should be noted for improvements in the new restoration. There is always a tendency for patients to prefer fixed over removable prostheses. It is the restorative dentist's responsibility to determine if this is feasible; facial support is an important decision in this regard.

Assessment of the patient's facial support with and without the denture in place, with the patient facing forward and in profile, should be photographed so that the clinician can compare the images in order to determine which type of prostheses would be more suitable (Figs. 15.2, 15.3, 15.4 and 15.5).

Facial support, if inadequate, is obtained mainly by the buccal flange of a removable restoration. Lip support is derived from the alveolar ridge shape and cervical crown contours of the anterior teeth. Resorption of the edentulous maxilla proceeds cranially and medially, and this often results in a retruded position of the anterior maxilla.

When evaluating anterior teeth in proper relation to the lip, the position of the anterior teeth is often anterior to the alveolar ridge. Depending on the severity of the resorption, there can be a discrepancy between the ideal location of the teeth and the ridge. This, in turn, leads to a discrepancy of the anticipated position of the implants

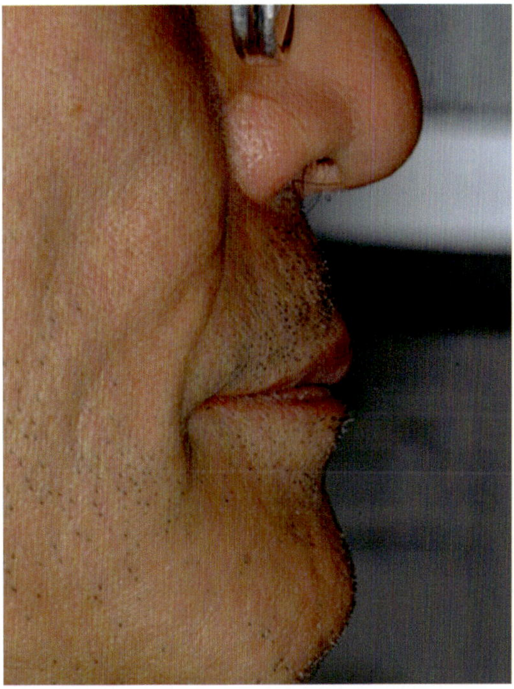

Fig. 15.2 Profile view with lip support without denture

in relation to the teeth. This discrepancy must be taken into consideration to achieve a prosthesis that satisfies the parameters of adequate speech, lip support, hygiene, sufficient tongue space and patient acceptance. Carl Misch [5] first proposed the classification system that we use today to classify the pink and white balance for partial- and full-arch implant-supported restorations.

Misch proposed five groups: FP1, FP2 and FP3. FP1 is the replacement of only the tooth. FP2 replaces the crown and a portion of the root with tooth-coloured material and very little (if any) pink. FP3 is the prosthetic replacement of both the gingiva and tooth tissue, i.e. the teeth and the artificial gingiva, when providing an implant restoration. RP 4 and RP 5 pertain to patients with moderate to advanced resorption where a fixed restoration cannot be provided. In this instance, an implant-supported overdenture with a flange of an implant and mucosa-supported overdenture with a flange are provided (Fig. 15.6).

Patients often favour a fixed restoration over a removable if possible. This becomes quite difficult if the anticipated positions of the teeth and implant result in a large horizontal discrepancy. Several options must be considered before finalizing implant placement.

If the horizontal discrepancy is quite large, options include the following:

1. Alveolectomy and a deeper implant placement to allow the contours of the restoration to satisfy the parameters of lip support and hygiene. Without bone

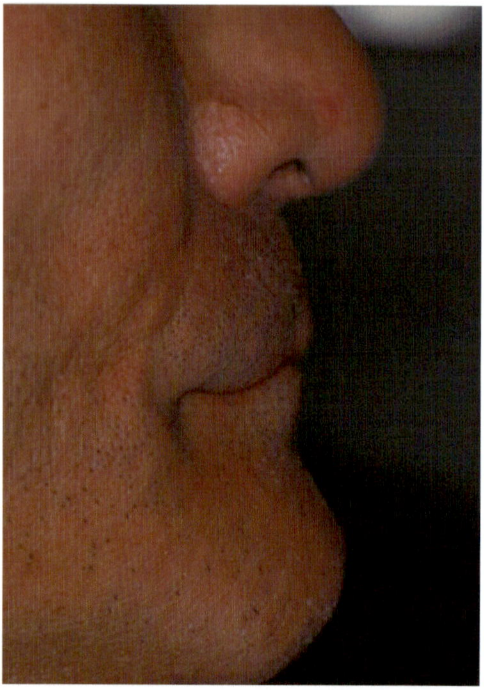

Fig. 15.3 Profile view with lip support with denture; lip looks over-supported. This patient may be a candidate for a fixed restoration on implants

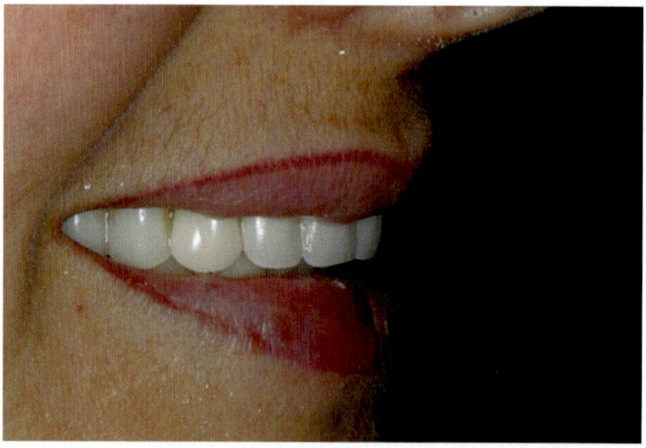

Fig. 15.4 Profile view with lip support with denture. This patient will require a flange to satisfy aesthetic parameters

reduction, undesirable contours in the restoration are developed, which make it very difficult for the patient to maintain hygiene (Fig. 15.7).

2. Le Fort 1 osteotomy—Most patients are reluctant to undergo this type of surgery.
3. Use of a removable flange and fabrication of an implant-supported overdenture.

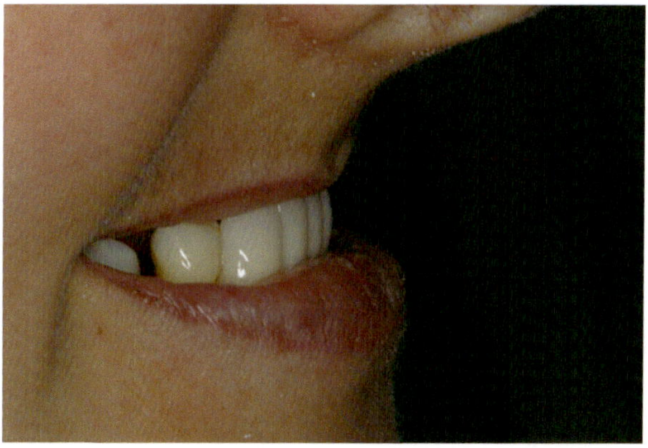

Fig. 15.5 Profile view with lip support without denture. Note the collapse of the lip. This patient may require a flange for aesthetic lip support

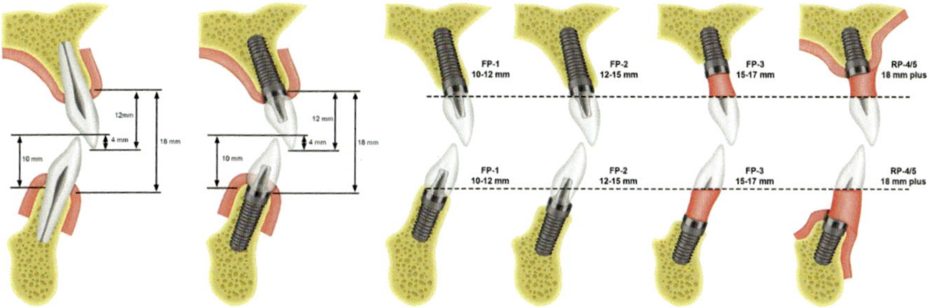

Fig. 15.6 Restorative space requirements

15.2.2 Smile Line and Lip Length

The movement of the upper lip during speech and smiling should be evaluated. Tjan et al. [6] described the average smile as having the position of the upper lip such that 75–100% of the maxillary incisors and interproximal gingival are displayed. In a high smile line, additional gingival was exposed, and in a low smile line, less than 75% of the maxillary anterior teeth are displayed. Lip length should also be evaluated because it influences the position of the maxillary anterior teeth. In a patient with a short upper lip, the maxillary anterior teeth will be exposed in repose (Fig. 15.8), whereas in patients with a long upper lip, the anterior teeth will usually be covered (Fig. 15.9).

Dentate patients with a terminal dentition may present with excessive gingival display. Causes of excessive gingival display include but are not limited to:

1. Vertical maxillary excess

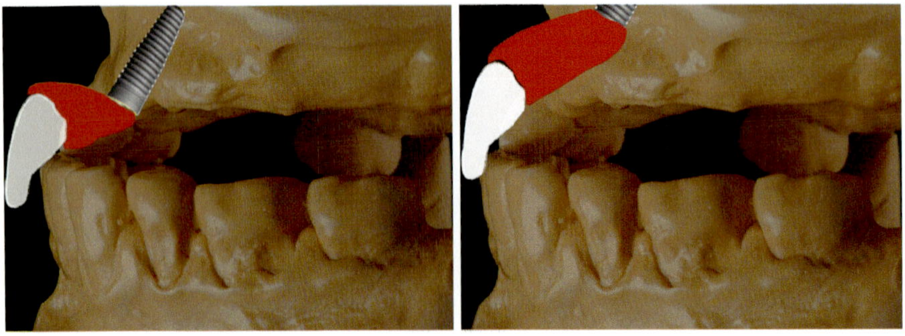

Fig. 15.7 A horizontal discrepancy between the implant position and the position of the incisal edge may necessitate deeper implant placement

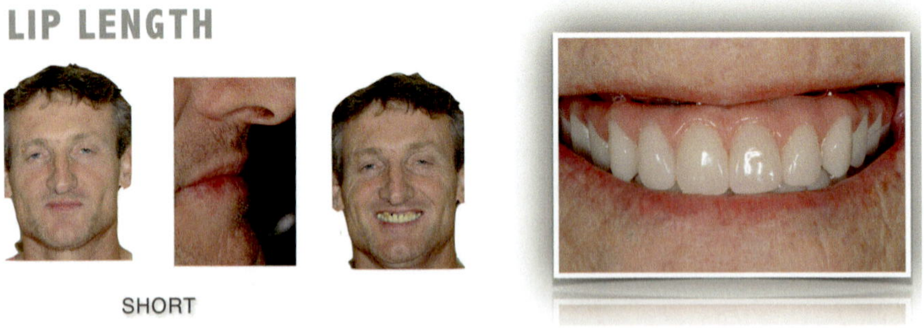

Fig. 15.8 Patients with a short lip and high smile line display the transition zone

2. Short upper lip
3. Hyperactive upper lip
4. Dentoalveolar extrusion
5. Delayed passive eruption
6. Multiple aetiologies [7]

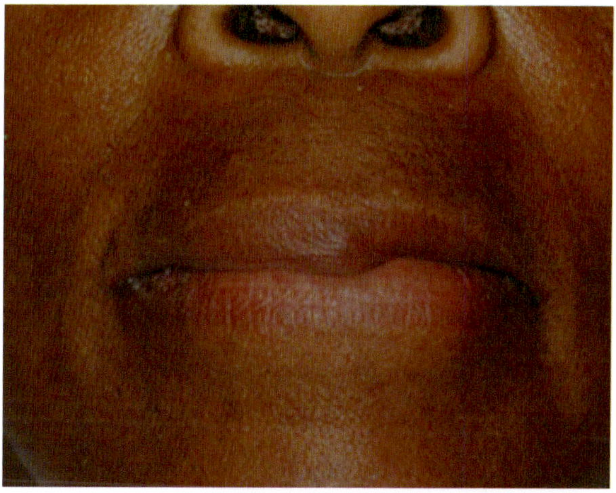

Fig. 15.9 Low smile line and long lip

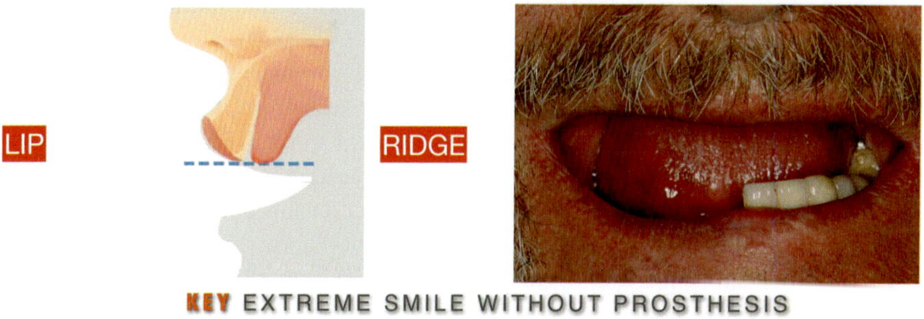

Fig. 15.10 Edentulous patient smiling. Ridge is not visible

The clinician must have an adequate diagnosis prior to embarking upon a treatment plan.

Edentulous patients should be asked to smile with and without the denture in place (Figs. 15.10 and 15.11). If the soft tissue of the edentulous ridge cannot be seen, the transition between an implant-supported prosthesis and the residual ridge crest will not be visible, resulting in flexibility for colour matching and the contour change of the prosthesis at the junction of the soft tissue. If the alveolar ridge crest is displayed whilst smiling, the aesthetics can be very challenging because the junction between the restoration and the gingival complex will be visible and bear aesthetic consequences. If the patient has minimal resorption, conventional metal ceramic restorations or zirconia-based restorations supported by implants can be planned and the existing soft tissue can be developed to enhance aesthetics. However, if an implant-supported denture (hybrid/profile prosthesis) is being planned, the alveolar ridge display will detract from the aesthetics. In situations like this, alveolectomy as part of a proactive protocol must be considered prior to implant placement. If alveolectomy is not performed, the restorative outcome will display the transition zone, which, ultimately, is very difficult to retreat. Alveolectomy must

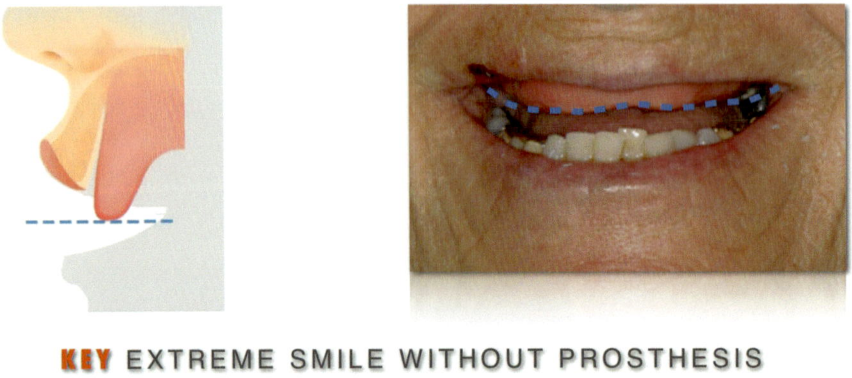

Fig. 15.11 Ridge displayed when a patient is smiling. This situation is aesthetically challenging since the interface between the gingival and restoration is visible

only be performed when there is an indication for it, and the minimum amount of bone must be removed to satisfy the aesthetic objectives [8–10].

The contours of the restorations must be planned from the outset. The emergence profile of the restorations should be straight as it exits from the gingival margin. Often, this requires alveolectomy to create sufficient space. The restorative dentist requires this space to develop adequate mechanics, aesthetics and cleansability. This space creation must be communicated to the surgeon through the use of a bone reduction guide, and it becomes the surgeon's responsibility to provide this space [11]. One misconception about graft-less protocols is that they always require a significant amount of bone reduction. Bone reduction must have a rationale, and the minimum bone reduction must be done to satisfy the requirements of implant placement and fabrication of a biomechanically sound restoration [12].

Rationales for bone reduction include but are not limited to:

1. Adequate buccolingual width of bone to place implants
2. Adequate space for hygiene
3. Adequate space for biomechanics of the restoration
4. Adequate space so that the patient can clean the undersurface
5. Hiding of transition zone
6. Improved emergence of the restoration

15.3 Intraoral Examination

15.3.1 Incisal Edge Position

The maxillary incisal edge position is determined utilizing the principles taught in complete denture fabrication. Traditional guidelines tell us that when the patient makes the F sound, the incisal edge should touch the vermillion border of the lower lip. Once the incisal edge position has been established, the length for the central incisors is determined. On average, the length of the central incisors is 10.5 mm [13, 14]; this can be longer in elderly patients who exhibit gingival recession.

The axial inclination of the central incisor should be placed to provide adequate support for the upper lip. Once the crown length, angulation and coronal form have been determined, the distance between the cervical crown margin and residual bone crest can be assessed [4]. To determine if a fixed or removable restoration would be appropriate, a wax try-in is done without a flange. For a fixed restoration, the clinical crown should ideally end up at the soft tissue level of the alveolar ridge. In this situation, minimal resorption would have occurred, inter-arch space will be favourable and an optimal tooth-lip relationship is present (Fig. 15.12). When a large vertical distance exists between the cervical aspect of the tooth and the alveolar ridge, and the tooth-lip relationship is favourable, pink ceramic may be utilized to disguise the tooth length and a fixed restoration is still possible. Note in Figs. 15.13 and 15.14 that for this patient, prosthetic gingiva can be placed without a ridge lap with adequate lip support and there is no exposure of the junction between the prosthesis and the mucosa. When there is both a vertical and horizontal discrepancy between the ideal position of the tooth and the alveolar ridge, and the tooth-lip relationship is not optimal, this may be an indication for use of a removable prosthesis. The flange will provide adequate lip support, and the teeth can be positioned appropriately to satisfy the parameters of aesthetics.

The mandibular incisal edge is positioned for function. The clinician must provide shallow guidance, sufficient to provide posterior disclusion in both protrusive and lateral excursions. Anterior guidance must be smooth and distributed among as many anterior teeth as possible.

15.3.2 Thickness of the Mucosa

The mucosal quality can be assessed by palpation or sounding or with the help of radiographs. Often, in edentulous patients, the interdental papillae are absent. When

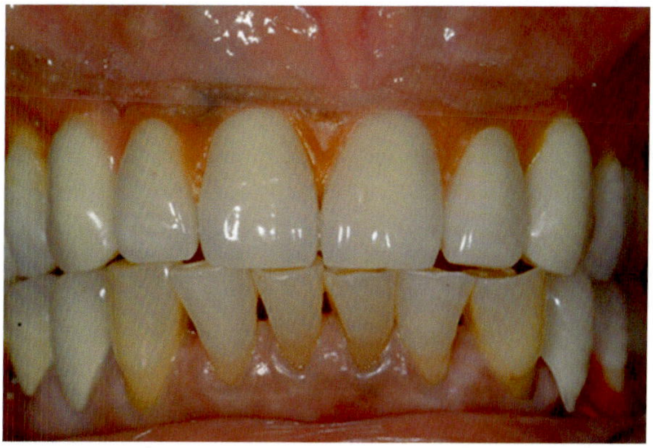

Fig. 15.12 Minimal bone resorption displaying a tooth-only defect

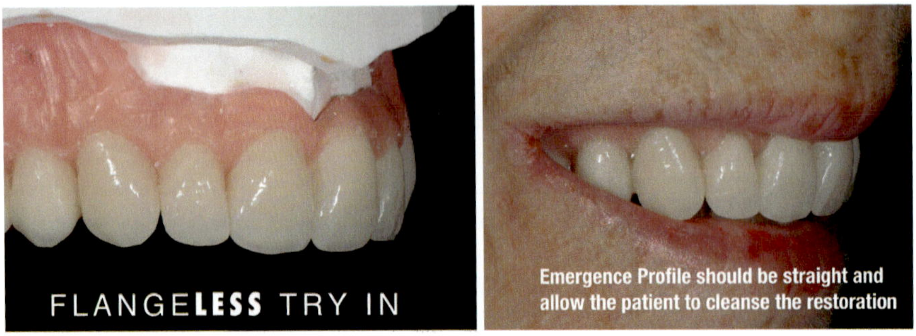

Fig. 15.13 Moderate resorption. Requires a flangeless try-in

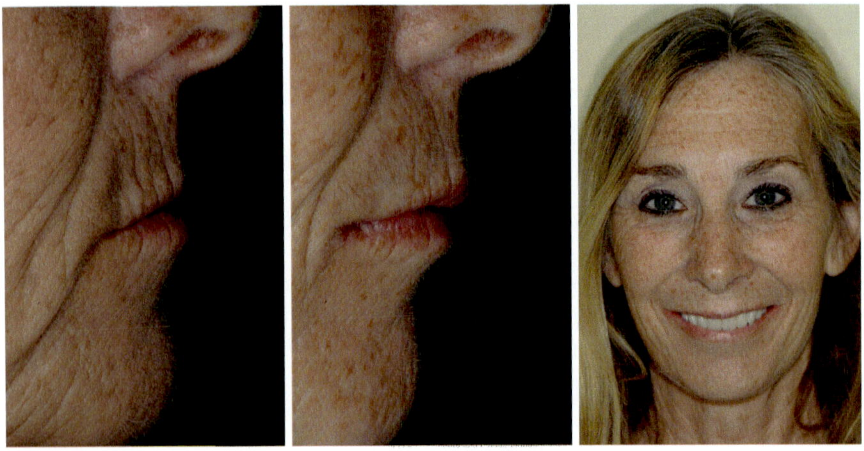

Fig. 15.14 Lip support and smile line evaluation with diagnostic try-in

adjacent teeth are lost, the interseptal bone disappears and the bone remodels. What is often the result is a flattened papilla. The papilla height is also depressed since there is lack of interproximal contacts.

When papillae are lost, it is very difficult if not impossible to regenerate it. Patients must be told that to achieve the papillary architecture that existed prior to the extraction of their teeth is unlikely. This illusion is created by manipulating the soft tissues with ovate pontics and varying the position of the interproximal contact. On occasion when implants are in the incorrect position, soft tissue is replaced by utilizing gingival coloured ceramics (Figs. 15.15 and 15.16). It is imperative that the patient preview the final result through the use of provisional restorations. In some instances, there is excessive hard and soft tissue loss, and the appearance of interdental papilla can only be recreated through the use of gingival coloured ceramics or acrylic resin (Figs. 15.17 and 15.18). A thick mucosa is easier to mould for an inter-implant papilla than a thin mucosa. Thick mucosa can also help hide abutment margins and facilitates correct emergence of the clinical crown. In some cases where

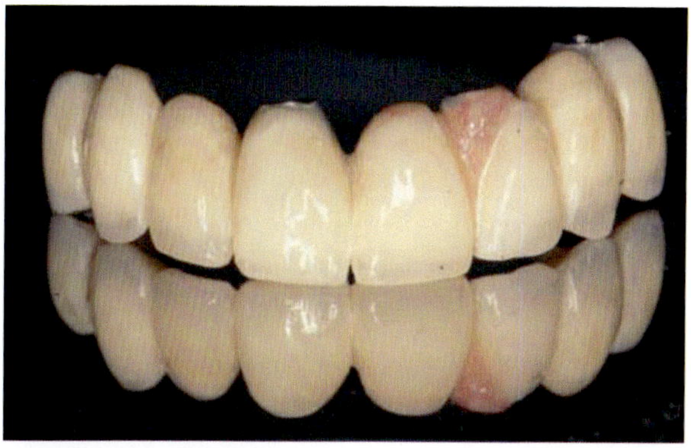

Fig. 15.15 Implant placed in interproximal area, between maxillary left central and lateral incisors. Pink acrylic resin has been used to disguise the discrepancy

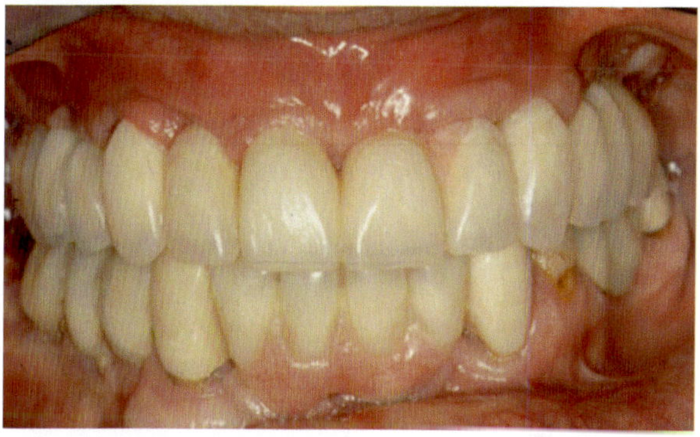

Fig. 15.16 Provisional restoration in the mouth to determine if the patient is accepting of pink acrylic resin

angulated abutments are required, the mucosa can facilitate in hiding the pronounced titanium collar. If the patient presents with very thin tissue, consideration must be given to soft tissue grafting in order to change the tissue type to a more favourable one.

15.3.3 Bone Quality and Quantity

Upon consideration of bone quantity, bone quality, resorptive patterns and maxillomandibular relationship, it usually becomes apparent that the actual amount of bone available for placement of implants in the edentulous maxilla may not only be limited but may also be present in areas remote from the original site of the natural teeth. In the premaxilla, the tooth position may be much further forward than the implant position, and this may pose certain biomechanical disadvantages. In the posterior maxilla, the resorption pattern may be so severe that a crossbite relationship may have to be utilized or alternatively the tooth position may have to be cantilevered facially so as to recreate the vertical and horizontal tooth relationships that existed prior to extraction.

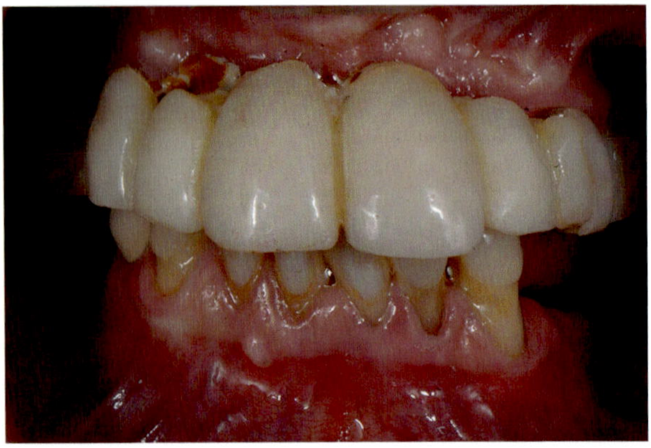

Fig. 15.17 Patient with terminal dentition demonstrating periodontal bone loss

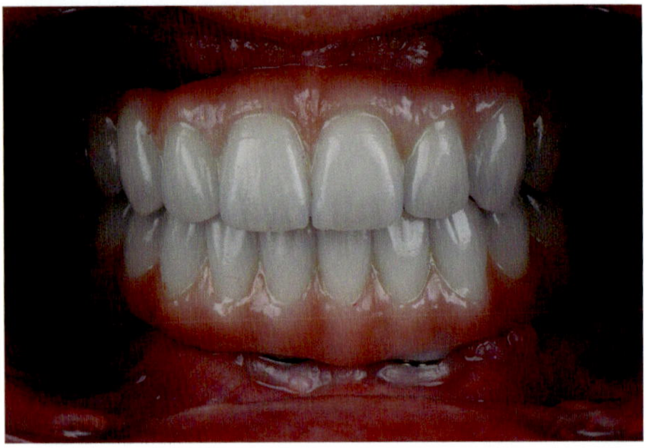

Fig. 15.18 Definitive restoration for patient in Fig. 15.17. Pink porcelain was utilized to close interdental spaces and provide improved aesthetics and speech

The clinician's ability to evaluate the maxillary bone both quantitatively and qualitatively makes this one of the most challenging sites for successful implant placement.

Visual examination with and without the denture in place will give the clinician an idea of the lip and facial support required and some idea as to whether a fixed or removable restoration would be more appropriate. However visual examination cannot reveal sufficient information about the location, volume, width and degree of mineralization of the bone under the soft tissues [15]. Computed tomography scans and tomograms reveal the three-dimensional architecture of the bone and provide the surgeon with precise representation of the availability and location of bone. Clinically, Lekholm and Zarb [14] have proposed a classification of jaw shape and quality, which is useful when planning treatment for the edentulous maxilla. They classified edentulous maxillae and mandibles into five shapes according to the degree of resorption, shape A, having minimal resorption, and shape E, being severely resorbed. Bone quality was classified into four patterns (1 through 4) depending on the amount and type of cortical bone present (Figs. 15.19 and 15.20). In the edentulous maxilla, type 3 or type 4 bone quality is often found. This quality

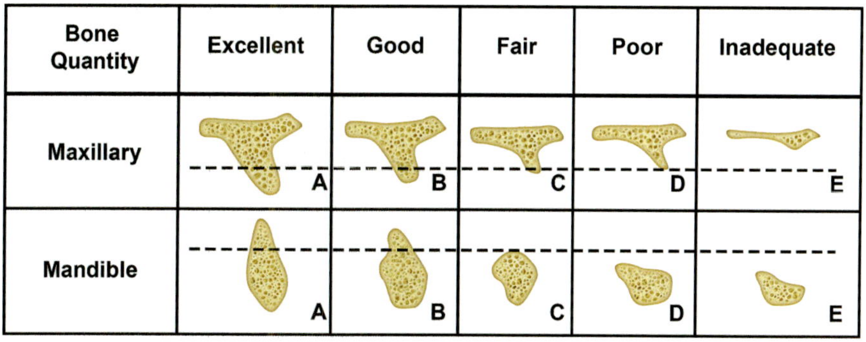

Fig. 15.19 Cross section of bone resorption pattern according to Lekholm and Zarb [14]

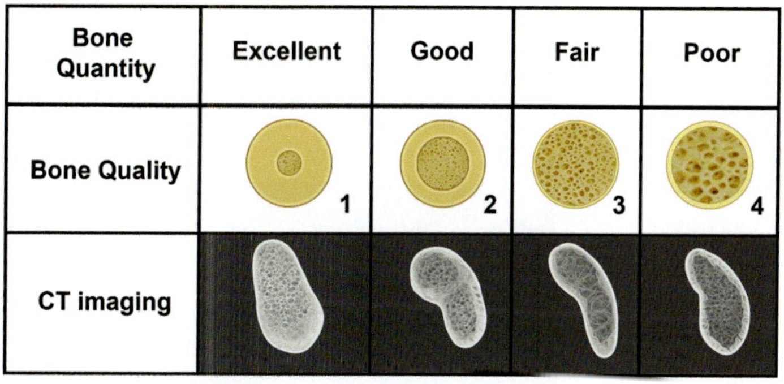

Fig. 15.20 Diagram indicating the quality of bone according to Lekholm and Zarb [11]

of bone often dictates over engineering at the time of implant placement. Additional implants are placed when the surgeon experiences bone of poor quality, the rationale being if one implant were to fail, the restorative dentist would still be able to progress with the anticipated prosthesis.

To obtain maximal benefit from such a scan, a radiographic template is highly recommended [4]. Titanium pins or gutta percha markers should be incorporated into an acrylic resin duplicate of the diagnostic denture set-up (Figs. 15.21 and 15.22). The markers are oriented perpendicular to the occlusal plane and should end apically at the height of the prospective clinical crown margin [16].

CT scans are extremely useful in evaluating the trajectory of the bone in the posterior maxilla. When a patient has been edentulous for a significant period of time, pneumatization of the sinuses prevents implant placement. Maxillary sinus lift procedures are frequently performed to create adequate bone volume for predictable implant placement [16]. The donor site varies depending on the volume of bone required. Bone from the iliac crest is often harvested when both sinuses require augmentation. Augmentation of the sinuses via iliac bone crest grafting can be a traumatic procedure, and patients often request alternative options. With information from the CT scan, implants can be inclined to avoid the maxillary sinuses [10],

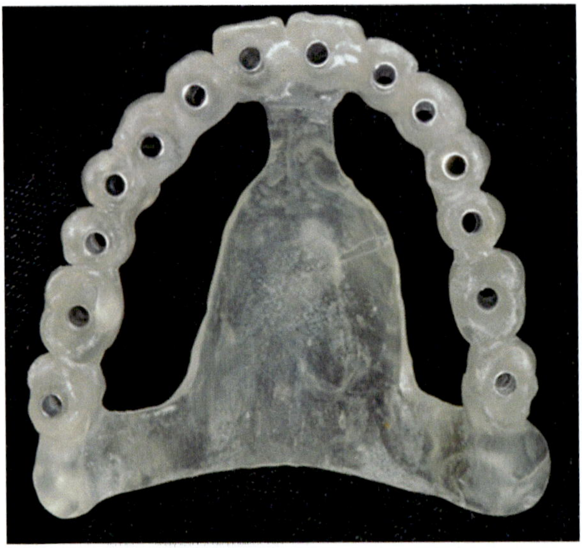

Fig. 15.21 Restrictive surgical guide with titanium pins

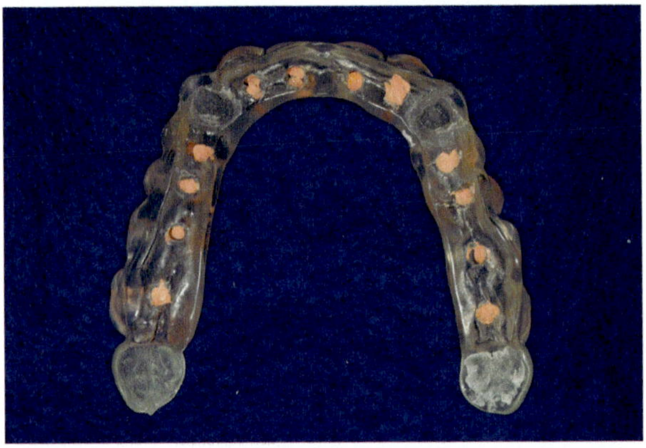

Fig. 15.22 Radiographic guide with gutta percha markers

or alternative procedures that utilize existing anatomical sites that offer reduced morbidity and minimal invasion of the existing structures can be utilized.

Zygomatic implants can be placed to engage the zygomatic bone inferolateral to the orbital rim and provide anchorage for a fixed prosthesis in conjunction with anterior implants [17]. Implants can also be placed in the maxillary tuberosity to provide support.

A systematic process must be undertaken when evaluating bone quantity in the edentulous maxilla. Three-dimensional radiography and virtual planning software have made the diagnosis and treatment planning predictable. Bedrossian has described the delineation of maxilla into three zones for a simplified treatment planning [18]. A treatment plan can be developed by the clinician after determination of presence of sufficient bone in the three zones of the maxilla. The alveolar bone of the anterior maxilla from canine to contralateral canine is designated as zone 1, the premolar region as zone 2 and the molar region as zone 3. Zone 4 is reserved for the zygomatic process.

If zones 1, 2 and 3 have available bone volume, then preferred number of axial implants should be placed. The greater the number of implants, the greater the possibility for segmentation of the prosthesis. If bone exists in zones 1 and 2, and the patient refuses a sinus augmentation procedure, then tilted posterior implants in combination with axial or tilted anterior implants can be considered. If zone 1 is the only area of available bone, then the zygomatic process or pterygoid plate implants can be considered for posterior support and axial or tilted implants for anterior support. If complete atrophy of the maxilla is evident with unavailability of bone in all three zones of the maxilla, then two zygomatic implants bilaterally may be used to provide support for the prosthesis. The reason for tilting of implant up to 45° is to avoid placement of implants in anatomic structures such as the maxillary sinus, nasal cavity or mental foramen. By bypassing these structures, bone grafting procedures are avoided or minimized.

15.3.4 Inter-arch Space

Jaw shape has a significant influence on prosthesis design. The resorption of alveolar bone has been a considerable issue in prosthodontics for as long as clinicians have tried to replace missing intraoral structures.

To accommodate adequate designs, different types of restorations require different dimensional tolerances. Accurately mounted casts are critical in assessing prosthetic space limitations. Spatial constraints must be considered as a matter of practicality. The limiting factor in edentulous patients is the available inter-arch space [4].

Insufficient restorative space is the most common error when planning full-arch restorations. Inadequate space results in either premature failure of the restoration or changing the treatment plan from one restoration to another to accommodate the space requirements.

Conventional screw-retained implant prostheses have been constructed with 10–12 mm between the edentulous ridges and the opposing occlusal plane. It provides sufficient space for the bulk of restorative material and also permits a prosthesis design to establish aesthetics and hygiene (Fig. 15.6).

Guidelines for space requirements for ceramic-based restorations are 10–13 mm for a screw-retained ceramic-based restorations and 14–16 mm for acrylic resin/titanium-based restorations. A conventional overdenture requires additional space. Guidelines for space requirements are between 14 and 16 mm in the anterior part of the maxilla. Space is required for acrylic resin, prosthetic teeth and titanium substructure. Heat-processed resin requires 2–3 mm to provide adequate strength as a denture-based material [12]. Space is also required for the prosthetic tooth, and there should be sufficient acrylic resin around the teeth for mechanical stability. In the maxilla, it is advisable to splint implants when used for overdenture prostheses,

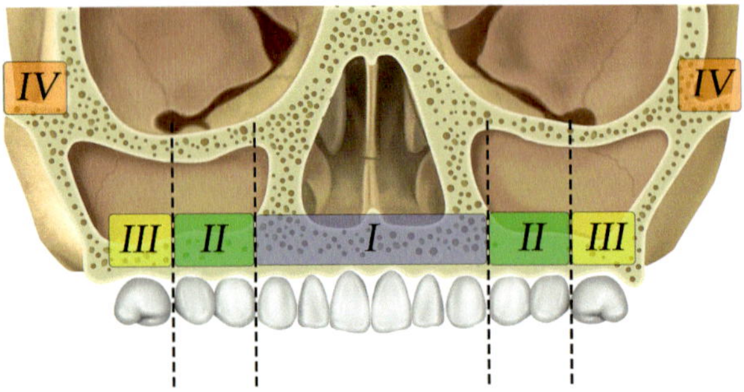

Fig. 15.23 Diagnostic bone evaluation for treatment planning

and as a result, 2–3 mm of space may be required to accommodate the necessary bulk for the tissue bar and any retaining clips (Fig. 15.23).

If space is limited, re-establishing a patient's vertical dimension or altering the opposing occlusion should be considered [4].

Clinicians should select the material that requires the least bone removal and satisfies the requirements of aesthetics, contour and biomechanics. Acrylic titanium restorations are very rarely done in the maxillary arch due to the amount of restorative space and bone removal required. They should be reserved for the mandibular arch when opposing a maxillary denture.

15.4 Treatment Planning

The long-term success of implant rehabilitation of the edentulous maxilla is dependent on the consideration of all the factors previously discussed. Treatment planning must address these diagnostic findings. Treatment planning must also address the patient's original complaints and meet the patient's expectations. The patient needs to have a relatively good idea of what the final outcome is likely to be. A compromised anatomical presentation can be difficult to perform procedures to improve the anatomical situations; with each procedure, perfect outcomes may not occur; going through a lengthy expense and treatment only to achieve a result which is aesthetically inferior to a complete denture can be hugely disappointing.

Patient communication at the outset is of utmost importance. To avoid any unexpected surprises, a great amount of time must be devoted to educating the patient about the relative advantages, disadvantages and limitations of proposed treatment.

Informed consent becomes important. The patient must fully understand and acknowledge the limitations of the proposed treatment, including possibility of implant failure. The patient must understand that treatment plan modifications may be required and the fact that placement of additional implants may be necessary. Informed consent must constitute the surgical risks of treatment and also the shortcomings of treatment to adequately address the patient's chief complaint and expectations.

In treatment planning, the following factors must be considered:

1. Aesthetics and patient desires
2. Type of support
3. Amount of resorption and inter-arch space
4. Number of implants
5. Implant distribution
6. Tissue-fitting surface
7. Economics

15.4.1 Aesthetics and Patient Desires

Meeting patient expectations is paramount when treatment planning. As discussed, earlier patients prefer to discard their removable appliance in favour of a fixed alternative. The clinician must know early in treatment if this is possible. Promising a patient a fixed reconstruction when diagnostic considerations are present otherwise may result in a disappointed patient. Patients are also satisfied with the aesthetic appearance of a complete denture. In particular, the appearance of the soft tissues is uniform, and interdental papillae between denture teeth are reproduced well with pink acrylic resin (Fig. 15.24). When a patient then transitions to a fixed reconstruction, interdental papilla between implants is often absent. An illusion of interdental papilla can be created by altering the position of the contact point between adjacent teeth and utilizing interproximal stain and a longer proximal contact (Fig. 15.25).

15.4.2 Type of Support

Essentially with the edentulous maxilla, there are two categories of prostheses, fixed and removable. Fixed prostheses include metal ceramic- and zirconia-based restorations supported by implants, and depending on the severity of the bone resorption, some pink porcelain may be required to simulate gingival contours. In the removable category, we have implant-supported overdentures and implant-retained and

Fig. 15.24 Denture and pink ceramics provide excellent aesthetics

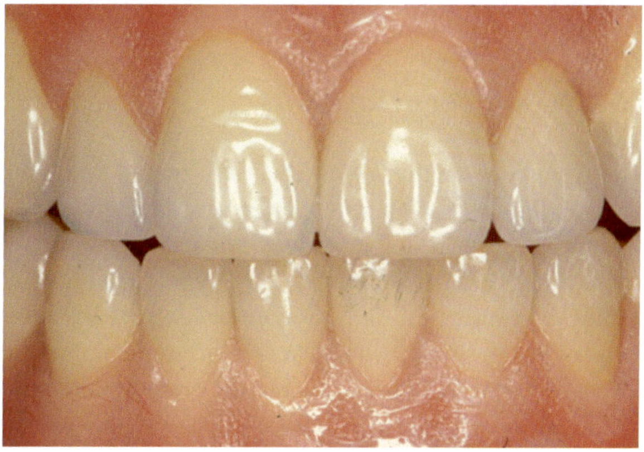

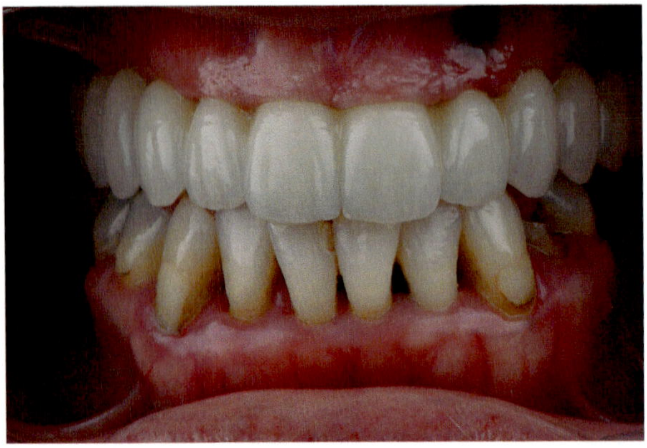

Fig. 15.25 Difficult-to-generate papilla in a full-arch implant restoration. Technicians create illusion with chroma inter-proximally and longer proximal contacts

tissue-supported overdentures. A removable prosthesis can be secured by different methods including bar and clip, magnet, ball attachments or use of a precision-milled or spark-eroded components.

The diagnostic factors previously discussed will allow the clinician to decide which type of prostheses will be more suitable.

15.4.3 Amount of Resorption and Inter-arch Space

This parameter dictates the type of prosthesis to be fabricated. The clinician needs to evaluate if the patient exhibits minimal, moderate or advanced resorption. Each type of prosthesis has a unique dimensional tolerance as previously discussed. Patients who exhibit minimal or moderate resorption are candidates for a fixed restoration, provided that parameters of facial and lip support are satisfied. Patients with advanced resorption can be satisfied aesthetically by fabrication of a removable prosthesis with a flange; this replaces necessary support that has been lost as a result of resorption. If patients in this category request a fixed restoration, they will need to understand that extensive grafting procedures will be required and even after that the aesthetic outcomes may not meet their expectations.

15.4.4 Number of Implants

There are many authors which have discussed treatment concepts for restoration of the edentulous maxilla with a fixed prosthesis. Recommendations have been made with respect to anticipated prosthesis designs and implants. Placement of 6–8 implants (10–15 mm in length) is recommended for a fixed implant prosthesis with cantilever pontics [16, 17]. Recommendations have also been made with regard to removable prostheses on implants; 4–6 implants have been recommended for both an implant and an implant- and tissue-supported restoration [13, 17].

Deciding on the number of implants to place is not governed by a formula and is dependent on multiple factors. The number of implants to place in each patient is determined by:

1. Quality of bone
2. Anticipated force to be placed on the restoration
3. Relationship between the shape of the residual ridge and the dental arch form

15.4.4.1 Quality of Bone

Frequently, type 3 and 4 bones are encountered in the maxilla. On occasion, the quality of the bone is such that conventional drills cannot be used to place the implant, and osteotomes are required to develop the site to receive the implant. The success of implants in the maxilla is less certain than in the edentulous mandible. When the quality of bone is not optimal, often the surgeon and restorative dentist consider placing additional implants. These implants are placed to allow the restorative dentist to continue with the anticipated prosthesis should one or two implants fail. Over-engineering in the maxilla can be advantageous, but consideration should also be given to the costs that may be encountered should all the implants integrate. Often, the restorative dentist will have to purchase additional abutments, and the costs of these will need to be passed onto the patient.

When the patient has had posterior teeth missing for a considerable length of time, the maxillary sinuses pneumatize, and often there is insufficient bone for implant placement in these areas. If the patient refuses to undergo additional augmentation procedures, the concept of the shortened dental arch can be utilized, and fewer implants are placed.

15.4.4.2 Anticipated Force to Be Placed on the Restoration

Part of the extraoral examination should also involve analysis of the patient's build and facial musculature. The masseter muscles should be observed for any hypertrophy that may be present. Bruxers often present with a pronounced antegonial notch, and this can be indicative of the likely force to be placed on the restorations. In these types of patients, it is wise to "over-engineer" and place additional implants for added support and distribution of force.

The opposing occlusion must also be evaluated. Patients are likely to exert less force if the implant restorations are opposed by a complete denture as compared to the force that can be exerted when the patient has a natural dentition.

The more the anticipated force on the implant restorations, the more implants should be allowed for.

15.4.4.3 Relationship Between Shape of Residual Ridge and the Dental Arch Form

Three typical arch forms are prevalent, square, ovoid and tapering. The edentulous maxillary residual ridge may also have three arch forms. Aesthetic requirements may require a dental arch different from the residual ridge form. The dental arch form is determined by the final tooth positions in the premaxilla and not from the residual ridge form. The final tooth position may need to be cantilevered to the facial in the definitive prostheses.

In a dental square arch, lateral and central incisors are not cantilevered facially, compared with the canine position. Mandibular excursions and occlusal forces may be reduced on the canine implants. As a result, implants in the canine position may suffice especially if they are splinted to posterior implants. The four pontics between the canines create reduced forces because forces are lowest in the incisor region and the square arch form has less cantilevered occlusal forces to the incisors (Figs. 15.26 and 15.27).

In a dental ovoid arch, there should be three implants in the premaxilla, not two as the square arch form (Figs. 15.28 and 15.29). Sometimes, this may require bone augmentation. For an ovoid dental arch form, planning for implants in the canine positions and at least one additional implant preferably in the central incisor region is important. The additional implant in the incisor region resists the additional forces created by this arch form, and biomechanically, the prosthesis design will be more stable as there will be less stress on the abutment screws.

The restoration of a tapering arch form places the greatest stresses on the anterior implants, especially when the pontics replace the incisors (Figs. 15.30 and 15.31). The anterior teeth are cantilevered facially from the incisor position with increased forces in maximum intercuspation and in excursions. In this case, four implants need to be placed in the premaxilla to replace the six anterior teeth. The worst-case scenario is a patient with a tapered dental arch form to be restored on a square residual ridge form; four implants are then required to compensate for the anterior tooth position. In this case, bone grafting may be required.

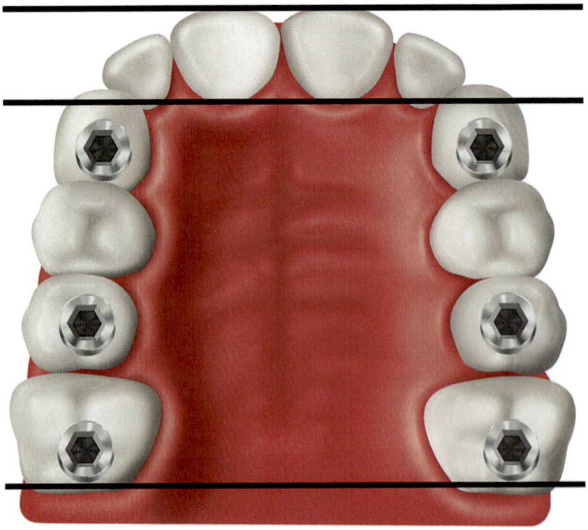

Fig. 15.26 Square arch form necessitating six implants

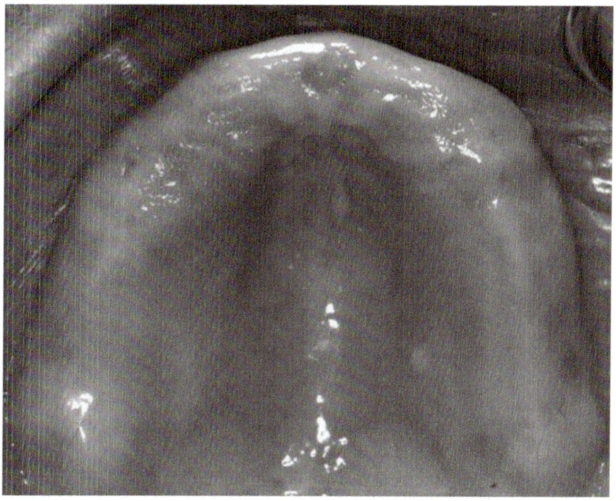

Fig. 15.27 Clinical square arch form

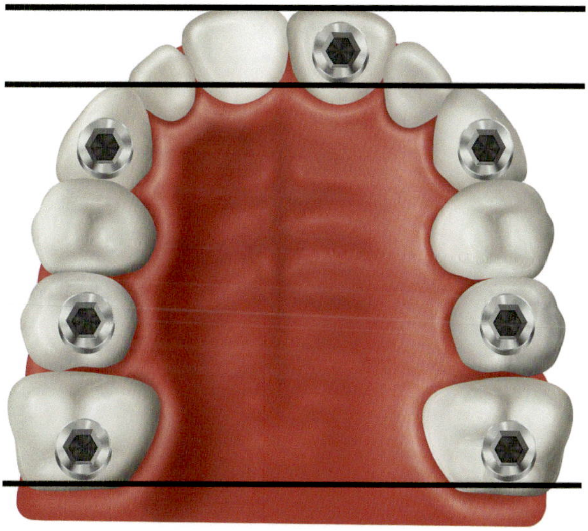

Fig. 15.28 Ovoid arch form; an additional implant is required in the premaxilla to biomechanically stabilize the prosthesis

15.4.5 Implant Distribution

Implant distribution and placement are critical in order to obtain optimum emergence profile for the definitive restorations as well as enable the patient to maintain adequate hygiene. For a patient who presents with minimal resorption and is treatment planned for ceramo-metal or zirconia-based restorations on implants, precise placement of implants is imperative and should be facilitated by the use of a surgical guide based on the diagnostic wax-up. Implants placed in interproximal positions can cause problems from both an aesthetic and hygiene perspective.

For those patients who display moderate resorption but still qualify for a fixed restoration with the use of pink porcelain, implant placement is not critical, but

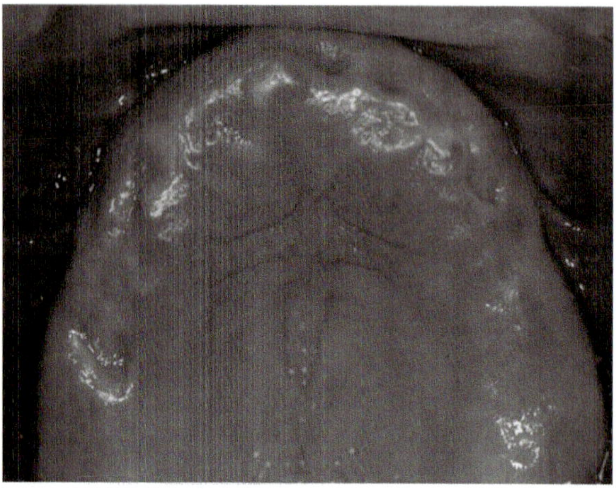

Fig. 15.29 Clinical ovoid arch form

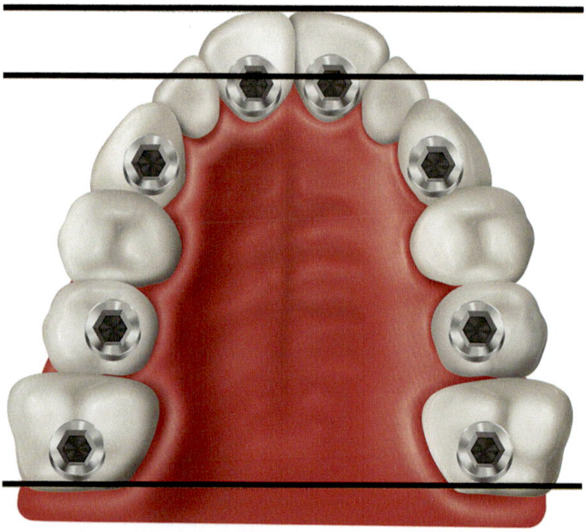

Fig. 15.30 Tapering arch form; an additional two implants are required to stabilize the prosthesis

implant distribution is. Implants placed in interproximal tooth positions will not impact the aesthetics since this will be disguised by the use of pink porcelain. Implant distribution is critical since implants will need to be placed so the load can be shared equitably. Splinting the implants is also advantageous since this improves the biomechanics of the prosthesis design.

In implant-supported overdentures, placement is not critical but distribution is. Implants need to be placed with a sufficient anteroposterior spread so that load can be distributed equitably, and cantilever length minimized.

In implant- and tissue-supported overdentures, both implant placement and distribution become critical. Implants need to be placed so that when a bar is constructed, there is an axis of rotation at the distal aspect of the tissue bar. The

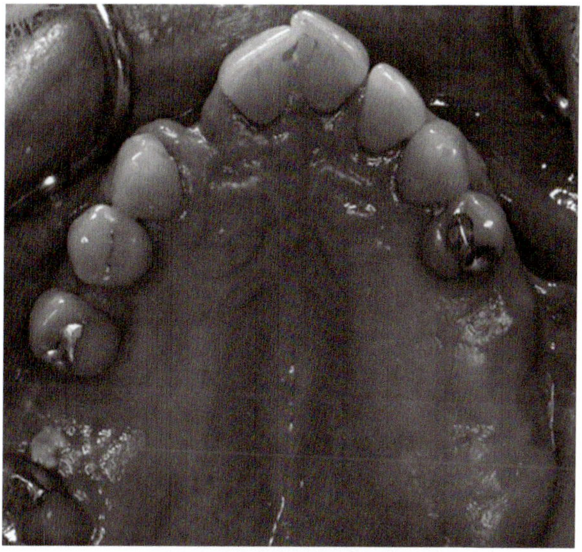

Fig. 15.31 Clinical tapered arch form

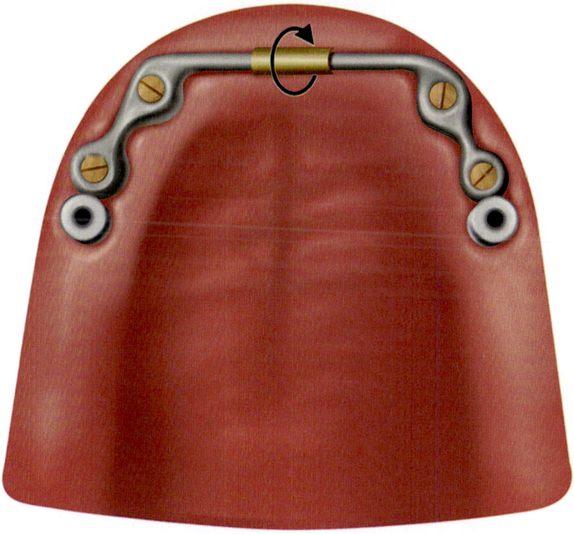

Fig. 15.72 Ideal design of implant- and tissue-supported overdentures; this rests on the anterior bar allows free rotation of the overdenture in the distal axis

distribution of implants should also be such that adequate room is available for the rest. Biomechanically, the AP spread should allow the load to be distributed over a wide area; when occluding over the bar, the load is borne by the implants; when loaded in the posterior, the prosthesis is free to rotate around the distal axis of rotation [19–21]. The anterior rest on the tissue bar serves as an indirect retainer (Fig. 15.72).

15.4.6 Tissue-Fitting Surface

As in any aspect of restorative dentistry, the provisional is key to the success of the definitive restoration. From a patient perspective, the communication of aesthetics and phonetics is important. From a clinician's perspective, biomechanics, occlusion and cleansability are key areas of concern. The original hybrid prostheses were designed to provide a "highwater" design. This was done predominantly to facilitate oral hygiene. Today, patients often complain of food entrapment with these types of designs. The provisional/immediate load prosthesis must satisfy the following criteria:

1. Reduce food entrapment—Following 3 months of healing, the acrylic provisional should be relined so that it compresses the tissue surface and creates a concave tissue surface allowing a convex restoration surface.
2. Provide cleansable contours by developing the tissue as outlined above.
3. Eliminate speech impairment. The t and d sounds relate to the palatal aspects of the maxillary prosthesis, and this area can be adjusted to accommodate for that. The "S" sound is developed utilizing the closest speaking space, and this should also be corrected in the provisional prior to proceeding to the definitive restoration.
4. The tissue contact should be intimate, but accessible to oral hygiene procedures.
5. The tissue surface should be highly polished (Figs. 15.32 and 15.33) [22].

15.4.7 Cost

Restoration of the edentulous maxilla is costly whichever method is used to restore the patient. Fixed reconstructions require more laboratory assistance and implant parts and hence are a lot more expensive.

However, cost needs to be considered not only during fabrication of the prosthesis but also during maintenance. Overdentures seem to have more post-insertion maintenance than their fixed counterparts [23]. If this is consistent, it could be questioned whether an economic indication for choosing an overdenture could be

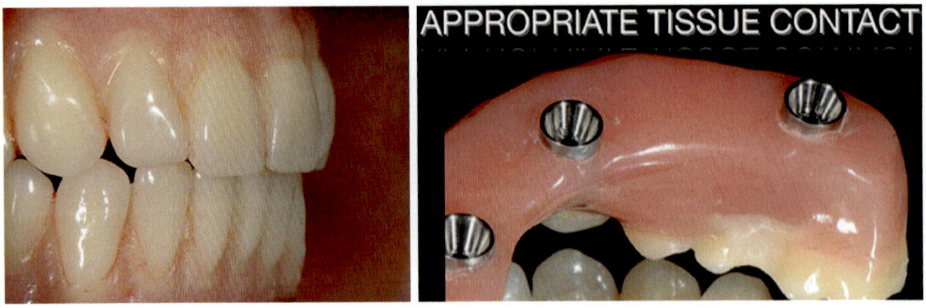

Fig. 15.32 Undersurface of the restoration should be highly polished and convex

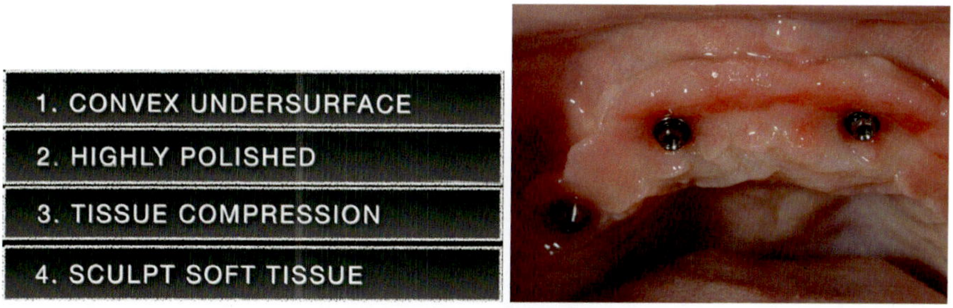

Fig. 15.33 The provisional restoration is used to sculpt the tissue

Fig. 15.34 Maxillary occlusal view

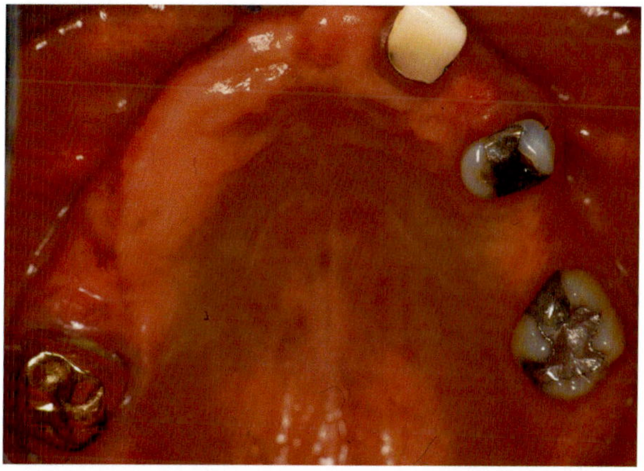

justified when there is sufficient bone to support implants for a fixed prosthesis. The patient must be made aware that maintenance costs for removable prostheses on implants will be higher than that of a fixed prosthesis.

The following case presentations will serve to reinforce diagnosis and treatment planning. Technical details of prosthesis fabrication will also be addressed.

Case 1: Ceramo-Metal Restorations on Implants

This 67-year-old female was seeking replacement of her current removable partial denture with fixed restorations. Her specific complaint was the instability of the denture as well as the class III tooth relationships of her mandibular anterior teeth (Figs. 15.34, 15.35 and 15.36).

On clinical and radiographic examination of teeth, a diagnosis of lack of posterior support was made. There was also insufficient bone in the posterior maxillary and mandibular areas for placement of implant-supported restorations.

The objectives of treatment included providing the patient with implant-supported restorations in both maxilla and mandible as well as orthodontically

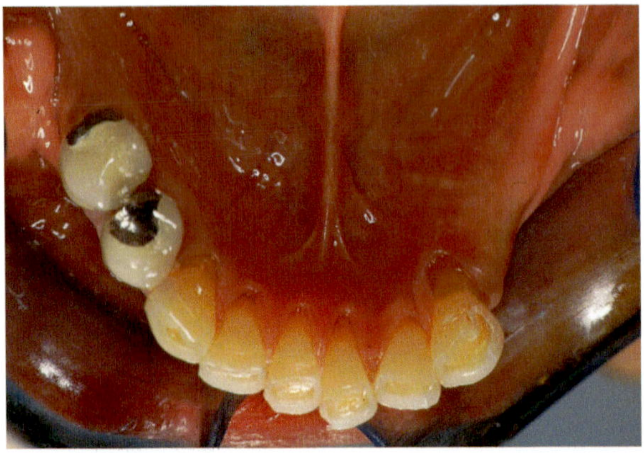

Fig. 15.35 Mandibular occlusal view

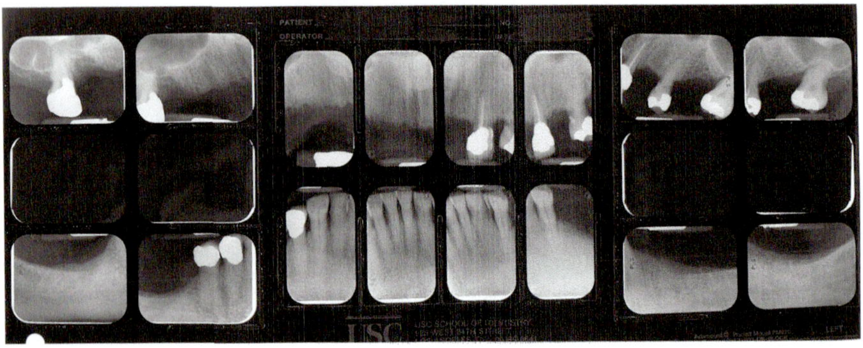

Fig. 15.36 Full-mouth periapical radiographs; note the failing maxillary dentition

retracting the mandibular anterior teeth to provide for a more class I horizontal and vertical tooth relationship.

When significant numbers of teeth are missing, the orthodontist is at a disadvantage because of lack of anchorage to effect the desired tooth movement. The literature has shown that dental implants can be used as anchors for both orthodontic and orthopaedic movement [23–25]. By utilizing an interdisciplinary approach, implants can be used to provide anchorage and then be restored as implant-supported restorations.

Diagnostic evaluation included evaluation of all the factors that had previously been discussed. The treatment plan was to fabricate a fixed ceramo-metal prosthesis supported by implants for the patient.

With these objectives in mind, a treatment plan was formulated which required communication between the surgeon, orthodontist and prosthodontist.

The first stage was to complete a bilateral maxillary sinus lift with bone augmentation as well as onlay grafting of the mandibular posterior sextants.

Implants are usually placed prior to the start of orthodontic treatment, which can be difficult since the post-orthodontic position of the teeth needs to be determined beforehand. An orthodontic set-up was completed on the cast to determine the post-orthodontic position of the teeth (Figs. 15.37 and 15.38). Using this set-up, a surgical template was fabricated to communicate the positioning of the implants to the surgeon (Figs. 15.39 and 15.40). The maxillary and mandibular implants were placed (Figs. 15.41 and 15.42) [24–26]. The implant in position of tooth #21 (mandibular left first premolar) could not be ideally positioned due to the distal root inclination of tooth #22 (mandibular left cuspid).

Once osseointegration had been established, provisional restorations fabricated from polymethyl methacrylate (PMMA) were placed on the implants (Fig. 15.43). These restorations simplified the attachment of the orthodontic appliance, restored occlusal function, improved aesthetics and provided posterior vertical support and served as blueprints for the definitive implant-borne restorations [26].

Orthodontic brackets were attached directly to the provisional restorations using PMMA, and orthodontic treatment was begun immediately. Using nickel titanium wires, a sustained orthodontic load was applied to effect lingual movement of teeth #22 (33), #23 (32), #24 (31), #25 (30) and #26 (42) (Fig. 15.44). On completion of orthodontic treatment, a second set of provisional restorations were fabricated since the vertical and horizontal relationships of the anterior teeth were now a more class I relationship (Fig. 15.45). Placement of the definitive restorations was facilitated by the existing provisional restorations; these restorations were used to communicate

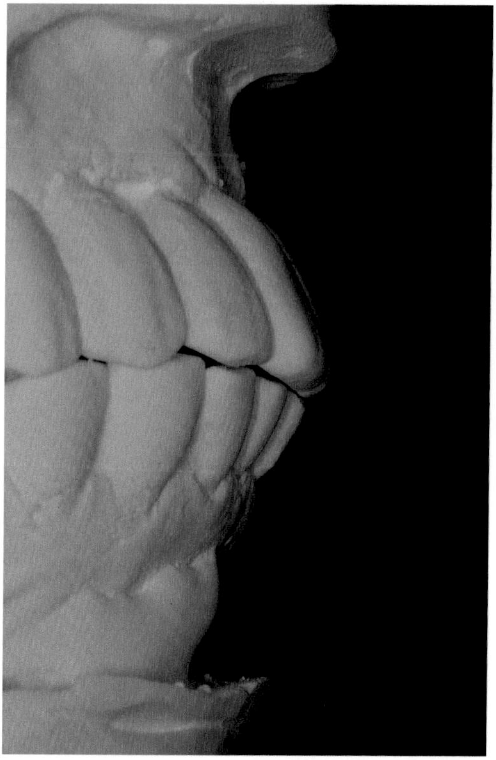

Fig. 15.37 Pre-orthodontic casts

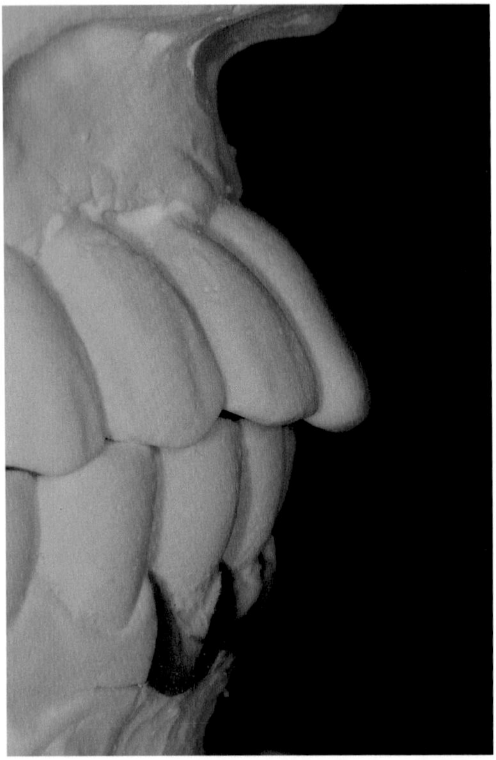

Fig. 15.38 Orthodontic set-up on casts illustrating lingual position of mandibular incisors

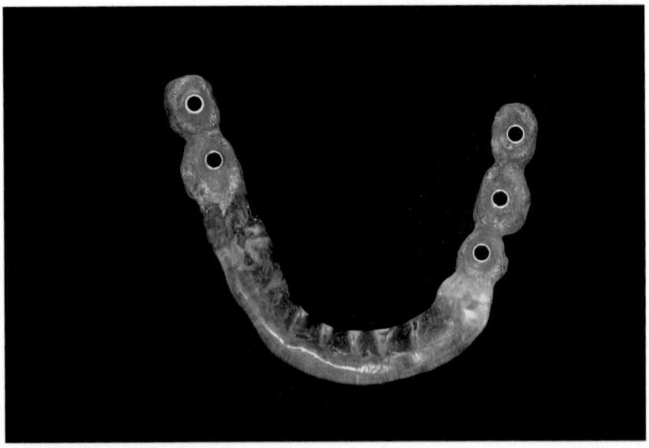

Fig. 15.39 Mandibular surgical guide

aesthetic and functional information to both patient and laboratory technician for a predictable outcome (Figs. 15.46, 15.47, 15.48 and 15.49).

A summary of treatment planning considerations is listed below.

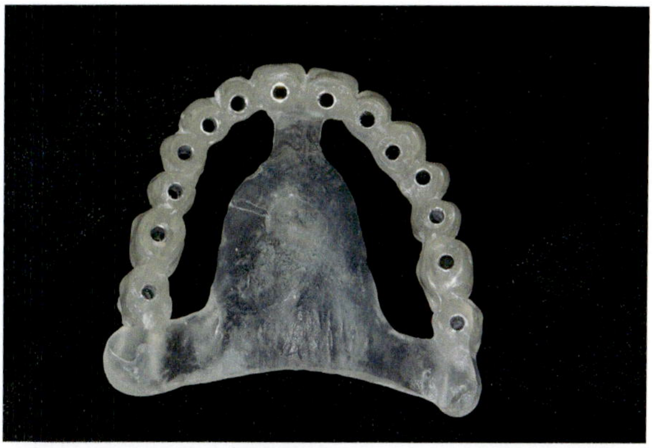

Fig. 15.40 Maxillary surgical guide

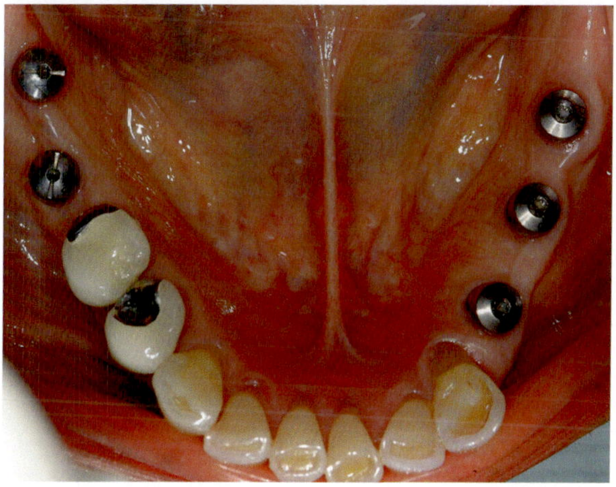

Fig. 15.41 Mandibular implant placement

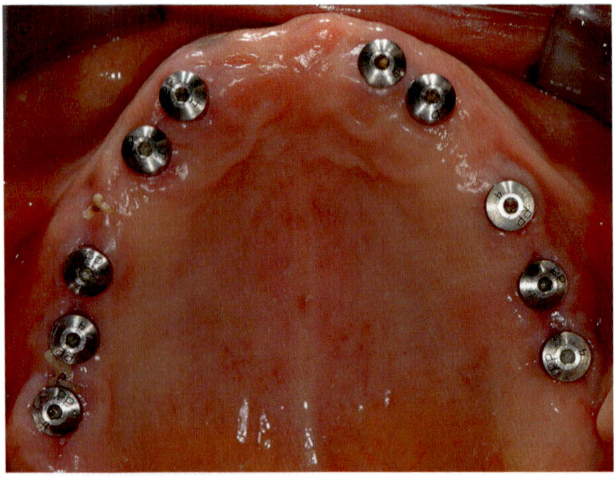

Fig. 15.42 Maxillary implant placement

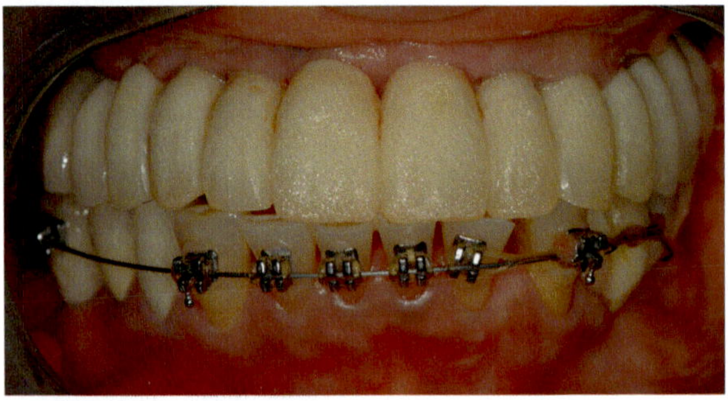

Fig. 15.43 First set of provisional restorations

Fixed ceramo-metal prosthesis	Treatment planning
Aesthetics	Patient has adequate facial and lip support
Type of support	Implant supported
Resorption and inter-arch space	Minimal resorption, 10 mm inter-arch space
Number of implants	Minimum 6 if bone quality and arch form adequate
Implant placement and distribution	Critical
Cost	Most expensive

Case 2: Zirconia Prostheses with Pink Ceramic

A 33-year-old gentleman presented with a failing dentition. He was on multiple medications that resulted in a reduction in salivary flow. His request was to obtain

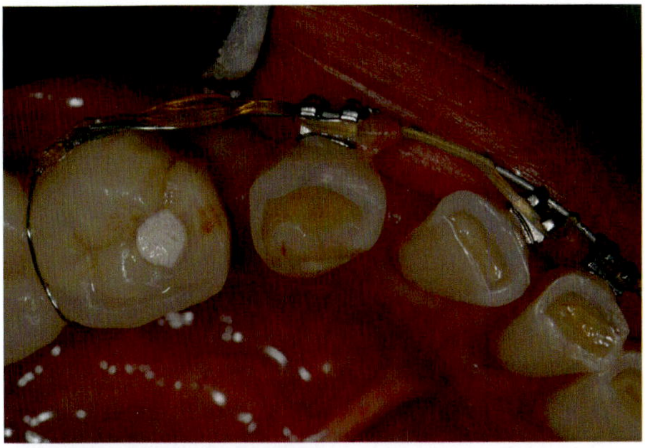

Fig. 15.44 Occlusal view showing retraction of mandibular anterior teeth

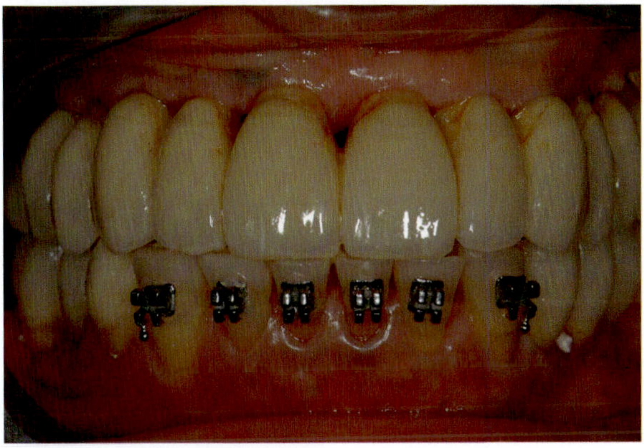

Fig. 15.45 Second set of provisional restorations; patient complained of black triangle between maxillary central incisors; this was to be modified in the final prosthesis

fixed permanent restorations on dental implants. He had an important life event in 4–6 weeks and requested a fixed restoration on dental implants during that period.

A thorough clinical evaluation was performed.

The following observations were made:

1. Pneumatized sinuses posterior to first premolars
2. Severe wear on his teeth
3. Irregular mandibular occlusal plane
4. Lack of posterior support
5. Mandibular molars with vertical fracture and of poor prognosis

The key decision-making parameters in this patient were the following:

1. **How many implants should be placed in the maxilla?**

   The patient presented with severe wear, large masseters and a history of sleep apnoea. It is the author's opinion that adhering to a specific treatment protocol

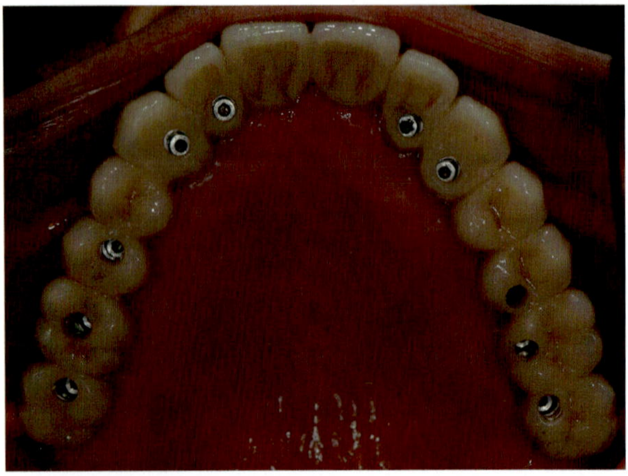

Fig. 15.46 Occlusal view of maxillary provisional restorations

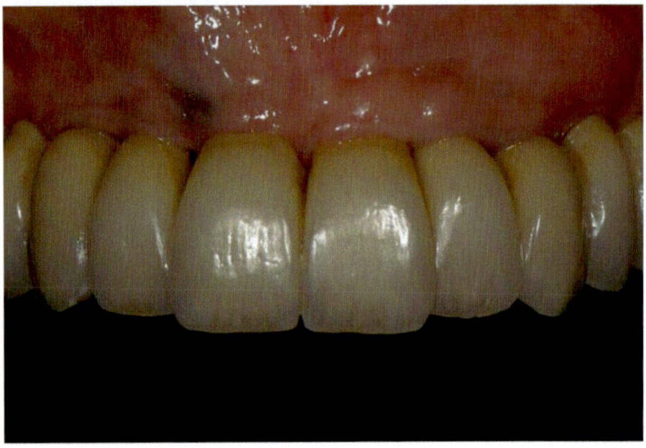

Fig. 15.47 Maxillary anterior view of completed restorations

involving placement of four implants would not be insufficient in terms of stress distribution and anteroposterior spread.

2. **Should the patient be grafted or should zygomatic implants be placed?**

   The patient is in his early 30s. Currently, there is sufficient bone to place implants utilizing a tilted protocol in the first premolars. This would allow the cantilever of one additional tooth. In patients who have signs of excessive force on their teeth, cantilevers should be avoided. The decision to increase the AP spread would require either bilateral sinus lifts and bone augmentation or zygomatic implants on each side. Both approaches would be clinically acceptable. It was decided to pursue the route of bilateral sinus lifts due to the patient's age. During the interim phase, a fixed provisional could still be provided on four implants, thus satisfying the patient's concerns.

3. **How do we address the mandibular occlusal plane?**

   The first molars were to be extracted in favour of implant placement. Orthodontics to correct the mandibular occlusal plane would be discussed with the patient to harmonize the anterior guidance.

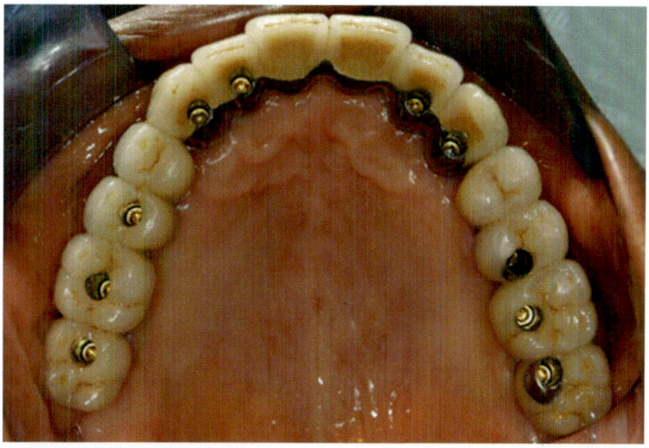

Fig. 15.48 Maxillary occlusal view of completed restorations

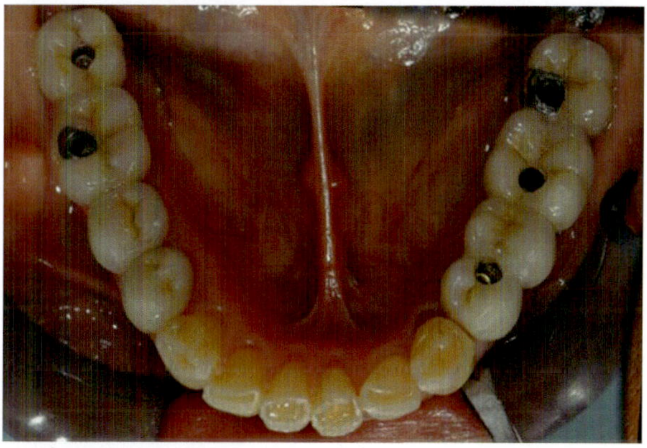

Fig. 15.49 Mandibular occlusal view of completed restorations

Prosthodontic Diagnosis

1. Incisal edge position—On clinical examination, there was insufficient display of the maxillary incisal edge. The occlusal plane was also canted to the patient's right. Teeth in the mandibular arch had over-erupted because of no occlusal contact (Figs. 15.50 and 15.51).
2. Restorative space—The treatment plan included a minimally layered zirconia restoration.
3. Lip support—The patient's lip was well supported.
4. Smile line—The patient had a low smile line, and this would not pose a problem in hiding the transition zone.
5. Contours and emergence—Space creation to develop appropriate contours, and emergence was required.
6. Tissue contact—Following extraction of the teeth and creation of adequate restorative space, shaping the restorative contours for a convex undersurface is attainable. The provisional restorations were to be used to compress the tissue and create a concave tissue surface.

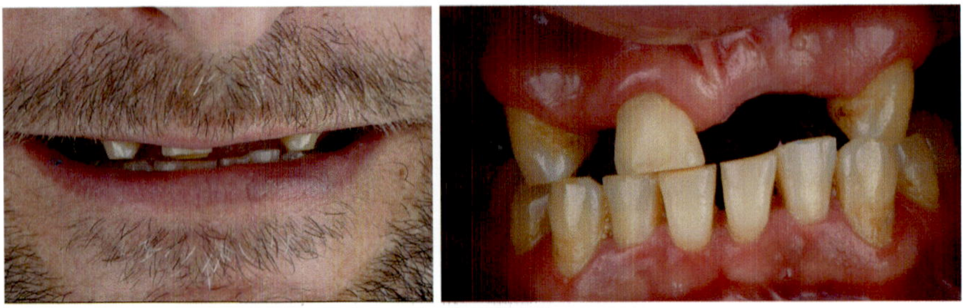

Fig. 15.50 Preoperative situation of patient desiring implant-supported restorations

Fig. 15.51 Patient's smile

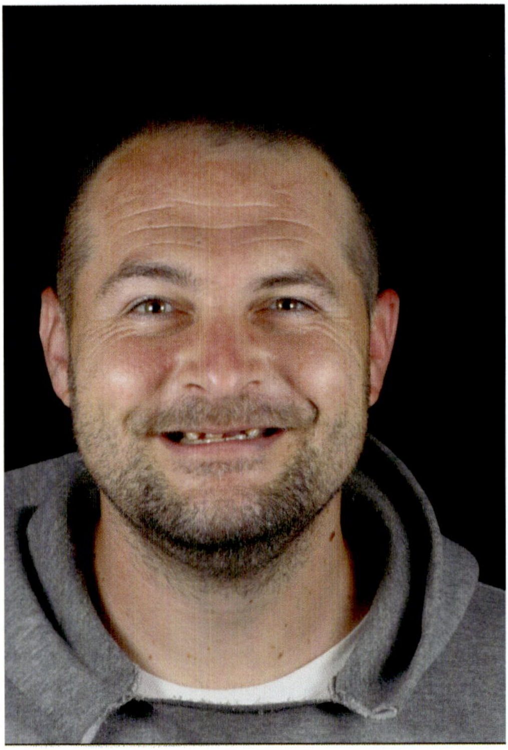

7. Occlusion—Occlusion must be addressed in the immediate load provisional to protect the implants in the weakest quality bone from excessive loads. In the definitive restoration, occlusion must be organized to distribute the loads over a wide an area as possible.

Surgical Evaluation

Clinical evaluation of patient showed excessive wear, vertical cracks in the mandibular first molars and lack of restorative space. Patient had a low lip line and long

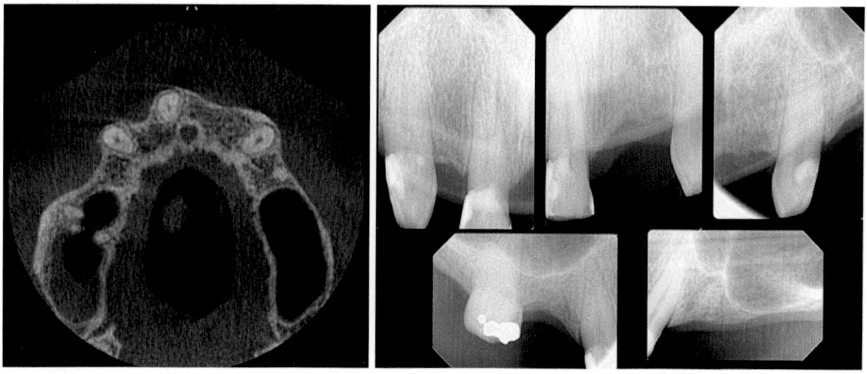

Fig. 15.52 Radiographs and CBCT section showing pneumatized sinuses

lip. One millimetre of gingival show on maximal smiling was noted. Gingival tissues were healthy.

Radiographic and CT evaluation of patient showed pneumatized sinuses posterior to maxillary first premolars and inadequate buccolingual width in the anterior maxilla where teeth had been extracted (Fig. 15.52). The mandible showed sufficient bone in width and height for implant placement in the mandibular molar region.

Surgical Treatment Plan

Space: The lack of inter-arch space in this case will have to be managed through minor bone reduction in the maxilla. This is done to create space for the zirconia-based restoration. Bone reduction is also done to ensure that there is an adequate buccolingual width of bone for implant placement. Bilateral sinus lifts and bone augmentation would be executed at the same time. The goal was to provide additional sites for dental implant placement. In the mandible, the first molars would be extracted, and implants placed immediately and allowed to integrate prior to restoration.

Spread: Four implants would be placed in the maxilla. The distal implants would be tilted to maximize the anteroposterior spread as much as possible.

Stability: The patient exhibits sufficient bone volume in the anterior maxilla as well as mandible. There are no large defects noted; therefore, underprepared osteotomies with gradual enlargement of the preparations will be undertaken. An aggressively threaded implant design will be utilized.

Surgical Treatment

The patient was treated in an office setting. Local anaesthesia supplemented with a very mild sedation was utilized. All maxillary teeth except those indexed by the surgical stent were removed. Surgical stent was indexed on the remaining maxillary teeth, and bone was reduced to allow for at least 12 mm of inter-arch space in the maxillary arch. The remaining teeth were removed, and the maxillary arch was recontoured as minimally as possible to provide sufficient width for implant

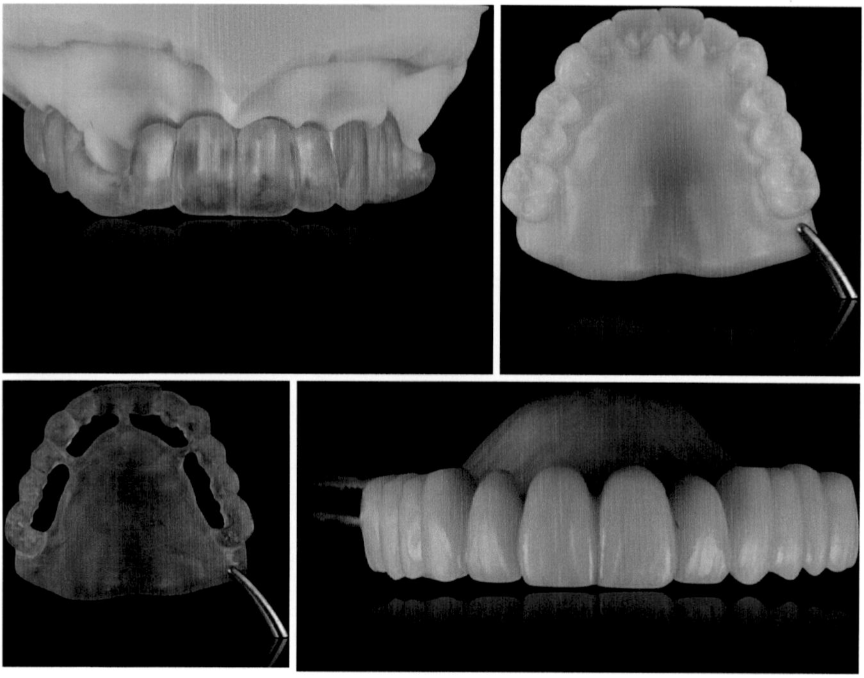

Fig. 15.53 Digital workup and milling of surgical guides and provisional restoration

placement. Bilateral sinus lifts were performed, and bone augmentation was completed. First molars were extracted in the mandible and single implants placed immediately. All implants in the maxilla were inserted at torque value of no less than 35 N. Multi-unit abutments were placed, and primary closure was achieved. A provisional fixed acrylic prosthesis was fabricated immediately following the surgical phase of treatment and secured to the implants on the day of surgical implant placement. Patient tolerated the anaesthesia and dental procedures very well and healed uneventfully. Post-graft healing additional implants were placed in the maxillary molar region.

Prosthodontic Sequence

The patient was scanned, and provisional restorations and surgical guides were milled (Fig. 15.53). Provisional restorations were fabricated at the correct vertical dimension for a direct pickup procedure. Vertical dimension was determined prior to implant placement and a record taken. Bone reduction guides were fabricated to communicate restorative space required.

A direct technique for immediate loading was employed, mounted and processed, and finished in the laboratory. The prostheses were adjusted to leave a 1 mm space between the prostheses and the tissue. Occlusion was adjusted for shimstock hold on the anterior teeth and shimstock drag on the posterior teeth. This is not scientifically based but designed on the basis of biomechanical principles. The further back the implants are placed in the maxilla, the poorer the quality of bone. The

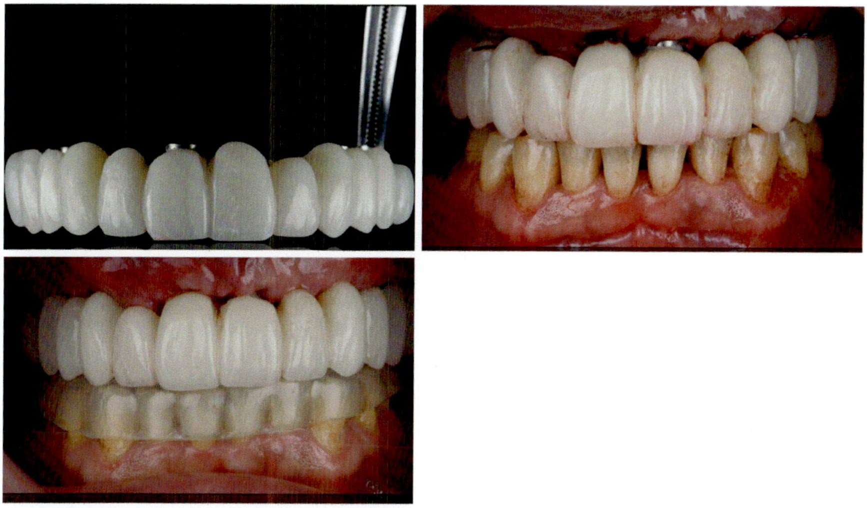

Fig. 15.54 Day of surgery; four dental implants are placed anterior to the sinus. Bilateral sinus lifts and bone augmentation completed. Provisionals loaded on four implants

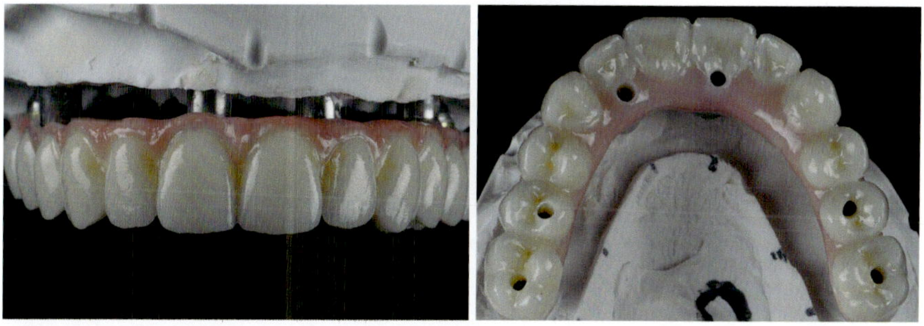

Fig. 15.55 Additional two implants placed in sinus bone graft and integrated. Definitive zirconia restoration fabricated on six implants

further back the occlusion, the higher the occlusal forces. It is the author's recommendation to limit the load on posterior teeth in immediate load full-arch restorations. Vertical dimension was verified on the delivery of the restoration. A soft night guard was provided post-surgery (Fig. 15.54). The patient was referred to an orthodontist to correct the mandibular occlusal plane whilst the grafts were healing and implants integrating.

Splinted open-tray impressions, jaw relation records and a trial restoration were inserted to verify aesthetics and phonetics.

The trial restoration was utilized to fabricate an acrylic prototype utilizing CAD software. Computer-aided milling was performed.

The definitive restorations included a minimally layered zirconia-based maxillary restoration with layered pink ceramics (Fig. 15.55).

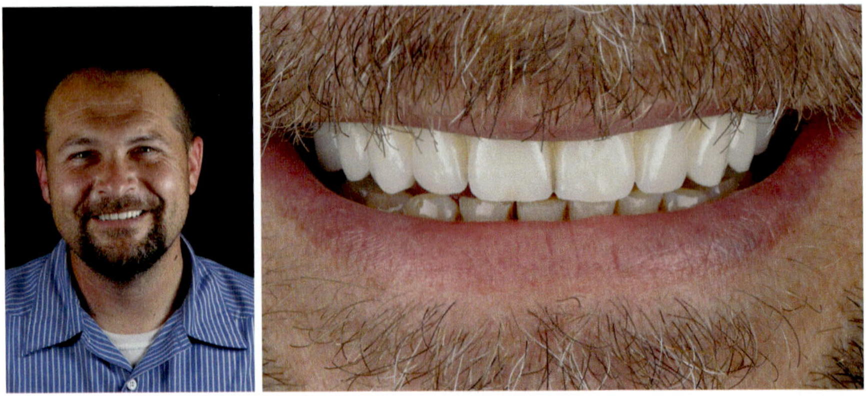

Fig. 15.56 Smile view

Fig. 15.57 Intraoral view of definitive restorations and corrected mandibular occlusal plane

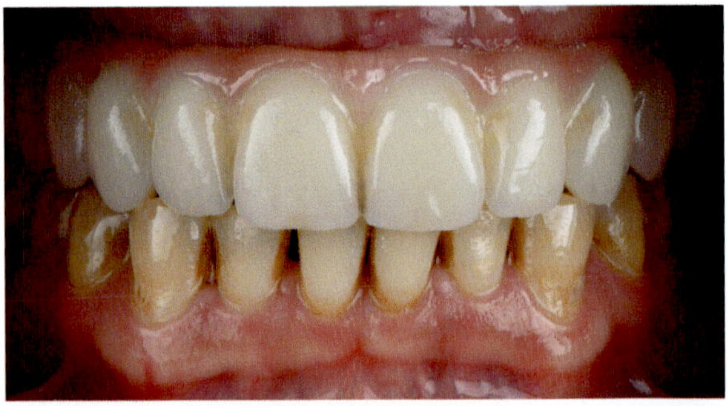

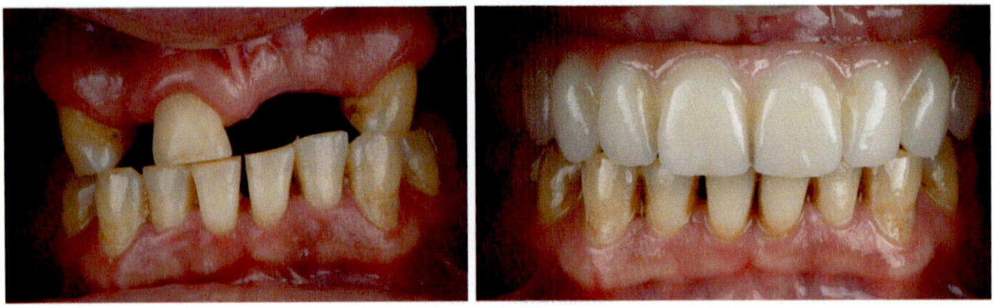

Fig. 15.58 Before and after

The prosthesis was delivered adjusting the undersurface to ensure positive pressure. Dynamic occlusion was adjusted for canine guidance. Static occlusion was adjusted to ensure shimstock hold on canines and premolars. Shimstock drag can occur on anterior teeth. Single-tooth monolithic restorations were fabricated for implants in the mandibular first molar regions (Figs. 15.56, 15.57, 15.58 and 15.59).

Screws were torqued according to the manufacturer's specifications, and access holes were sealed using Teflon and composite resin.

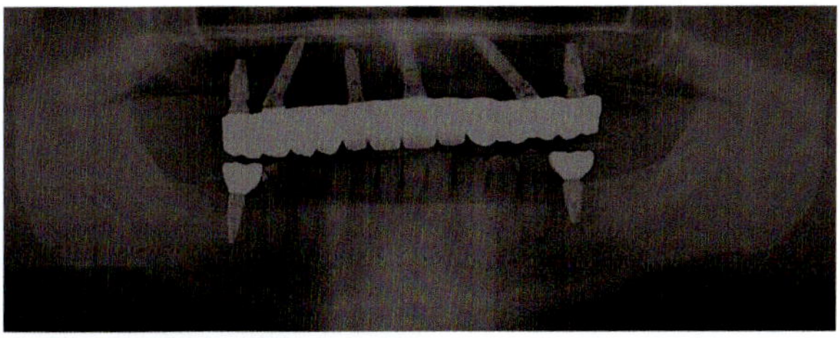
Fig. 15.59 Final panoramic radiograph

A night-time appliance was provided, and maintenance instructions were provided.

This particular case highlights diagnosis and treatment planning. The clinician is faced with a choice of grafting or graft-less. Both approaches would be acceptable. Grafting is still a useful treatment modality and should not be disregarded. Often, clinicians espouse to a totally graft-less practice and will not graft under any circumstance. This approach should be avoided. The patient deserves to be made aware of the treatment options available, advantages and disadvantages, longevity and possible complications that may arise.

The clinician should be astute in diagnosis and treatment planning to provide the patient with a course of treatment that is rational and biomechanically sound and has every possible chance of success.

Fixed zirconia prosthesis with pink ceramic	Treatment planning
Aesthetics	Patient has adequate facial and lip support
Type of support	Implant supported
Resorption and inter-arch space	Moderate resorption, >10 mm inter-arch space
Number of implants	Minimum 6 if bone quality and arch form adequate
Implant placement and distribution	Placement not critical, distribution is
Cost	Most expensive

Case 3: Implant-Supported Overdenture

Implant-supported overdentures are fabricated when excessive tissue defects prevent the use of a fixed prosthesis or when the quality and/or the amount of bone will not permit the ideal placement of the implants to provide adequate support for a fixed restoration.

Overdentures may be implant supported or implant retained, and tissue supported.

Space requirements for implant-supported overdentures are greater than that of fixed restorations on implants. A minimum of 13 mm of space from the opposing dentition is needed. This space is required for the metal framework, heat-processed acrylic resin and prosthetic tooth.

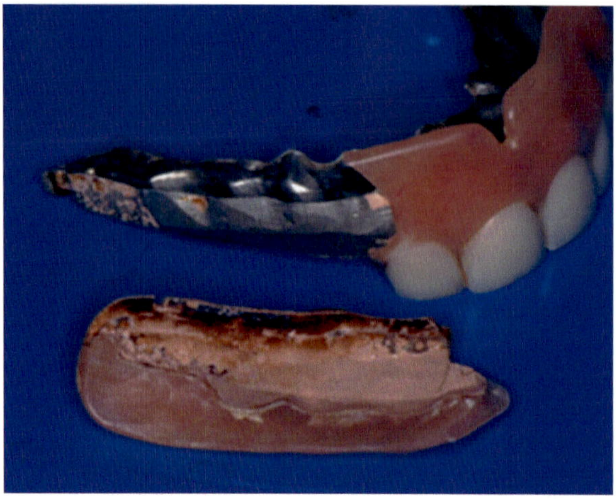

Fig. 15.60 Acrylic resin fracturing off framework. This is quite common in implant-supported overdentures

As far as implant number and position are concerned, a minimum of six implants well distributed around the arch is recommended. Other factors influencing the number of implants utilized will include bone quality and dental arch form. An advantage of overdentures is that facial support can be provided with the flange, and implant placement is not so critical. One disadvantage with implant-supported overdentures is the maintenance required. Often, patients can exert far greater forces with an implant-supported denture, and this can result in the acrylic resin fracturing off the framework (Fig. 15.60).

A 45-year-old male presented with a failing maxillary implant-supported denture. The primary bar had worn, and the prosthesis was lacking in retention. The prosthesis had also worn and was fractured in multiple areas. The patient was treatment planned for a spark erosion-type prosthesis. This type of restoration incorporates a primary bar and an overlying suprastructure, which is housed in the denture. Implant impressions were made, and jaw relations and a tooth try-in were performed. Aesthetics, phonetics and lip support were verified. The bar was fabricated utilizing spark erosion technology. This bar had a 2-degree taper and incorporated receptacles for a swivel latch attachment, and additional auxiliary retention was also included. A superstructure was spark eroded to fit on top of the framework and allow precision locking of the swivel lock into the receptacle incorporated in the bar. Following silicoating, a denture wax-up was processed onto the bar using heat-processed acrylic resin. With a sufficient number of implants, support does not have to be gained from the palate, and the patient can benefit from greater perception of taste and temperature change (Figs. 15.61, 15.62, 15.63, 15.64, 15.65, 15.66, 15.67, 15.68, 15.69, 15.70 and 15.71).

Implant-supported overdenture	Treatment planning
Aesthetics	Flange required for adequate lip and facial support
Type of support	Implant supported
Resorption and inter-arch space	Severe resorption 13–15 mm inter-arch space

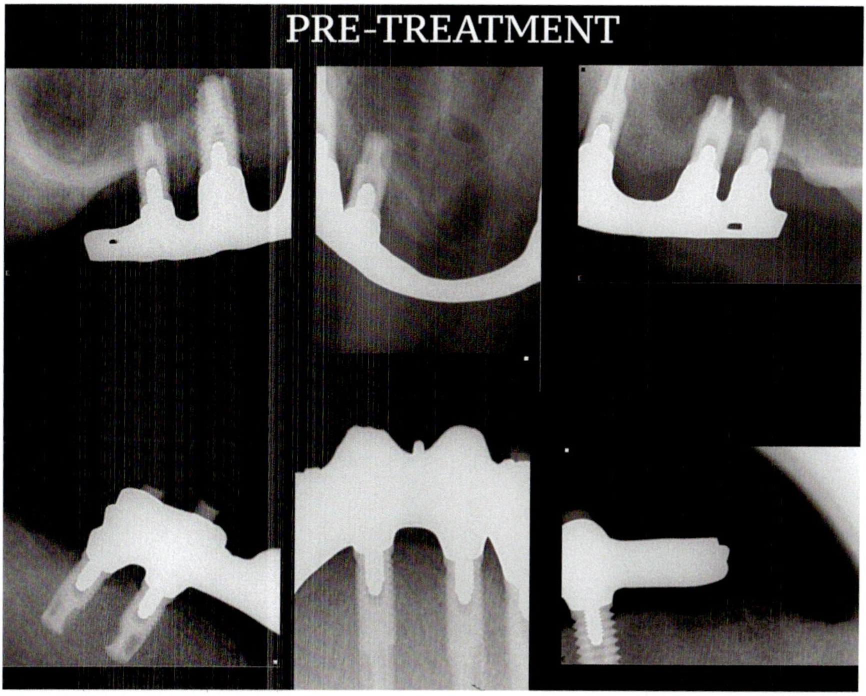

Fig. 15.61 Radiographs of implant and implant bar in situ

Implant-supported overdenture	Treatment planning
Number of implants	Minimum 6 if bone quality and arch form adequate
Implant placement and distribution	Implants should be well distributed
Cost	Less expensive than ceramo-metal prostheses. More maintenance costs

Case 4: Implant- and Tissue-Supported Overdenture

When designing implant overdentures for the maxilla, a configuration of implant placement/bar design is required which will require free rotation of the prostheses.

In the maxilla, a minimum of four implants is required. Even with the use of four implants, it is advised to gain support from the palate. Space requirements are like implant-supported overdentures with 13–15 mm being required. Implant placement requires a straight line connection between the anterior two implants, so a bar can be fabricated. This bar should not encroach on the palate as this may result in increased bulk of the denture in this area that may subsequently affect speech. Patients accepting this type of prosthesis should be warned ahead of time that there will be resiliency associated with the prosthesis on biting down. Patients going

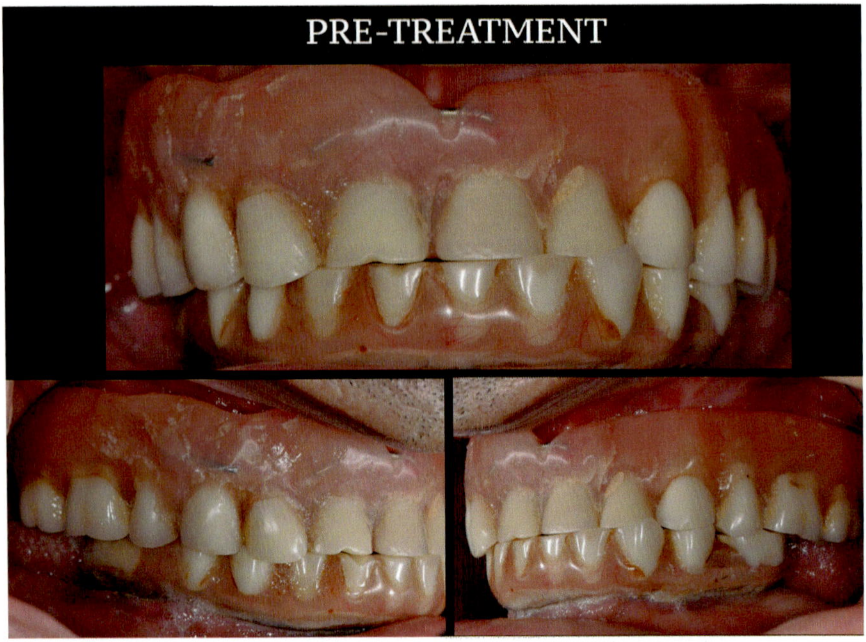

Fig. 15.62 Failing maxillary and mandibular prosthesis. Note fracture and wear

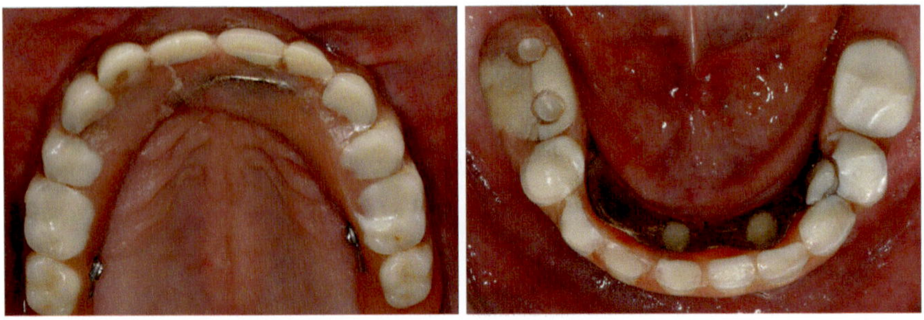

Fig. 15.63 Occlusal view demonstrating wear

through extensive therapy often have unrealistic expectations and may be better off with additional implant placement and fabrication of a fully implant-supported restoration.

Use of more than two implants complicates the design of the overdenture in that sometimes the bar configuration does not allow free rotation of the prostheses.

ERA attachments are positioned adjacent to the distal implants. These attachments permit the overlying prosthesis to be compressed into the mucoperiosteum in the extension areas. As a result, the denture-bearing tissues absorb the occlusal forces (Fig. 15.72) [27]. The clip needs to be non-retentive, so the denture is free to rotate around the axis of the ERA attachments. Sometimes, when this rotation is not

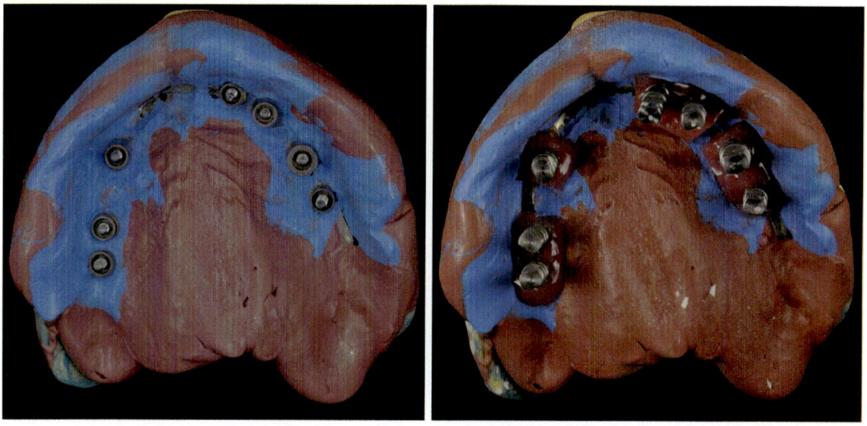

Fig. 15.64 Impressions at fixture level and implant analogues attached

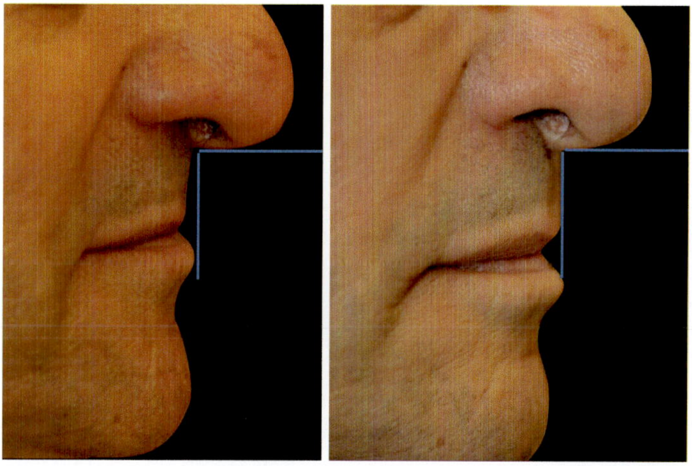

Fig. 15.65 Lip support with and without wax try-in in place

allowed, damage to the clip results. In this instance, the anterior clip provided indirect retention (Figs. 15.73 and 15.74) [28].

A 52-year-old male presented requesting increased stability of his maxillary denture. All treatment options were offered to the patient. As a result of lack of facial support and limited finances, an implant-retained and tissue-supported overdenture was treatment planned.

Four implants were placed; these implants maximized the anteroposterior spread. A cast bar was fabricated and verified for passive fit on the implants. The configuration of the bar was such that it would allow free rotation of the overlying prosthesis. Once passive fit was confirmed, a master cast was fabricated by picking up the bar

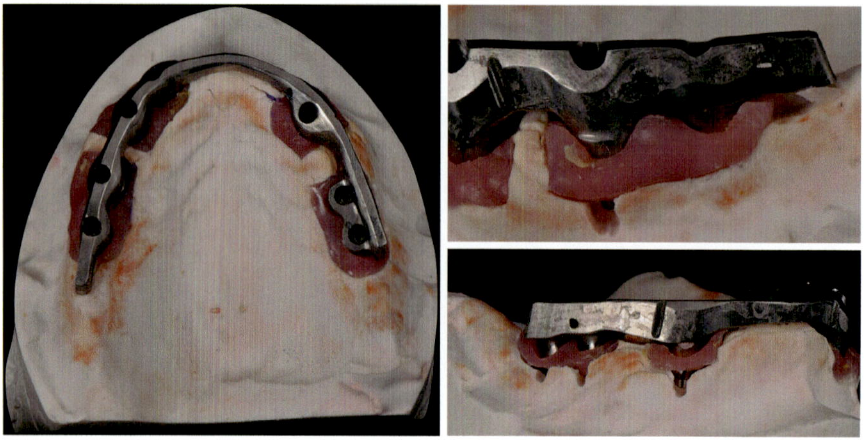

Fig. 15.66 Maxillary bar with retention mechanism

Fig. 15.67 Diagram illustrating that two types of retention mechanism are incorporated into implant-supported bars. There are receptacles for the swivel latches and vertical cylindrical slots to help stabilize the prosthesis

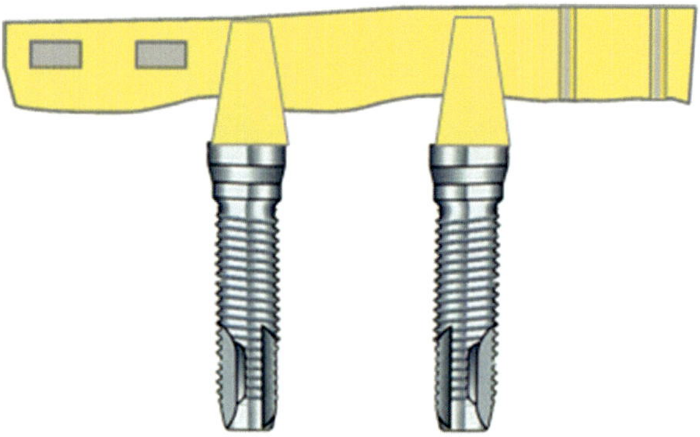

in a border-moulded impression. A cast framework was supported by the bar onto which heat-cured acrylic resin was processed (Figs. 15.75, 15.76, 15.77 and 15.78).

Implant-supported overdenture	Treatment planning
Aesthetics	Flange required for adequate lip and facial support
Type of support	Implant and tissue supported
Resorption and inter-arch space	Severe resorption 13–15 mm inter-arch space
Number of implants	Minimum 4
Implant placement and distribution	Implants should be well distributed
Cost	Less expensive than ceramo-metal prostheses. More maintenance costs

Implant rehabilitation of the edentulous maxilla is one of the most challenging endeavours facing the restorative dentist. Comprehensive evaluation and precise evaluation of the patient's needs, followed by appropriate treatment planning, provide the restorative dentist with the platform to satisfy patient expectations [15].

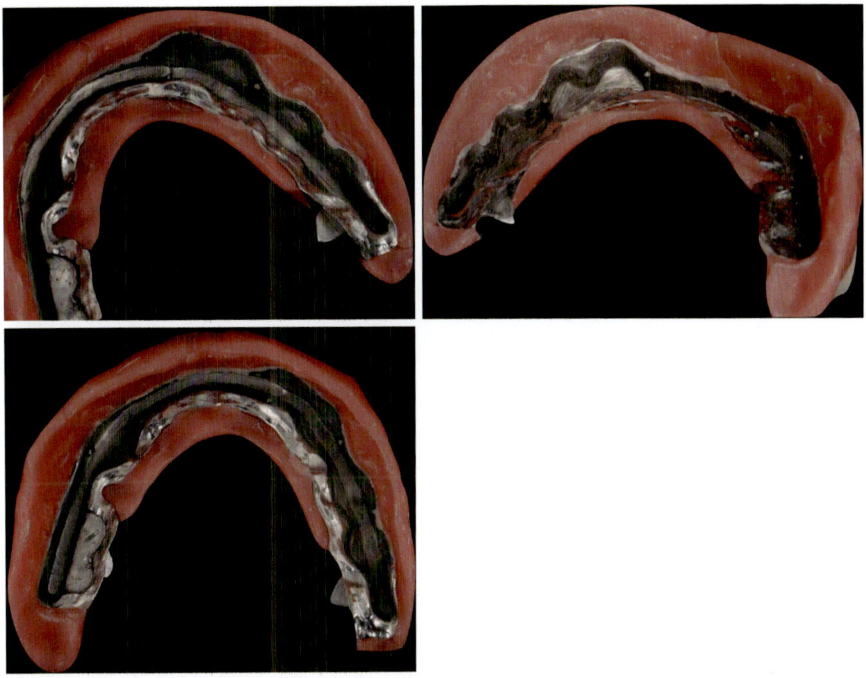

Fig. 15.68 Intaglio of prosthesis demonstrating suprastructure; note the swivel latches in the posterior and vertical resistance pins distributed throughout the restoration

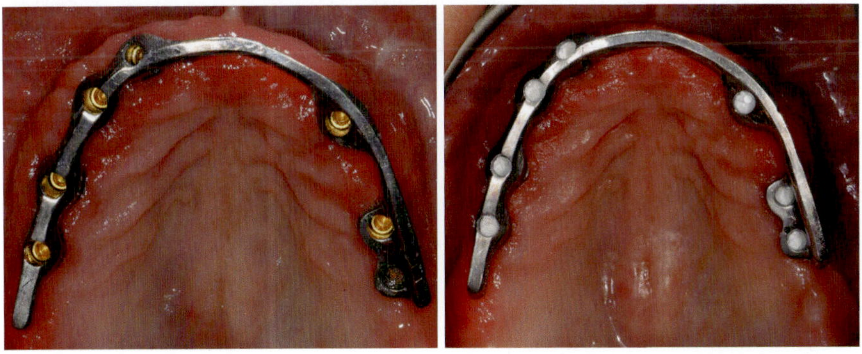

Fig. 15.69 Bar in situ

Communication is required between restorative dentist and surgeon to ensure optimal placement of implants. Only with precision in implant placement can aesthetics in the final prosthesis be provided (Fig. 15.79).

Patient's transitioning from a complete denture to a fixed reconstruction will have high expectations, and clear communication is critical at the outset so that realistic expectations are set, and patients' objectives are met. Nothing is more

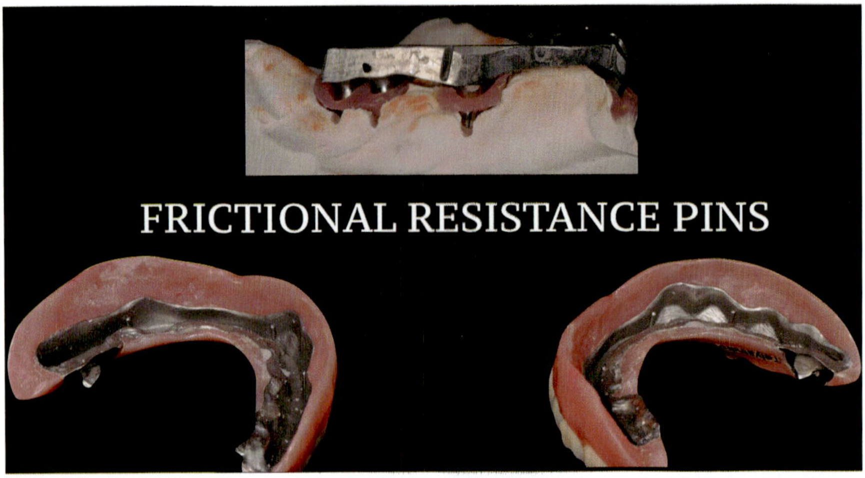

Fig. 15.70 Demonstration of frictional resistance pins and intaglio of prosthesis

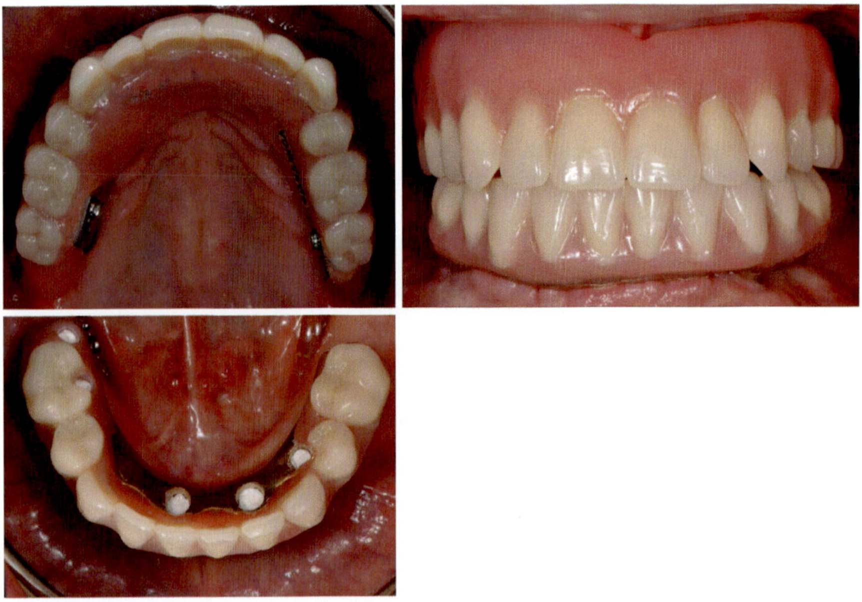

Fig. 15.71 Definitive prostheses in situ. Maxillary implant-supported removable overdenture. Mandibular fixed implant-supported denture/hybrid

disappointing for both patient and clinician going through a lengthy expensive treatment only to have a less than optimal outcome.

Whether planning for a fixed or removable prosthesis, attention to detail is required at every step. When all sequences of treatment are executed appropriately,

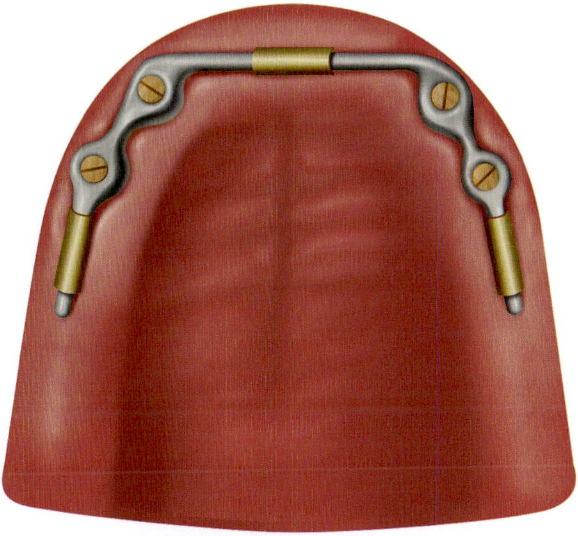

Fig. 15.73 This design will not allow free rotation of the overdenture. The clips will require regular maintenance

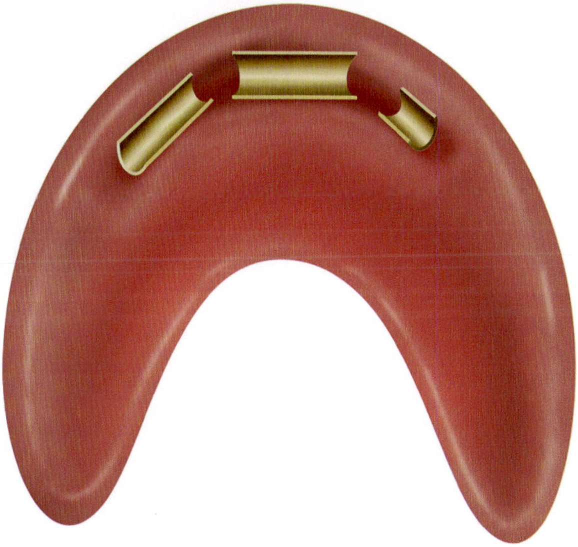

Fig. 15.74 Internal of overdenture; this distribution of clips will not allow rotation of the overdenture and will not allow equitable distribution of support between the implants and the mucosa

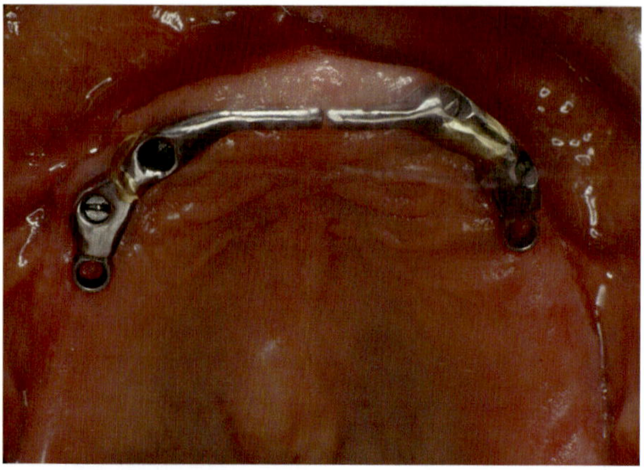

Fig. 15.75 Occlusal view showing implant bar; often, this bar is made in two sections, joined intraorally and soldered. Note the distal ERA attachments

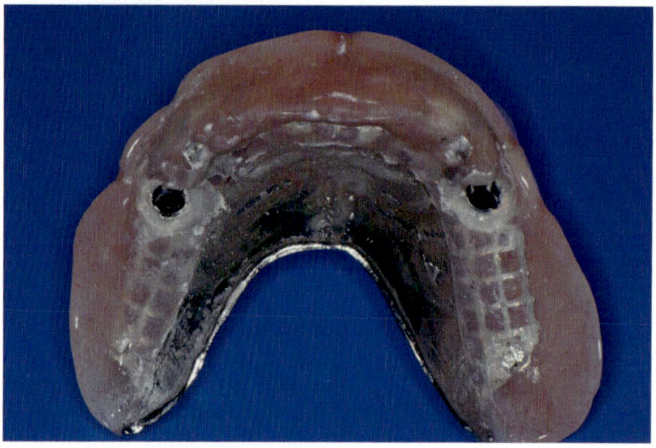

Fig. 15.76 The maxillary denture is fabricated with spacers for the ERA attachments. Note that the support is also required from the palate

implant rehabilitation of the edentulous maxilla is one of the most gratifying procedures for both the restorative dentist and the patient.

Case 5: Zirconia Restorations on Implants Replacing a Tooth-Only Defect with Bilateral Sinus Lifts

The following patient presentation illustrates the philosophy of minimally invasive implant therapy for full-arch implant rehabilitation utilizing digital technologies.

A 62-year-old female presented seeking a solution to her failing maxillary dentition. Her teeth had been compromised due to periodontal disease. She also presented with a previous history of dental implant failure (Figs. 15.80 and 15.81).

On clinical and radiographic examination, her maxillary dentition was deemed to be of poor prognosis. She had an inadequate amount of bone in the maxillary left quadrant due to bone loss and pneumatization of the maxillary sinus. The patient was treatment planned for maxillary full-arch implant rehabilitation with sinus bone augmentation in her maxillary left quadrant.

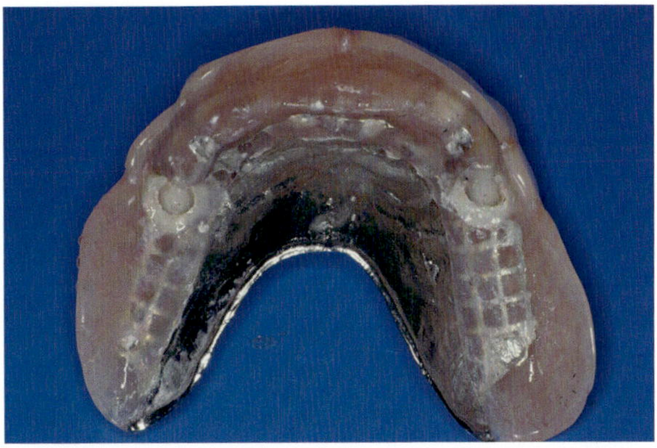

Fig. 15.77 The spacers are removed, and the attachments are picked up in the mouth; space is also created to allow free rotation of the denture around the anterior clip

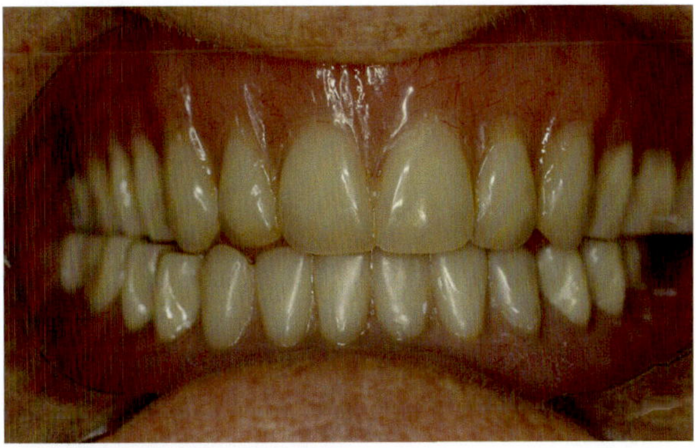

Fig. 15.78 Final maxillary denture intraorally; this denture is implant and mucosa supported

The patient's concerns were the following:

1. She did not want to wear a removable appliance at any point during the treatment process.
2. She wanted the teeth to look and feel like her own.
3. She wanted teeth back to the second molar.

Considerations in implementing care were the following:

1. History of periodontal disease and previous implant failure
2. History of diabetes
3. Preservation of bone
4. Being able to provide implant bridgework which resembles her existing dentition without pink ceramics
5. Transitioning the patient with fixed restoration during the entire treatment process

The above considerations required a more cautious approach in treatment planning and execution. Immediate loading of the implants was eliminated in favour of

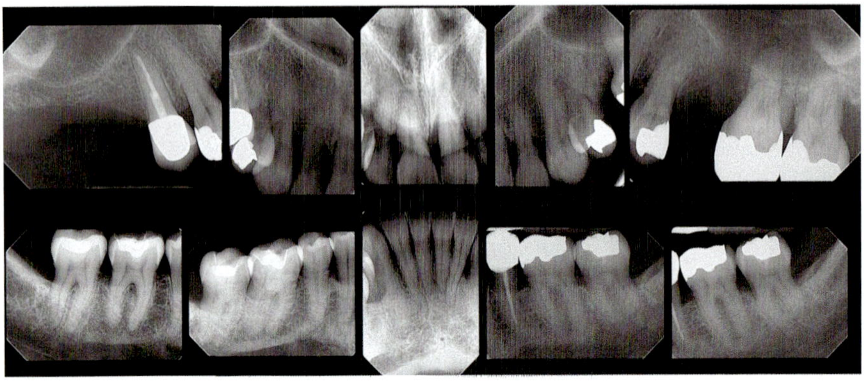

Fig. 15.79 Preoperative radiographs

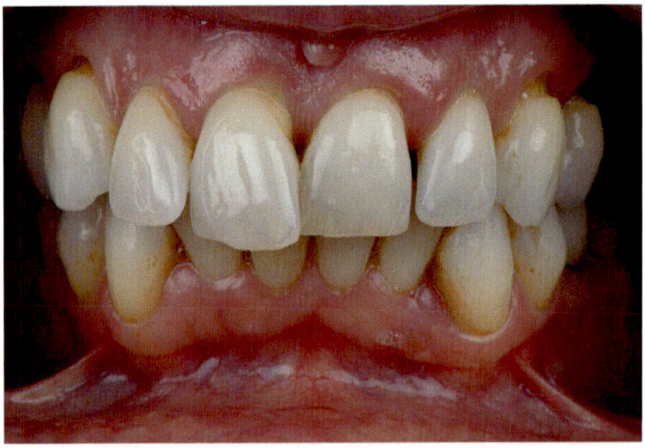

Fig. 15.80 Buccal view of patient showing minor crowding and deep vertical overlap

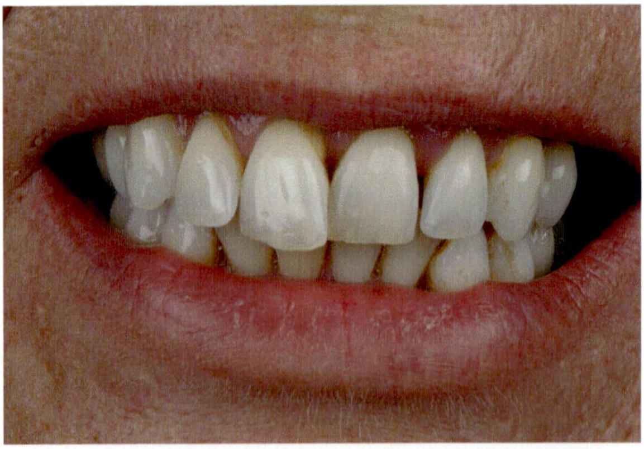

Fig. 15.81 Smile view of patient showing display of gingiva when smiling

healing and conventional load. Immediate loading of implants should only be done after a thorough evaluation of the risk factors involved and not performed dogmatically.

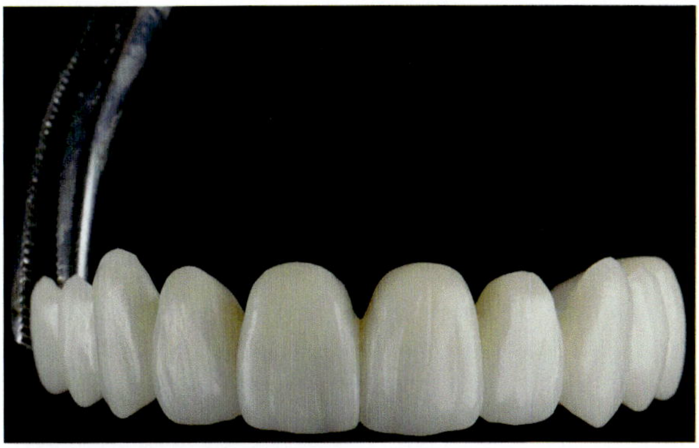

Fig. 15.82 Digitally milled shell provisionals from PMMA puck. (Ivoclar ProArt)

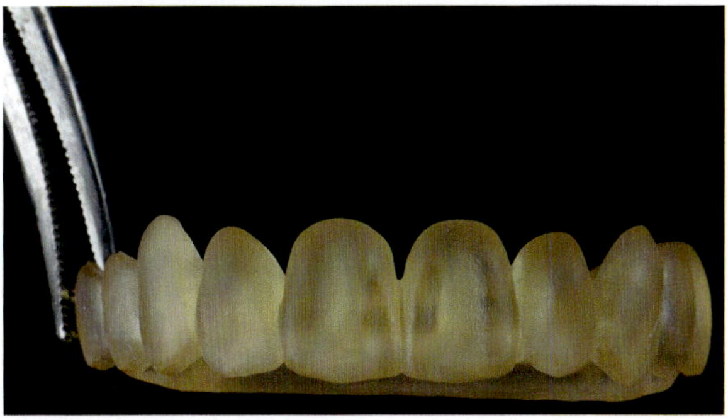

Fig. 15.83 Printed tooth-supported surgical guides

Treatment Plan and Sequence

1. Intraoral scans were completed (Trios 3 Shape Technologies), and shell provisionals were milled (ProArt CAD, Ivoclar Vivadent), utilizing key strategic teeth which would anchor the restoration whilst implants were integrating (Figs. 15.82 and 15.83).
2. Sinus lift and bone augmentation were completed on the patient's upper left quadrant. Extraction of strategic teeth and placement of dental implants were also done. Strategic teeth would be prepared to support a provisional restoration so that implants would not be loaded. This decision was made due to a history of failed implants and history of diabetes (Figs. 15.84 and 15.85).
3. Placement of implants in the maxillary left quadrant.
4. On integration, implant impressions would be made to fabricate an implant-supported provisional. This would be segmented (Fig. 15.86).
5. Extraction of remaining teeth and grafting of extraction sites with a bone xenograft to maintain ridge height and width. Delivery of segmented provisionals.
6. Tissue maturation and stabilization.
7. Fabrication of prototype to verify aesthetics, phonetics and occlusion (Figs. 15.87, 15.88 and 15.89).

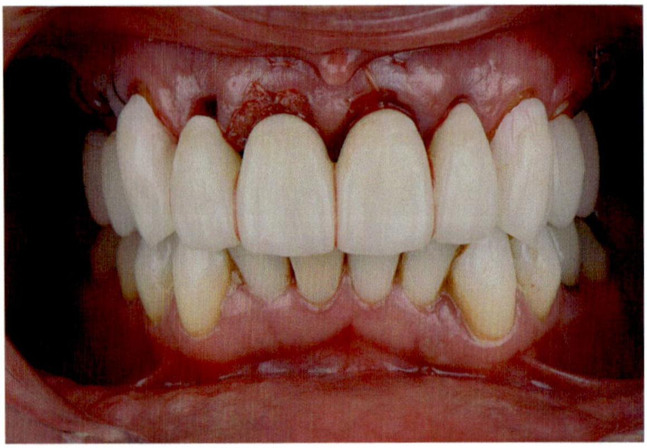

Fig. 15.84 Day of surgery; strategic teeth have been extracted, implants are placed and bone allograft is placed in extraction sockets. Shell provisionals relined

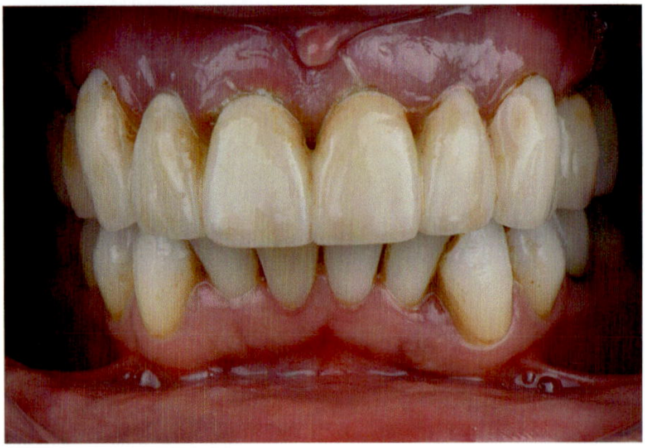

Fig. 15.85 Post-operative characterized provisional

8. Fabrication of segmented zirconia restoration supported by implants (Figs. 15.90, 15.91, 15.92 and 15.93).
9. Maintenance.

By completing the above sequence, the following objectives were met:

1. Transitioning the patient through fixed provisional restorations at all times
2. Preservation of bone
3. Eliminating the risk associated with immediate loading in a patient that has a history of previous implant failure
4. Minimizing risk in a patient who has periodontal disease and type 2 diabetes
5. Placement of more than four implants and segmentation of the restoration
6. Utilization of technology to make treatment more efficient

Zirconia-based restorations	Treatment planning
Aesthetics	Tooth-only defect, no bone reduction
Type of support	Implant supported

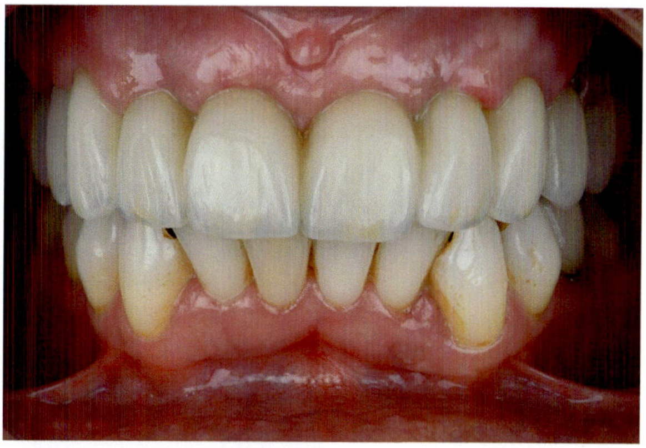

Fig. 15.86 Strategic teeth have been extracted, and milled implant-supported provisional is placed

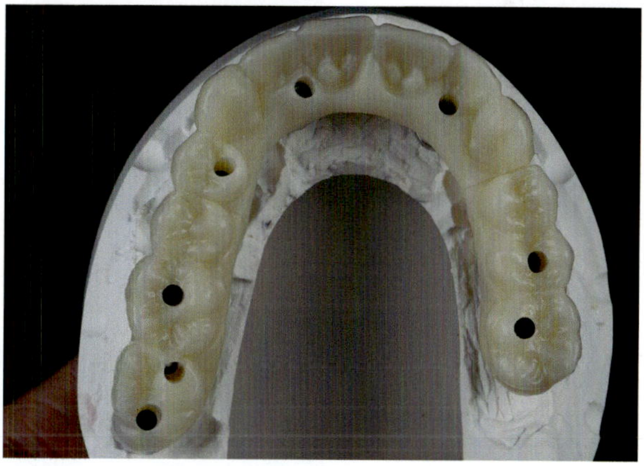

Fig. 15.87 Milled prototype from acrylic puck fabricated in three segments

Zirconia-based restorations	Treatment planning
Resorption and inter arch space	Minimal resorption 11–13 mm
Number of implants	6–8
Implant placement and distribution	Implants should be well distributed and ideally placed
Cost	Less expensive than ceramo-metal prostheses

Case 6: Zirconia Restorations on Implants with an All on 4™ Concept Replacing a Tooth-Only Defect

Often, patients refuse additional grafting procedures, and there is insufficient bone to be able to place more than four implants in each arch. In these clinical situations, the patient must be made aware of the advantages and disadvantages of such

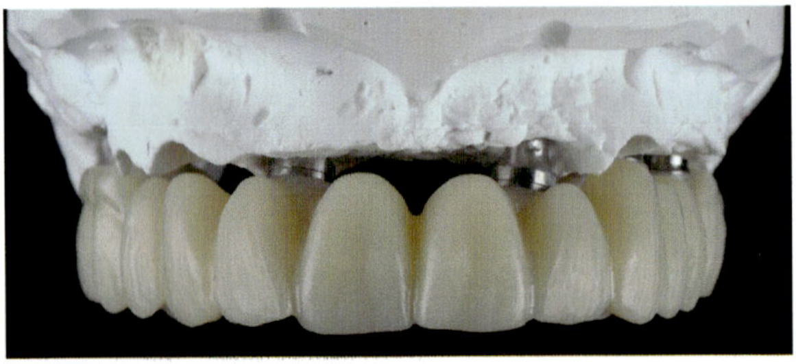

Fig. 15.88 Anterior view of milled prototype showing segmentation of prosthesis and anteroposterior spread of implants

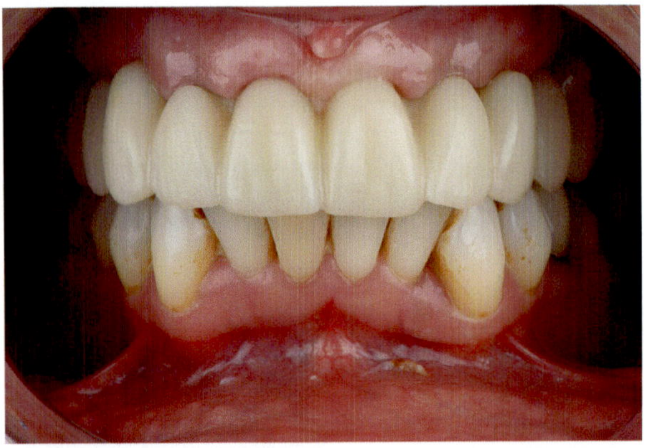

Fig. 15.89 Anterior view of adjusted prototype

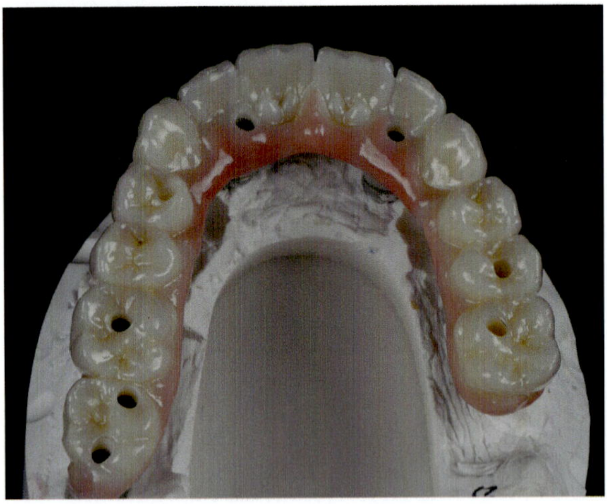

Fig. 15.90 Occlusal view of minimally layered zirconia prosthesis fabricated in three segments. (Ceramics by Artem Asemov)

treatment protocols and must be fully aware of the clinical and financial consequences of implant failure.

The following patient presentation illustrates the philosophy of minimally invasive implant therapy for full-arch implant rehabilitation utilizing four implants in each arch using digital technologies.

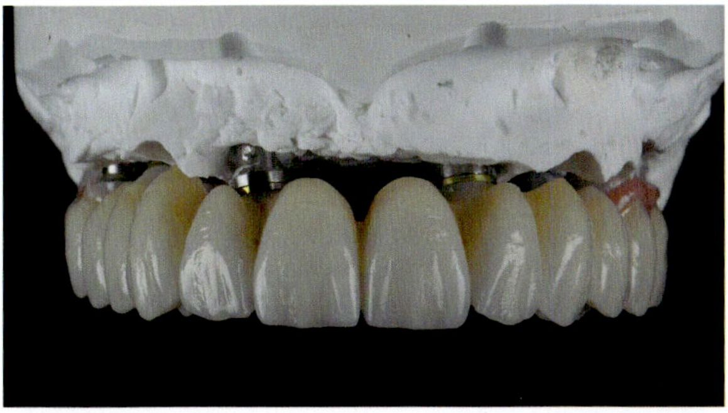

Fig. 15.91 Minimally layered zirconia prosthesis

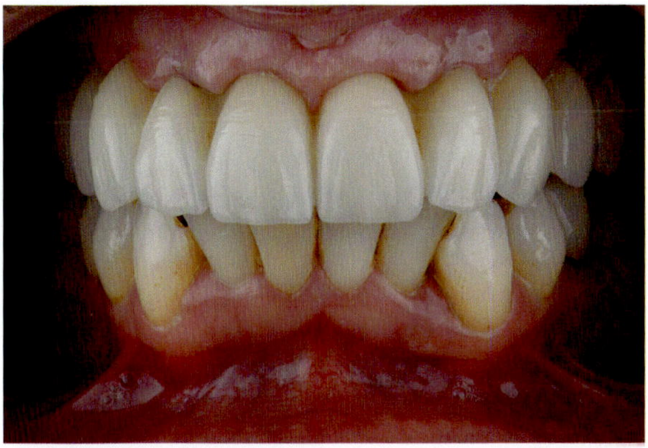

Fig. 15.92 Intraoral view of minimally layered zirconia prosthesis

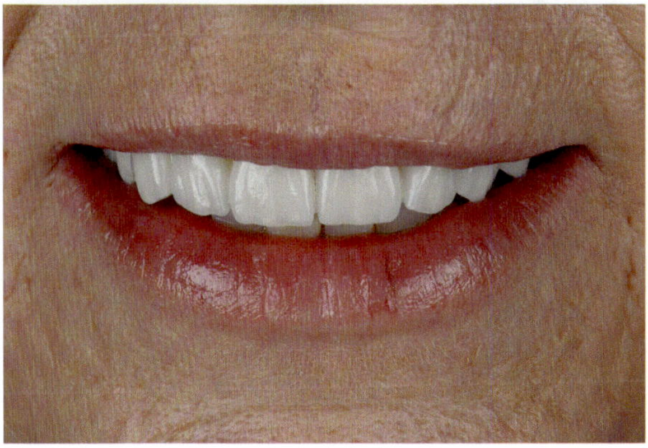

Fig. 15.93 Smile view of restoration in situ

A 71-year-old female presented seeking a solution to her failing maxillary and mandibular dentition. A detail medical and dental evaluation was performed. Specific concerns in treatment planning were multiple medications that resulted in the patient being xerostomic. The patient's teeth had been compromised due to caries and periodontal disease (Figs. 15.94, 15.95, 15.96 and 15.97).

The following diagnosis was made:

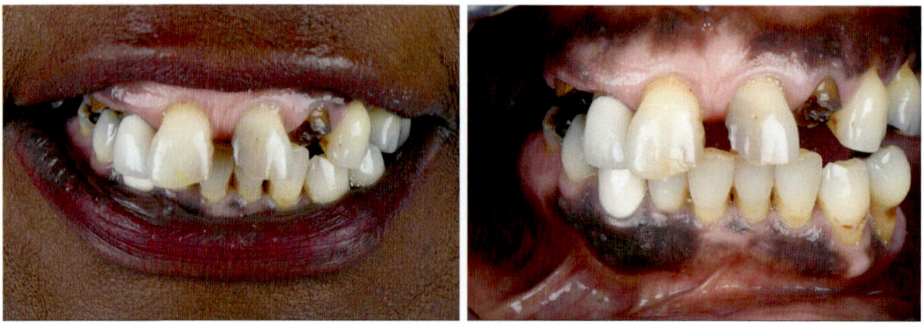

Fig. 15.94 Preoperative clinical view of smile and retracted intraoral view

Fig. 15.95 Full face

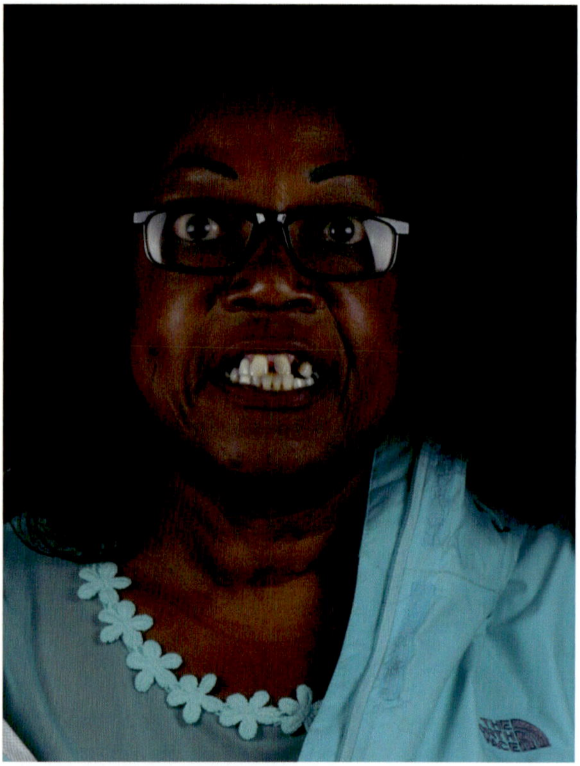

1. Caries
2. Periodontal disease
3. Lack of posterior support
4. Bimaxillary protrusion

On clinical and radiographic examination, her maxillary and mandibular dentition was deemed to be of poor prognosis.

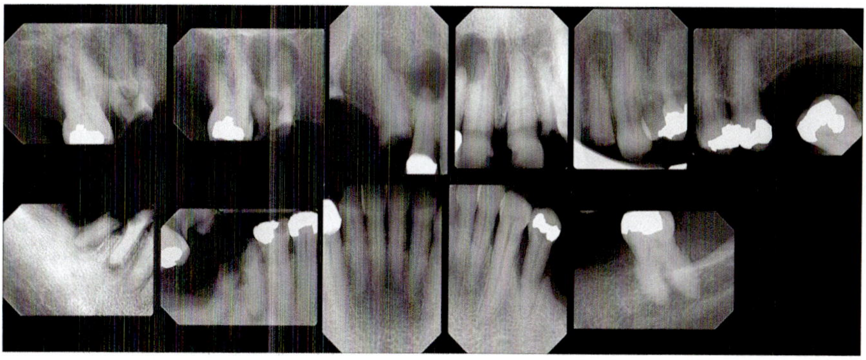

Fig. 15.96 Periapical radiographs

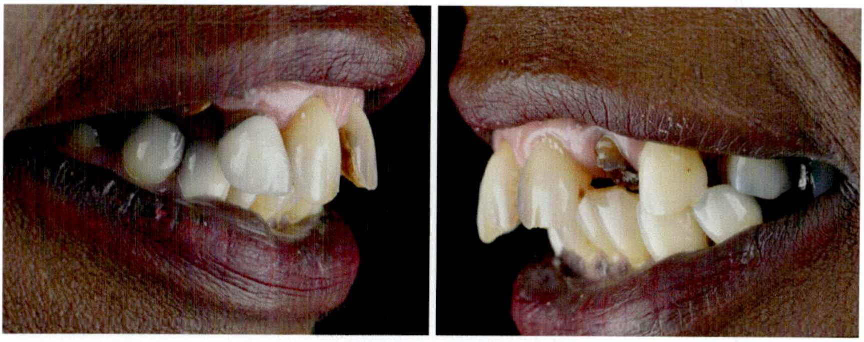

Fig. 15.97 Lateral view of smile showing over-eruption and flaring

The following clinical issues required attention:

1. Lack of bone in the posterior maxilla
2. Over-eruption of teeth compromising restorative space
3. Flaring of teeth
4. High smile line with excessive gingival display

The patient's concerns were the following:

1. The patient did not want to wear a removable appliance at any point during the treatment process.
2. The patient wanted to address the bimaxillary protrusion.
3. The patient refused grafting procedures.

Considerations in implementing care were the following:

1. Multiple medications causing the patient to be xerostomic.

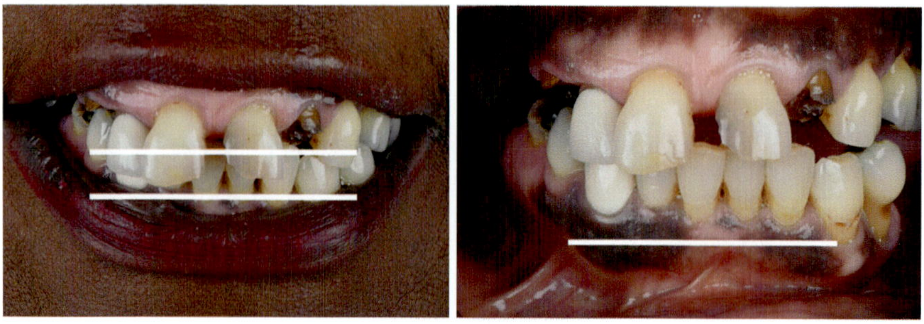

Fig. 15.98 White lines showing anticipated positioning of maxillary and mandibular incisal edge

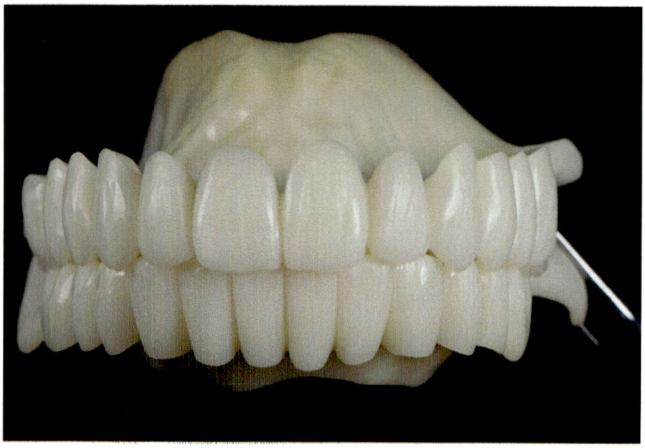

Fig. 15.99 Milled provisional

2. The patient's smile line exhibited excessive gingival display and a short lip. It is the author's opinion that bone reduction and use of pink prosthetics in these types of clinical situations are contraindicated (Fig. 15.98).
3. Preservation of bone.
4. Providing an FP1 prosthesis and addressing the bimaxillary protrusion: This would entail palatal placement of dental implants and carefully selecting a pre-angled multi-unit abutment to ensure appropriate emergence profile.
5. Providing an anteroposterior spread that is optimal. Placement of implants that do not compromise connector size for the definitive restorations.
6. Minimal alveolar bone recontouring to shift the maxillary occlusal plane up and to lower the mandibular occlusal plane.
7. Transitioning the patient with fixed restoration during the entire treatment process.

The above considerations required a more cautious approach in treatment planning and execution.

Treatment Plan and Sequence

1. Intraoral scans were completed (Trios 3 Shape Technologies), and shell provisionals were milled (ProArt CAD, Ivoclar Vivadent) (Fig. 15.99).

2. The patient was treated surgically and prosthetically in 1 day, utilizing laboratory-fabricated static surgical guides. No guided surgery was performed per se. The surgical guides were stabilized on retained teeth, and osteotomies of the anterior implants were performed. Four implants were placed in the maxilla and four in the mandible. Multi-unit abutments were secured, and soft tissue closure was achieved. Deep sedation with profound local anaesthesia was used to remove all teeth except ones needed for stability of bone reduction and surgical stent. A tooth-supported surgical guide was provided to ensure accurate three-dimensional placement of implants in the maxilla. This required careful depth placement so that a pre-angled multi-unit abutment could be selected with a minimum collar height. This would allow correction of the flaring of the teeth as well as an optimal emergence profile. Alveolectomy was completed in the mandible to provide appropriate restorative space and correct the mandibular incisal edge position. The mandibular bone was reduced minimally to create a platform for implant placement. The patient was informed that the mandible may require pink prosthetics. The patient's provisional immediate load prostheses were fabricated on the same day as implant placement. The patient tolerated the procedure well and healed uneventfully.
3. A direct technique for immediate loading was employed. Vertical dimension, centric relation and occlusal plane were verified. After protection of the surgical sites with rubber dam, temporary cylinders were first picked up in the maxillary prosthesis. Patient was guided into centric relation, and a similar pickup of temporary cylinders was performed in the mandibular provisional restoration. The prostheses were removed and transferred to the dental laboratory where the prostheses were processed and finished. The prostheses were adjusted to compress the tissue by 2 mm and to develop the pontic sites from the outset. Twelve teeth were provided in the maxilla and ten teeth in the mandible. Occlusion was adjusted for shimstock hold on anterior teeth and shimstock drag on the posterior teeth to reduce forces in the posterior in this particular situation due to implant positioning and immediate loading. Vertical dimension was verified on delivery of the restoration. Extraction of remaining teeth and grafting of extraction sites with a bone xenograft were done to maintain ridge height and width. Delivery of splinted provisionals was also done (Figs. 15.100, 15.101, 15.102 and 15.103).

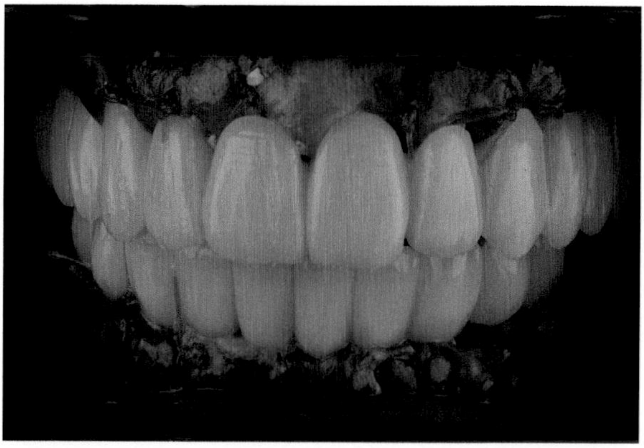

Fig. 15.100 Immediate load provisional restorations in situ

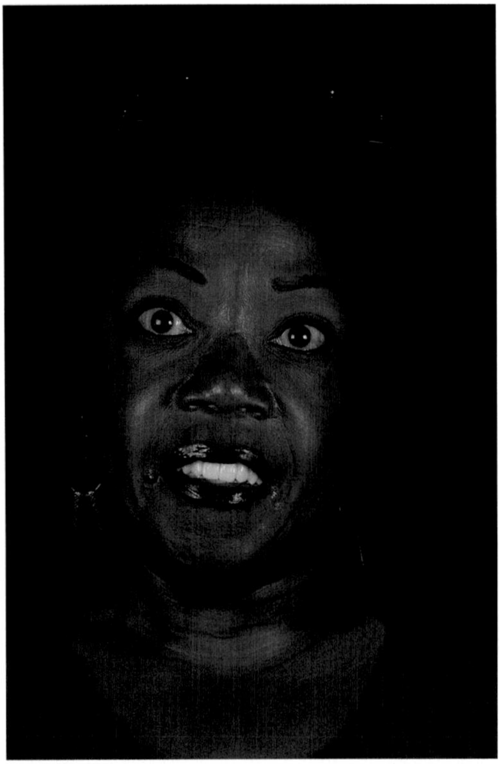

Fig. 15.101 Smile view showing tooth display. Increased length can be adjusted in provisionals

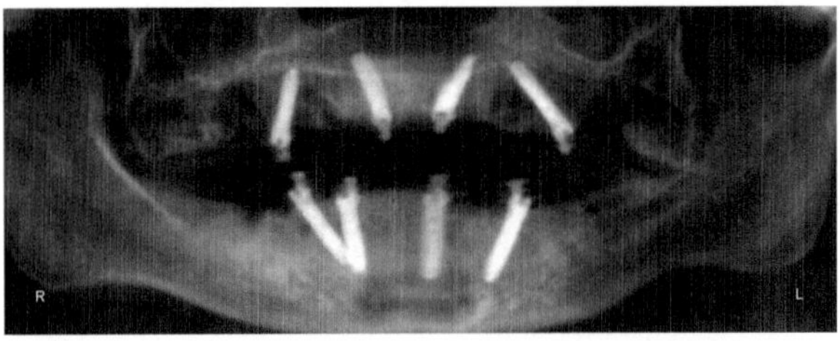

Fig. 15.102 Panoramic view of implant placement

4. Tissue maturation and stabilization.
5. Post-integration, an additional provisional restoration was fabricated to ensure verification of aesthetics, phonetics and tissue compression (Fig. 15.104).
6. Splinted open-tray impressions, jaw relation records and tooth try-ins were performed. Additional provisional restoration was fabricated. Aesthetics, phonetics and soft tissue contours were further developed in the provisional restoration.
7. Minimally layered zirconia restorations were fabricated for both maxilla and mandible. Occlusion was provided on polished zirconia. Tissue-contacting surface was designed in polished zirconia (Figs. 15.105, 15.106, 15.107 and 15.108).

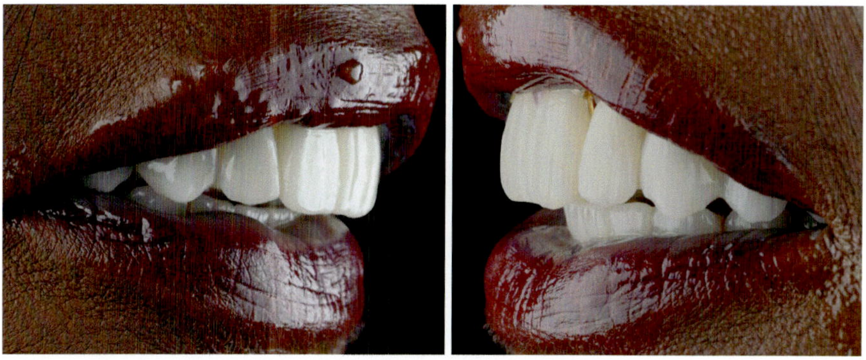

Fig. 15.103 Lateral view of provisionals

Fig. 15.104 Anterior view of second set of provisionals fabricated

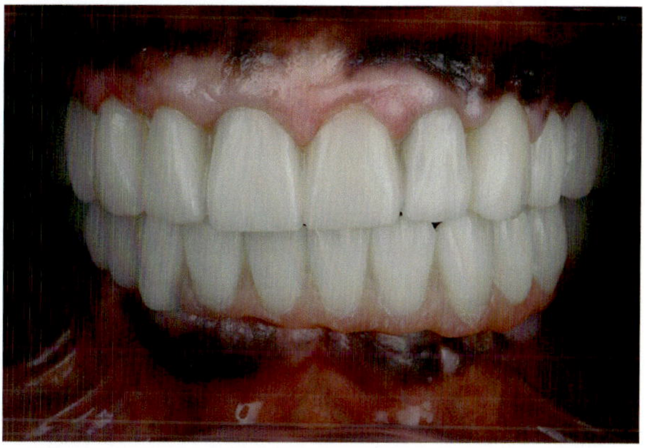

8. The prosthesis was delivered adjusting the undersurface to ensure positive pressure. Dynamic occlusion was adjusted for canine guidance. Static occlusion was adjusted to ensure shimstock hold on canines and premolars. Shimstock drag occurred on the anterior teeth and no contact was seen on the cantilevers (Fig. 15.109).
9. Screws were torqued according to the manufacturer's specifications, and access holes were sealed using Teflon and composite resin.

By completing the above sequence, the following objectives were met:

1. Transitioning the patient through fixed provisional restorations at all times
2. Preservation of bone and fabrication of an FP1 prosthesis in the maxilla
3. Restoration of posterior support
4. Satisfying the patient's aesthetic concerns and solving the issue of bimaxillary protrusion
5. Utilization of technology to make treatment more efficient prosthetically

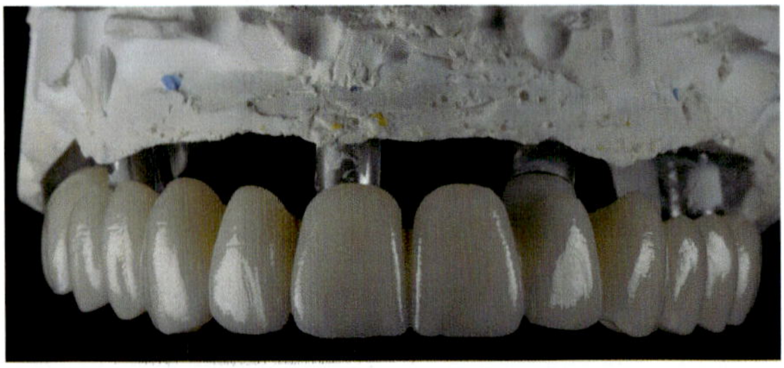

Fig. 15.105 Anterior intraoral view of minimally layered zirconia prosthesis

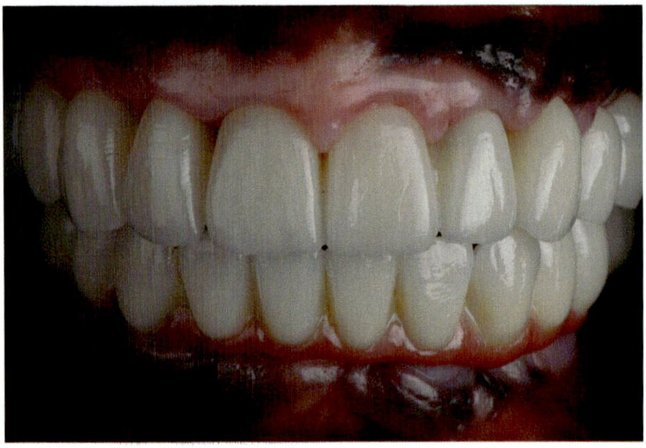

Fig. 15.106 Layered restorations in situ

Zirconia-based restorations	Treatment planning
Aesthetics	Provide desired lip support
Type of support	Implant supported
Resorption and inter arch space	Severe resorption 11–15 mm inter-arch space
Number of implants	Minimum 4
Implant placement and distribution	Implants should be well distributed
Cost	Less expensive than ceramo-metal prostheses. More maintenance costs

Case 7: Full-Mouth Implant Rehabilitation Utilizing Zygomatic Implants for Posterior Anchorage

Patient was a 73-year-old female with no significant medical conditions.

The patient's clinical and radiographic data were gathered to determine the appropriate method to satisfy the surgical requirements.

The patient presented in an edentulous state. The patient reported that she had been told that dental implants were not possible in her maxillary arch without extensive grafting procedures. She denied grafting in the maxilla. She reported absolute dissatisfaction with her existing dentures and a lack of confidence in the treatment process in general. She was frustrated with the previous care provided and wanted a more definitive result with a fixed restoration. She demanded that transition to fixed

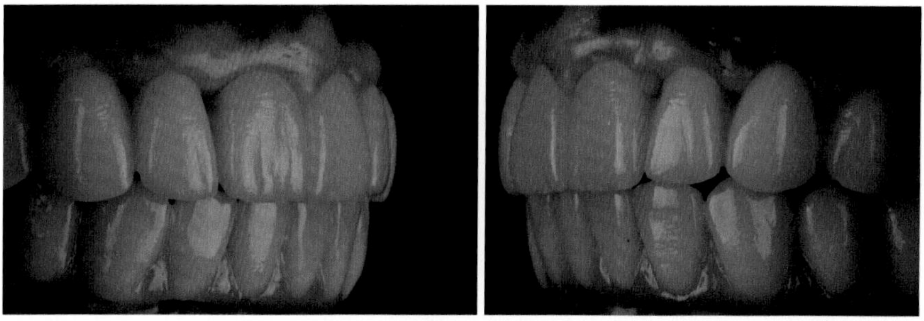

Fig. 15.107 Lateral view depicting change in occlusal plane, flaring and incisal edge positions

Fig. 15.108 Smile view of restoration in situ

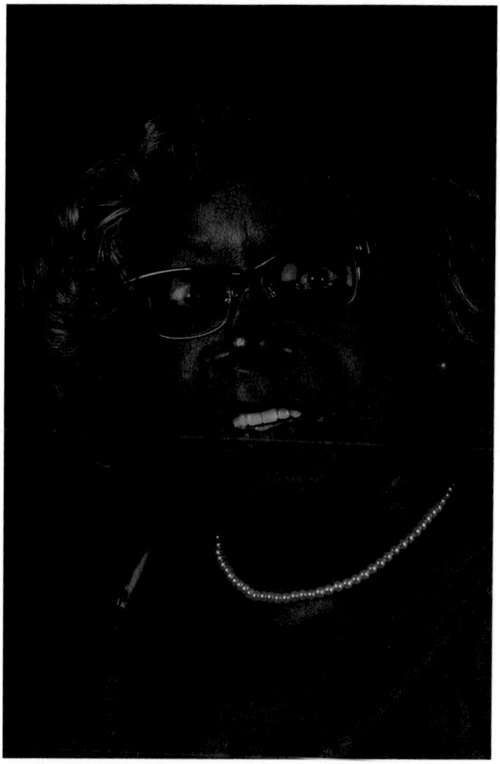

restorations be completed with minimal time spent in dental offices and without any grafting.

Clinical examination of the patient revealed significant lack of lip support by the existing bony structures of the maxilla. The edentulous ridge was not visible during smiling with the denture removed (Figs. 15.110, 15.111 and 15.112).

Panoramic and cross-sectional images of the maxilla and mandible were obtained and showed significant atrophy of both arches. The maxilla exhibited large

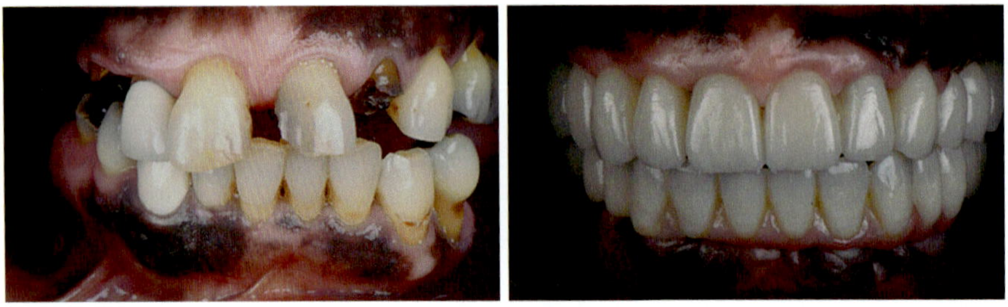

Fig. 15.109 Pre- and post-operative views following rehabilitation. (Ceramics by Artem Asemov)

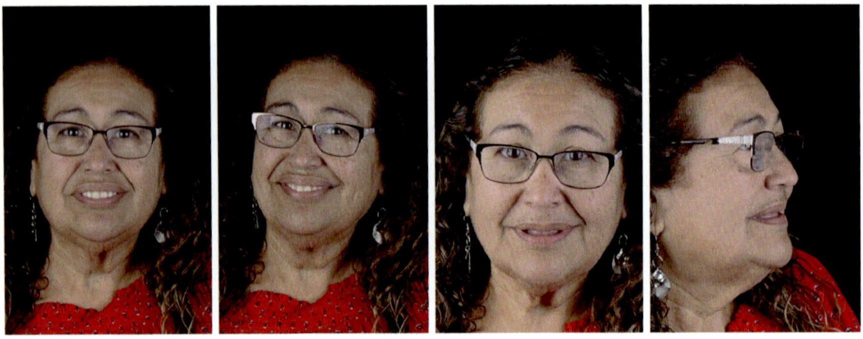

Fig. 15.110 Preoperative view of patient with and without existing dentures

pneumatized sinuses occupying the majority of the maxilla and a retained maxillary third molar. There was significant atrophy of the premaxilla with 7–8 mm of alveolus remaining below the floor of the nose. There was minimal bone remaining in the molar and premolar regions. The mandible showed moderate amount of resorption with 10 mm of bone above the inferior alveolar nerve and with sufficient width throughout (Figs. 15.113 and 15.114).

Surgical Treatment Plan

1. Patient is a healthy 73-year-old with no absolute contraindications for oral surgical procedures. Mild sedation with profound local anaesthesia was utilized to perform the procedure in a safe and comfortable manner.
2. Space: The patient has undergone moderate alveolar atrophy with perhaps alveoloplasty at the time of the existing implant placement. 41 mm of inter-arch space was measured clinically. The patient was treatment planned for a zirconia prosthesis in both arches There was sufficient space for the proposed restoration. No further space creation via bone reduction was necessary. It was determined due to severe atrophy of the maxilla and superior position of the implants that an appropriate contour to the prosthesis can be achieved to provide lip support without a horizontal shelf formation; therefore, no further bone reduction is necessary to place implants.

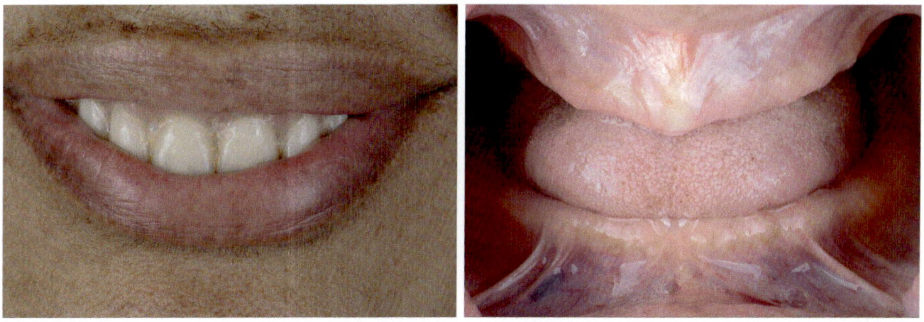

Fig. 15.111 Denture fabricated with incisal edge too coronally positioned. Patient complaining of incisal edge touch vermillion border excessively during F sound

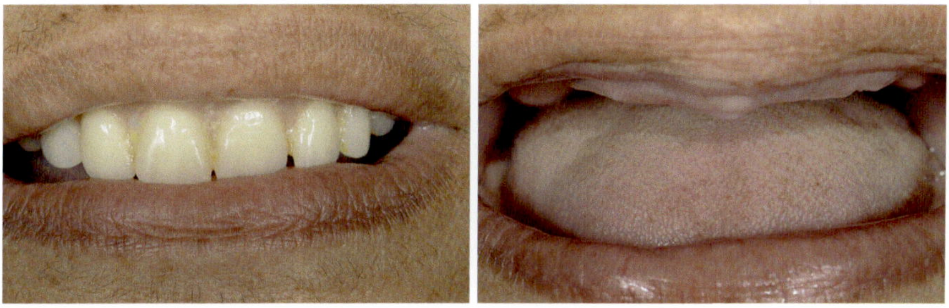

Fig. 15.112 Display of the ridge on smiling. May require some bone recontouring

3. Spread: The challenge in this patient is the lack of bone in the posterior zones of maxilla. The patient had denied grafting; an alternative placement scheme was devised with posterior support provided by bilateral zygomatic implants. The mandible would be treated with a conventional graft-less procedure. Two implants would be placed just anterior of the mental foramen and two axial implants in the anterior midline of the mandible.
4. Stability: The zygoma is an extremely dense bone structure that will provide excellent stability to the zygomatic implants. There is sufficient ridge to allow for anchorage of the crestal portion of the zygomatic implants. The anterior implants would be placed with the apical portion in the very dense lateral nasal wall-pyriform rim of the maxilla.

Prosthetic Evaluation

On clinical examination, the dentures lacked retention and stability. There was an abundance of keratinized mucosa.

From a diagnostic perspective, the following factors were evaluated.

1. Incisal edge position—The patient was unhappy with the aesthetics of the existing dentures. The maxillary incisal edge position appeared to be too low. A

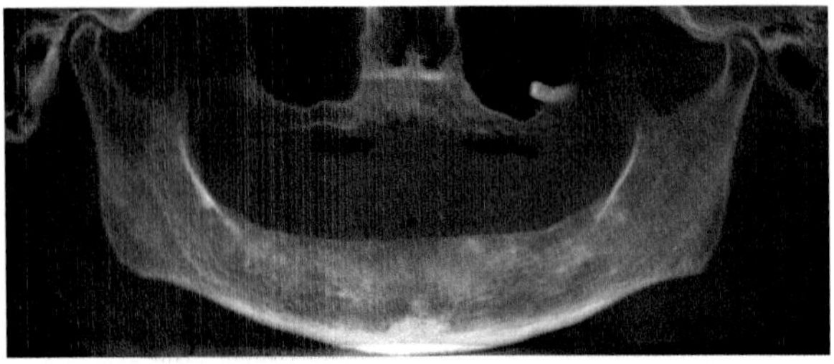

Fig. 15.113 Panoramic radiograph showing pneumatized sinuses and retained third molar

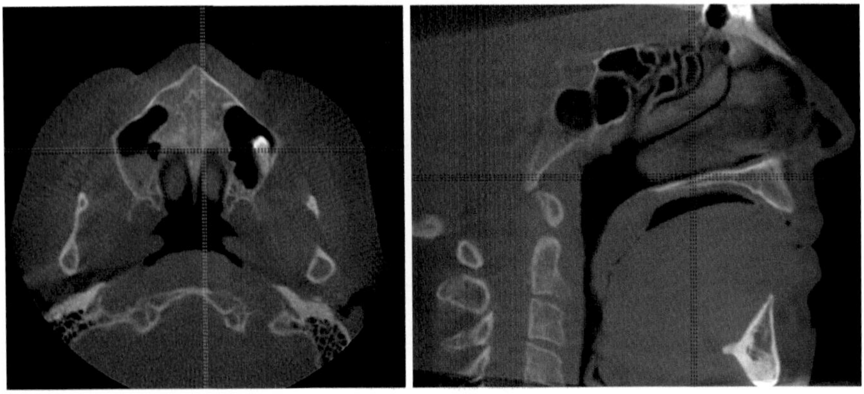

Fig. 15.114 CBCT cross section

diagnostic denture set-up was to be done to evaluate any modifications in aesthetics (Figs. 15.115 and 15.116).

2. Restorative space—Due to the severe bone resorption, restorative space would be available for any material combination.
3. Lip support—The patient had a severe lack of lip support and a concave facial profile when the dentures were removed. This is one of the factors that would pose a challenge in providing the patient with a fixed restoration. Due to the fact that the patient was unwilling to go through additional grafting procedures, alternative clinical strategies would need to be evaluated such as alveolectomy and tilting of the anterior implants so the contour of the restoration could be developed so that it was maintainable.
4. Smile line—With the dentures removed, the alveolar ridge was not visible so hiding the transition zone would not pose a problem.
5. Contours and emergence—The horizontal discrepancy between the implant position and where the patient desired the teeth aesthetically posed a significant challenge. Using shorter implants, tilting the anterior implants and starting the emergence profile higher up would help create some space for contour development.
6. Tissue contact—The existing tissues must be made healthy prior to any surgical procedures. Soft relining of the patient's existing denture needs to be carried out to achieve this. Due to the extensive resorption and available space, shaping the

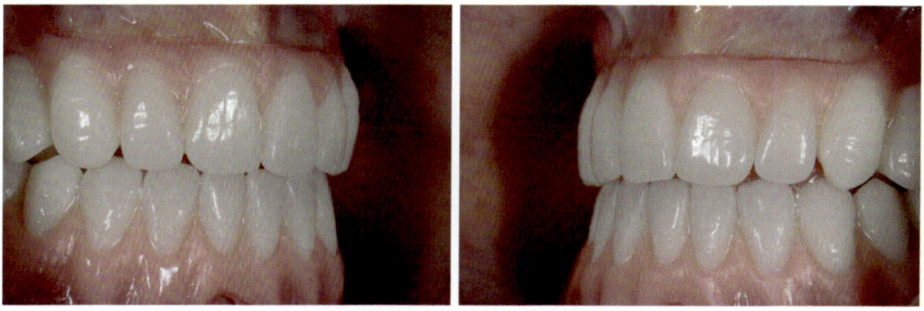

Fig. 15.115 Flangeless try-in

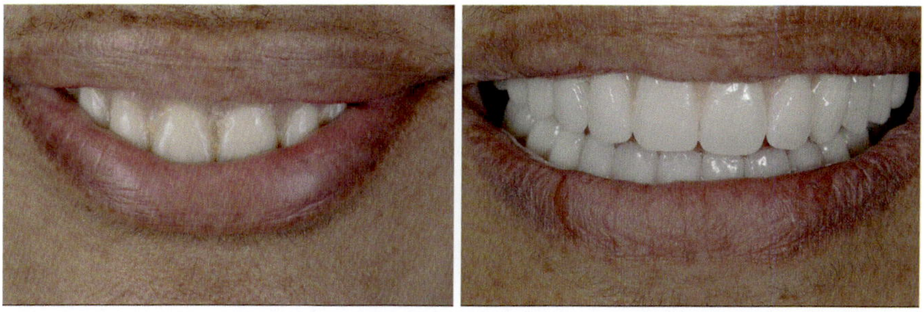

Fig. 15.116 Aesthetic evaluation in comparison to her previous denture

restorative contours for a convex undersurface is attainable. This will allow the patient to maintain the prosthesis.

7. Occlusion—Occlusion must be addressed in the immediate load provisional to protect the implants in the weakest quality bone from excessive loads. In the definitive restoration, occlusion must be organized to distribute the loads over a wide an area as possible.

Prosthodontic Sequence

Immediate dentures at the correct vertical dimension were fabricated for a direct pickup procedure. Vertical dimension was determined prior to implant placement and a record made (Figs. 15.117 and 15.118).

A direct technique for immediate loading was employed. Vertical dimension, centric relation and occlusal plane were verified. After protection of the surgical sites with rubber damn, temporary cylinders were first picked up in the maxillary prosthesis. Patient was guided into centric relation, and a similar pickup of temporary cylinders was performed in the mandibular provisional denture. The prostheses were removed and transferred to the dental laboratory where the prostheses were processed and finished. The prostheses were adjusted to leave a 1 mm space between the prostheses and the tissue. Ten teeth were provided, and there were no cantilevers. Occlusion was adjusted for shimstock hold on the anterior teeth and shimstock

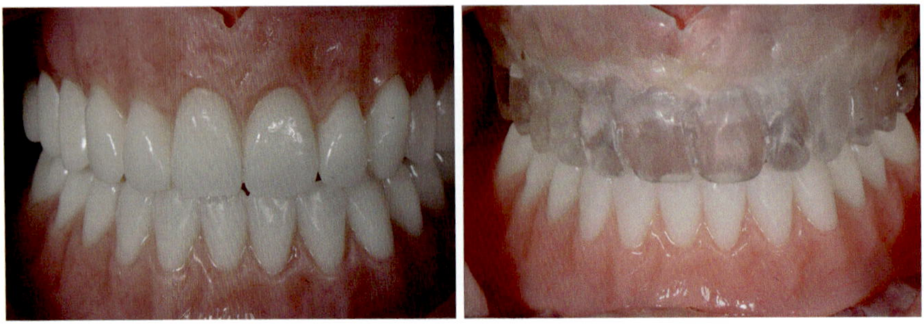

Fig. 15.117 Dentures and surgical guides ready

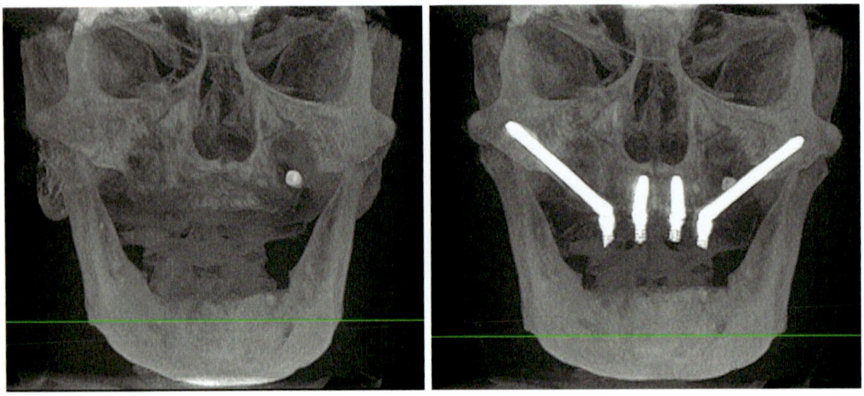

Fig. 15.118 Four implants placed in the maxilla. Posterior implants are zygomatic implants

drag on the posterior teeth. Vertical dimension was verified on delivery of the restoration (Figs. 15.119, 15.120 and 15.121).

Splinted open-tray impressions, jaw relation records and a trial restoration were inserted to verify aesthetics and phonetics.

The trial restoration was utilized to fabricate a monolithic zirconia restoration in both maxilla and mandible (Fig. 15.122).

The prostheses were delivered adjusting the undersurface to ensure positive pressure. Dynamic occlusion was adjusted for canine guidance. Static occlusion was adjusted to ensure shimstock hold on canines and premolars. Shimstock drag occurred on the anterior teeth, and no contact was seen on the cantilevers (Figs. 15.123, 15.124 and 15.125).

Screws were torqued according to the manufacturer's specifications, and access holes were sealed using Teflon and composite resin.A night-time appliance was provided, and maintenance instructions were provided.

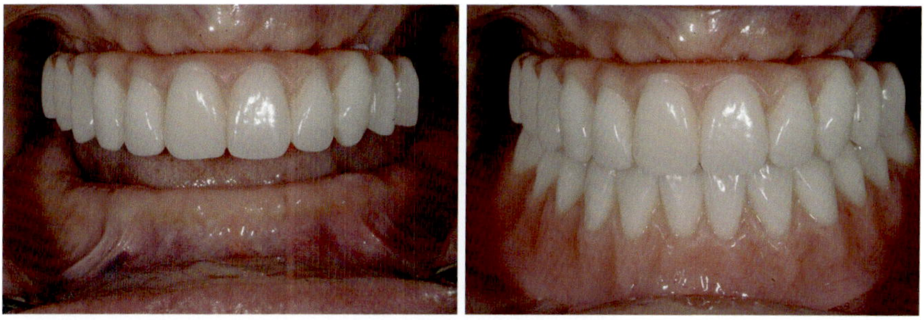

Fig. 15.119 Maxillary arch demonstrating fixed provisional restoration against opposing denture

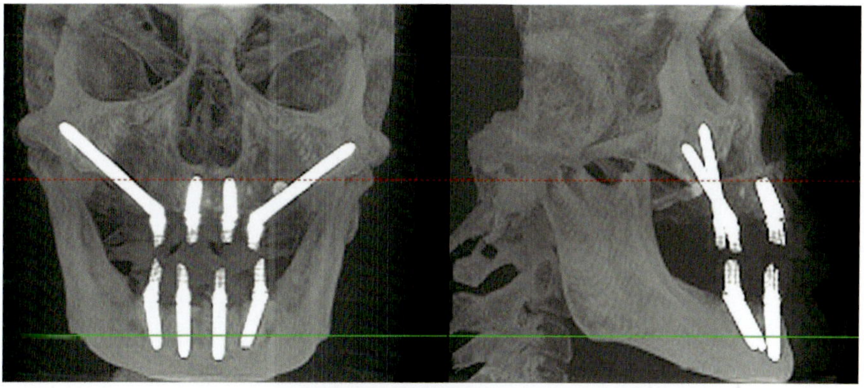

Fig. 15.120 Four implants placed in the mandibular arch

Fig. 15.121 Maxillary and mandibular fixed provisional restorations after 4 months in situ. Oral hygiene must be emphasized

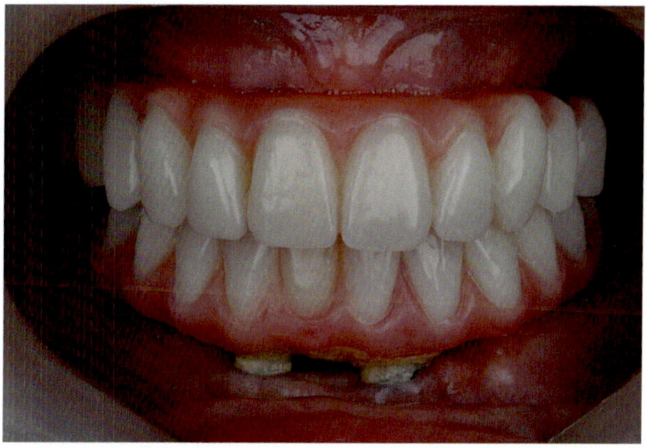

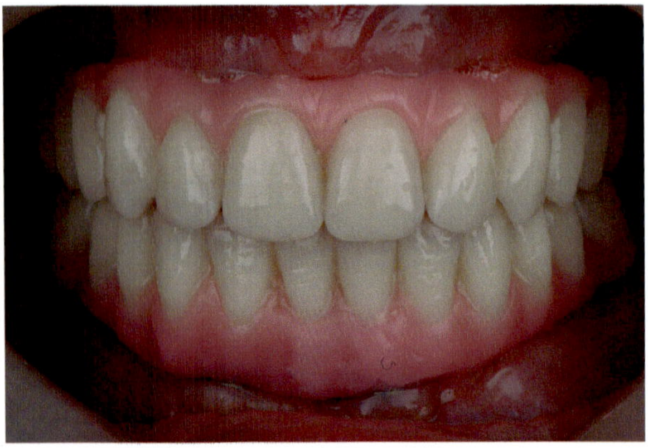

Fig. 15.122 Aesthetic wax try-in used to fabricate prototypes

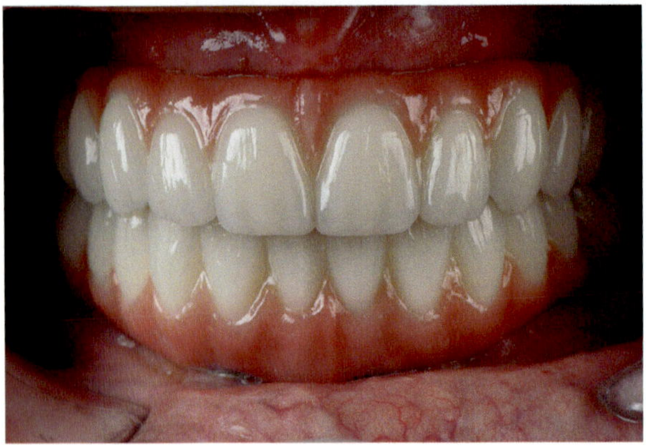

Fig. 15.123 Definitive zirconia restorations

Zirconia-based restorations on zygomatic implants	Treatment planning
Aesthetics	Lip support will be required
Type of support	Implant supported
Resorption and inter-arch space	Severe resorption 16 mm inter-arch space
Number of implants	Minimum 4
Implant placement and distribution	Implants should be well distributed
Cost	Less expensive than ceramo-metal prostheses

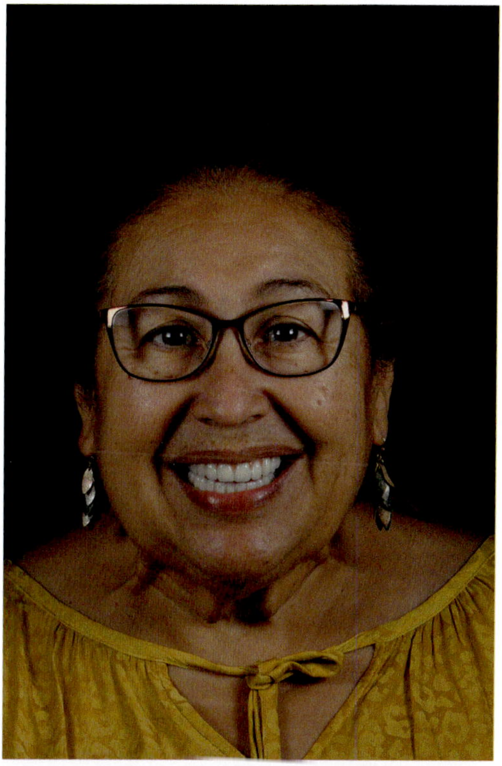

Fig. 15.124 Final smile view

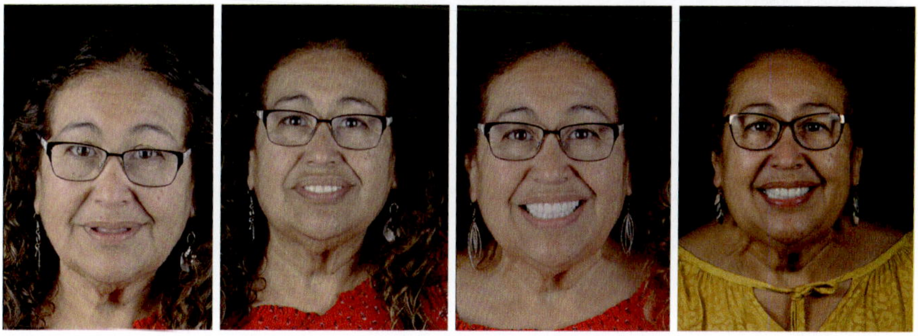

Fig. 15.125 Patients transition from dentures to implant-supported restorations utilizing a graftless workflow

Acknowledgements The patient treatment in case 1 was provided by Dr. Paolo Corrado. The patient treatment in case 3 was provided by Dr. Dan Lin.

References

1. Branemark PI, Hansson BO, Adell R, Breine U, Lindstrom J, Hallen O, et al. Osseointegrated implants in the treatment of the edentulous jaw. Experience from a 10 year period. Scand J Plast Reconstr Surg Suppl. 1977;16:1–132.
2. Tallgren A. The reduction in face height of edentulous and partially edentulous subjects during long term denture wear: a longitudinal roentgenographic cephalometric study. Acta Odontol Scand. 1966;24:195–239.
3. Maló P, de Araújo Nobre M, Lopes A, Ferro A, Botto J. Clin Implant Dent Relat Res. 2019;21(4):565–77.
4. Zitzmann NU, Marinello CP. Treatment plan for restoring the edentulous maxilla with implant supported restorations: removable overdenture versus fixed partial denture design. J Prosthet Dent. 1999;82(2):188–96.
5. Misch CE, Goodacre CJ, Finley JM, Misch CM, Marinbach M, Dabrowsky T, English CE, Kois JC, Cronin RJ Jr. Consensus conference panel report: crown-height space guidelines for implant dentistry-Part 1. Implant Dent. 2005;14(4):312–8.
6. Tjan AH, Miller GD, The JG. Some esthetic factors in a smile. J Prosthet Dent. 1894;51:24–8.
7. Silberberg N, Goldstein M, Smidt A. Excessive gingival display—etiology, diagnosis, and treatment modalities. Quintessence Int. 2009;40(10):809–18.
8. Att W, Bernhart J, Strub JR. Fixed rehabilitation of the edentulous maxilla: possibilities and clinical outcome. J Oral Maxillofac Surg. 2009;67(11 Suppl):60–73.
9. Capelli M, Zuffetti F, Del Fabbro M, Testori T. Immediate rehabilitation of the completely edentulous jaw with fixed prostheses supported by either upright or tilted implants: a multicenter clinical study. Int J Oral Maxillofac Implants. 2007;22(4):639–44.
10. Block MS, Haggerty CJ, Fisher GR. Nongrafting implant options for restoration of the edentulous maxilla. J Oral Maxillofac Surg. 2009;67(4):872–81.
11. Krekmanov L, Kahn M, Rangert B, et al. Tilting of posterior mandibular and maxillary implants for improved prosthesis support. Int J Oral Maxillofac Implants. 2000;15(3):411.
12. Henry PJ. A review of guidelines for implant rehabilitation of the edentulous maxilla. J Prosthet Dent. 2002;87:281–8.
13. Balshi TJ, Wolfinger GJ, Balshi SF. Int J Oral Maxillofac Implants. 1999;14(3):398–406.
14. Lekholm U, Zarb GA. Patient selection and preparation in Branemark P-I. In: Zarb GA, Albrektsson T, editors. Tissue-integrated prostheses: osseointegration in clinical dentistry. Chicago: Quintessesnce Publ Co; 1985. p. 199–209.
15. Bosse LP, Taylor TD. Problems associated with implant rehabilitation of the edentulous maxilla. Dent Clin North Am. 1998;42(1):117–27.
16. Wicks RA. A systematic approach to definitive planning for osseointegrated implant prostheses. J Prosthodont. 1994;3(4):237–42.
17. Rawal S, Balshi TJ, Jivraj S, Birdi B. Evolution of full-arch implant prosthodontics: from analog protocols to digital workflows. Compend Contin Educ Dent. 2019;40(9):578–85.
18. Bedrossian E. Rescue implant concept: the expanded use of the zygoma implant in the graftless solutions. Oral Maxillofac Surg Clin North Am. 2011;23(2):257–76.
19. Naert I, DeClercq M, Theuniers G, et al. Overdentures supported by osseointegrated fixtures for the edentulous mandible. A 2.5 year report. Int J Oral Maxillofac Implants. 1988;3:191–6.
20. Dudley J. Maxillary implant overdentures: current controversies. Aust Dent J. 2013;58(4):420–3.
21. Di Francesco F, De Marco G, Capcha EB, Lanza A, Cristache CM, Vernal R, Cafferata EA. Patient satisfaction and survival of maxillary overdentures supported by four or six splinted implants: a systematic review with meta-analysis. BMC Oral Health. 2021;21(1):247.
22. Eckert SE, Hueler G, Sandler N, Elkattah R, McNeil DC. Immediately loaded fixed full-arch implant-retained prosthesis: clinical analysis when using a moderate insertion torque. Int J Oral Maxillofac Implants. 2019;34(3):737–44.

23. Patodia C, Sutton A, Gozalo D, Font K. Cost and complications associated with implant-supported overdentures with a resilient-attachment system: a retrospective study. J Prosthet Dent. 2022;128(2):181–6.
24. Chiche FA, Leriche MA. Multidisciplinary implant dentistry for improved esthetics and function. Pract Periodont Aesthet Dent. 1998;10(2):177–86.
25. Smalley W, et al. Osseointegrated titanium implants for maxillofacial protraction in monkeys. Am J Orthod Dentofacial Orthop. 1988;94:285–95.
26. Douglas J, Killinay D. Dental implants used as orthodontic anchorage. J Oral Implantol. 1988;13:28–38.
27. Chee WWL. Considerations for implant overdentures. J Calif Dent Assoc. 1992;20:25–8.
28. Lewis S. Implant retained overdentures. Compendium. 1993;14(10):1270–83.

Treatment Planning the Edentulous Mandible

16

Saj Jivraj and Winston Chee

16.1 Introduction

The mandibular denture is a difficult prosthesis to manage; many articles and techniques have been written about improving the efficacy of the restoration from differing impression techniques to tooth form [1, 2]. Despite these efforts, there remains a population of patients who cannot function adequately using this type of restoration. Presently, some feel that the complete denture prosthesis is below the standard of care and that the most basic restoration for the edentulous mandible should be an implant-retained overdenture with two implants placed in the anterior mandible [3] (Figs. 16.1 and 16.2).

From a diagnostic perspective, several parameters need to be evaluated before deciding upon the type of prosthesis that is most appropriate for the patient. The following considerations pertain to restorative treatment planning.

Diagnostic considerations include, but are not limited to:

1. Display and positioning of the mandibular incisal edge
2. Facial proportions
3. Restorative space
4. Contours and emergence
5. Tissue contact
6. Opposing occlusion
7. Tissue and quality of saliva
8. Ridge form

S. Jivraj (✉)
Private Practice, Anacapa Dental Art Institute, Oxnard, CA, USA

W. Chee
Advanced Prosthodontics, Herman Ostrow School of Dentistry, University of Southern California, Los Angeles, CA, USA

W. Chee, S. Jivraj (eds.), *Treatment Planning In Implant Dentistry*, BDJ Clinician's Guides, https://doi.org/10.1007/978-3-031-68726-6_16

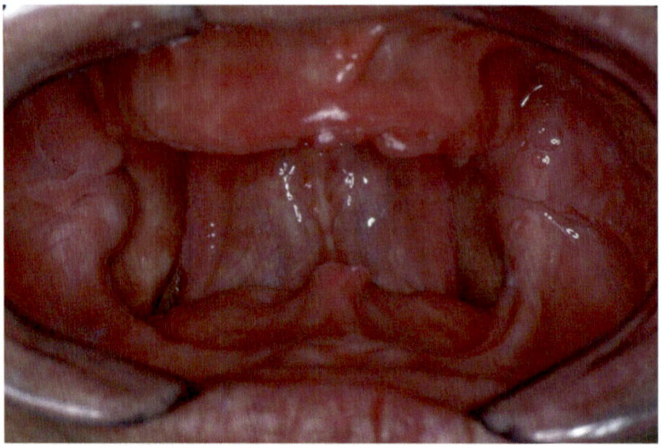

Fig. 16.1 Severely resorbed mandibular ridge with genial tubercles extending above the level of the ridge

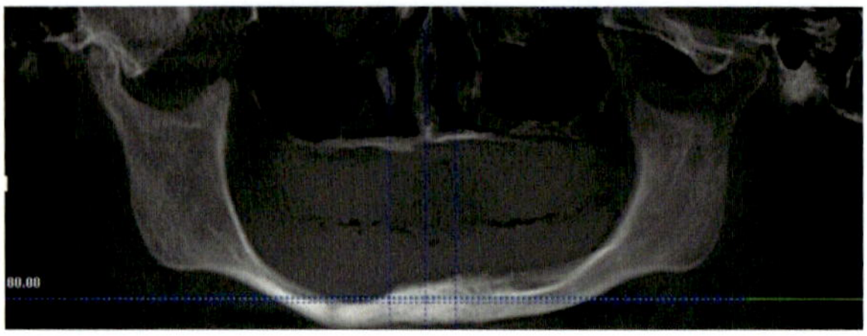

Fig. 16.2 Orthopantomogram illustrating resorption of mandibular arch with inferior dental canal close to the ridge crest and adequate bone to place implants in the anterior mandible

16.1.1 Position of the Mandibular Incisal Edge

The maxillary incisal edge is positioned for aesthetics and phonetics. The mandibular incisal edge is positioned for function. The clinician must provide shallow guidance, sufficient to provide posterior disclusion in both protrusive and lateral excursions. Anterior guidance must be smooth and distributed amongst as many anterior teeth as possible [4].

A thorough evaluation must be made of the existing mandibular incisal edge position. When patients are missing posterior teeth and have been diagnosed as having lack of posterior support, the mandibular incisal edge is often in the incorrect position. Conventional prosthodontic guidelines will place the mandibular incisal edge just at the level of the lower lip with 0.5–1.0 mm of the incisal edge visible. Guidelines in relation to the lower mandibular occlusal plane can also be sought from anatomical landmarks such as the retromolar pad.

The impact of ageing on the facial tissues may result in increased mandibular incisal edge display. The lack of opposing teeth in the maxillary arch may also result in over-eruption of the mandibular anterior dentition.

The over-eruption of teeth brings with it an excess of bone, which often is of inadequate width to place dental implants. Often, the clinician is faced with the dilemma of "To extract or not to extract". This decision is based on several factors which include but are not limited to the following (Figs. 16.3, 16.4 and 16.5):

1. Extent of over-eruption and restorative procedures requires positioning the teeth correctly.
2. Extent of over-eruption and presence of posterior teeth for orthodontic anchorage.
3. Patients' predisposition to caries.
4. Patients' desires and costs.
5. Presence of bone in the posterior mandible. If there is severe bone resorption, the clinician is faced with the decision of having only suitable bone for implant placement in the anterior mandible.

16.1.2 Facial Proportions

Loss of mandibular teeth may bring with it diminished facial proportions in the lower third of the face. Re-establishing this with a prosthetic is part of the clinician's responsibility. Decisions will need to be made in regard to occlusal vertical dimension and space required for the restoration (Fig. 16.6) [5].

16.1.3 Restorative Space

Insufficient restorative space is the most common error when planning full-arch restorations. Inadequate space results in either premature failure of the restoration or changing the treatment plan from one restoration to another to accommodate the space requirements.

To accommodate adequate designs, different types of restorations require different dimensional tolerances [7]. Accurately mounted casts are critical in assessing prosthetic space limitations. Spatial constraints must be considered as a matter of practicality. The limiting factor in edentulous patients is the available inter-arch space. Adequate restorative space is critical, and guidelines exist depending upon the type of prosthesis being treatment planned. There must be adequate space for

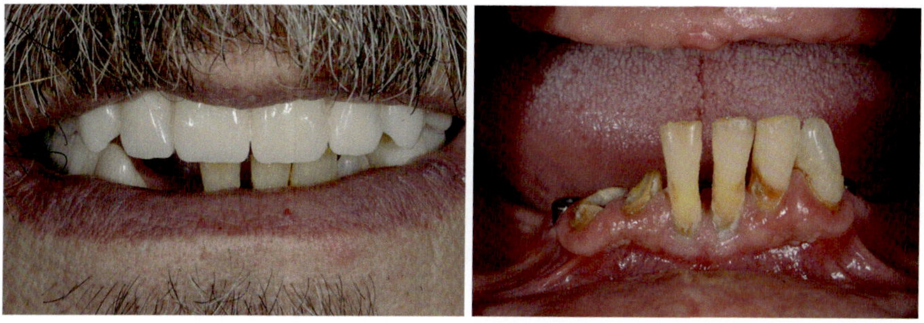

Fig. 16.3 Clinical picture of over-erupted mandibular teeth compromising restorative space

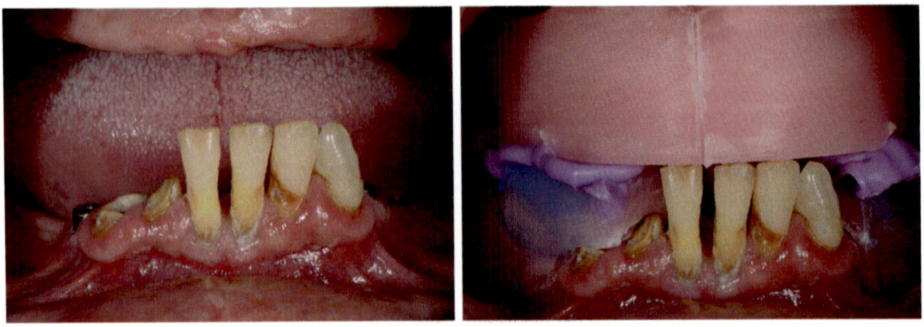

Fig. 16.4 Jaw relation records of patient in Fig. 16.3. The level of the anticipated teeth must be communicated to the laboratory

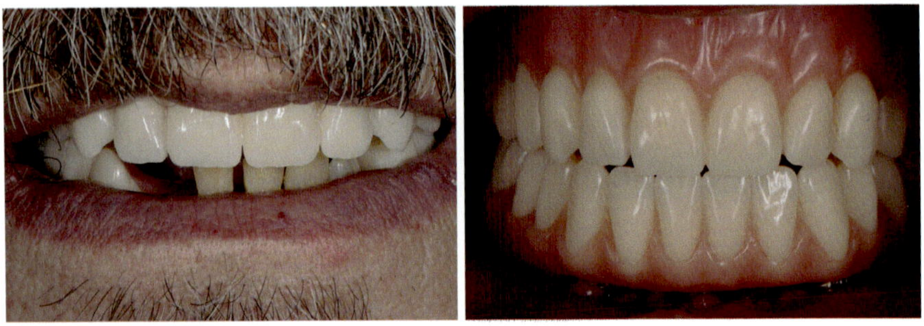

Fig. 16.5 Maxillary denture and mandibular immediately loaded implant-supported prosthesis for patient in Figs. 16.3 and 16.4

bulk of restorative material that also permits a prosthesis design to establish aesthetics and hygiene. If space is limited, re-establishing a patient's vertical dimension or altering the opposing occlusion should be considered.

Guidelines for space requirements for ceramic-based restorations are 10–13 mm for a screw-retained ceramic-based restorations and 14–16 mm for acrylic resin/titanium-based restorations. Clinicians should select the material that requires the least bone removal and satisfies the requirements of aesthetics, contour and biomechanics (Figs. 16.7 and 16.8).

16.1.4 Contours and Emergence

The contours of the restorations must be planned from the outset. The emergence profile of the restorations should be straight as it exits from the gingival margin. Often, this requires alveolectomy to create sufficient space. The restorative dentist requires this space to provide a restoration that satisfies the requirements of mechanics, aesthetics and cleansability. This space creation must be communicated to the surgeon through the use of a bone reduction guide, and it becomes the surgeon's responsibility to provide this space. Bone reduction must have a rationale, and the

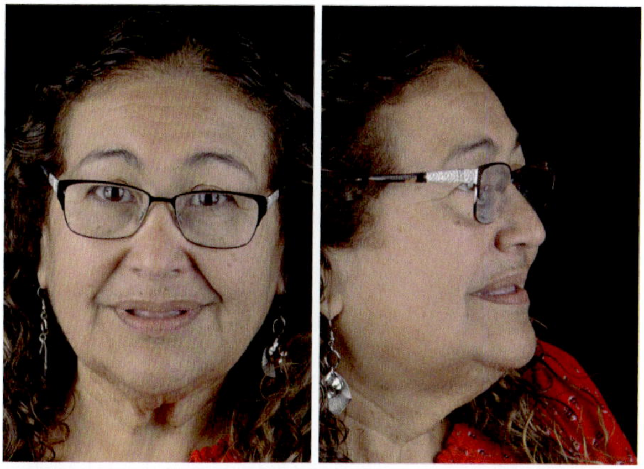

Fig. 16.6 Ramifications of tooth loss on facial support

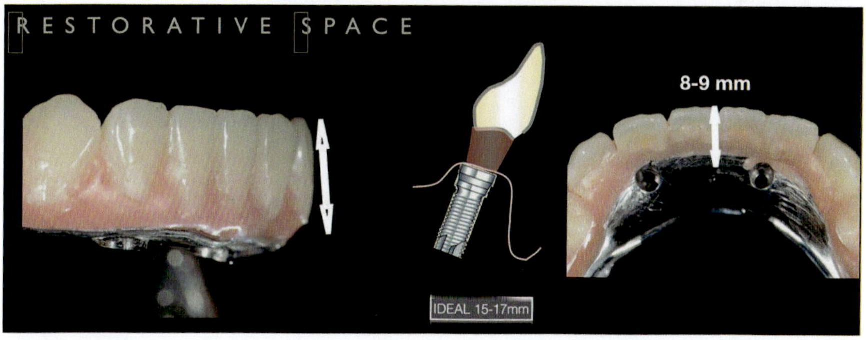

Fig. 16.7 Restorative space required for acrylic resin titanium prosthesis

minimum bone reduction must be done to satisfy the requirements of implant placement and fabrication of a biomechanically sound restoration (Fig. 16.9).

Rationales for bone reduction include but are not limited to:

1. Adequate buccolingual width of bone to place implants
2. Adequate space for hygiene
3. Adequate space for biomechanics of the restoration
4. Adequate space so that the patient can clean the undersurface
5. Improved emergence of the restoration

16.1.5 Tissue Contact

Historically fixed restorations in the mandible had been restored with the high-water design. This included abutments of a specific height which resulted in the restoration being 3–4 mm above the tissue. This facilitated oral hygiene, but the inconvenience for the patients was food entrapment.

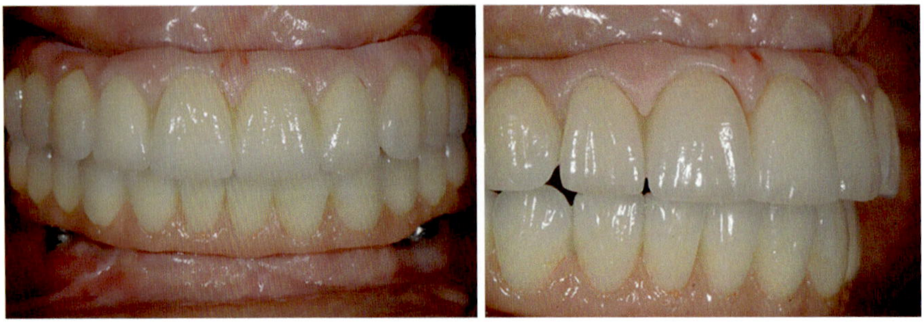

Fig. 16.8 Lack of restorative space resulted in a porcelain fused to cobalt chrome framework restoration for the mandible

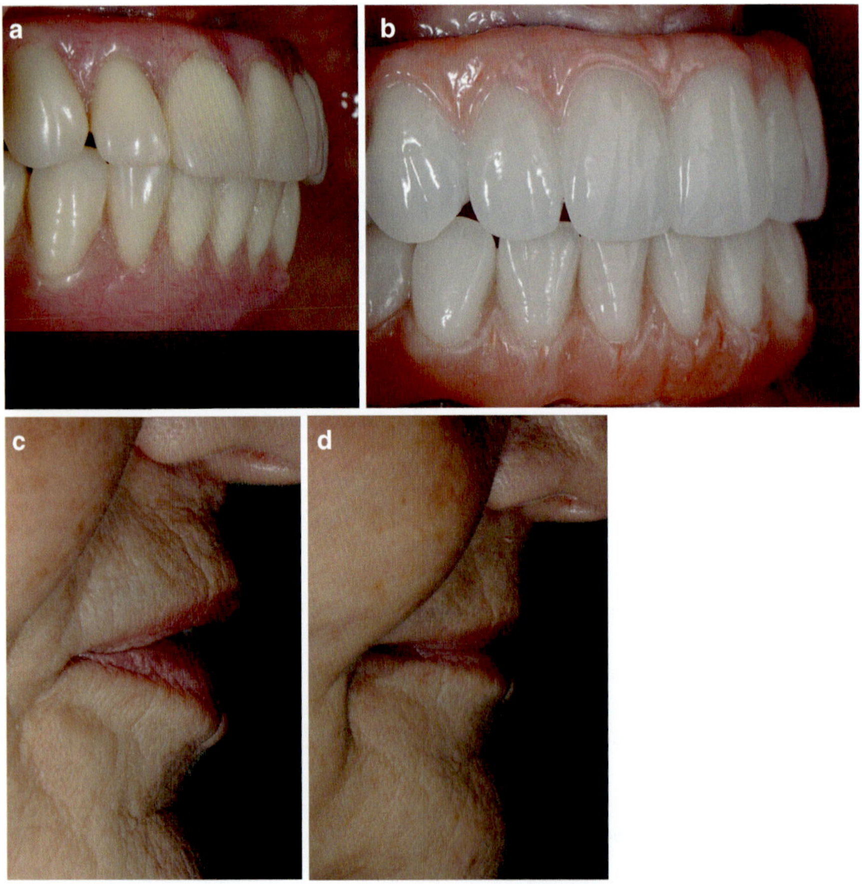

Fig. 16.9 Lip over-supported by restoration. Correction made

As in any aspect of restorative dentistry, the provisional is key to the success of the definitive restoration. From a patient perspective, the communication of aesthetics and phonetics is important. From a clinician's perspective, biomechanics, occlusion and cleansability are key areas of concern. The provisional/immediate load prosthesis must satisfy the following criteria:

1. Reduce food entrapment—Following 3 months of healing, the acrylic provisional should be relined so that it compresses the tissue surface and creates a concave tissue surface allowing a convex restoration surface (Fig. 16.10).
2. Provide cleansable contours by developing the tissue as outlined above.
3. The tissue contact should be intimate, but accessible to oral hygiene procedures.
4. The tissue surface should be highly polished (Fig. 16.11).

16.1.6 Opposing Occlusion

Often when restoring, a single-arch restorative space becomes an obstacle. When the patient has been missing teeth for several years, the teeth in the opposing arch over-erupt and compromise restorative space. Treatment planning must include strategies to create space. This may be through reshaping, restoring, repositing or removing teeth. The most conservative option should be chosen.

16.1.7 Tissue and Quality of Saliva

The clinician should evaluate the patient's medical history for any medications that may cause xerostomia. A documented dental history must investigate how the patient lost their teeth and will provide the clinician with risk factors. If caries was the cause, partly due to medication-induced xerostomia, the choice between fixed and removable restorations must be made very carefully. A visual inspection of the tissue is a critical pre-determinant before deciding upon the type of prosthesis to fabricate. Patients who suffer from xerostomia are not good candidates for an

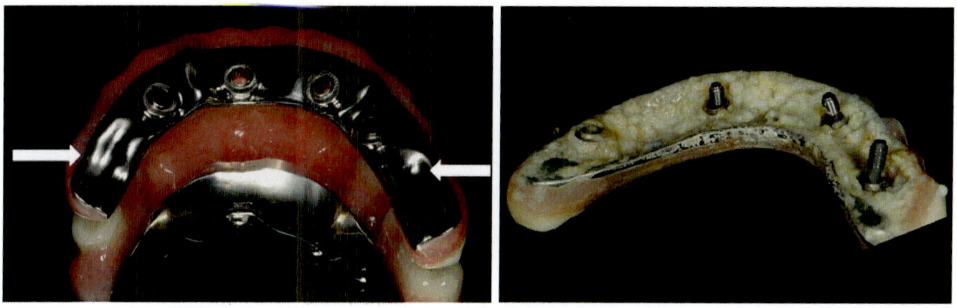

Fig. 16.10 Undersurface of restoration not amenable to cleansing

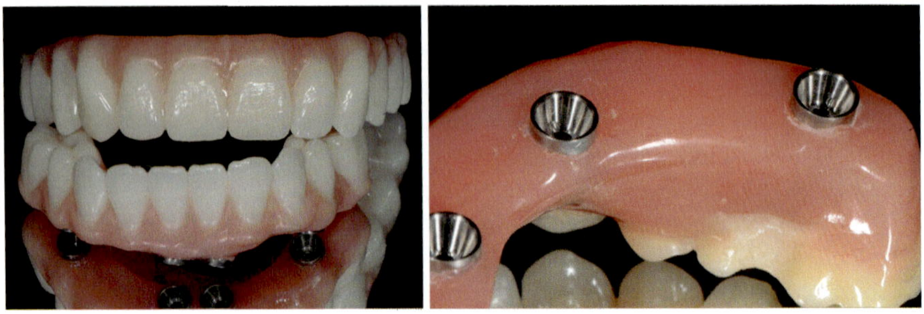

Fig. 16.11 Undersurface should be convex and highly polished

implant- and mucosa-supported restoration due to the irritation that the flanges may cause.

16.1.8 Ridge Form

The anatomical situation of the residual ridge has a bearing on the stability and retention that can be achieved for a removable appliance. Both the height and shape of the residual ridge play a part. In implant- and mucosa-supported overdentures, posterior ridge form plays a critical role in providing lateral stability. If the posterior ridge form is flat, it is the author's opinion that implant- and mucosa-supported removable overdentures are often contraindicated; this is due to mobility of the prosthesis even though connected to implants. Patients are dissatisfied with their expectations for stability of the prostheses and pain on occluding in mucosal supported areas.

Treatment choices for the mandible include but are not limited to the following:

1. No treatment
2. Conventional dentures
3. Implant-retained and mucosa-supported overdentures
4. Screw-retained fixed implant-supported dentures in zirconia or titanium acrylic
5. Implant-supported restorations in metal ceramic or zirconia

This chapter attempts to describe the treatment planning aspects of therapy rather than the technical aspects. The discussion will be based on patient needs and desires, anatomical presentation of patients, cost-benefit analysis, maintenance and post-operative visits.

16.2 The Implant-Retained and Mucosa-Supported Overdenture

This type of restoration is ideal for patients who complain of looseness and mobility of the mandibular denture but not of pain or soreness of the mucosa with the use of a mandibular complete denture. The complete overdenture prosthesis is made to full extensions as conventional complete dentures usually are. This is to maximize areas of support for the prostheses. The function of the implants in this type of restoration is primarily to aid in retention of the prosthesis and not for support of the restoration. Studies have shown that over the long term, implants supporting this type of restoration have a high success rate [4–6]. In the simplest form, two implants are placed between the mental foramina; the function of the genio-glossus muscle and the fact that the mandibular anterior teeth are usually the last teeth to be lost lead to usually having sufficient bone to place implants in this area even though the rest of the alveolus may be severely resorbed (Fig. 16.12). Unless the implants are very short (8 mm or less) or they are severely divergent (more than 20°), they need not be splinted. A low-profile attachment with easily replaceable retainers should be used (Figs. 16.13, 16.14 and 16.15). At present, the most efficacious attachment is the locator attachment manufactured by Zest Attachments, San Diego, CA. This attachment is marketed by other implant companies also, e.g. 3i (Implant Innovations Inc., Palm Beach, Florida, USA). Advantages of this particular attachment are that it is made for many implant systems; it comes in varying heights to accommodate soft tissue thicknesses and has a low profile. The retention can be varied with the choice of plastic-retentive elements which are easily replaced. One portion of the attachment is screwed directly into the implant body; this abutment is selected to fit the thickness of the mucosa and depth of the implant with the goal to have the attachment as low as possible yet expose the retentive element. Advantages of this type of restoration are (1) reduced number or implants, (2) ability to convert existing removable prosthesis and (3) ease of repair of prostheses.

Disadvantages of this type of restoration are that (1) implants cannot diverge too much (less than 20°), (2) prostheses still require support from mucosa and (3) periodic maintenance is required to replace attachments and to compensate for

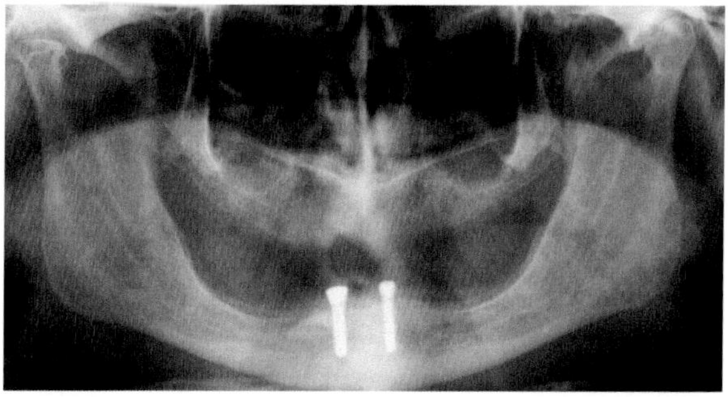

Fig. 16.12 Panoramic radiograph showing two dental implants placed in the anterior part of the mandible

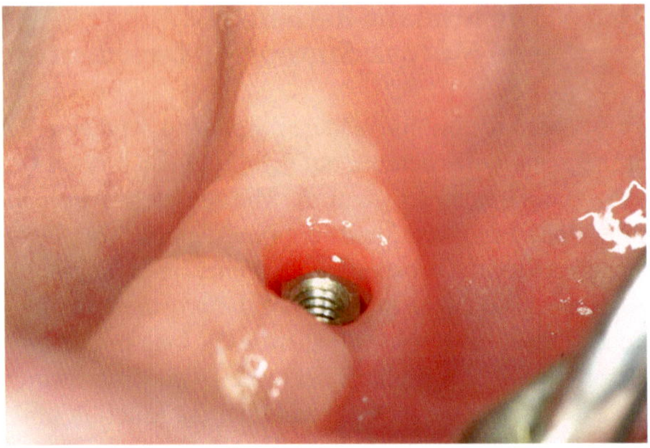

Fig. 16.13 Depth of tissue should be measured prior to selecting locator

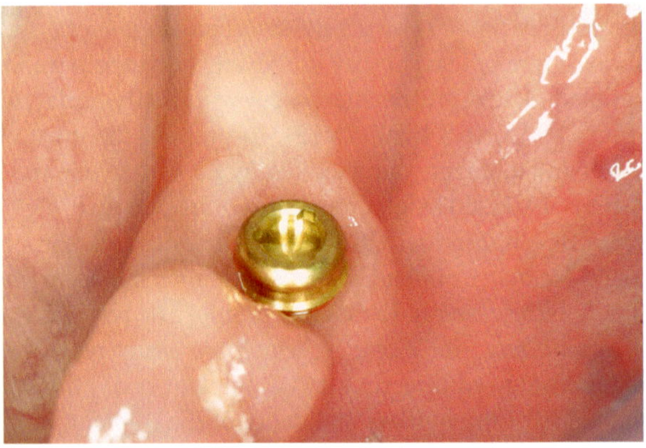

Fig. 16.14 Locator should be selected so that it is 1.5 mm above tissue surface

continued resorption of bone in posterior areas (Figs. 16.16, 16.17, 16.18, 16.19, 16.20, 16.21, 16.22 and 16.23).

Adequate inter-occlusal space must be present so that a sufficient bulk of acrylic resin can resist fracture; areas where the attachments are will be weakened to accommodate the attachments. 10 mm or more is desirable. Figures 16.24, 16.25 and 16.26 illustrate a poorly planned overdenture restoration; it is evident that there is insufficient space available for all the implant components. The resulting overdenture will be thin having minimal bulk of acrylic resin resulting in a prosthesis that is weak and prone to breakage.

Since the object of this prosthesis is to be tissue borne, only one axis of rotation should exist for this type of prostheses. If the prosthesis is not designed to move freely about an axis, then premature replacement of the attachments will be required or breakage of components will ensue with only two implants; this objective is achieved automatically (Figs. 16.27 and 16.28). Figures 16.29, 16.30 and 16.31 illustrate poorly designed overdenture prostheses; a tissue bar with multiple axes of rotation was fabricated resulting in repeated breaking of the attachments and ultimately breaking of the prostheses. This occurred due to stresses during function

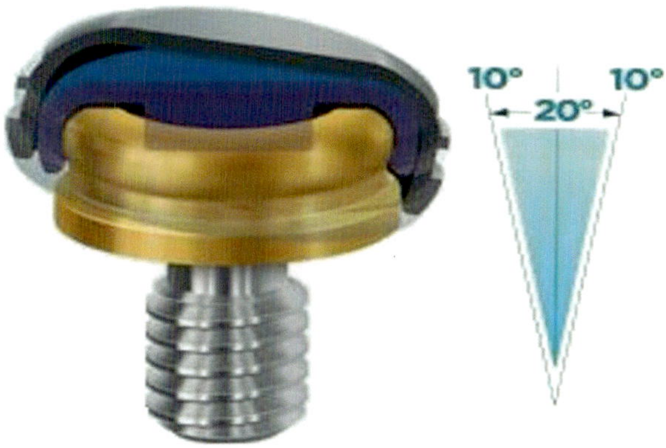

Fig. 16.15 Locator retention mechanism within 20° of divergence

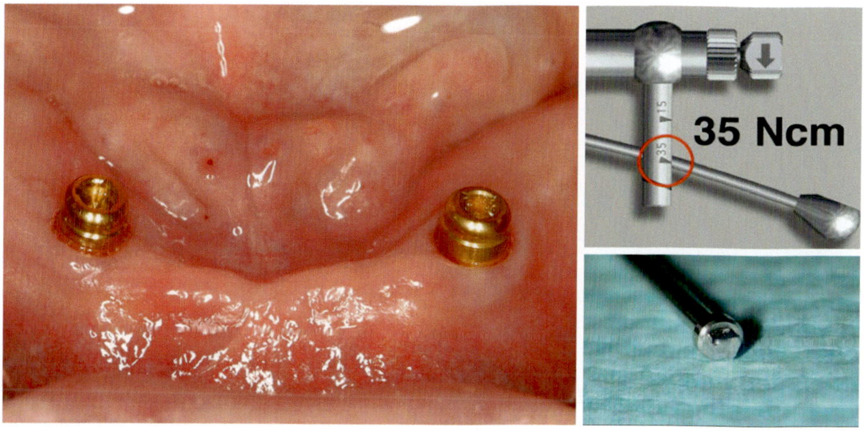

Fig. 16.16 Locators torqued into place

caused by torquing of the prostheses over the tissue bar. This type of prostheses is not meant to be fully supported by the implants, and some freedom of motion is required to share the load with the mucosa. When implants are too divergent or short and require more implants placed, the prostheses and tissue bar must be designed to freely rotate about one axis. Failure to do so will cause premature wear of components or breakage [7].

Figures 16.32, 16.33, 16.34 and 16.35 illustrate a patient who had four short implants placed in the anterior mandible; a tissue bar was fabricated to splint the implants and distribute the stress amongst them, attachments were placed distal to the posterior implants to create one rotation axis and the prostheses was relieved to rotate freely about this axis. Figure 16.36 demonstrates the stability of the implant-retained overdenture; the prostheses remain stable though the tongue is protruded.

Though costs of implant-retained overdentures are increased over conventional complete dentures when this service is provided, there is growing evidence that patients who receive this type of prostheses benefit with better function, nutrition

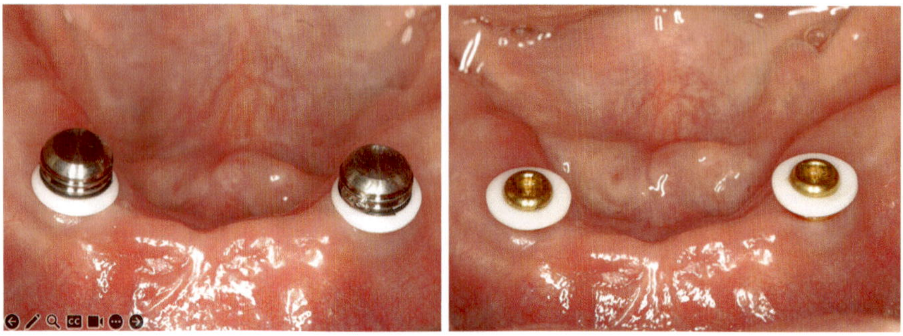

Fig. 16.17 Locator housings and silicone block-out rings placed

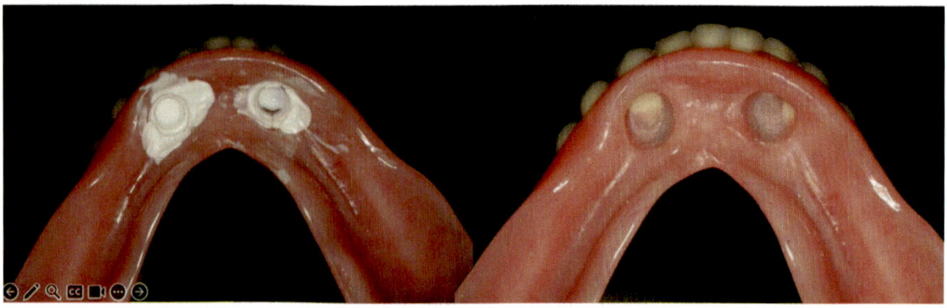

Fig. 16.18 Area of implants marked with fit checker and room made

and general well-being [8–15]. An important issue with this type of restoration is that patients must be informed that they will still have a removable prosthesis, that the mucosa under the denture bases will still be loaded and that there will be continuous maintenance required of the prostheses once delivered. The maintenance will include regular relines of the prostheses, regular replacement of attachments, oral hygiene and prophylaxis of the implants and possible breakage of components [15–20]. Patients must be informed of these facts prior to beginning treatment; adjustments are most frequent during the first year of usage and will continue. Another consideration of providing this type of restoration is to consider the effect on the maxillary arch; it has been shown that there is increased resorption of the anterior maxilla and mandibular posterior ridges with long-term use of the implant-retained overdenture. Possibly, this is due to the increased bite forces generated directly over the implants in the anterior mandible. Regular relines are indicated to maintain an even occlusal contact between the maxillary and mandibular prostheses [21–24].

There are also reports in the literature about immediately loading implants with overdentures; though this is possible, caution should be taken with patient selection and mode of restoration. Most of the studies with overdenture restorations immediately loaded have multiple implants splinted with a tissue bar. This increases the cost of the procedure and makes maintenance more difficult [25, 26].

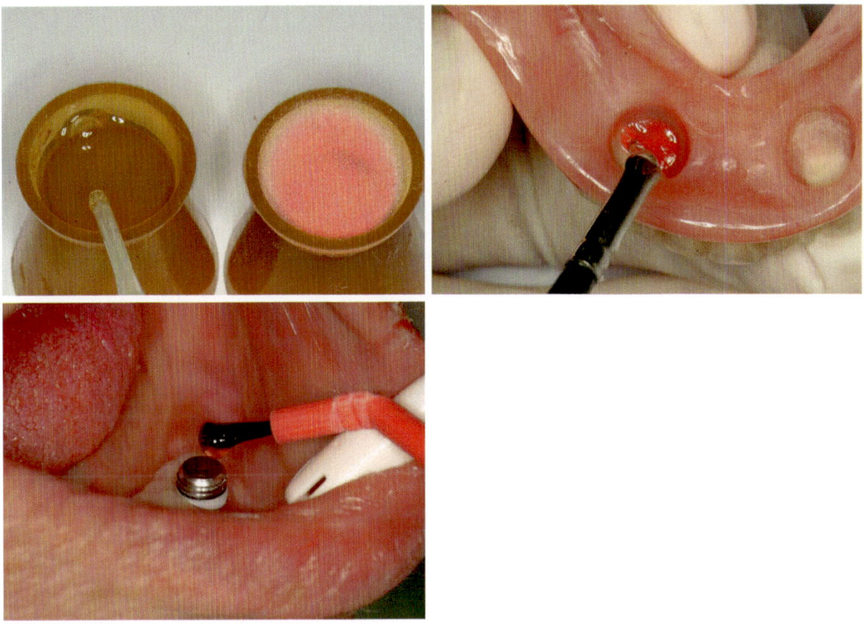

Fig. 16.19 Pickup using cold-cured acrylic resin

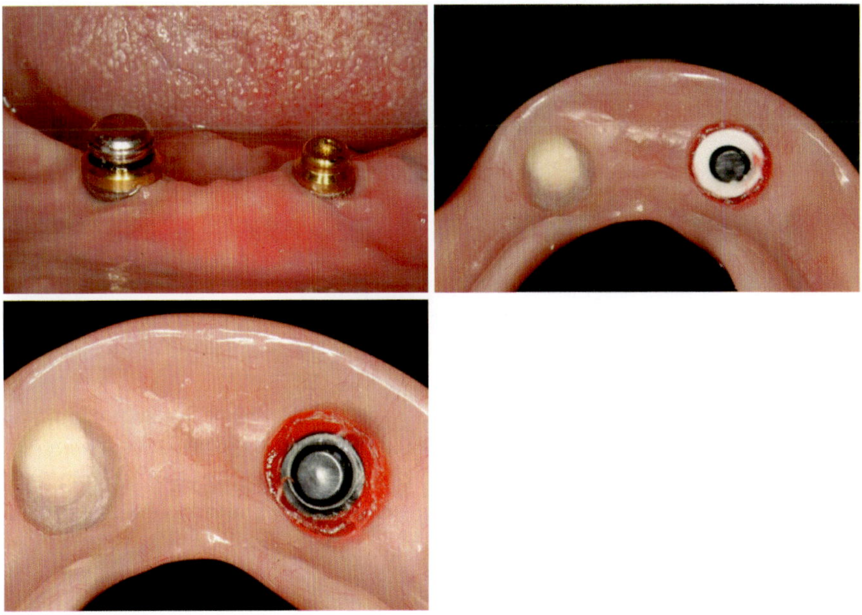

Fig. 16.20 Locator picked up one at a time

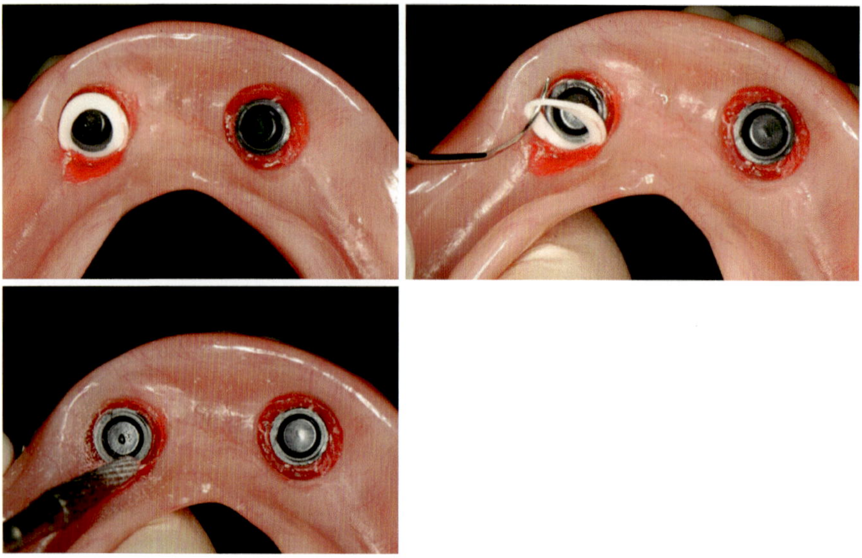

Fig. 16.21 Silicone ring removed, undersurface polished

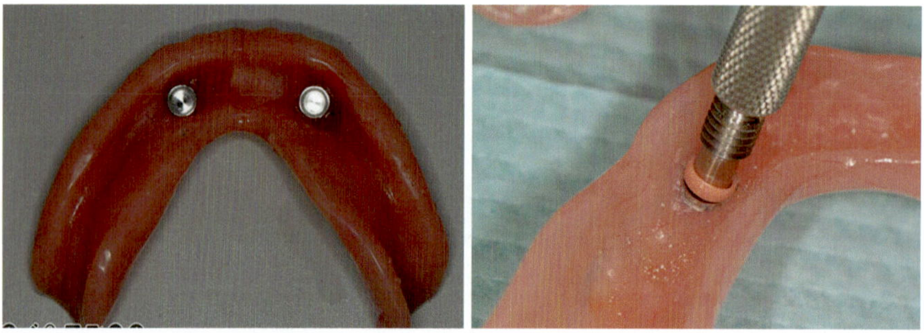

Fig. 16.22 Blanks removed and retention mechanism inserted

The number of implants to be placed and the type of retentive mechanism are predicated on patient- and clinician-related factors. An opposing dentate occlusion may necessitate more implants for prosthetic stability. A recent 5-year randomized clinical trial revealed no statistically significant differences in patient satisfaction, implant survival or maintenance with one or two implants retained and mucosa-supported overdentures. A metal reinforcement for a solitary anchor design was recommended.

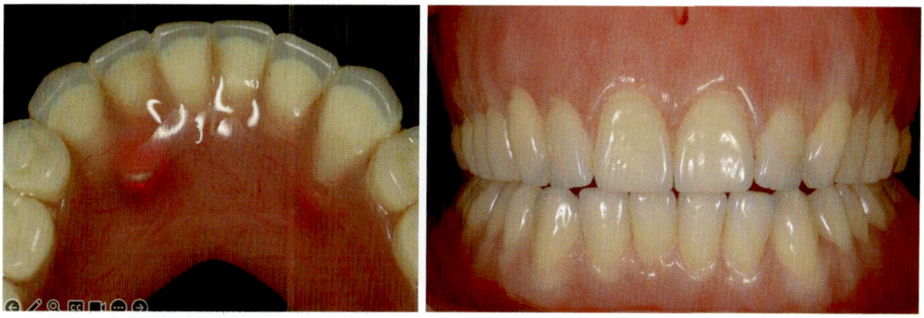

Fig. 16.23 Final denture in place

Fig. 16.24 Casts should always be mounted in the diagnostic phase to insure that sufficient inter-occlusal space is available

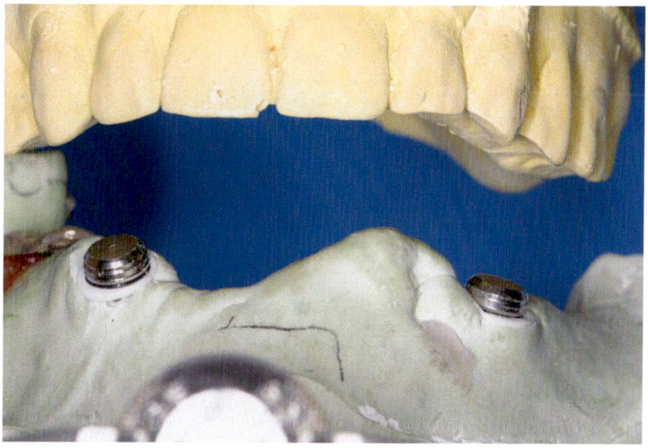

16.2.1 Fixed Implant-Supported Denture

When the anatomical presentation of the patient will allow an overdenture restoration and more than two implants are possible, treatment choices can be expanded to fixed implant-supported restorations. The implant-retained and -supported overdenture has little indication in the mandibular arch when four or more implants are placed. The fixed implant-supported denture is a restoration that requires 4–6 implants that are traditionally placed between the mental foramina. These implants are sufficient to support a fixed restoration with cantilevers posterior to the terminal implants (Figs. 16.37 and 16.38). This type of restoration is dependant totally on the implants for support and can be provided for all edentulous patients who have sufficient bone and inter-arch space to receive implants in the anterior mandible. With age changes and the many medications that reduce saliva flow, removable prostheses can become increasingly uncomfortable for xerostomic patients to wear. Since the fixed implant-supported denture does not load the mucosa, patients who experience pain when using conventional complete denture prostheses are well suited to this type of restoration (Fig. 16.39). In addition, this type of restoration has the most documentation over a long term [27, 28].

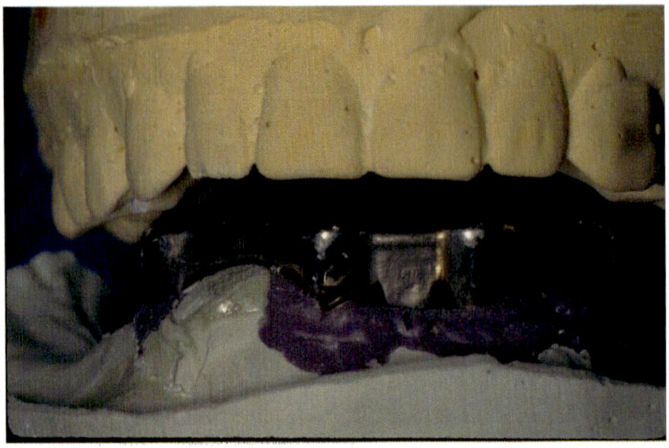

Fig. 16.25 Mounted casts indicating insufficient room for the implant components and the tissue bar

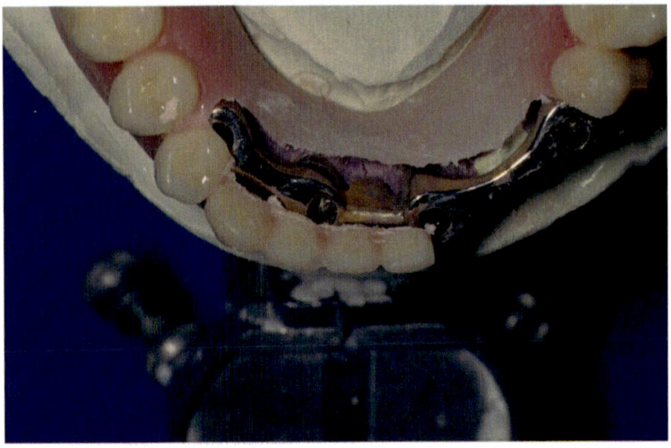

Fig. 16.26 Occlusal view of casts showing minimal space for the overdenture prosthesis components over the tissue bar

Costs for this type of restoration are initially higher than overdenture prostheses. However, the satisfaction of patients is also higher, combined with fewer postoperative visits for adjustments and unscheduled appointments; this prosthesis becomes an attractive choice for the treatment of edentulous patients [29, 30]. In addition, there is documentation available supporting the equivalent success of implants between the delayed and immediate loading protocols for providing this type of restoration [10, 31–35]. It is the author's first choice to restore edentulous mandibles with this prosthesis using the immediate loading protocol (Fig. 16.40). Postoperative visits are markedly reduced after insertion of the implants and provisional restoration, and patient satisfaction and comfort are increased over conventional loading protocols. Even when providing overdenture prostheses to patients, care should be taken so that the implants placed for the overdenture prostheses do not preclude placement of additional implants to support a fixed-type prosthesis.

Treatment planning for this type of restoration begins with a patient interview, followed by a clinical examination and a review of radiographs; a panoramic radiograph is useful to determine the availability of bone to receive implants in the anterior mandible. A CBCT scan of the area to receive implants is mandatory to determine the buccolingual proportions of the bone and proximity of neurovascular

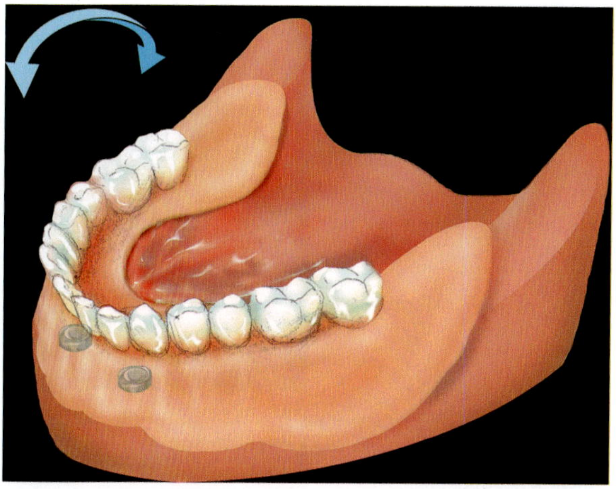

Fig. 16.27 When there is one axis of rotation, the prostheses can freely move and share the load with the mucosa, and the implants serve to retain the prostheses

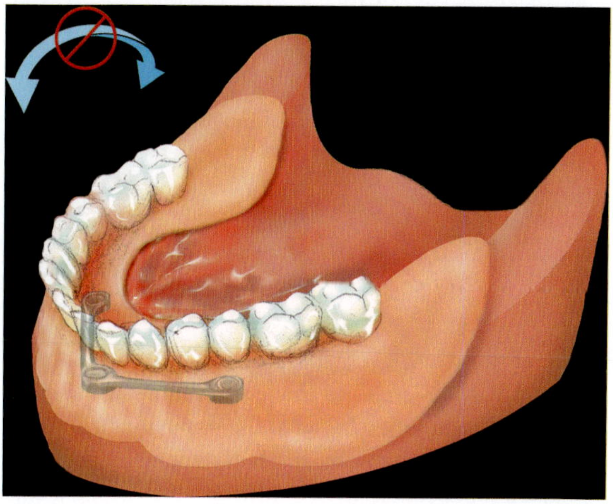

Fig. 16.28 When there is no axis of rotation, the prostheses will bind and torque the tissue bar and implants, which leads to failure of the components

structures. A minimum of 12–15 mm of inter-occlusal space from the platform of the implant to the opposing occlusion is required for the implant components, framework and teeth. If insufficient space presents, then consideration to increasing the vertical dimension, ostectomy or fixed metal ceramic restorations requiring less inter-occlusal space must be considered.

A surgical guide is constructed based on the patient's existing complete denture or dentition if the teeth are in an acceptable position. Then implant surgery can proceed. Four to six implants are placed between the mental foramina in as exaggerated arch form as possible; the more the anterior posterior spread, the longer the cantilever can be made. It is always the clinician's objective to minimize or eliminate the cantilever as much as possible [35–37]. In vitro and in vivo experiments have demonstrated that most stress is placed on the terminal implant when occlusal forces are applied to the cantilever. These two factors dominate in determining the

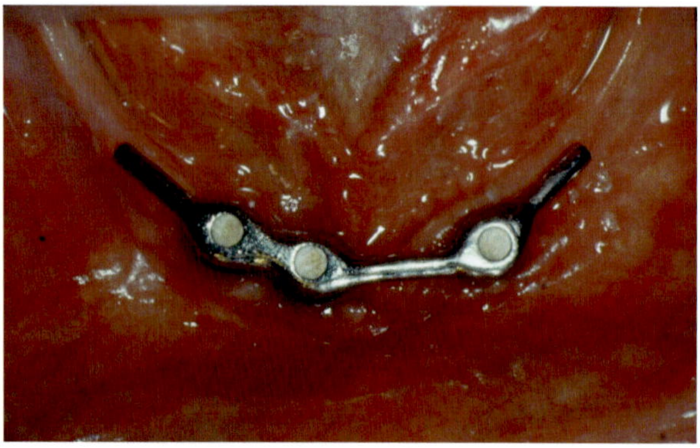

Fig. 16.29 Intraoral view of poorly designed tissue bar

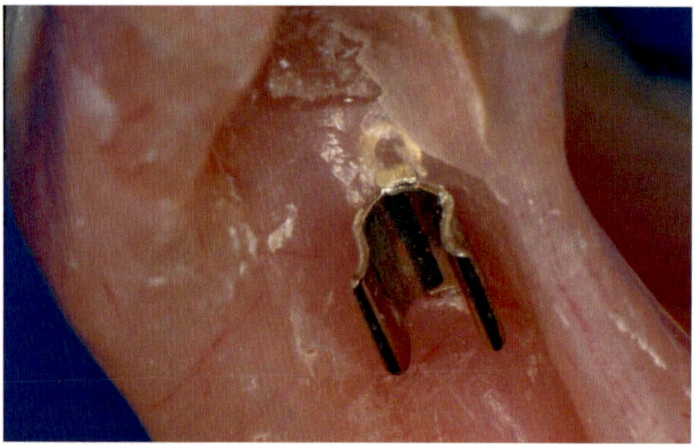

Fig. 16.30 Broken attachment clip from prostheses over tissue bar in Fig. 16.29

length of the cantilever, the anterior posterior spread, the area of the distributed implants and the length of the terminal implant (Figs. 16.41 and 16.42). Cantilever length is also modified by what the opposing occluding arch is, i.e. a complete denture, natural dentition or implant-supported restoration. Increased loading will demand a reduced length of cantilever. If too long a cantilever is placed, mechanical failure of the implant components of the prostheses is a common sequela (Figs. 16.43 and 16.44). To reduce the loading of the terminal implant, some have advocated placing short implants distal to the mental foramina and connecting all the implants [36–42].

Mandibular flexure may be a consideration in treatment planning for a fixed implant-supported prosthesis. It is a phenomenon that occurs simultaneously with mandibular movements and may affect changes in the shape of the mandible. Multiple authors have reported increased biomechanical stress at the prosthetic and implant levels, poor passivity, distortion of the impression, discomfort during function, porcelain chipping, screw loosening and fracture. A recent study [43] reported that the mandible showed clinically significant shortening and tightening from the maximum intercuspation to the maximal opening position. This is an initial study with a limited sample size, and further investigation is necessary. Considering the amount of tightening and shortening caused by mandibular flexure, it may have

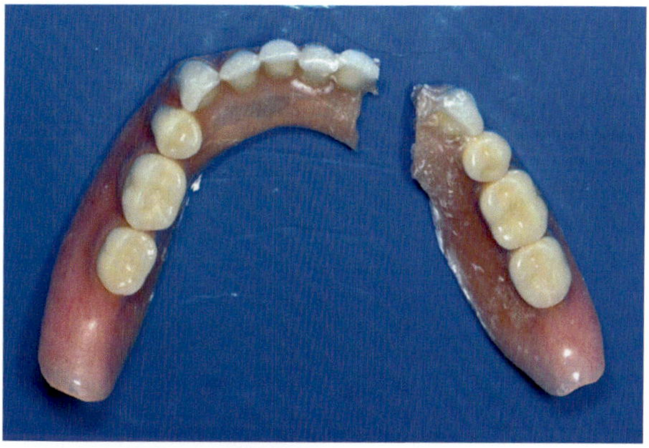

Fig. 16.31 Broken prosthesis constructed over tissue bar in Fig. 16.29

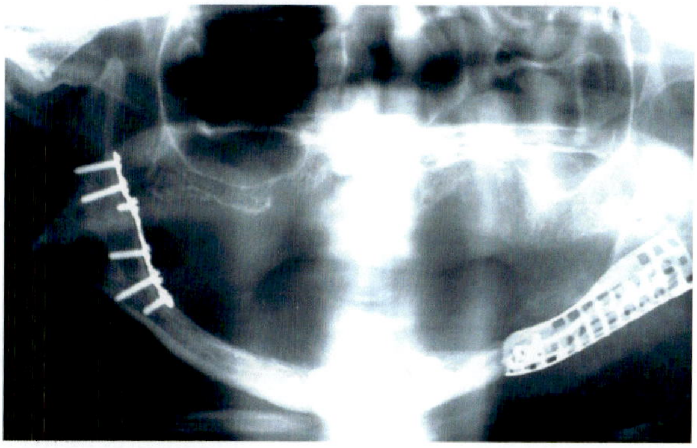

Fig. 16.32 Radiograph of severely resorbed mandible with fractures on left and right sides; inferior dental nerve has been severed bilaterally; the patient has difficulty using a conventional prosthesis; four short implants are inserted in the anterior mandible

relevance in treatment planning, particularly in the case of a rigid long-span screw-retained prosthetic superstructure where implants are connected anterior and posterior to the mental foramen. Solutions to this may be to split the prosthesis in the midline or use a material which is sufficiently rigid so that it negates the effect of mandibular flexure.

Once implants have been placed, they can (1) have cover screws placed and submerged under the mucosa (two stages), (2) have healing caps placed and have mucosa sutured around them (single stage) and (3) be immediately loaded. There are sufficient publications documenting the safety and efficacy of immediately loading splinted in the anterior mandible, making this the standard protocol of the authors. Resonance frequency analysis (RFA) measurements of implants placed in the anterior mandible indicate that the implants are stable on placement and continue to remain stable through osseointegration. Success rate studies have shown that the success of immediately loading implants in this location is similar to the delayed conventional protocol. The only modification made is that no cantilevers are used on the provisional [44, 45]. With immediately loading the implants, a 3–4-month healing period and confirmation of osseointegration, impressions of the integrated implants can proceed for the definitive restoration. Alternatively, if the patient

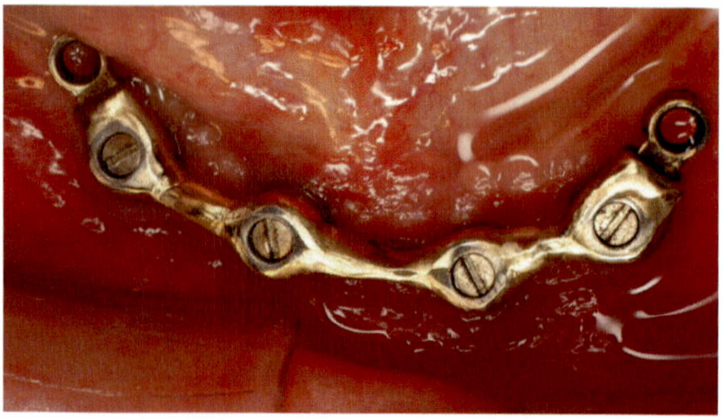

Fig. 16.33 Tissue bar constructed for the patient in Fig. 16.32 to maintain only one axis of rotation in order that the prosthesis has freedom of rotation and the attachments are placed distal to the last implant

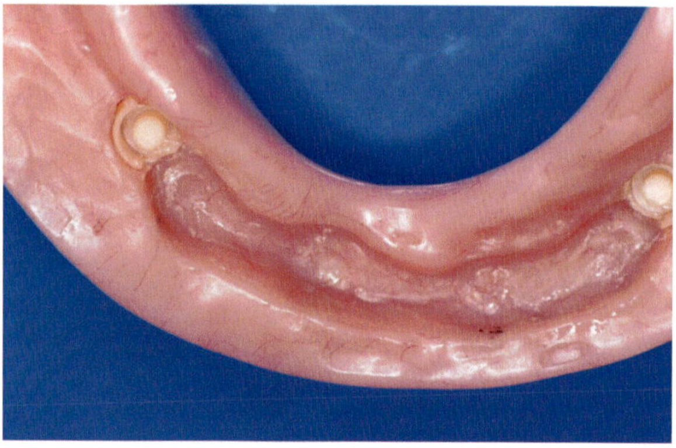

Fig. 16.34 Tissue surface of prostheses made over tissue bar in Fig. 16.33

is satisfied with the tooth position and function of the provisional restoration, analogues can be attached to the provisional restoration and set in a plaster cast, and then an index of the tooth positions from the buccal and lingual can be made with putty silicone. At this time, the cast can be mounted against the maxilla using the provisional restoration. Thus, implant positions, jaw registration and tooth positions are established in one visit. Digital technology through scanning combined with analogue techniques can also make the time to the definitive restorations more efficient.

Using the scans, framework construction can begin with care taken that there is sufficient room for teeth and acrylic resin. Attention must be paid to the dimensions of the framework—knowing that most stress is concentrated at the cantilever, this area of the framework is made larger, and an L beam shape is formed to maximize rigidity of the framework with large cavities for retention of the acrylic resin (Figs. 16.45, 16.46, 16.47 and 16.48). Another approach to reduce mechanical failure and to decrease the length of the cantilever is to place implants distal to the mental foramen and connect them (Fig. 16.49). The framework is fabricated through CAD/CAM technology which is tried in for passivity, and teeth are set to occlude with the opposing arch. Following this, acrylic resin and teeth are processed on to the framework.

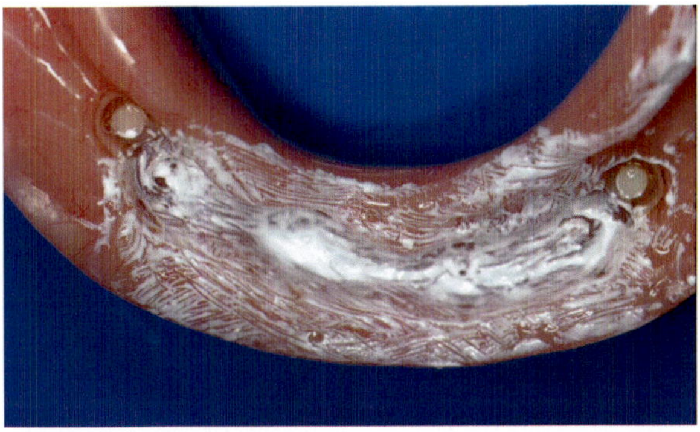

Fig. 16.35 The prosthesis in Fig. 16.34 is adjusted to rotate freely with the help of disclosing paste

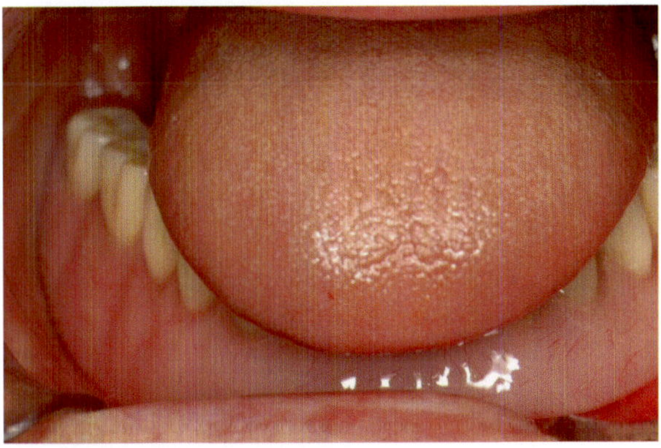

Fig. 16.36 The prosthesis for the patient in Fig. 16.32 inserted; it remains stable throughout when the patient protrudes her tongue

Framework materials range from gold alloys and silver palladium alloys to titanium. Gold and silver alloys are cast onto pre-machined cylinders. Due to the rising cost of gold and the advent of CAD/CAM technology, gold is rarely used as a framework material in this regard and has been superseded by titanium frameworks. Titanium frameworks are milled by implant manufacturers or laboratories with suitable milling machines; the authors' experience with titanium frameworks is that while they fit well, the relationship to the teeth and the contours are less than desirable and often need customization.

Framework designs for a full-arch, one-piece, implant-supported acrylic resin and titanium-based restoration have changed significantly since the transition from gold frameworks to titanium. Different manufacturers have different designs available, and despite technological advances, frameworks still do not replicate the characteristics familiar to gold frameworks. With titanium frameworks, a few key parameters become important:

1. Bulk for strength
2. Adequate access for oral hygiene
3. Minimal display of metal
4. Retention for acrylic

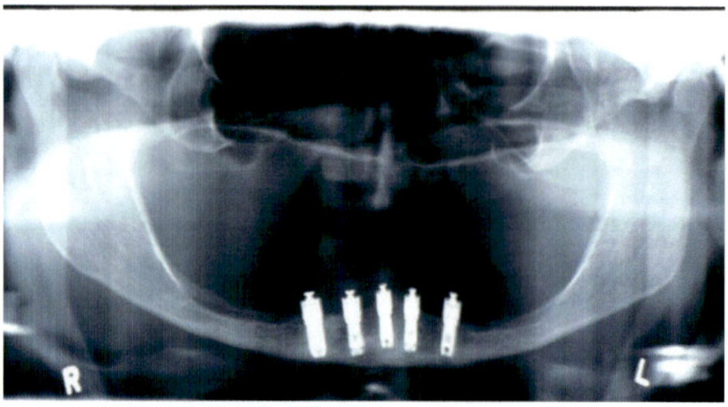

Fig. 16.37 Radiograph of implants placed in the anterior mandible to support a hybrid restoration

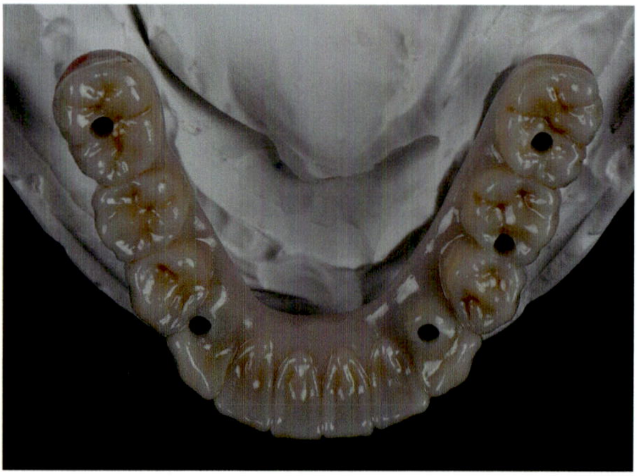

Fig. 16.38 Cantilevers in a hybrid restoration should always be minimized

5. Adequate space for acrylic resin
6. Adequate strength in the cantilever section
7. Attention to cross-sectional area (Fig. 16.50)

When considering these parameters, there are mainly two types of framework designs to support acrylic resin teeth. One of these designs is the "minimalist" framework where acrylic is wrapped around the bar and encompasses it 360° including the intaglio surface. One advantage is that it can be relined, but little is known about its longevity in terms of biomechanics. Anecdotally, numerous colleagues have experienced fractures of this type of framework. Failures may be due to excessive cantilever or inadequate bar shape, and further studies need to explore these issues. The second type of framework may include I- or L-shaped bar designs to maximize rigidity. One advantage of this design is that due to the shape of the titanium framework requiring less bulk of material in any one dimension, adequate space and retention for acrylic resin can be achieved which maximizes thickness in the cantilever area. The evidence base is also lacking with this design.

The authors have had clinical experience of repeated fracture of teeth, acrylic resin delamination and denture teeth wearing in a mandibular implant-supported

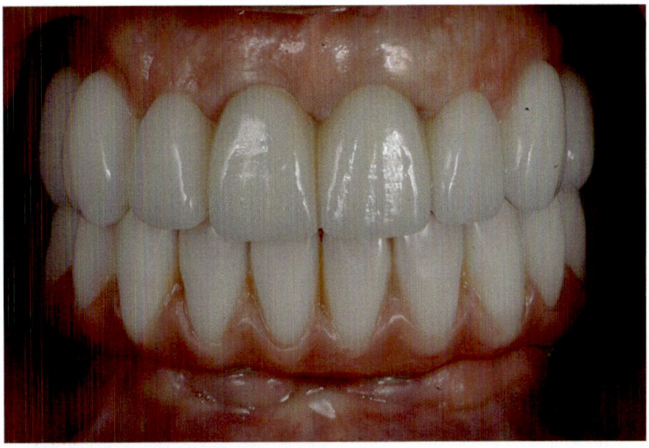

Fig. 16.39 Mandibular hybrid restoration in situ, showing favourable contours

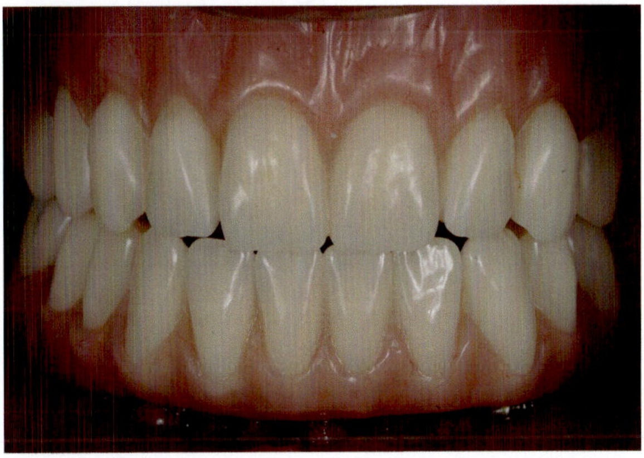

Fig. 16.40 Intraoral view of immediately placed provisional restoration when hybrid restorations are placed for immediate loading; if possible, the fit surfaces are always above the level of the mucosa to facilitate placement of the provisional restoration and minimal disturbance to the surgical site

prosthesis. This is a result of the nature of the material and the forces that can be generated with a fully implant-supported restoration.

Another possible option is to utilize technology in the manufacturing of acrylic to titanium restorations such as milling acrylic around an embedded titanium framework utilizing polychromatic monolithic acrylic. This type of restoration may eliminate many of the potential complications of traditional denture teeth bonded to titanium with processed acrylic such as delamination of teeth and fracture of acrylic veneering materials.

Acrylic resin titanium implant-supported fixed dentures are recommended when opposing a maxillary denture due to similar restorative materials wearing against each other. When the patient has an existing maxillary natural dentition, the clinician may choose a more robust material such as monolithic zirconia. These provide better wear resistance, are less prone to fracture and can be fabricated with smaller dimensions, so that the patient has additional room for the tongue. The clinical process is similar except that an acrylic prototype is tried in to verify occlusion prior to the definitive restoration in zirconia being fabricated (Fig. 16.51a–c).

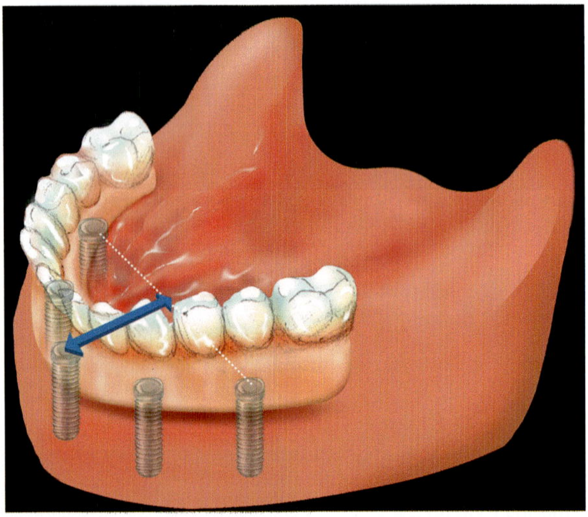

Fig. 16.41 The distribution of implants will dictate the length of the cantilever; the length of the cantilever is equal to the length indicated in the diagram, which is the anteroposterior spread of the implants

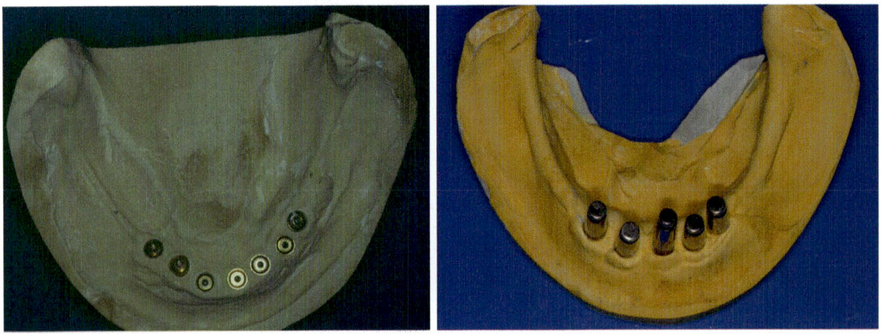

Fig. 16.42 (**a**, **b**) Two master casts showing different AP spreads and allowing different lengths of cantilever

16.2.2 Metal Ceramic/Zirconia Fixed Units

When patients present with many of the teeth unrestorable for periodontal or structural reasons, there are times when removing these teeth in order to provide implant-supported restorations becomes the most predictable option. As the alveolar housing is still present with teeth present, there will be minimal bone resorption; this would contraindicate the use of implant-supported fixed denture due to insufficient space. In these situations, all the principles of restoring teeth in the anterior and posterior quadrants which have been described in earlier chapters must apply.

For this type of restoration, more implants are required to support the restoration for biomechanical, technical and ease of maintenance issues. The bulk of the frameworks are smaller; therefore, cantilevers should be avoided; metal ceramic units distort during fabrication; therefore, shorter segments are easier to fit, and repairs and maintenance are easier with short spans.

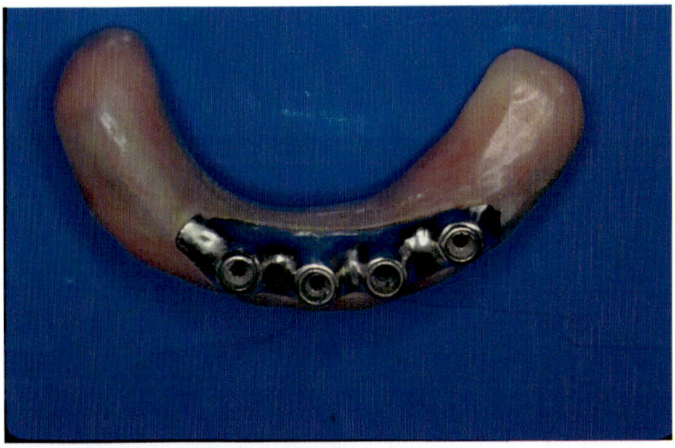

Fig. 16.43 Tissue surface of a hybrid prosthesis with poorly distributed implants and too large a cantilever

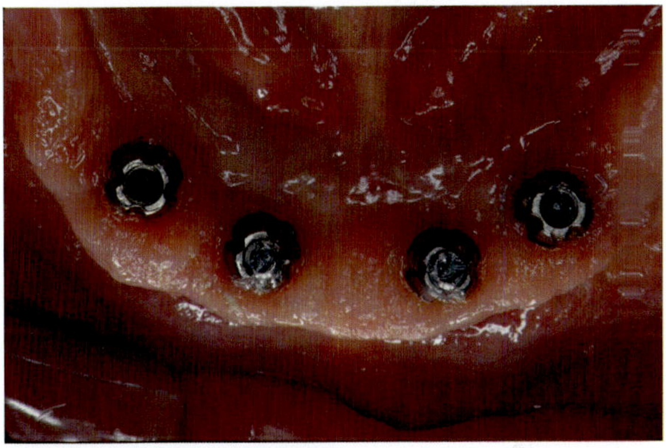

Fig. 16.44 Implants supporting prostheses in Fig. 16.43; note the fractured screws in the anterior two implants caused by excessive loading due to cantilever length

Another reason why more implants and full-arch restorations should be avoided is mandibular flexion. Many reports have addressed the dimensional changes of the mandible during jaw activity as a result of masticatory muscle action [46]. The theoretical implications of mandibular flexion argue against one-piece full-arch restorations. Considerable buccolingual forces on opening and closing will be applied to the restoration and the restoration-abutment interface.

The treatment planning guidelines are similar to what was discussed for the edentulous maxilla. The following parameters need to be evaluated:

1. Aesthetics—As patients age, the display of the mandibular anterior teeth increases. Aesthetics in this regard is appropriate placement of the mandibular central incisor and display of teeth in speech and smiling.
2. Inter-arch space—The inter-arch space requires 8–10 mm from the platform of the implant to the opposing occlusion. This allows appropriate tooth length and accommodation of vertical and horizontal overlap.
3. Number and distribution of implants—Deciding on the number of implants to place is not governed by a formula and is dependent on multiple factors. The number of implants to place in each patient is determined by:

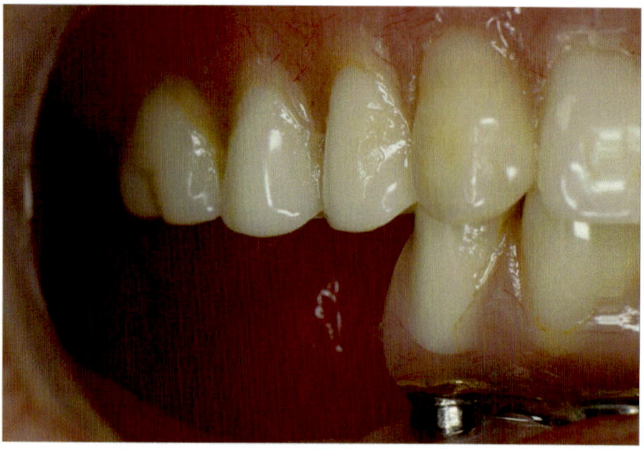

Fig. 16.45 Intraoral view of fractured hybrid restoration

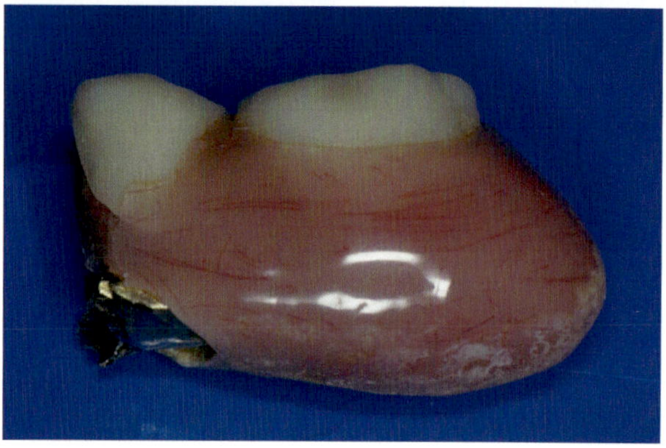

Fig. 16.46 Fractured fragment from Fig. 16.45

(a) Quality of bone
(b) Anticipated force to be placed on the restoration
(c) The segmentation of the units

Usually, three segments are fabricated, one replacing each posterior sextant and one anteriorly. Force estimations for each segment should be assessed based on the factors outlined above and the number of implants determined accordingly.

With this type of restoration, the implant position is more critical than the other two choices of restoration; therefore, the surgical guide and stabilization of the surgical guide are critical. Whenever possible, several teeth can be maintained to support and index the surgical guide; when this is not possible, temporary implants can be used to aid in stabilizing surgical guides or guided surgery protocols may be utilized [47–50].

Figures 16.52, 16.53, 16.54 and 16.55 illustrate an edentulous mandible restored with metal ceramic restorations; this patient was recently edentulated and presented with minimal bone resorption. Implants were placed using temporary implants to stabilize the surgical guide, and following this, the implants were immediately loaded with a provisional restoration. After confirmation of integration, the definitive metal ceramic restorations were delivered.

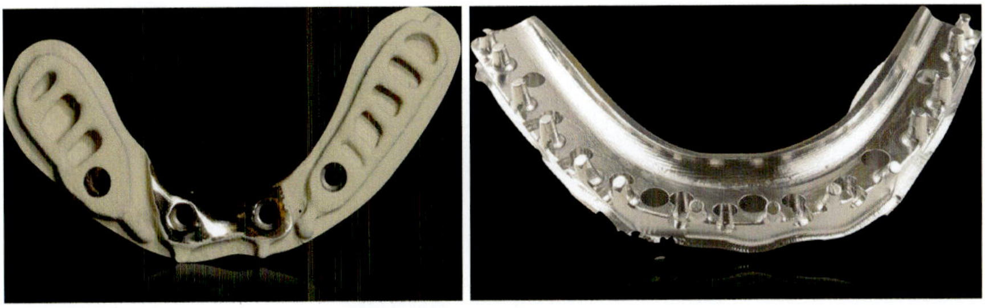

Fig. 16.47 Framework design illustrating acrylic retentive areas and dimensions required to resist fracture. Comparison of gold and titanium frameworks

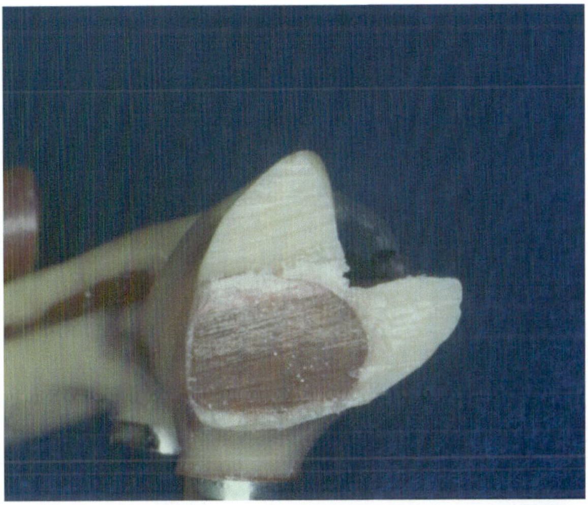

Fig. 16.48 L-shaped cross section of the framework to resist occlusal forces yet allow space for acrylic resin

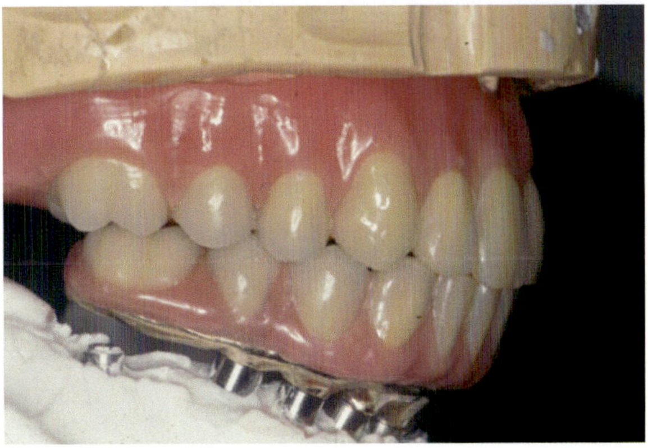

Fig. 16.49 Lateral view of maxillary denture and mandibular hybrid restoration on articulator; note the implant positioned below cantilever extension; a healing cap will be placed to make contact with the undersurface of the prosthesis intraorally to support the cantilever

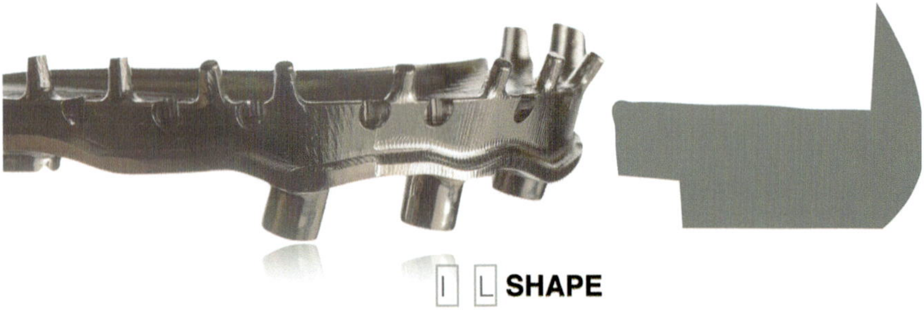

Fig. 16.50 Favourable cross section of framework

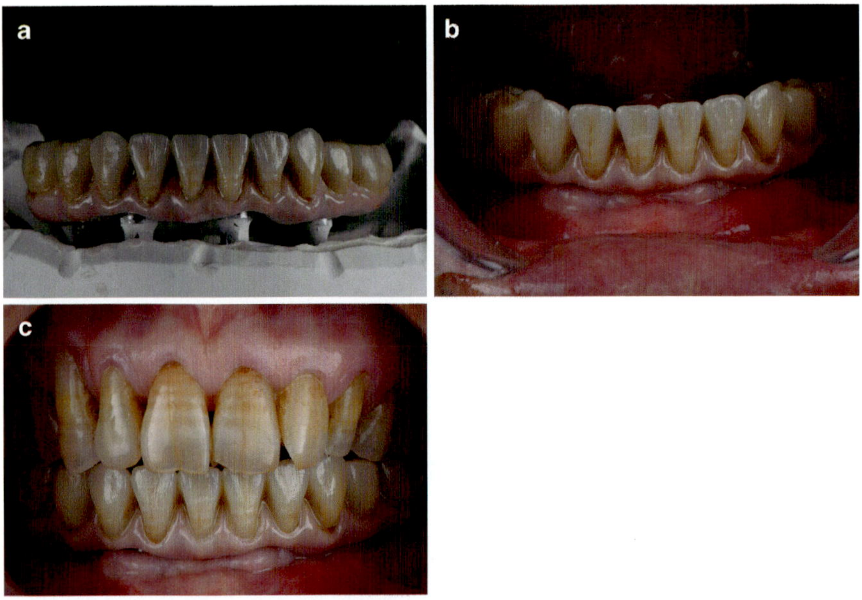

Fig. 16.51 (**a–c**) Monolithic zirconia restoration

Fig. 16.52 Eight implants have been placed in this patient utilizing a surgical guide indexed on temporary implants

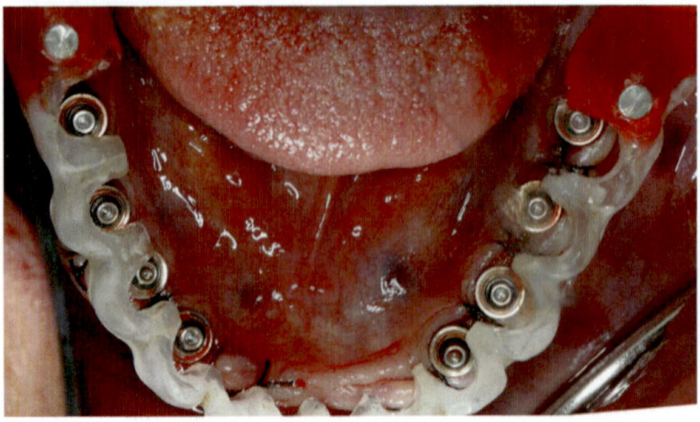

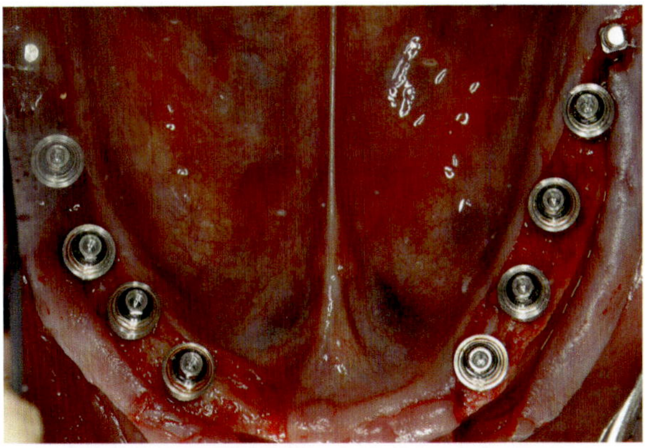

Fig. 16.53 Occlusal view showing ideal implant placement for screw-retained restorations. Note the temporary implants in the posterior where the surgical guide was indexed

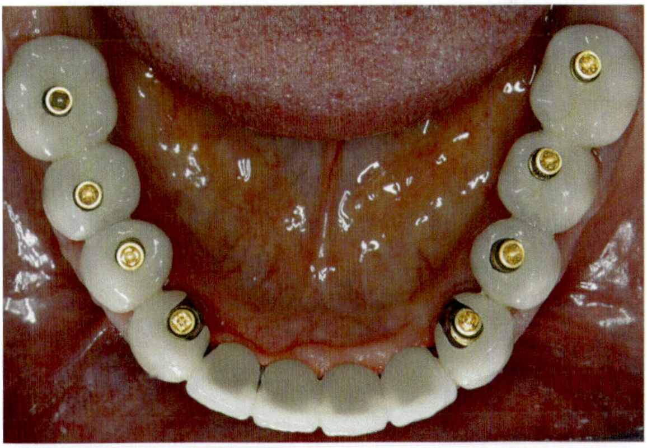

Fig. 16.54 Well-controlled implant placement resulting in ideal implant positions for screw retention. This restoration was segmented distal of the left and right canines

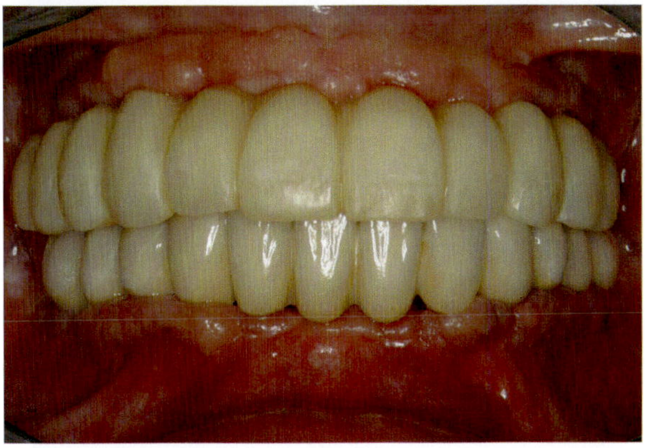

Fig. 16.55 Anterior view of restoration; note the minimal space available for restorations resulting in the choice of metal ceramic restorations to replace teeth in the mandibular arch

16.3 Milled Cobalt Chromium

Cobalt chromium frameworks have had a major resurgence in recent years. All the traditional problems with fit, bonding and corrosion related to cast designs have been eliminated with the inception of milled framework designs. These frameworks are then veneered with porcelains to create traditional porcelain fused to metal restorations. From an aesthetic point of view, metal ceramic prostheses can be created in a way that is more tooth-like than frameworks veneered with acrylics, especially after some years in function in the oral cavity (Fig. 16.56) [51].

CAD/CAM designs allow better control of ceramic thickness, passive frameworks, predictable ceramic bonding and less bending than high noble frameworks, especially in cantilevers. Cobalt chrome frameworks are particularly advantageous when less than 15 mm of restorative space is available, and a posterior cantilever is present. The restoration can withstand occlusal forces even at minimal thickness. The main attraction, however, seems to be the cost as compared to gold-based frameworks. The main disadvantages are laboratory based, as an industrial milling and sintering machine are required, with a skilled dental technician to utilize these newer technologies.

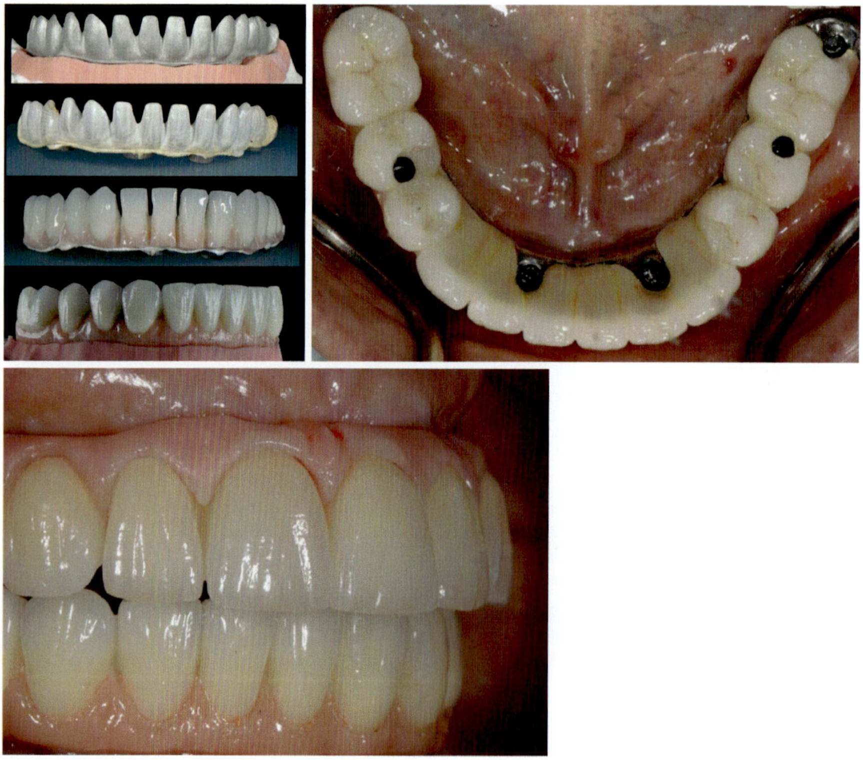

Fig. 16.56 Porcelain fused to cobalt chrome framework

16.4 Zirconia-Based Restorations

Zirconia frameworks have evolved significantly over the last 10 years and have become hugely popular as a restorative material for fully implant-supported restorations. The primary advantage of zirconia is that it is biocompatible and aesthetic and has great material strength. The tooth-like colour of zirconia makes it beneficial in aesthetic areas of the oral cavity, and the excellent wear characteristics make it advantageous in the posterior areas as well. These properties have resulted in the increased use of zirconia in the fabrication of these restorations.

Zirconia has a high flexural strength, which makes it suitable as a framework in veneered or full-contour reconstructions [51–55].

Zirconia frameworks can be designed according to the following parameters:

1. Monolithic
2. Minimally layered
3. Hybrid designs with individual lithium disilicate or zirconia crowns
4. Hybrid designs where a zirconia supra-structure is supported by a titanium framework

16.4.1 Monolithic

The advantage of monolithic zirconia is the reduction. In chipping, this occurs with minimally layered restoration. These structures are robust and can result in highly aesthetic restorations providing longevity as long as cantilever length and connector size are respected [55–57] (Figs. 16.57, 16.58 and 16.59).

16.4.2 Minimally Layered

It is possible to achieve strength and maximum aesthetics by minimal layering zirconia frameworks with veneering porcelain. However, a few clinical studies show that unsupported veneered ceramic has a higher risk of chipping. To take advantage of both the strength of zirconia and ideal aesthetics, it is recommended that frameworks be designed such that occlusal contact areas are in monolithic zirconia with minimal layering on the buccal surfaces in aesthetic areas. One caveat is that all veneered porcelain must be appropriately supported, with anatomically shaped design to the underlying zirconia framework. When focusing on this issue, questions often arise in regard to the flexural strength of full-contour zirconia alone and the flexural strength of porcelain-fused-to-zirconia systems. Clinicians have concerns about potential chipping and fracture of the veneering porcelain. Most studies will report that the veneering porcelain is the weak point in any multilayer system including traditional PFM techniques. Regardless of whether a noble metal or zirconia framework is being used, the overlying porcelain must be well supported. Shear bond strength of porcelain to zirconia has also been investigated; studies

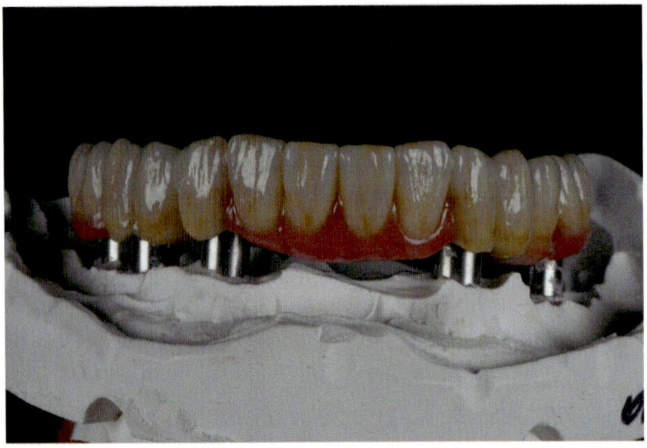

Fig. 16.57 Monolithic mandibular restoration

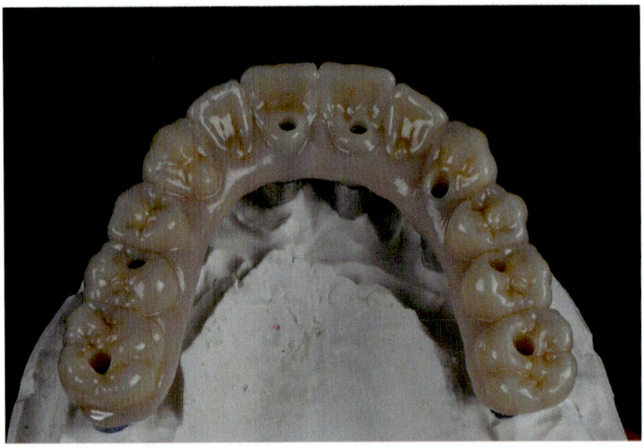

Fig. 16.58 Monolithic maxillary restoration

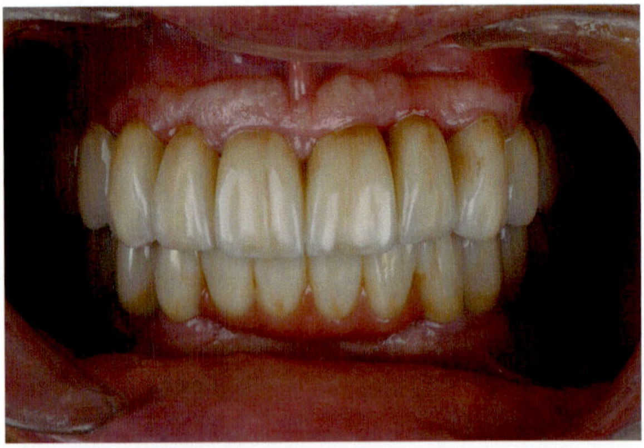

Fig. 16.59 Monolithic restorations in situ

show differences in bond strength depending on the veneering porcelain used and if the zirconia substructure is coloured or uncoloured. It is the authors' recommendation that when using a zirconia substructure, compatible veneering porcelains should be used and the heating and cooling cycles must be carefully controlled. Limiting the veneering porcelain and having a full-contour zirconia framework with zirconia occlusion are advantageous in this regard (Figs. 16.60, 16.61 and 16.62).

16.4.3 Hybrid Designs with Individual Ceramic Crowns

These types of restorations provide many advantages:

1. Maximal aesthetics since there are individual restorations especially with aesthetics in the interproximal areas.
2. Stress distribution due to underlying splinting and cross-arch stabilization of the implants.
3. Ease of dealing with restorative complications—If a single crown were to fracture, it can be replaced individually.

16.4.4 Hybrid Designs Where the Zirconia Supra-structure Is Supported by a Titanium Framework

The delivery of full-arch implant-supported restorations has been significantly advanced by the rapid introduction of innovative digital technologies into clinical practice. These technologies allow for greater ease, cost efficiencies and improved workflows. Intraoral scanning is one of these technologies that have significantly improved the acquisition of diagnostic data and clinical information required for the definitive restoration. It enables the clinician to execute a complex implant rehabilitation in a fewer number of visits.

Intraoral scanning for single-tooth implant restorations has been shown to be just as accurate as analogue techniques. Full-arch scans have not been as reliable and consistent. It was shown that the precision of full-arch scans decreases as the distance between the scanning abutments increases. This inaccuracy can be a result of

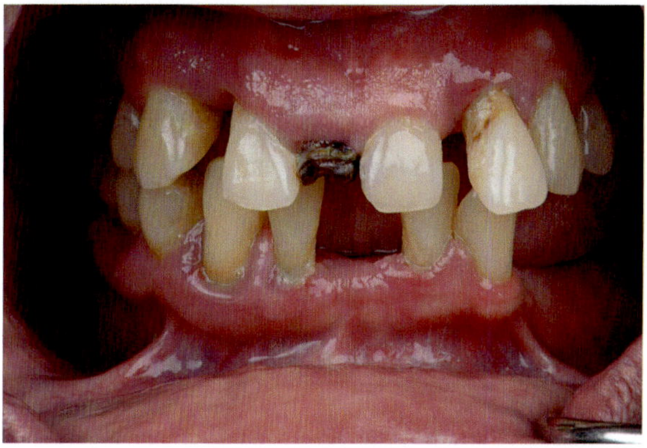

Fig. 16.60 Pre-op of patient

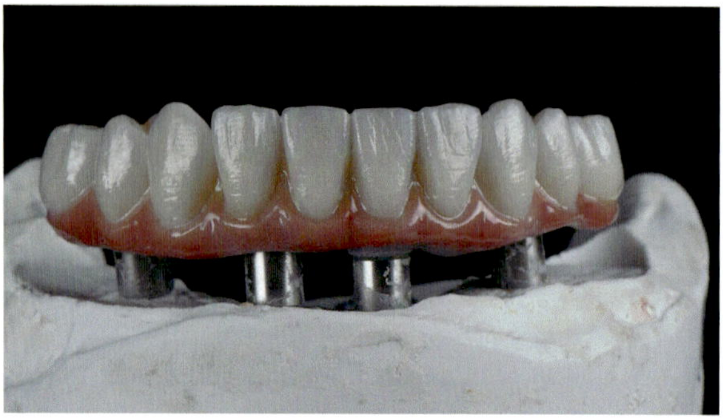

Fig. 16.61 Layered zirconia restorations for the patient in Fig. 16.60

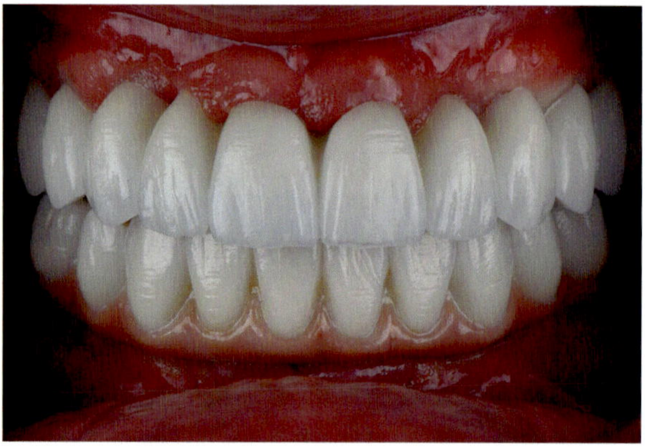

Fig. 16.62 Layered restorations in situ

scanning protocols, scan abutment designs and different technologies associated with different types of scanners. Recently, scan gauges have been introduced that standardize the scanning procedure. Scanning for full-arch implant restorations on multi-unit abutments is becoming a clinical reality [56–59] (refer to Chap. 8 for more details).

The manufacturing process has also benefited from technology with laboratories now able to complete the definitive restorations utilizing a full digital workflow.

Fabrication of full-arch zirconia restoration supported by a titanium substructure can be completed utilizing a full digital workflow [60].

These types of full-arch restorations may provide the following benefits:

1. Ease of fabrication—CAD/CAM technology
2. Passivity of the framework—Utilizing scan gauges and AI technology frameworks can be fabricated with a true digital model-less workflow. This can result in a clinically acceptable passive framework.
3. Implant/abutment interface—A titanium-to-titanium interface was used to minimize wear on the head of the implant. There is not zirconia touching the head of the fixture or even the multi-unit abutment. The clinician is also able to torque the prosthesis without creating undue stress in the zirconia framework.

4. Occlusion/wear—The framework can be fabricated with full-contour zirconia with minimal cutback or full-contour zirconia and stain. The occlusion is designed in zirconia for stability of occlusal contacts.
5. Strength of framework/veneering porcelain—The zirconia is supported by a titanium substructure which biomechanically enhances the restoration. Care must be taken to ensure that the thickness of zirconia is adequate.
6. Aesthetics—It is improved by minimal cutback and layering.
7. Delivery/retrievability—The entire restoration is screw retained and designed with retrievability in mind.

The clinical information is systematically organized and manipulated in CAD software to propose a design for the prosthesis. This design can be previewed, and corrections made. The clinician may choose to go directly to the definitive restorations in one visit if the provisional restorations satisfy the requirements of aesthetics, contour and phonetics.

It is recommended however that a clinical try-in of a printed resin prosthesis be done prior to definitive delivery to verify the clinician's requirements and the patient's satisfaction. The definitive restorations are fabricated via a CAD/CAM process where the framework is digitally designed and milled from a blank of commercially pure titanium via a computer numeric controlled machine. Such a process has shown to be efficient in producing accurate, customizable and durable frameworks. Today, even the supra-structure is fabricated through a CAD/CAM process to produce the veneering acrylic or zirconia prosthesis (Figs. 16.63, 16.64, 16.65, 16.66 and 16.67).

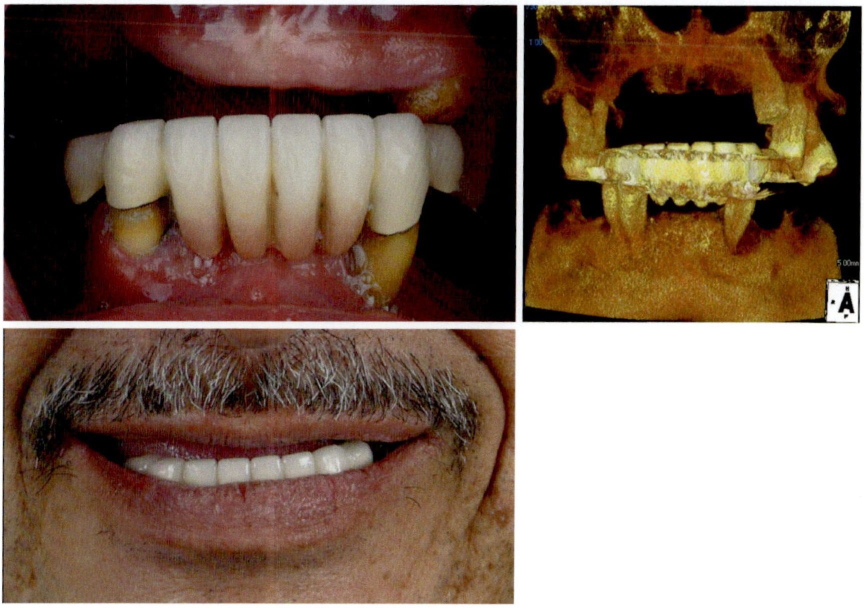

Fig. 16.63 Patient presents with a terminal dentition

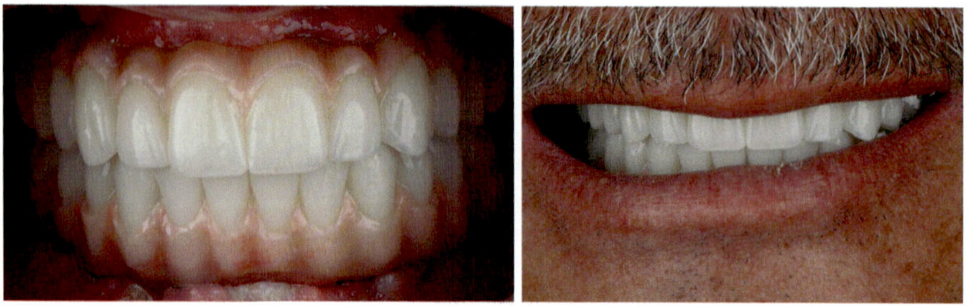

Fig. 16.64 After implants have integrated, provisional restorations are fabricated

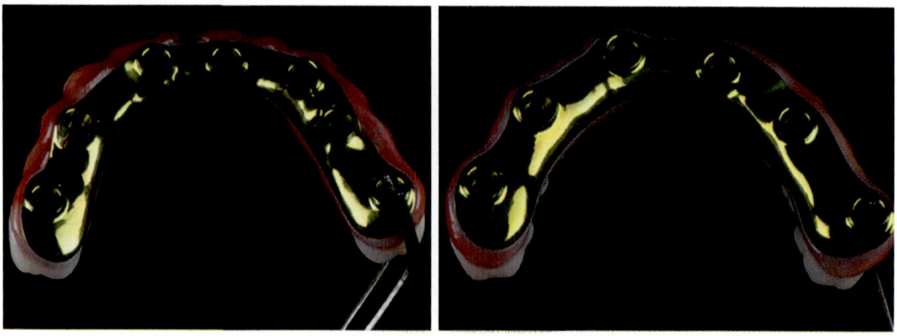

Fig. 16.65 Zirconia supported by a titanium framework

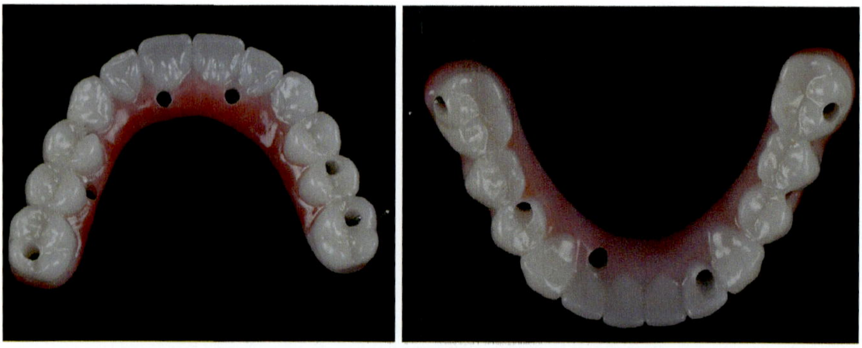

Fig. 16.66 Zirconia-titanium restorations showing AP spread of implants

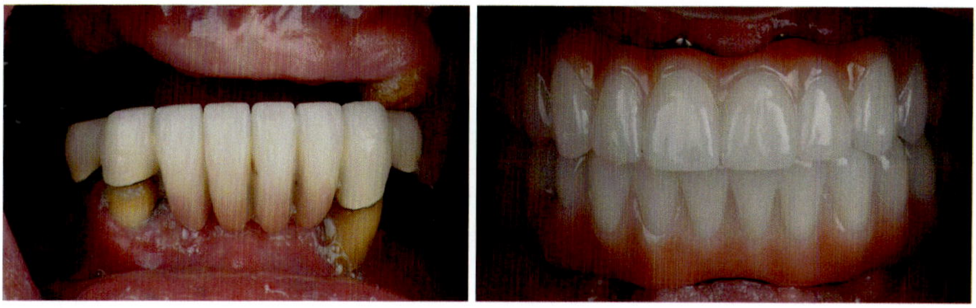

Fig. 16.67 Before and after full-mouth implant rehabilitation

16.5 Conclusion

There are three main choices for restoring the mandibular arch with implants, a minimalist approach with two implants to retain a removable prosthesis or a fixed restoration which may be a hybrid-type restoration or metal ceramic implant-supported restoration. The overdenture-type restoration is the least expensive initially; however, it requires more maintenance, and removable prosthesis continues to load tissues posterior to the implants.

The fixed types of prostheses will provide almost normal function and require minimal post-operative adjustments; the overdenture is more economical and very satisfactory for those patients who lack the muscular coordination to wear complete dentures but have no complaint of pain due to loading of the mucosa.

The choice between the hybrid and metal ceramic restorations primarily depends on the amount of bone loss that patients present with, secondarily, the cost of the metal ceramic units together with the increased number of implants may determine the type of restoration provided. Patients should be made aware that acrylic teeth on a hybrid-type restoration may need to be replaced every 5–6 years depending on the rate of wear, and this may have additional financial repercussions. Similarly, porcelain fracture is possible on the metal ceramic units.

Patient satisfaction and function are higher with the fixed options; the advantages and disadvantages of each must be discussed with patients prior to initiation of treatment.

References

1. Zarb GA. The edentulous milieu. J Prosthet Dent. 1983;49(6):825–31.
2. Zitzmann NU, Marinello CP. A review of clinical and technical considerations for fixed and removable implant prostheses in the edentulous mandible. Int J Prosthodont. 2002;15(1):65–72.
3. Feine JS, Carlsson GE, Awad MA, Chehade A, Duncan WJ, Gizani S, Head Heydecke G, Lund JP, MacEntee M, Mericske-Stern R, Mojon P, Morais JA, Naert I, Payne AG, Penrod J, Stoker GT, Tawse-Smith A, Taylor TD, Thomason JM, Thomson WM, Wismeijer D. The McGill consensus statement on overdentures. Mandibular two-implant overdentures as first choice standard of care for edentulous patients. Gerodontology. 2002;19(1):3–4.
4. Dawson P. Functional occlusion from TMJ to smile design. 1st ed. Elsevier; 2007.

5. Kaya KS, Türk B, Cankaya M, Seyhun N, Coşkun BU. Assessment of facial analysis measurements by golden proportion. Braz J Otorhinolaryngol. 2019;85(4):494–501.
6. Gotfredsen K, Holm B. Implant-supported mandibular overdentures retained with ball or bar attachments: a randomized prospective 5-year study. Int J Prosthodont. 2000;13(2):125–30.
7. Cordioli G, Majzoub Z, Castagna S. Mandibular overdentures anchored to single implants: a five-year prospective study. J Prosthet Dent. 1997;78(2):159–65.
8. Naert I, Gizani S, Vuylsteke M, van Steenberghe D. A 5-year randomized clinical trial on the influence of splinted and unsplinted oral implants in the mandibular overdenture therapy. Part I: Peri-implant outcome. Clin Oral Implants Res. 1998;9(3):170–7.
9. Chee WW. Considerations for implant overdentures. J Calif Dent Assoc. 1992;20(5):25–8.
10. Zitzmann NU, Sendi P, Marinello CP. An economic evaluation of implant treatment in edentulous patients-preliminary results. Int J Prosthodont. 2005;18(1):20–7.
11. Takanashi Y, Penrod JR, Lund JP, Feine JS. A cost comparison of mandibular two-implant overdenture and conventional denture treatment. Int J Prosthodont. 2004;17(2):181–6.
12. Thomason JM, Lund JP, Chehade A, Feine JS. Patient satisfaction with mandibular implant overdentures and conventional dentures 6 months after delivery. Int J Prosthodont. 2003;16(5):467–73.
13. Awad MA, Lund JP, Shapiro SH, Locker D, Klemetti E, Chehade A, Savard A, Feine JS. Oral health status and treatment satisfaction with mandibular implant overdentures and conventional dentures: a randomized clinical trial in a senior population. Int J Prosthodont. 2003;16(4):390–6.
14. Melas F, Marcenes W, Wright P. Oral health impact on daily performance in patients with implant-stabilized overdentures and patients with conventional complete dentures. Int J Oral Maxillofac Implants. 2001;16(5):700–12.
15. Morais JA, Heydecke G, Pawliuk J, Lund JP, Feine JS. The effects of mandibular two-implant overdentures on nutrition in elderly edentulous individuals. J Dent Res. 2003;82(1):53–8.
16. Heydecke G, Locker D, Awad MA, Lund JP, Feine JS. Oral and general health-related quality of life with conventional and implant dentures. Community Dent Oral Epidemiol. 2003;31(3):161–8.
17. Awad MA, Lund JP, Dufresne E, Feine JS. Comparing the efficacy of mandibular implant-retained overdentures and conventional dentures among middle-aged edentulous patients: satisfaction and functional assessment. Int J Prosthodont. 2003;16(2):117–22.
18. Attard NJ, Zarb GA. Long-term treatment outcomes in edentulous patients with implant overdentures: the Toronto study. Int J Prosthodont. 2004;17(4):425–33.
19. Chaffee NR, Felton DA, Cooper LF, Palmqvist U, Smith R. Prosthetic complications in an implant-retained mandibular overdenture population: initial analysis of a prospective study. J Prosthet Dent. 2002;87(1):40–4.
20. Payne AG, Walton TR, Walton JN, Solomons YF. The outcome of implant overdentures from a prosthodontic perspective: proposal for a classification protocol. Int J Prosthodont. 2001;14(1):27–32.
21. Walton JN, MacEntee MI. Problems with prostheses on implants: a retrospective study. J Prosthet Dent. 1994;71(3):283–8.
22. Payne AG, Solomons YF. Mandibular implant-supported overdentures: a prospective evaluation of the burden of prosthodontic maintenance with 3 different attachment systems. Int J Prosthodont. 2000;13(3):246–53.
23. Attard NJ, Zarb GA, Laporte A. Long-term treatment costs associated with implant-supported mandibular prostheses in edentulous patients. Int J Prosthodont. 2005;18(2):117–23.
24. Thiel CP, Evans DB, Burnett RR. Combination syndrome associated with a mandibular implant-supported overdenture: a clinical report. J Prosthet Dent. 1996;75(2):107–13.
25. Lechner SK, Mammen A. Combination syndrome in relation to osseointegrated implant-supported overdentures: a survey. Int J Prosthodont. 1996;9(1):58–64.
26. Jacobs R, Schotte A, van Steenberghe D, Quirynen M, Naert I. Posterior jaw bone resorption in osseointegrated implant-supported overdentures. Clin Oral Implant Res. 1992;3:63–70.

27. Narhi TO, Geertman ME, Hevinga M, Abdo H, Kalk W. Changes in the edentulous maxilla in persons wearing implant-retained mandibular overdentures. J Prosthet Dent. 2000;84(1):43–9.
28. Chiapasco M, Gatti C. Implant-retained mandibular overdentures with immediate loading: a 3- to 8-year prospective study on 328 implants. Clin Implant Dent Relat Res. 2003;5(1):29–38.
29. Payne AG, Tawse-Smith A, Thompson WM, Kumara R. Early functional loading of unsplinted roughened surface implants with mandibular overdentures 2 weeks after surgery. Clin Implant Dent Relat Res. 2003;5(3):143–53.
30. Adell R, Eriksson B, Lekholm U, Branemark PI, Jemt T. Long-term follow-up study of osseointegrated implants in the treatment of totally edentulous jaws. Int J Oral Maxillofac Implants. 1990;5(4):347–59.
31. Ferrigno N, Laureti M, Fanali S, Grippaudo G. A long-term follow-up study of non-submerged ITI implants in the treatment of totally edentulous jaws. Part I: Ten-year life table analysis of a prospective multicenter study with 1286 implants. Clin Oral Implants Res. 2002;13(3):260–73.
32. Attard NJ, Zarb GA. Long-term treatment outcomes in edentulous patients with implant-fixed prostheses: the Toronto study. Int J Prosthodont. 2004;17(4):417–24.
33. Becker W, Becker BE, Huffstetlert S. Early functional loading at 5 days for Branemark implants placed into edentulous mandibles: a prospective, open-ended, longitudinal study. J Periodontol. 2003;74(5):695–702.
34. Schnitman PA, Wohrle PS, Rubenstein JE, DaSilva JD, Wang NH. Ten-year results for Branemark implants immediately loaded with fixed prostheses at implant placement. Int J Oral Maxillofac Implants. 1997;12(4):495–503.
35. Balshi TJ, Wolfinger GJ. Immediate loading of Branemark implants in edentulous mandibles: a preliminary report. Implant Dent. 1997;6:83.
36. Chee W, Jivraj S. Efficiency of immediately loaded mandibular full-arch implant restorations. Clin Implant Dent Relat Res. 2003;5(1):52–6.
37. Tarnow DP, Emtiaz S, Classi A. Immediate loading of threaded implants at stage 1 surgery in edentulous arches: ten consecutive case reports with 1- to 5-year data. Int J Oral Maxillofac Implants. 1997;12(3):319–24.
38. Randow K, Ericsson I, Nilner K, Petersson A, Glantz PO. Immediate functional loading of Branemark dental implants. An 18-month clinical follow-up study. Clin Oral Implants Res. 1999;10(1):8–15.
39. English CE. Critical A-P spread. Implant Soc. 1990;1(1):2–3.
40. McAlarney ME, Stavropoulos DN. Theoretical cantilever lengths versus clinical variables in fifty-five clinical cases. J Prosthet Dent. 2000;83(3):332–43.
41. McAlarney ME, Stavropoulos DN. Determination of cantilever length-anterior-posterior spread ratio assuming failure criteria to be the compromise of the prosthesis retaining screw-prosthesis joint. Int J Oral Maxillofac Implants. 1996;11(3):331–9.
42. White SN, Caputo AA, Anderkvist T. Effect of cantilever length on stress transfer by implant-supported prostheses. J Prosthet Dent. 1994;71(5):493–9.
43. Londono J, Schoenbaum TR, Varilla Ortiz AV, Franco-Romero G, Villalobos V, Carosi P, Mijiritsky E, Pozzi A. Mandibular flexure and its significance: an in vivo cone beam-computed tomography proof-of-concept study. J Clin Med. 2023;12(12):4149.
44. Rodriguez AM, Aquilino SA, Lund PS, Ryther JS, Southard TE. Evaluation of strain at the terminal abutment site of a fixed mandibular implant prosthesis during cantilever loading. J Prosthodont. 1993;2(2):93–102.
45. McCartney JW. Cantilever rests: an alternative to the unsupported distal cantilever of osseointegrated implant-supported prostheses for the edentulous mandible. J Prosthet Dent. 1992;68(5):817–9.
46. Jemt T, Carlsson L, Boss A, Jorneus L. In vivo load measurements on osseointegrated implants supporting fixed or removable prostheses: a comparative pilot study. Int J Oral Maxillofac Implants. 1991;6(4):413–7.
47. Bischof M, Nedir R, Szmukler-Moncler S, Bernard JP, Samson J. Implant stability measurement of delayed and immediately loaded implants during healing. Clin Oral Implants Res. 2004;15(5):529–39.

48. Barewal RM, Oates TW, Meredith N, Cochran DL. Resonance frequency measurement of implant stability in vivo on implants with a sandblasted and acid-etched surface. Int J Oral Maxillofac Implants. 2003;18(5):641–51.
49. Goodkind RJ, Heringlake CB. Mandibular flexure in opening and closing movement. J Prosthet Dent. 1972;30:134–8.
50. Aalam AA, Reshad M, Chee WW, Nowzari H. Surgical template stabilization with transitional implants in the treatment of the edentulous mandible: a technical note. Int J Oral Maxillofac Implants. 2005;20(3):462–5.
51. Abduo J. Fit of CADCAM implant frameworks: a comprehensive review. J Oral Implantol. 2014;40:758–66.
52. Larsson C, Vult Von Steyern P. Implant supported full arch zirconia based mandibular fixed dental prostheses. Eight year results from a clinical pilot study. Acta Odontol Scand. 2013;71:1118–22.
53. Puri S, Parciak EC, Kattadiyil MT. Complete mouth reconstruction with implant supported fixed partial dental prosthesis fabricated with zirconia frameworks: a 4 year clinical follow up. J Prosthet Dent. 2014;112:397–401.
54. Cheng CW, Chien CH, Chen CJ, Papaspyridakos P. Complete mouth rehabilitation with modified monolithic zirconia implant supported fixed dental prosthesis and an immediate loading protocol: a clinical report. J Prosthet Dent. 2013;109:347–52.
55. Guess PC, Bonfante EA, Silva NR, Coelho PG, Thompson VP. Effect of core design and veneering technique on damage and reliability of Y-TZP-supported crowns. Dent Mater. 2013;29:307–16.
56. Miyazaki T, Nakamura T, Matsumura H, Ban S, Kobayashi T. Current status of zirconia restorations. J Prosthodont Res. 2013;57(4):236–61. https://doi.org/10.1016/j.jpor.2013.09.001. Epub 2013 Oct 18.
57. Preis V, Letsch C, Handel G, Behr M, Schneider-Feyrer S, Rosentritt M. Influence of substructure design, veneer application technique, and firing regime on the in vitro performance of molar zirconia crowns. Dent Mater. 2013;29:e113–21.
58. Mosharraf R, Rismanchian M, Savabi O, Ashtiani AH. Influence of surface modification techniques on shear bond strength between different zirconia cores and veneering ceramics. J Adv Prosthodont. 2011;3(4):221–8. https://doi.org/10.4047/jap.2011.3.4.221.
59. Kim JS, Raigrodski AJ, Flinn BD, Rubenstein JE, Chung KH, Mancl LA. In vitro assessment of three types of zirconia implant abutments under static load. J Prosthet Dent. 2013;109(4):255–63. https://doi.org/10.1016/S0022-3913(13)60054-2.
60. Pozzi A, Tallarico M, Barlattani A. Monolithic lithium disilicate full contour crowns bonded on CAD-CAM zirconia complete arch implant bridges with 3–5 years of follow-up. J Oral Implantol. 2015;41(4):450–8.

17 Material Considerations for Full Arch Implant-Supported Restorations

Saj Jivraj and Winston Chee

One of the most compelling advancements in restorative dentistry has been the clinical replacement of teeth using dental implants. In recent years, the field of prosthodontics has had significant advancements and growth due to advancements in digital planning, digital impressions, and CAD/CAM (Computer Aided Design/ Computer Aided Machining) technology. Today's patients have high expectations, and merely providing them with function and comfort may not be enough. In today's clinical environment, patients also want high aesthetic standards, faster treatment times, fewer visits, and less maintenance requirements. Many patients present with a terminal dentition and inquire about options that involve replacing their teeth with full arch fixed rehabilitations both for the provisional and definitive phase.

Today, full arch fixed implant-supported restorations can be designed using a variety of materials. Regretfully, the literature does not provide a solid evidence base in regard to which materials the clinician should choose. There is insufficient data to demonstrate that one design or set of materials is better than another. Most of the literature comprise case reports, which track a small number of patients over a constrained period of time and provide very biased information [1]. Although these reports do provide us with useful information, they cannot be classified as true evidence. The reality is that CAD/CAM technology is evolving and by the time clinicians have completed studies on a group of materials and followed them for a period of time, those materials become obsolete and newer improved materials or designs become available.

Despite technological advances, certain principles remain the same. The purpose of this chapter will be to give the reader clinical guidelines on how to design a framework and the various combinations of materials that are available.

S. Jivraj (✉)
Private Practice, Anacapa Dental Art Institute, Oxnard, CA, USA

W. Chee
Advanced Prosthodontics, Herman Ostrow School of Dentistry, University of Southern California, Los Angeles, CA, USA

W. Chee, S. Jivraj (eds.), *Treatment Planning In Implant Dentistry*, BDJ Clinician's Guides, https://doi.org/10.1007/978-3-031-68726-6_17

Design considerations for fabrication of the prosthesis include but are not limited to:

1. Screw access trajectory
2. Restorative space
3. Nature of opposing dentition
4. Aesthetic demands
5. Framework cross-sectional area for cantilevers and around screw channels
6. Ease of fabrication and passivity

17.1 Screw Access Trajectory

Screw retention offers clear benefits when planning a full arch splinted implant-supported restoration [2]. Among these advantages are the following:

1. The precision of fit of screw-retained restorations can be verified with radiographs using the Sheffield test [3].
2. Less time in delivery in comparison to cemented restorations [4].
3. Screw-retained restorations have total retrievability, which is advantageous for the following reasons:
   (a) Periodic maintenance—It is a relatively simple procedure to remove the prosthesis if necessary for access to fixtures and intermediary abutments.
   (b) Dealing with loosened screws—Access to screws is typically direct.
   (c) Fracture of the prosthesis—The prosthesis can easily be removed for repair.
   (d) Modification of the prosthesis—Can accommodate issues such as continued tissue remodeling.
   (e) Managing complications of the dental fixtures—Access for dealing with implant failure, peri-implant issues, infection is more readily available.

It can be seen from the above that designing a screw-retained restoration has a significant safety factor with regard to long-term maintenance of these prosthetics.

More and more often clinical situations present where screw access trajectory is often in an unfavourable position. In this scenario, the clinician has two options:

1. Use of pre-angled abutments—Pre-angled abutments do come with specific collar heights and this must be considered to maximize aesthetic outcomes.
2. Use of a two-part restoration with a primary framework that corrects implant trajectory and a secondary screw-retained suprastructure (Figs. 17.1, 17.2, 17.3, 17.4 and 17.5).

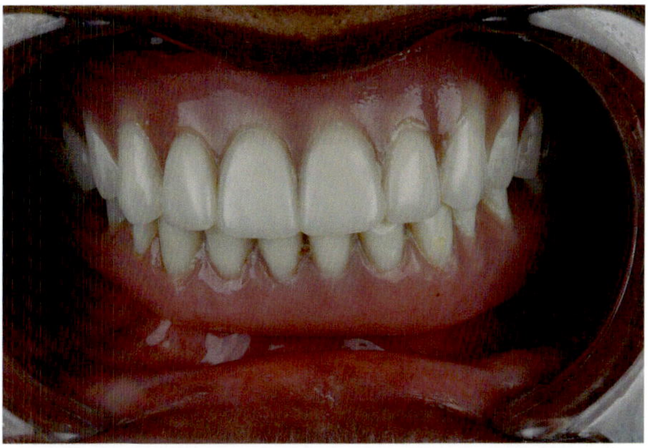

Fig. 17.1 Failing acrylic titanium restoration. Too bulky and teeth position too far forward because of implant trajectory

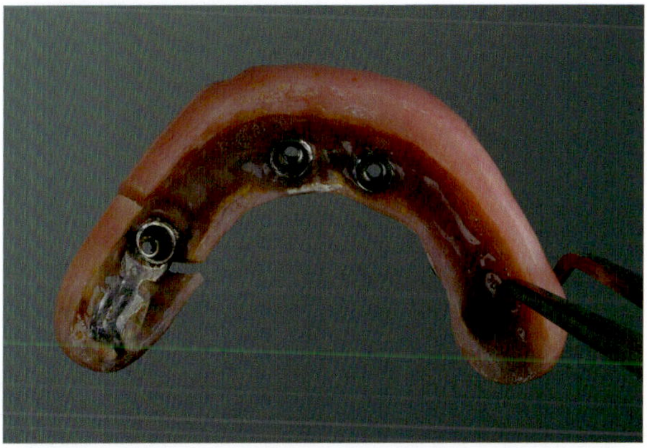

Fig. 17.2 Undersurface showing poor contours and bulk

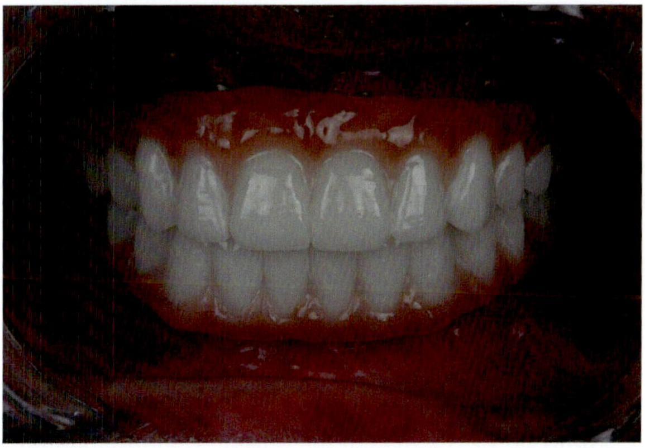

Fig. 17.3 Provisional restoration to satisfy contours and aesthetics

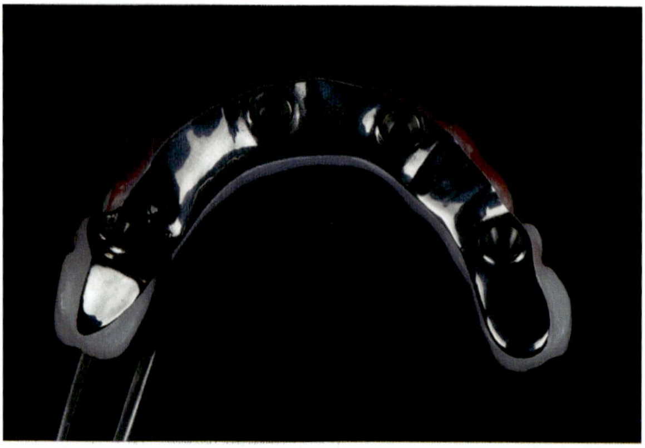

Fig. 17.4 Two-piece titanium zirconia restoration with convex contour milled in titanium

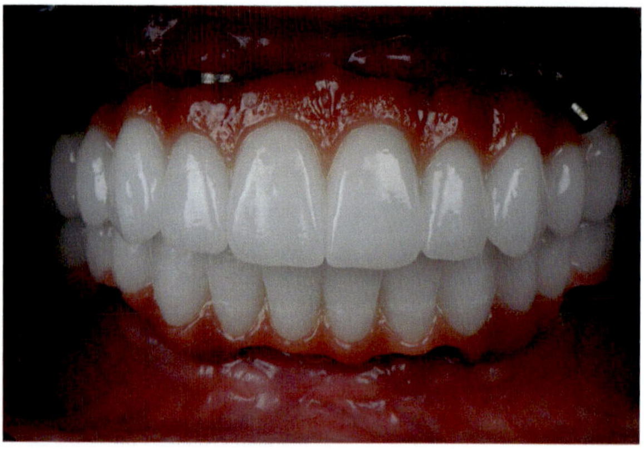

Fig. 17.5 Definitive restoration with correct emergence profile

17.2 Restorative Space

Lack of restorative space is one of the most common occurrences that can compromise a restoration [5]. Inadequate restorative space will result in two scenarios:

1. Restorative complications such as material failure leading to repair or replacement of the veneering materials or complete framework fracture leading to failure of the entire prosthetic restoration.
2. Changing the treatment plan from one restoration type to another to accommodate the space requirements.

Good communication between the surgical and restorative team prior to commencing therapy helps prevent both scenarios above. Restorative space is key, and this must be ascertained at the outset. The clinician must spend time on diagnostics to determine if the patient has mild, moderate, or severe resorption.

General guidelines for space requirements are the following:

1. Monolithic full contour zirconia fixed restorations require 10 mm or more of space from the head of the implant to the opposing dentition.

2. Porcelain fused to metal/zirconia fixed restorations requires 12 mm or more of space from the head of the implant to the opposing dentition.
3. Acrylic resin bonded to titanium fixed restorations will require 15 mm or more from the head of the implant to the opposing dentition.
4. Implant-supported overdentures will require 16 mm or more of space from the implant to the opposing dentition [6].

17.3 Nature of Opposing Dentition

Patients with implant-supported restorations have a reduced amount of proprioception. Patients are unable to determine how much force is being put on the restoration because of the lack of a pain stimulus [7]. With this in mind, there have been studies looking at various restorative materials and their effects not only on the implant-supported prosthesis, but on the opposing dentition as well. One such clinical study investigated the maintenance requirements in patients with differing opposing occlusion types, for example, implant-supported restorations vs. implant-supported restorations, implant-supported restorations vs. natural dentitions, and implant-supported restorations vs. complete denture wearers [8]. This study reported that the patients with implant vs. implant occlusions suffered a higher degree of fracture and greater wear of the occlusal surface (Fig. 17.6).

Another study focused on occlusal surface design using noble metals, feldspathic porcelain, and acrylic [9]. For stability of occlusal contact, clinicians have preferred a metallic occlusal surface rather than porcelain and acrylic; however, due to aesthetic concerns, patients often favour tooth-coloured materials. Historically, feldspathic porcelain has been the material of choice but more recently clinicians have utilized zirconia on the occluding surface of the restoration. One concern by clinicians has been the effect of zirconia on the opposing dentition. An in vitro study was conducted to evaluate the clinical validity of using a full contour zirconia occlusal surface. This study compared zirconia's wear capacity to that of feldspathic porcelain and it was reported that the antagonistic tooth wear was less in zirconia than

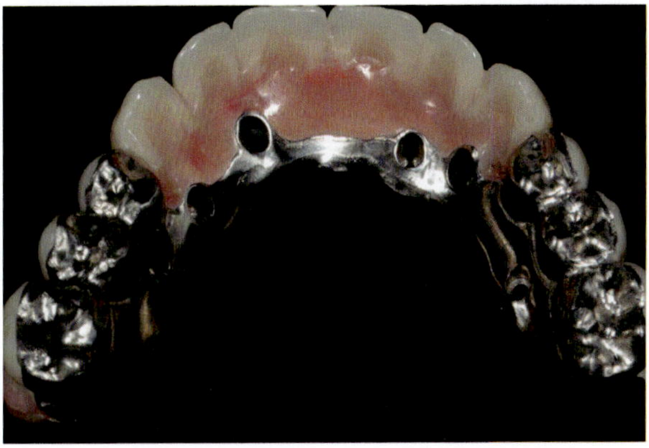

Fig. 17.6 Milling titanium occlusal surfaces can maintain the vertical dimension

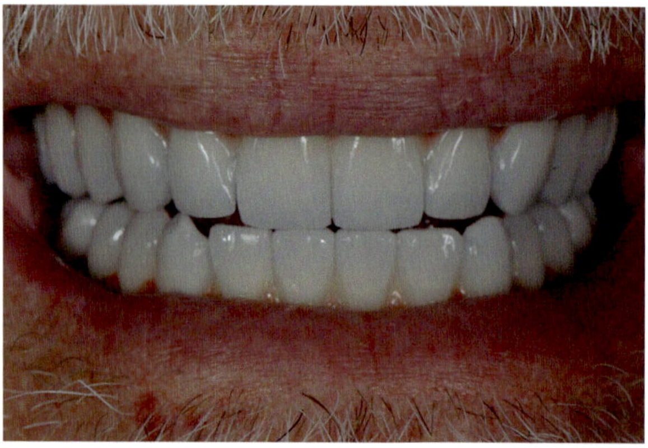

Fig. 17.7 Use of zirconia in the maxilla and acrylic resin titanium in the mandible has many advantages

feldspathic porcelain suggesting zirconia may be more beneficial for antagonistic tooth wear [10]. Wear from polished zirconia happens less than other ceramics because well-polished zirconia is smoother than the other ceramic materials. The data on this subject is limited, and further studies are required.

One clinical situation where the nature of the opposing dentition is of note is when designing fully implant-supported prostheses for the maxillary and mandibular arches together. It has been advocated to restore the maxillary arch with a zirconia-based ceramic prosthesis and an acrylic resin bonded to titanium prosthesis for the mandibular arch [11]. Advantages of using this opposing arch design include the following:

1. Maximum esthetics with minimal staining over time with the use of ceramics in the maxilla
2. Absence of reported, “clicking” by patients with opposing ceramic surfaces
3. Flexibility and resiliency in the system. This is not scientifically based
4. Reduced costs (Fig. 17.7)

One disadvantage would be increased wear of the mandibular acrylic-based restorations. This can be considered a controlled failure, and the patient must be made aware that the acrylic resin teeth will most likely need to be replaced every 5–7 years. There are times when patients present with high function, having opposing arches with the mandibular arch surfaces with acrylic, the softer material serves as a “fuse” to prevent chipping and breakage. Replacing the acrylic tooth surfaces is not too costly and is easily replaced.

17.4 Aesthetic Demands

Talented ceramists can produce high-level aesthetic results using both traditional noble metal alloy and zirconia frameworks. In regard to light transmission, both noble metal alloys and zirconia have been shown to be opaque [12]. Anecdotally many laboratory technicians report superior esthetic results with zirconia frameworks due to the ability to be able to colour the zirconia and be able to have a tooth-coloured framework rather than an opaque grey coloured framework which is usual with traditional high noble metal alloy frameworks.

When it comes to long-term colour stability and aesthetics, ceramic-based restorations with either high noble alloy or zirconia frameworks are superior to acrylic resin-bonded titanium restorations. As mentioned above, ceramics should be considered for maxillary restorations and acrylic resin titanium in the mandible when full mouth implant rehabilitation is contemplated.

17.5 Cantilevers

17.5.1 Framework Cross-Sectional Area for Cantilevers and Around Screw Channels

Specific attention needs to be paid to dimensions of the framework in the cantilever area and around screw access channels (Figs. 17.8 and 17.9). Specifically, the cross-sectional area of the chosen material must be sufficient enough to have strength and rigidity to perform in the intraoral environment. For screw channels, this is typically most important when considering the lingual or palatal cross-sectional area of the material. When focusing on cantilevers, connector size is critical for traditional noble metal alloys, titanium, and zirconia frameworks. While there is no specific data on the minimum dimensions required for these frameworks, if space is extremely limited, the authors prefer traditional noble metal frameworks. However, for the typical implant-supported restoration, patients who have undergone moderate to advanced resorption will have plenty of room to provide robust connectors with sufficient cross-sectional area. Literature on tooth supported zirconia-based restorations recommended a minimal connector size of 4 mm × 4 mm and it is the authors' preference to respect this 16 mm^2 area for implant frameworks as well in the area of channels or connectors [13].

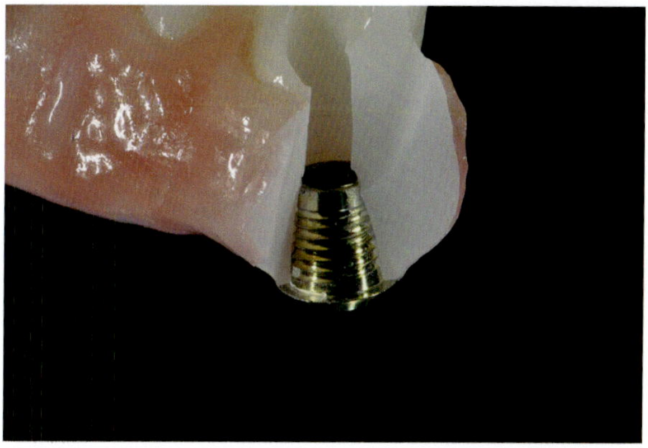

Fig. 17.8 Inadequate thickness of zirconia around abutment and screws access hole will result in fracture of the zirconia framework

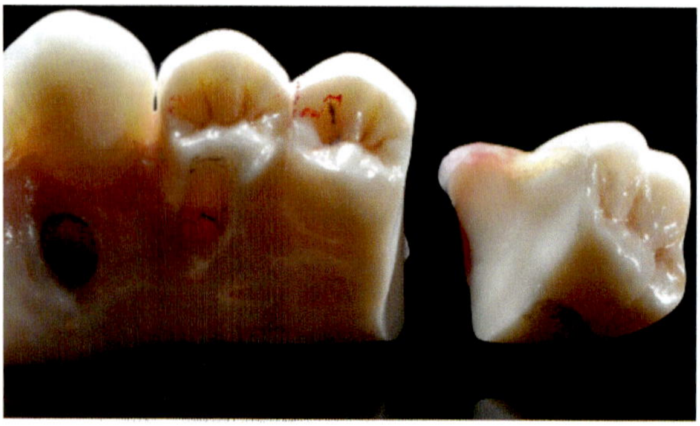

Fig. 17.9 Cantilevers should also be minimized in zirconia as this may result in fracture

There are few studies to guide clinicians on length of cantilever in the maxilla especially when utilizing the more contemporary materials such as zirconia. Length of cantilever has a significant effect on failure of these types of restorations; and in a meta-analysis, it has been shown that length of cantilever is more significant than the number of implants [14]. Deflection of the cantilever is related to its length; so minute increases in length have a significant impact on the fracture complications of restorations. Laboratory-based studies on zirconia have shown that

1. The longer the cantilever the lower the load to failure
2. The smaller the connector size the less load to failure
3. Failure usually occurred in the distal abutment wall and screw channel [15]
   Recommendations for cantilever include the following:
1. Limit distal cantilever
2. Limit buccal cantilever
3. Increase thickness of the framework in the cantilever section distal to the most distal implant and the areas that house the abutment and screw channel
4. Limit occlusion on the cantilever

17.6 Ease of Fabrication and Passivity

Traditional techniques in fabricating full arch implant-supported restorations involve waxing casting and application of a veneering material such as acrylic or porcelain. This approach has been adopted for many years and is considered the gold standard for fabrication of implant-supported restorations. The results achieved with these techniques have been predictable and successful [16]. Traditional techniques do require a high degree of skill and problems inherent with waxing and casting can lead to it being a laborious procedure, which is not only time consuming but can also add additional costs to treatment. In addition, when using gold in frameworks, many of the materials used expand or contract trying to compensate with the distortions, often those frameworks are cut and soldered to obtain a passive fit. With the increasing costs of gold clinicians have moved away from traditional techniques and have begun to employ more contemporary techniques using CAD/

CAM technology and materials such as zirconia and titanium. These techniques also require a high degree of skill but are less time consuming in the manufacturing process and due to the efficiencies gained from these techniques tend to be less costly than conventional fabrication procedures. Titanium frames fit well milled from a titanium puck, and zirconia frames are compensated from sintering distortion by cementing ti-bases to accommodate a good fit of the framework.

When using screw-retained splinted restorations, it has traditionally been extremely difficult to establish absolute passivity in an implant framework. Implant framework inaccuracies stem from a variety of factors, such as component machining tolerances, impression material distortion, die stone setting expansion, alloy and wax expansion and contraction, and distortion of the framework during heat treatment and porcelain application. Digital technologies have been developed to overcome some of these inaccuracies, but further studies are required to establish consistency before incorporating these technologies in a digital full arch workflow [17].

Common solutions to provide a passive framework have been sectioning and soldering or fabricating cement-retained restorations. Although cement-retained restorations have become increasingly accepted, they still have the disadvantage that they are not readily retrievable and studies have also shown that despite clinicians' best efforts, excess cement is often left behind which can result in biological complications [18]. Another approach to achieve a passive screw-retained framework has been use of the adhesive corrected implant frameworks where individual cylinders were cemented within the framework after it had been cast (KAL technique). This approach has merit in that it eliminates many of the current prosthetic and laboratory inaccuracies associated with traditional techniques [19].

With the utilization of CAD/CAM technology, many of the variables have been eliminated and frameworks can be produced with high precision [20] providing the operator has taken care in producing an accurate impression either from a material-based approach or optically, and the laboratory technician has exercised care in replicating it into either an analog cast or has created a digital file. Furthermore, due to the elimination of potential errors, the overall workflow has been simplified by utilization of CAD/CAM, which allows frameworks to be produced in fewer clinical steps with less labor in the dental laboratory [21].

There are several different materials that can be used to fabricate these CAD/CAM frameworks for implant-supported restorations, and these materials include but are not limited to:

1. Acrylic resin bonded or milled to titanium
2. High Performance Polymers—PEEK (Poly Ether Ether Ketone)
3. Milled cobalt chromium
4. Zirconia—Monolithic
   (a) Minimally layered
   (b) Hybrid design with zirconia frameworks and individually cemented crowns (Lithium disilicate or Zirconia)

17.7 Acrylic Resin Bonded or Milled to Titanium

With the transition from gold to titanium frameworks, full arch, one-piece, acrylic resin and titanium-based repair framework designs have undergone substantial modification [22]**. Although technological advancements have occurred, different manufacturers have proposed diverse designs, and frameworks still lack the typical qualities of gold frameworks. When using titanium frameworks, a few crucial factors become crucial.**

1. Bulk for strength
2. Adequate access for oral hygiene
3. Minimal display of metal
4. Retention for acrylic
5. Adequate space for acrylic resin
6. Adequate strength in the cantilever section
7. Attention to cross-sectional area

When considering these parameters, there are mainly two types of framework designs to support acrylic resin teeth. One of these designs is the "minimalist" framework where acrylic is wrapped around the bar and encompasses it 360° including the intaglio surface. One advantage is that it can be relined, but little is known about its longevity in terms of biomechanics. Anecdotally, numerous colleagues have experienced fractures of this type of framework. Failures may be due to excessive cantilever or inadequate bar shape and further studies need to explore these issues. The second type of framework may include I- or L-shaped bar designs to maximize rigidity. One advantage of this design is that due to the shape of the titanium framework requiring less bulk of material in any one dimension, adequate space and retention for acrylic resin can be achieved which maximizes thickness in the cantilever area. The evidence base is also lacking with this design. Although these frameworks have served many patients well, particularly in the edentulous mandible, success in the mandible does not automatically translate to success in the maxilla (Figs. 17.10, 17.11 and 17.12).

The authors have had clinical experience of repeated fracture of teeth, acrylic resin delamination, and denture teeth wearing in the anterior maxilla (Fig. 17.13).

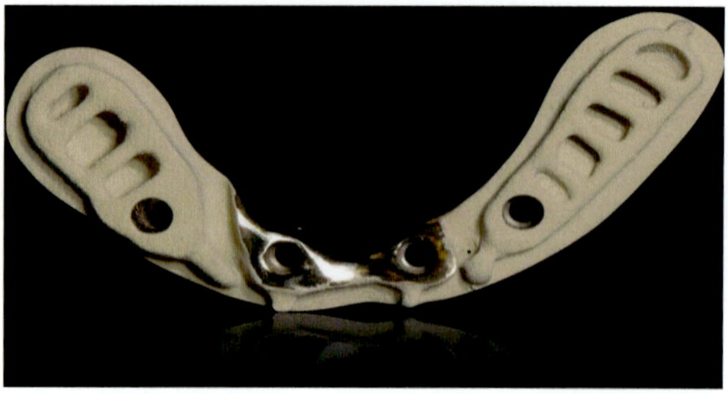

Fig. 17.10 Original characteristics of gold frameworks

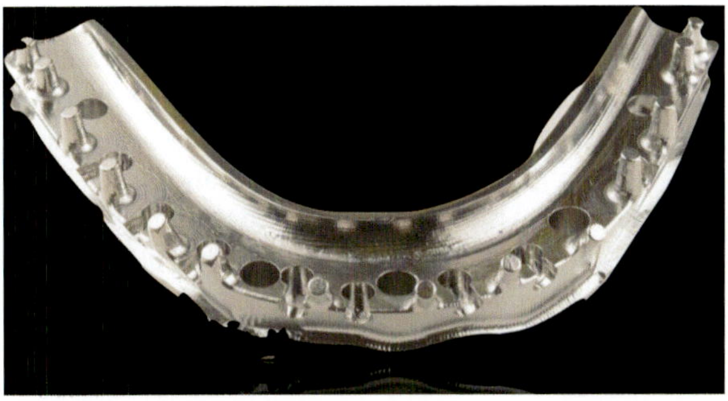

Fig. 17.11 Titanium frameworks with similar characteristics to original gold frameworks

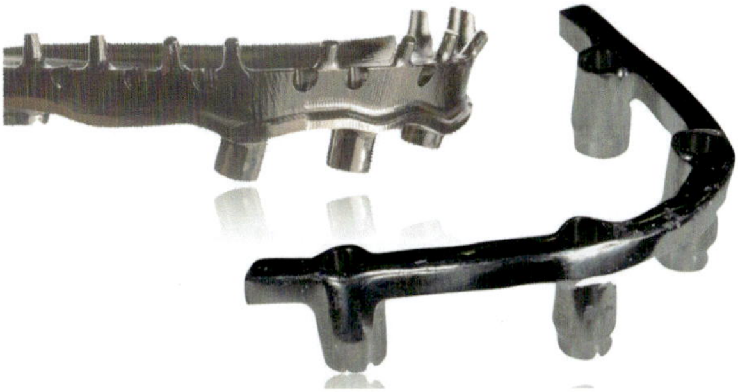

Fig. 17.12 Examples of wraparound and L-shaped frameworks

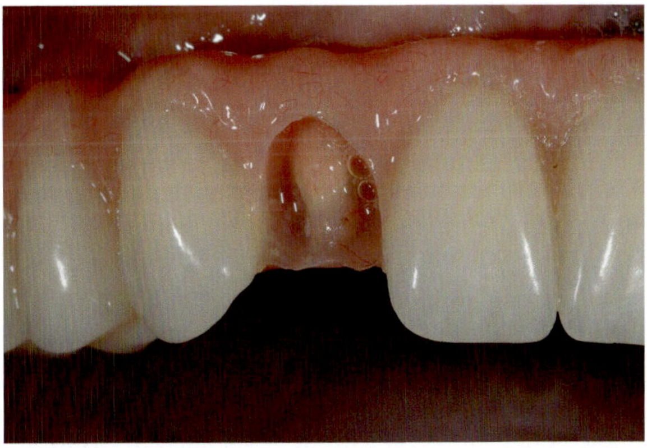

Fig. 17.13 Displacement of acrylic resin tooth from titanium framework

One possible factor for this clinical presentation could be the nature of force application in the maxillary anterior region, which is typically tensile in nature as opposed to the posterior maxillary region and the mandibular arch, which is mainly compressive in nature. This problem is exacerbated in patients who present with signs of bruxism. These patients are prone to accelerated wear of posterior teeth which will eventually lead to increased force and potential overload of the anterior teeth and result in fractures. In order to avoid premature damage to maxillary anterior denture teeth, one possible option is to extend the metal framework onto the occlusal surfaces. The fabrication of prototypes with selective and controlled cutback procedures will allow accurate copy milling and incorporating metal posterior occlusal surfaces into the framework. Another possible option is to utilize new processes in the manufacturing of acrylic to titanium restorations such as milling acrylic around an embedded titanium framework utilizing polychromatic monolithic acrylic [23]. This type of restoration may eliminate many of the potential complications of traditional denture teeth bonded to titanium with processed acrylic such as delamination of teeth and fracture of acrylic veneering materials. The evidence base is lacking with these newer technologies, and further research needs to be conducted in these areas.

These various designs and technologies can be used in high- and low-force situations. As noted previously, in high-force situations, the teeth will wear much more quickly and will potentially need to be replaced as part of long-term maintenance. Although it is possible to make attractive restorations with denture teeth, the pink acrylic does lose its sheen over time and can accumulate greater amounts of stain compared to ceramic.

17.8 High Performance Polymers: PEEK

The reason for the recent enthusiasm surrounding PEEK has been its potential for use as a metal alternative. Perhaps the most interesting property of PEEK for use as a framework material is its Young's elastic modulus (4GPa), which allows the PEEK substructure to more closely match the biomechanical characteristics of the jaw's natural bone (2–12 GPa). Unusually, PEEK is well positioned in that it is strong and resistant to repetitive cyclical loading cycles, yet is slightly elastic, lightweight, and able to dissipate stress forces placed on it. It is these "bone-like" properties that offer PEEK as a more biomechanically engineered substructure material [24]. It is postulated that the shock absorbing properties of this material may result in less stress being transferred to the bone implant interface. There is no evidence to support such a claim although theoretically it may seem reasonable. The Young's elastic modulus of PEEK (4 GPa) is similar to the acrylics (2 GPa) and being a lot lower than titanium (100 GPa), but still retaining sufficient stiffness for rigidity of structure. However, unlike acrylic, PEEK also has sufficient strength (120 MPa flexural strength versus 40 MPa for acrylic) and excellent flexural fatigue resistance to cyclic loads that make it fit for the purpose of long-term restorations. PEEK's resistance to failure from flexural fatigue may be of interest to potentially address some of the technical complications associated with cantilever design, and lab-based tests have been published that show resistance to failure with distal cantilevers of up to 19 mm length [25]. PEEK as a permanent framework material has become an option in recent times through the availability of CAD-CAM forms. However, clinical data is typically limited at present to case studies [26–28] although the first formal clinical studies are starting to become available [29].

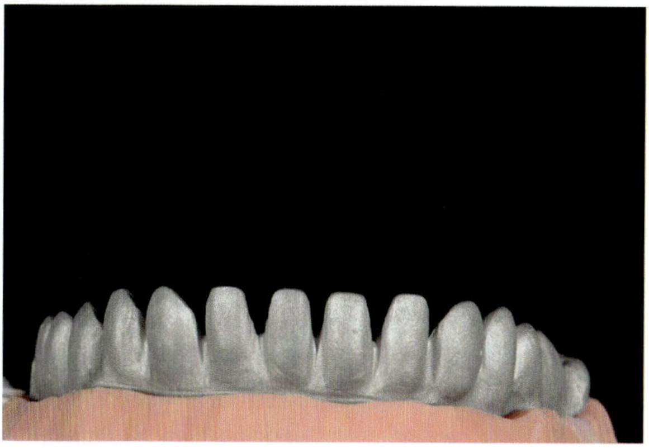

Fig. 17.14 Milled cobalt chromium framework

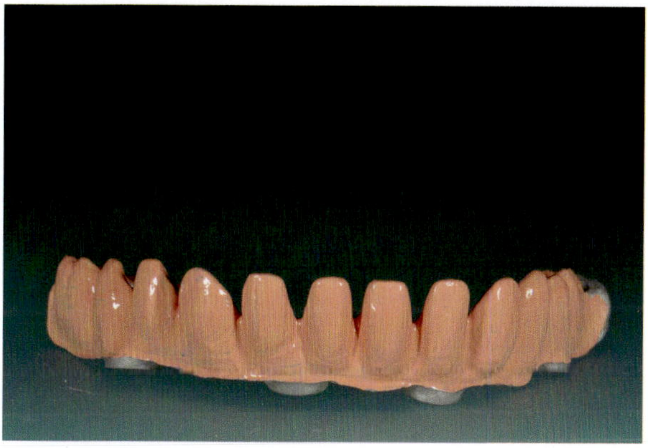

Fig. 17.15 Opaque must be applied appropriately to mask grey colour of metal

17.9 Milled Cobalt Chromium

There has been a significant resurgence of cobalt chromium frameworks in recent years. The introduction of milled framework designs has solved all of the conventional issues with fit, ceramic layering and space, bonding, and corrosion associated with casted systems [29]. Traditional porcelain fused to metal restorations is made by veneering porcelains over these frames (Figs. 17.14, 17.15, 17.16 and 17.17).

CAD-CAM designs allow better control of ceramic thickness, passive frameworks, predictable ceramic bonding, and less bending than high noble frameworks, especially in cantilevers. Cobalt chrome frameworks are particularly advantageous when less than 15 mm of restorative space is available and a posterior cantilever is present. The restoration can withstand occlusal forces even at minimal thickness [29]. The main attraction, however, seems to be the cost as compared to gold-based frameworks. The main disadvantages are laboratory based, as an industrial milling and sintering machine is required, with a skilled dental technician to utilize these newer technologies.

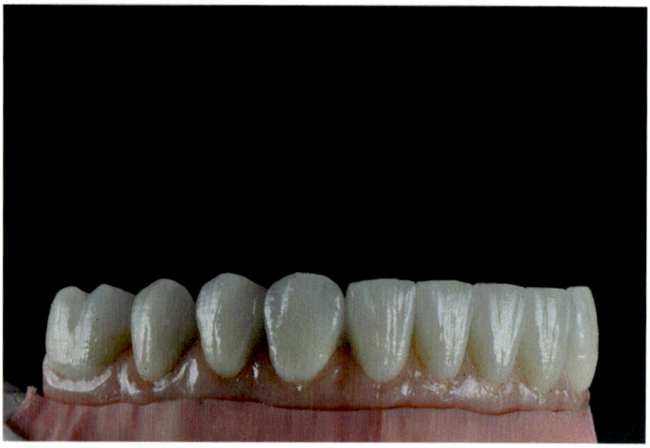

Fig. 17.16 Completed ceramics on cobalt chromium framework

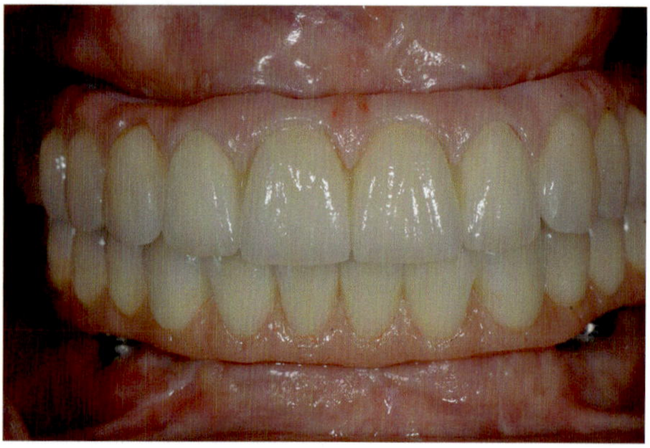

Fig. 17.17 Intraoral view of mandibular restoration in Fig. 17.16

17.10 Zirconia

Over the past 10 years, zirconia frameworks have evolved significantly and have gained immense popularity as a restorative material for restorations that are entirely implant-supported. The main benefits of zirconia are its high material strength, biocompatibility, and aesthetics [30]. Zirconia is advantageous in aesthetic sections of the oral cavity due to its tooth-like hue, and it is also advantageous in posterior locations due to its great wear qualities. Because of these qualities, zirconia has become mainstream in fabrication of full arch implant-supported restorations.

Clinical reports have evaluated restorations with a zirconia structure supported by implants and have provided some insight [31].

Zirconia has a high flexural strength, which makes it suitable as a framework in veneered or full contour reconstructions. Some technical complications are likely to occur, these include but are not limited to

1. Chipping of the veneering ceramic
2. Debonding of the titanium inserts
3. Catastrophic failure of the framework

To reduce the risk of complications, there are a myriad of details the clinician and laboratory technician must respect.

Zirconia frameworks can be designed according to the following parameters:

1. Monolithic zirconia
2. Minimally cut back zirconia with ceramic layering
3. Hybrid designs with individual lithium disilicate or zirconia crowns
4. Hybrid designs with a primary titanium bar with overlying zirconia framework which may be layered or monolithic utilizing intraoral scanning and CAD-CAM protocols

17.11 Monolithic

From an evidence-based perspective, long-term data (10 years plus) to support monolithic full contour frameworks at this time is lacking. This statement should not be a considered a deterrent, but caution must be exercised during case selection (Figs. 17.18 and 17.19).

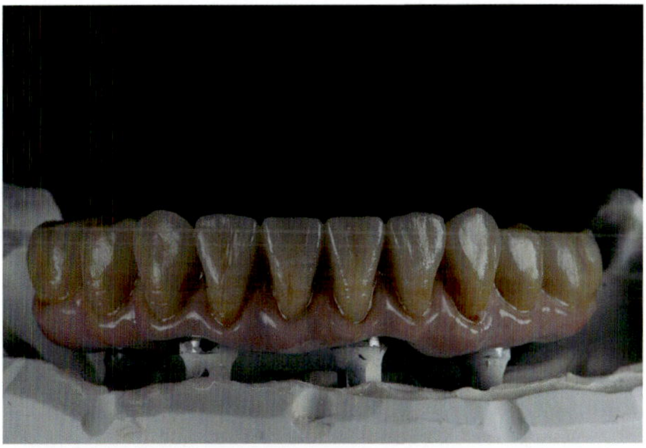

Fig. 17.18 Monolithic zirconia framework with staining

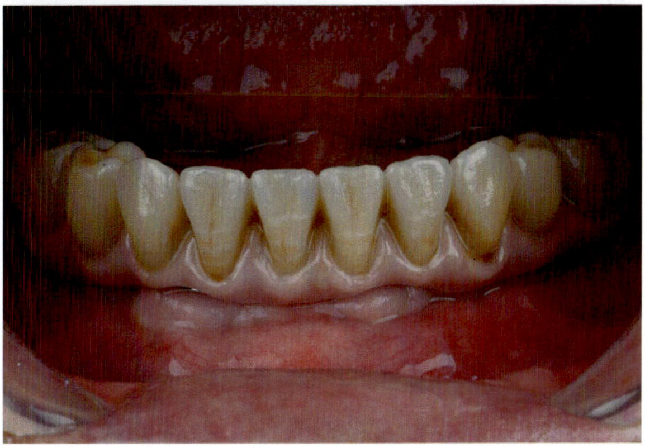

Fig. 17.19 Clinical picture of monolithic zirconia with pink ceramic layering in situ

17.12 Minimally Layered

It is possible to achieve strength and maximum esthetics by minimal layering zirconia frameworks with veneering porcelain [32]. However, a few clinical studies show that unsupported veneered ceramic has a higher risk of chipping [33]. To take advantage of both the strength of zirconia and ideal aesthetics, it is recommended that frameworks be designed such that occlusal contact areas are in monolithic zirconia with minimal layering on the buccal surfaces in aesthetic areas. One caveat is that all veneered porcelain must be appropriately supported, with anatomically shaped design to the underlying zirconia framework [34]. When focusing on this issue, questions often arise in regard to the flexural strength of full contour zirconia alone and the flexural strength of porcelain fused to zirconia systems. Clinicians have concerns about potential chipping and fracture of the veneering porcelain. Most studies will report that the veneering porcelain is the weak point in any multilayer system including traditional PFM techniques [35]. Regardless of whether a noble metal or zirconia framework is being used, the overlying porcelain must be well supported [36]. Shear bond strength of porcelain to zirconia has also been investigated, studies show differences in bond strength depending on the veneering porcelain used and if the zirconia substructure is coloured or uncoloured [36]. It is the authors' recommendation that when using a zirconia substructure compatible veneering porcelains should be used and the heating and cooling cycles must be carefully controlled. Limiting the veneering porcelain and having a full contour zirconia framework with zirconia occlusion is advantageous in this regard (Figs. 17.20, 17.21, 17.22, 17.23, 17.24, 17.25 and 17.26).

One important design consideration with these zirconia restorations is the decision to incorporate cantilever or not. Cantilevers in implant dentistry are valuable for sites where anatomic structures such as the maxillary sinuses exclude the ideal placement of dental implants and are being used more often for graft-less procedures. They may, however, negatively affect the biomechanics of implant restorations and may result in mechanical and/or biologic problems. Presently, evidence is limited concerning breakage of cantilevered zirconia implant frameworks. This

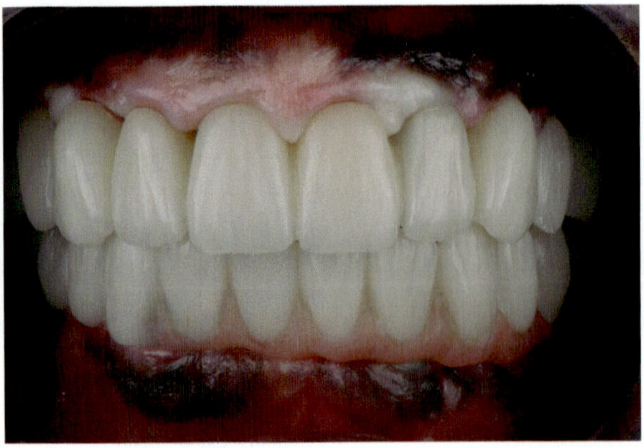

Fig. 17.20 Acrylic prototypes are tried intraorally to verify occlusion and contours

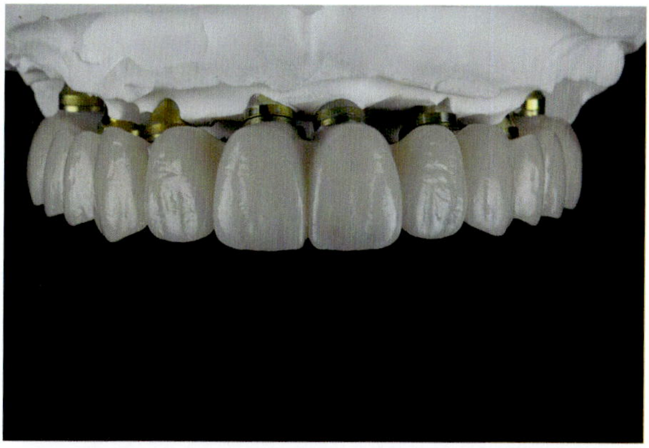

Fig. 17.21 Maxillary acrylic prototype to be tried intraorally

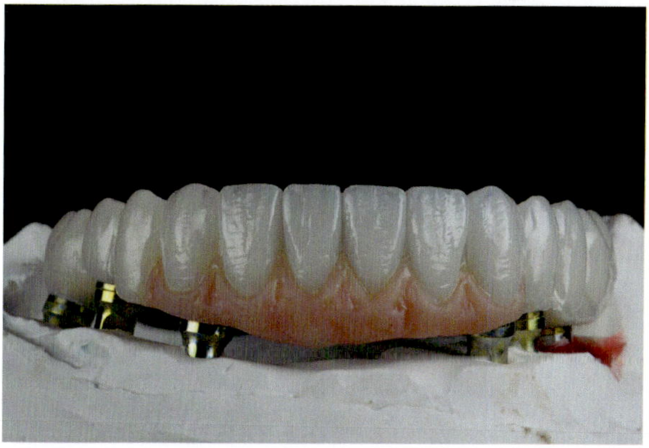

Fig. 17.22 Mandibular acrylic prototype to be tried intraorally

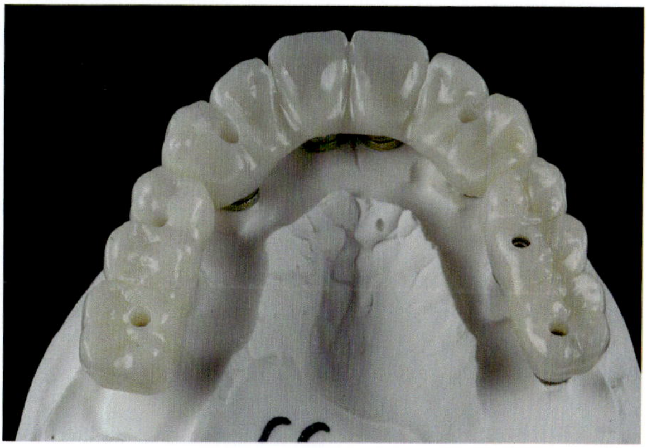

Fig. 17.23 Maxilla has been designed in three sections, occlusion design in zirconia. Anterior bridge combination screw retained and cemented design due to trajectory of anterior implants

evidence is mainly limited to anecdotal and expert clinical reports. Well-designed, clinically relevant laboratory studies are needed to establish the mechanical properties of zirconia cantilevered frameworks.

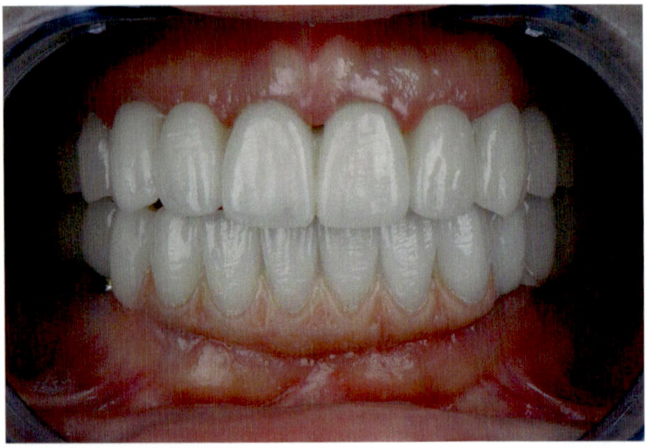

Fig. 17.24 Provisionals intraorally. (Lab work by Artem Asemov)

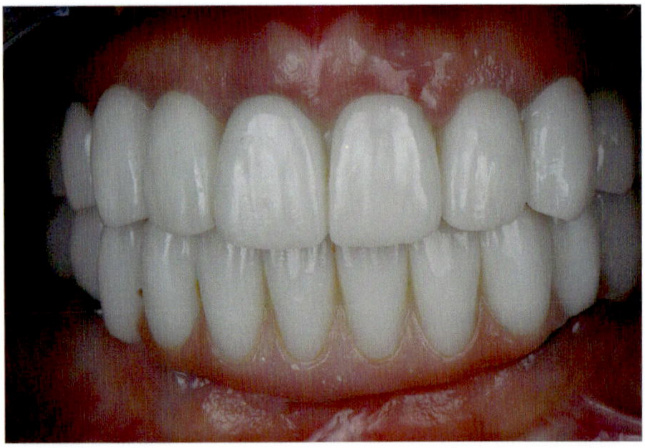

Fig. 17.25 Minimally layered ceramics intraorally

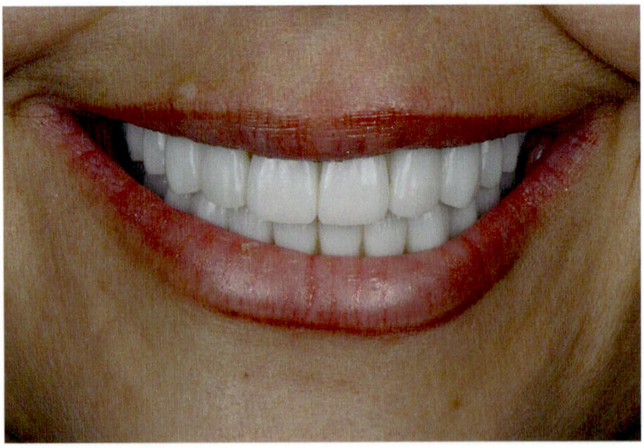

Fig. 17.26 Patients smile

When designing zirconia-based implant frameworks, the following should be considered:

1. Maximize connector dimensions, buccal lingually and occlusal gingivally.
2. Minimize distal cantilever length.
3. Minimize buccal cantilever.
4. Ensure very light occlusal contacts in the cantilever region.
5. Thicken the chimney around the most distal implant, and thicken the buccal and lingual walls around the chimney of the implant.
6. Ensure monolithic zirconia is well polished. Studies have shown it to be kind to the opposing occlusion.
7. Minimal post-sintering adjustment. This will also help with preserving the strength of the material and avoiding accelerated ageing failures in the presence of saliva.
8. Design for retrievability. This allows simple detachment of the appliance and the chance to service the restoration or treat any implant-related problems. With proper implant placement, this can be achieved in most situations when treating the edentulous arch.
9. If restoring to the head of the fixture, the literature supports the use of a titanium insert. This increases the maximum load bearing capacity of the restoration. It also compensates for the three-dimensional distortion that occurs post-sintering. Zirconia abutments have been designed with a titanium component that has been fused or cemented to the zirconia. The unique design feature is that it permits titanium-to-titanium contact at the abutment implant interface, and it results in the same high degree of predictability associated with conventional metal abutment implant connections [37].

17.13 Hybrid Designs with Individual Ceramic Crowns

These types of restorations provide many advantages:

1. Maximal aesthetics since there are individual restorations especially with aesthetics in the interproximal areas.
2. Stress distribution due to underlying splinting and cross arch stabilization of the implants.
3. Ease of dealing with restorative complications—If a single crown was to fracture, it can be replaced individually (Figs. 17.27, 17.28, 17.29, 17.30 and 17.31).

Ideally they should be designed with the screw access trajectories in a favourable position so the restoration can be readily serviced at hygiene appointments. However, despite the clinician's best intentions, anatomic limitations may not allow screw-retained implant placement in the anterior maxilla, even after correction with angled abutments. In these situations, a "hybrid" between a monolithic design and individual cemented restoration may solve a challenging problem created by anterior implant trajectory [38].

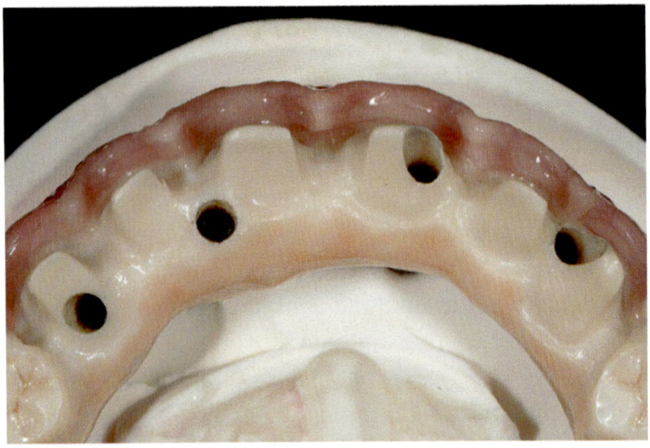

Fig. 17.27 Hybrid design, when screw access holes are not ideally located, individual crowns can be made and luted

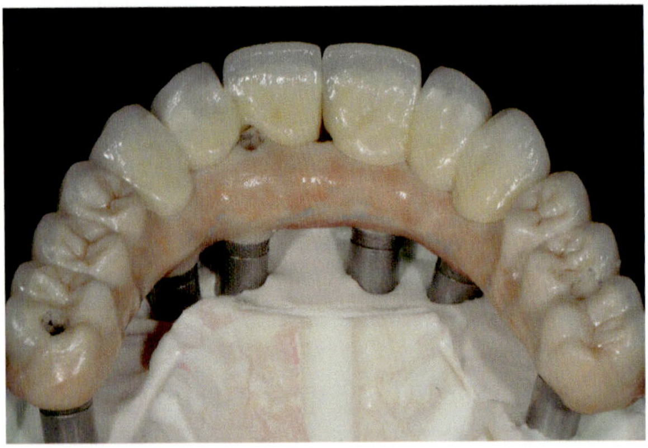

Fig. 17.28 Individual crowns in zirconia replacing maxillary anterior teeth

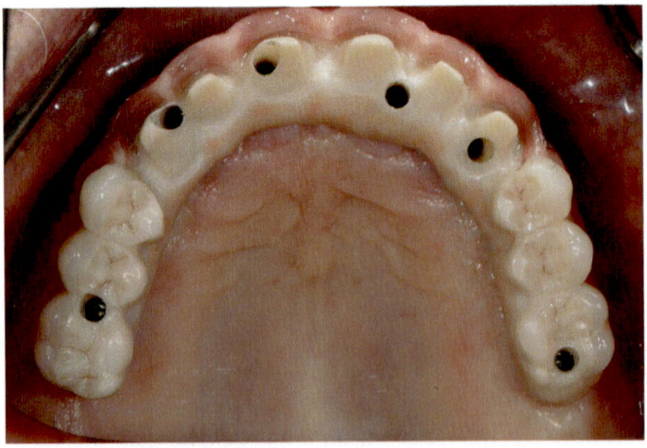

Fig. 17.29 Framework try-in intraorally

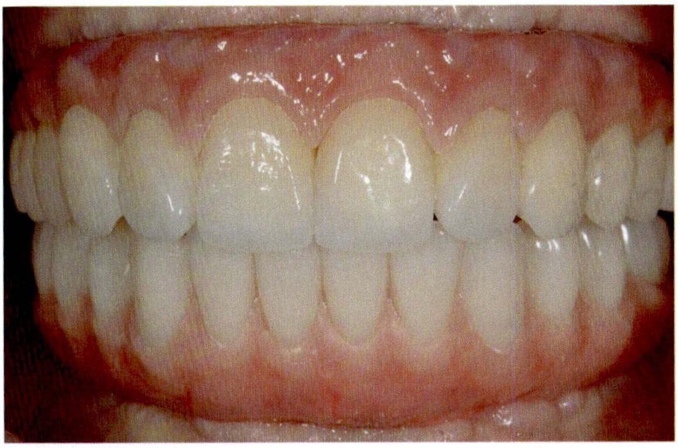

Fig. 17.30 Maxillary hybrid zirconia restoration opposed by acrylic titanium restoration

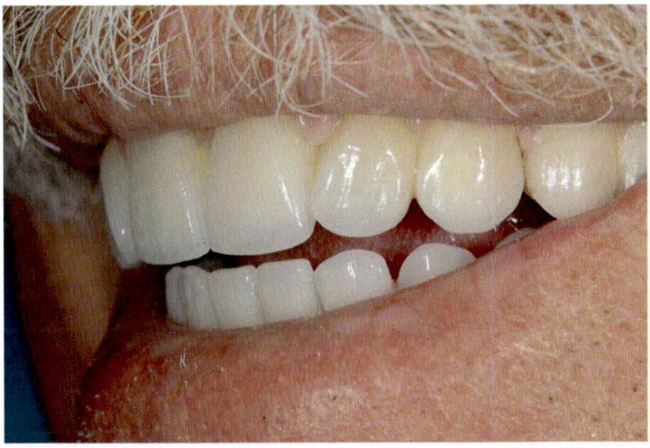

Fig. 17.31 Smile view of restorations in Fig. 17.30

Hybrid designs with individual crowns also have many disadvantages, especially when the screw access holes are not accessible.

1. Retrievability becomes an issue.
2. Practically, the time it takes to deliver the restoration is elevated. Dealing with complications also becomes time consuming.
3. Often clinicians use composite to replace the missing gingiva. The aesthetics of pink composite over time is not optimal. Composite also inherently chips especially in the area where the papillae have been designed.
4. Laboratory fees are higher due to the time taken to fabricate the restoration.

17.14 Hybrid Designs with a Primary Titanium Bar and Overlying Zirconia Framework Utilizing Intraoral Scanning and CAD-CAM Protocols

The delivery of full arch implant-supported restorations has been significantly advanced by the rapid introduction of innovative digital technologies into clinical practice. These technologies allow for greater ease, cost efficiencies, and improved workflows. Intraoral scanning is one of these technologies that has significantly improved the acquisition of diagnostic data and clinical information required for the definitive restoration. It enables the clinician to execute a complex implant rehabilitation in a fewer number of visits.

Intra oral scanning for single tooth implant restorations has been shown to be just as accurate as analogue techniques. Full arch scans have not been as reliable and consistent. It was shown that the precision of full arch scans decreases as the distance between the scanning abutments increases. This inaccuracy can be a result of scanning protocols, scan abutment designs, and the different technologies associated with different types of scanners. Recently, scan gauges have been introduced that standardize the scanning procedure. Scanning for full arch implant restorations on multi-unit abutments has become a clinical reality.

The protocols to scan include but are not limited to

1. A more controlled path for the scanner to follow reducing the amount of scan head movements.
2. Allowing more than one scannable feature on the gauge to be deleted if tolerance of scan captured is less than the known gauge measurement.
3. Inclusion of an alignment procedure where the scan information is analysed using an increased point cloud data set for its reference to the planes present in the gauge design.

The manufacturing process has also benefited from technology with laboratories now able to complete the definitive restorations utilizing a full digital workflow.

Fabrication of full arch zirconia restoration supported by a titanium substructure can be completed utilizing a full digital workflow.

These types of full arch restorations may provide the following benefits:

1. Ease of fabrication—CAD-CAM technology.
2. Passivity of the framework—Utilizing scan gauges and AI technology frameworks can be fabricated with a true digital model-less workflow. This can result in a clinically acceptable passive framework.
3. Implant/abutment interface—A titanium-to-titanium interface was used to minimize wear on the head of the implant. There is not zirconia touching the head of the fixture or even the multi-unit abutment. The clinician is also able to torque the prosthesis without creating undue stress in the zirconia framework.
4. Occlusion/wear—The framework can be created with full contour zirconia with minimal cut back or full contour zirconia and stain. The occlusion is designed in zirconia for stability of occlusal contacts.
5. Strength of framework/veneering porcelain—The zirconia is supported by a titanium substructure which biomechanically enhances the restoration. Care must be taken to ensure the thickness of zirconia is adequate.
6. Esthetics—Is improved by minimal cut back and layering.
7. Delivery/retrievability—The entire restoration is screw retained and designed with retrievability in mind.

The clinician must provide the following information to the laboratory:

1. Intraoral scanning of gauges in specific pathways
2. Scanning of the tissues intraorally
3. Scanning of the provisional restorations with gauges extra-orally and scanning maximum intercuspation intraorally
4. Clinical photographs
5. Prescription of the desired changes

The clinical information is systematically organized and manipulated in CAD software to propose a design for the prosthesis. This design can be previewed, and corrections made. The clinician may choose to go directly to the definitive restorations in one visit if the provisional restorations satisfy the requirements of esthetics, contour, and phonetics.

It is recommended however that a clinical try-in of a printed resin prosthesis be done prior to definitive delivery to verify the clinician's requirements. The definitive restorations are fabricated via a CAD-CAM process where the framework is digitally designed and milled from a blank of commercially pure titanium via a computer numeric controlled machine. Such a process has shown to be efficient in producing accurate, customizable, and durable frameworks. Today even the suprastructure is fabricated through a CAD-CAM process to produce the veneering acrylic or zirconia prosthesis.

The following patient presentation will illustrate the digital workflow.

The patient presented with a terminal dentition and treatment was planned for a maxillary and mandibular implant-supported restoration (Fig. 17.32). Bilateral sinus lifts were performed in the maxilla, and 7 root form implants were placed in the maxilla and 6 in the mandible (Paltop Dynamic, Keystone Dental Group) (Fig. 17.33). Provisional restorations were fabricated to optimize esthetics, form and function (Fig. 17.34). The advantages of a full digital workflow include but are not limited to

1. No impressions.
2. Clinician can complete the definitive restoration in two visit post integration.
3. Aesthetics can be verified with a 3D printed try-in and modifications can be made.
4. No sophisticated equipment is required. The practitioner can utilize their existing intraoral scanner to capture all the data required (Fig. 17.35).

The following data is required:

1. Proprietary scan gauges are placed and scanned (Fig. 17.36).
2. The soft tissue is scanned (Fig. 17.37).
3. The undersurface of the provisional is scanned (Fig. 17.38).
4. The patient is asked to occlude into maximum intercuspation, and a right and left bite scan is performed (Fig. 17.39).

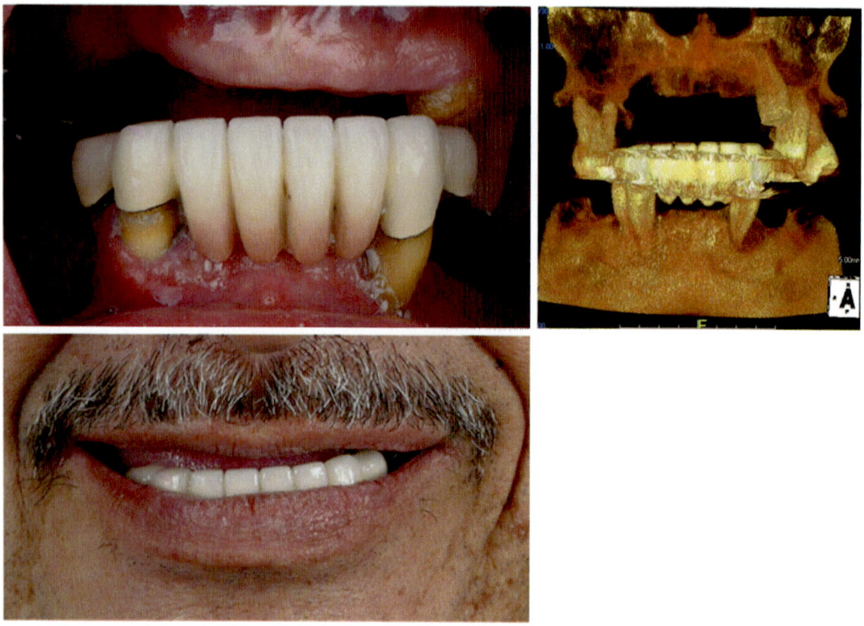

Fig. 17.32 Pre-operative situation of a terminal dentition has been treatment planned for maxillary and mandibular implant-supported restorations

Fig. 17.33 After bilateral sinus lifts 7 Paltop dynamic implants placed in the maxilla and 6 in the mandible

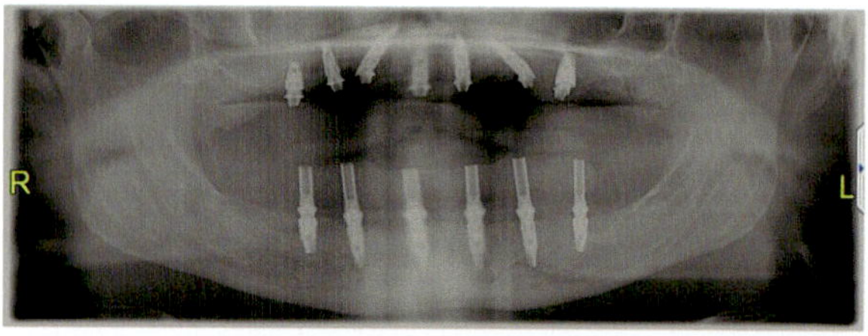

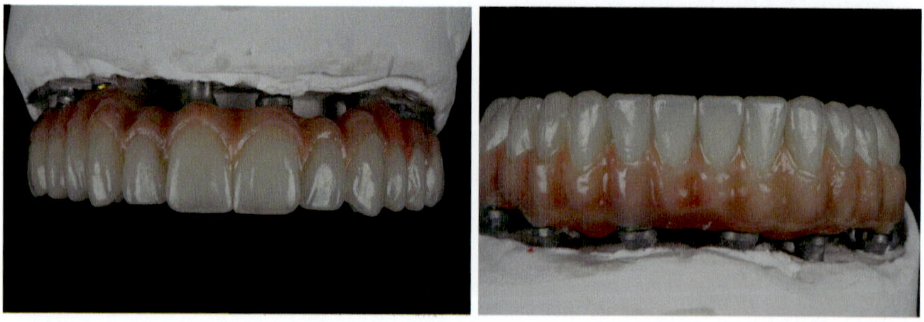

Fig. 17.34 Provisional restorations fabricated

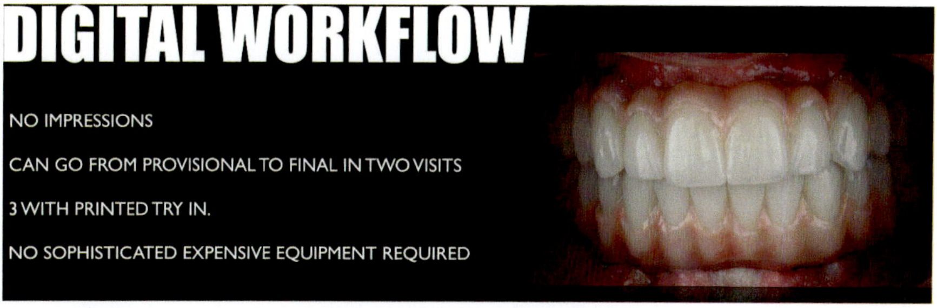

Fig. 17.35 Advantages of a digital workflow

Fig. 17.36 An example of scan gauges scanned in the mouth. (Osteon Technologies)

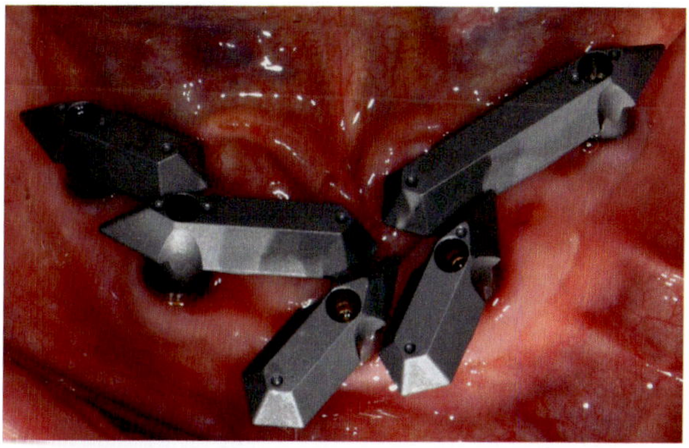

Fig. 17.37 An example of soft tissue scan

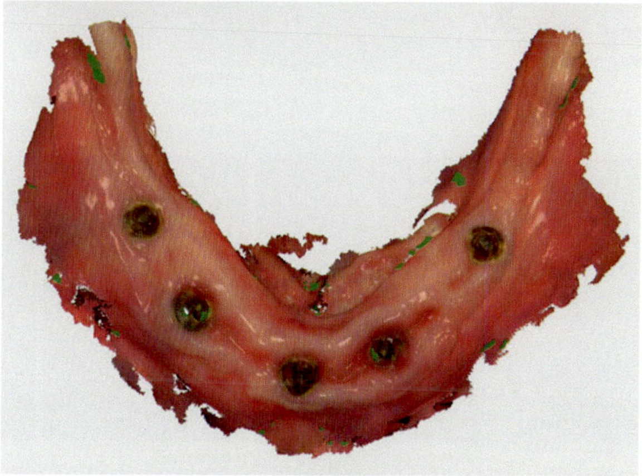

The following photos are also submitted with the scans:

1. Provisionals in the mouth
2. Smile
3. Full face (Fig. 17.40)

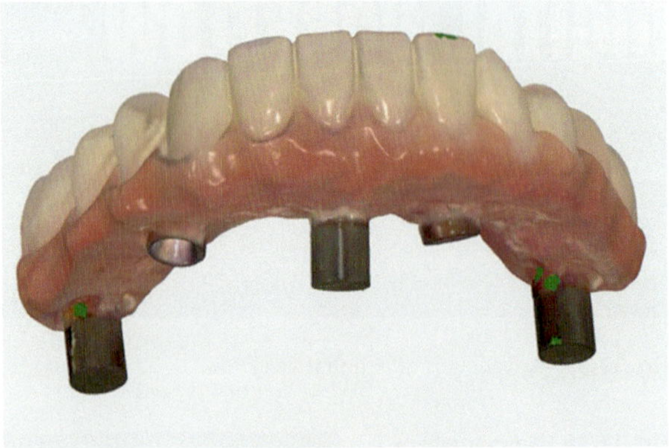

Fig. 17.38 An example of scanning of a provisional restoration undersurface

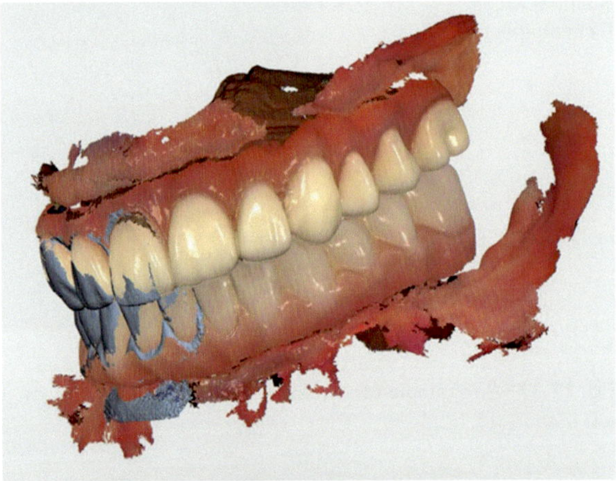

Fig. 17.39 An example of scanning the prosthesis in the mouth and recording occlusal relationships

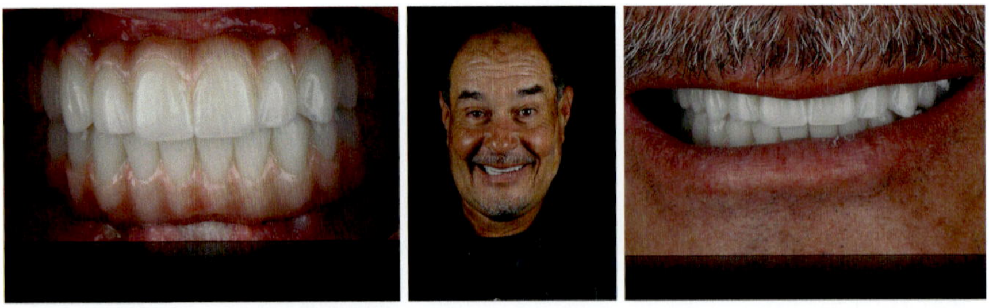

Fig. 17.40 Photos submitted to Osteon

The all the data is uploaded to CAD software, and a proposed design is created for approval by the clinician (Figs. 17.41 and 17.42).

One approved, a primary titanium substructure is milled to support an overlying zirconia framework. These two materials are bonded together utilizing a resin cement (Fig. 17.43).

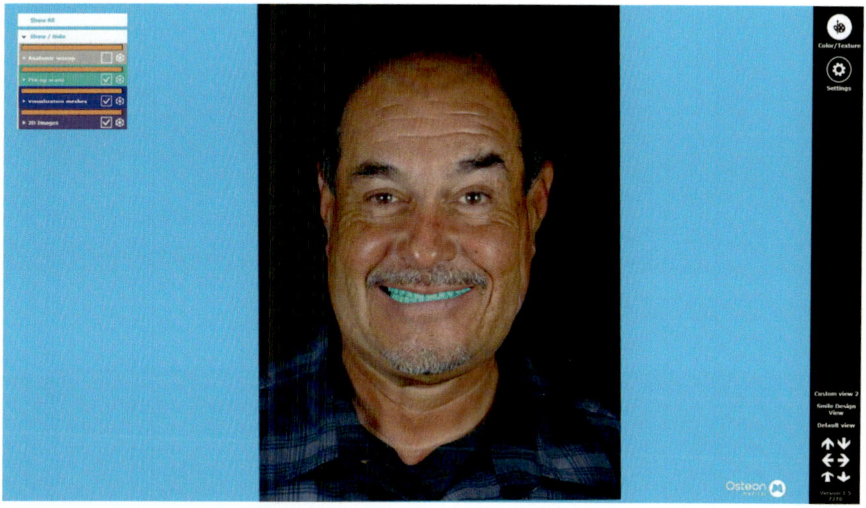

Fig. 17.41 CAD design

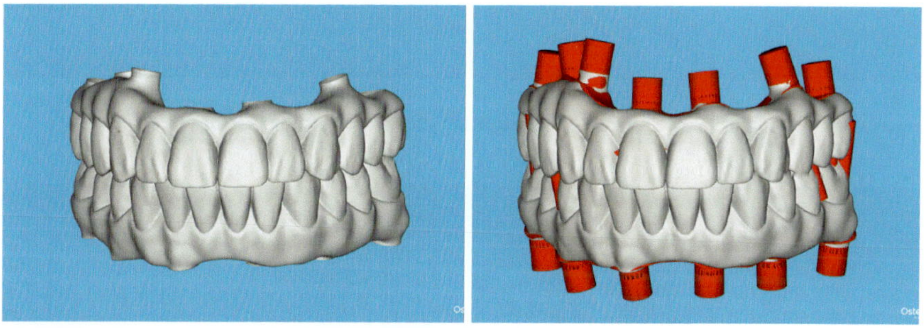

Fig. 17.42 Restoration proposals of both substructure and suprastructure

The undersurface of the restoration and contours are convex and cleansable (Fig. 17.44).

The definitive restorations are delivered, and screws torqued to manufacturers recommendations (Figs. 17.45, 17.46, 17.47, 17.48, 17.49, 17.50, 17.51, 17.52 and 17.53).

Manufacturers often promote the digital workflow to the clinician in a way that makes full arch implant reconstruction seamless. The clinician should be aware that full mouth reconstruction on implants is based on diagnosis, and digital technologies are just a tool to assist us in reaching our end goal. The clinician still has many decisions to make which include:

1. Tooth position
2. Centric relation
3. Vertical dimension

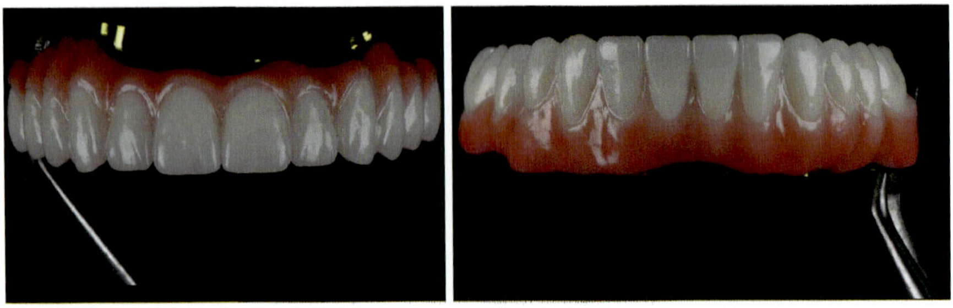

Fig. 17.43 Combination titanium/zirconia restoration

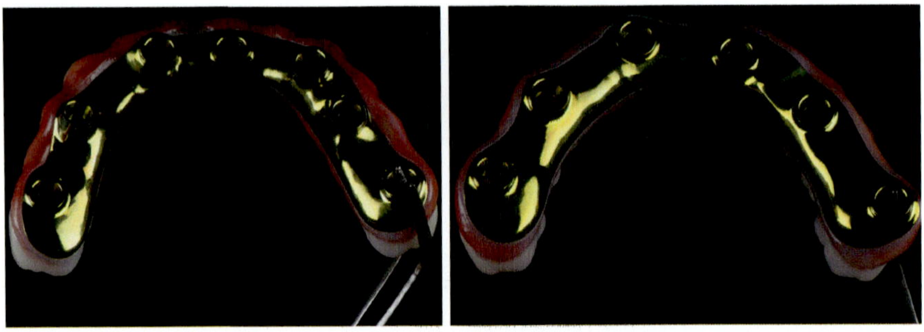

Fig. 17.44 Undersurface or restoration illustrating convex cleansable surface

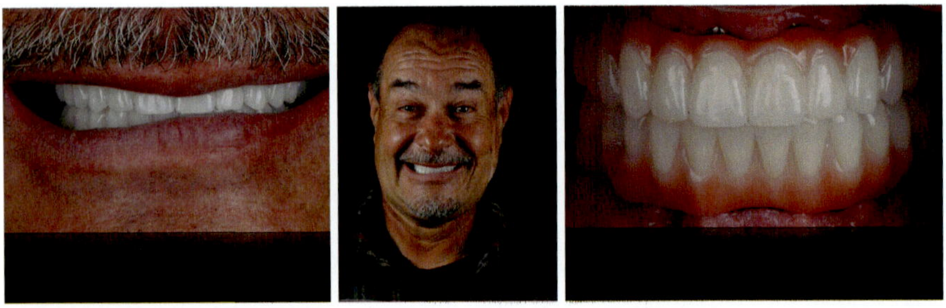

Fig. 17.45 Definitive restorations delivered

4. Envelope of function
5. Assessment of passivity
6. Soft tissue compression required
7. Aesthetics
8. Verification that the digital model is accurate based on the scan

Although model-less digital technologies appear to be appealing they do not have as long a clinical track record and a like-to-like comparison cannot be made to the conventional workflow. They have been advocated for use in situations when minimal bone reduction is performed, and the clinician is planning for an FP1 type

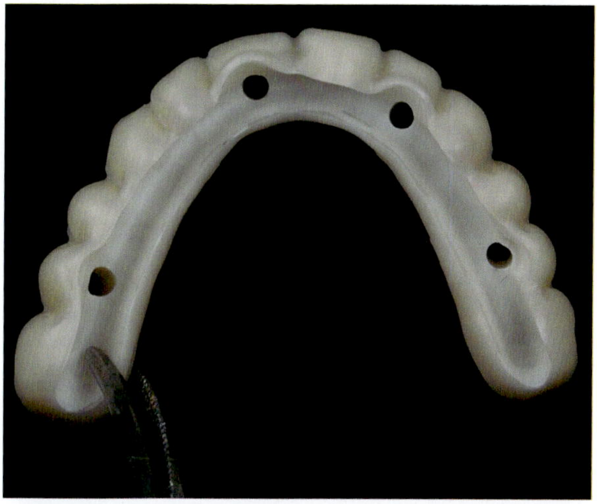

Fig. 17.46 Zirconia overlay

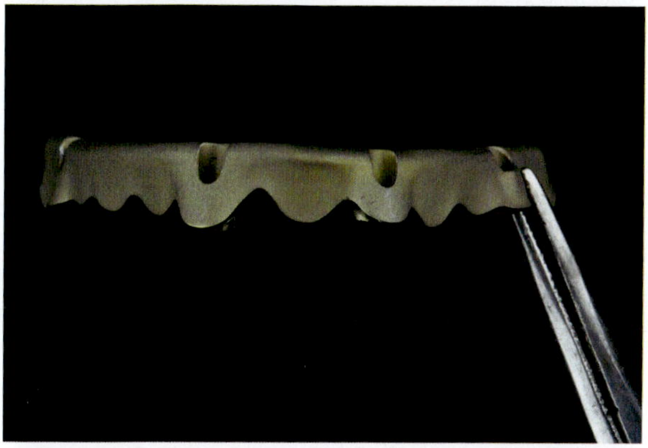

Fig. 17.47 Milled titanium substructure

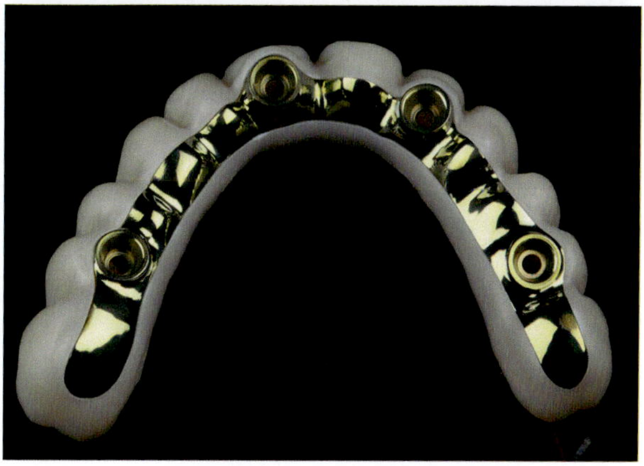

Fig. 17.48 Titanium is bonded to the zirconia overlay with a resin cement

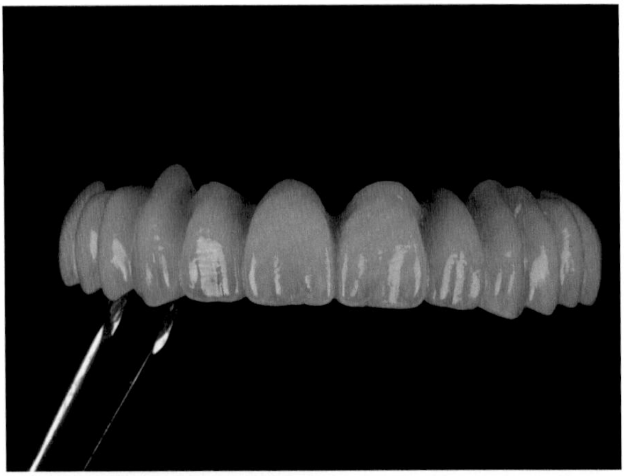

Fig. 17.49 FP1 type prosthesis designed to compress tissue. (Ceramics by Artem Asemov)

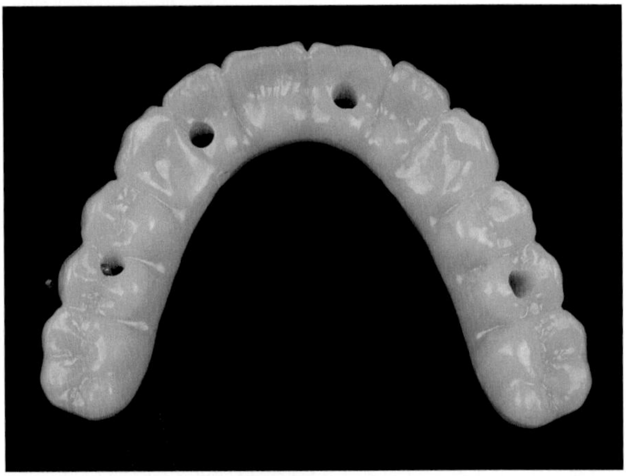

Fig. 17.50 Occlusion in polished zirconia

of restoration. There is once again no scientific basis for these claims. Manufacturers often make claims to fit a combined titanium/zirconia restoration in a space of 6–8 mm. The clinician once again has to think about minimal material thicknesses for long-term strength (Fig. 17.54).

Often clinicians pay the price for overzealous manufacturer claims. This results in patient and clinician disappointment. The astute practitioner should critically evaluate all manufacturer claims and not implement technologies which have not been tried and tested. If they do, the patient should be well informed, and the clinician should be prepared to absorb any costs associated with complications (Figs. 17.55, 17.56 and 17.57).

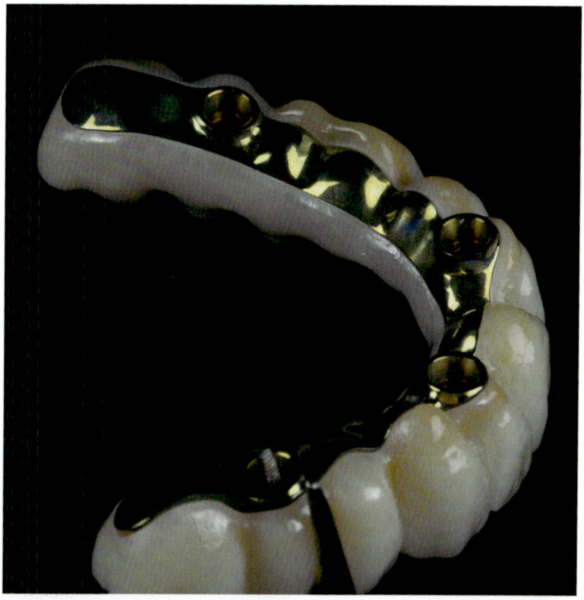

Fig. 17.51 Undersurface of restoration

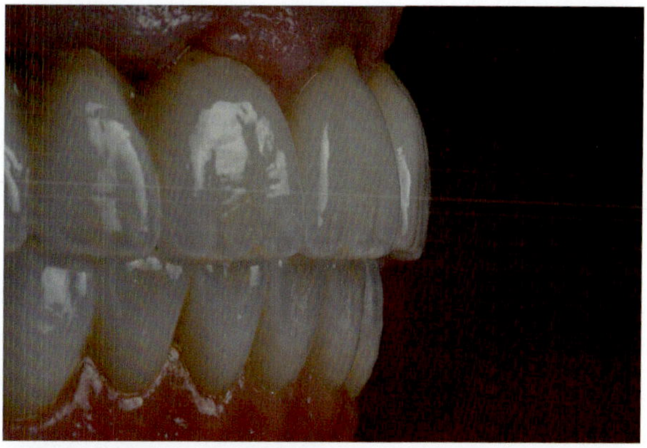

Fig. 17.52 Lateral view showing compression against tissue

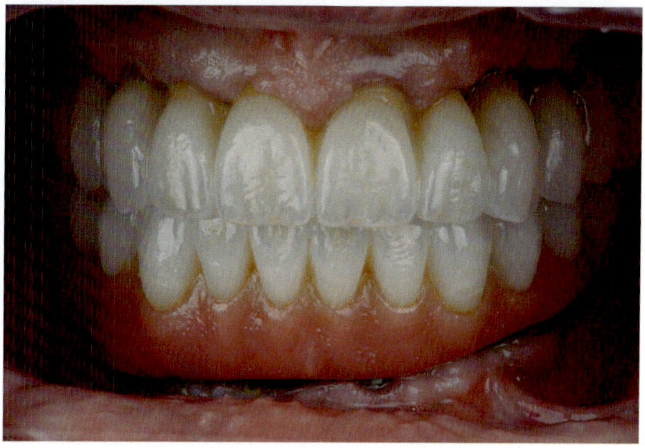

Fig. 17.53 Intraoral view of FP1 restoration in the maxilla and FP3 in mandible

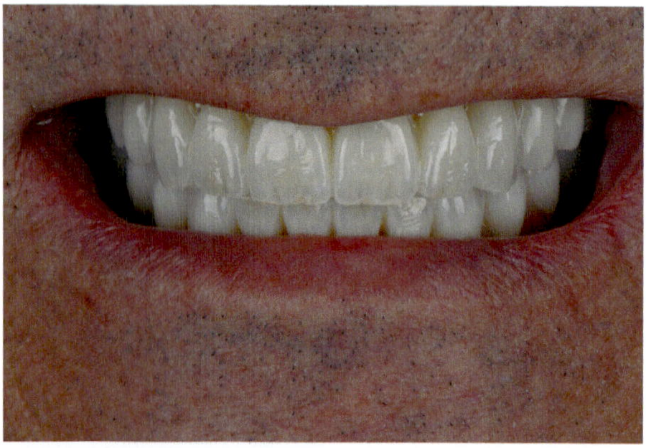

Fig. 17.54 Smile view of restoration in Fig. 17.52

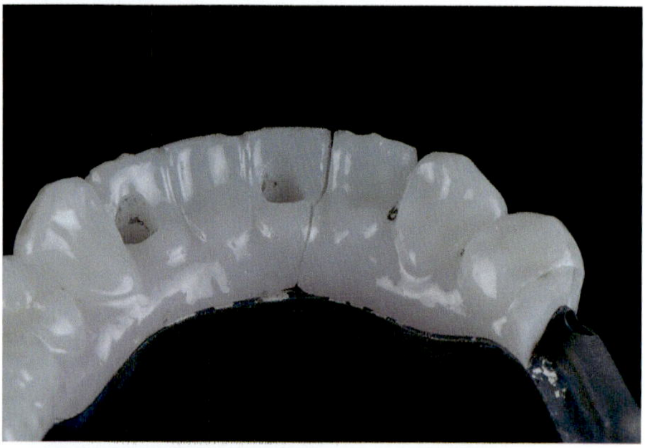

Fig. 17.55 Fractured zirconia suprastructure

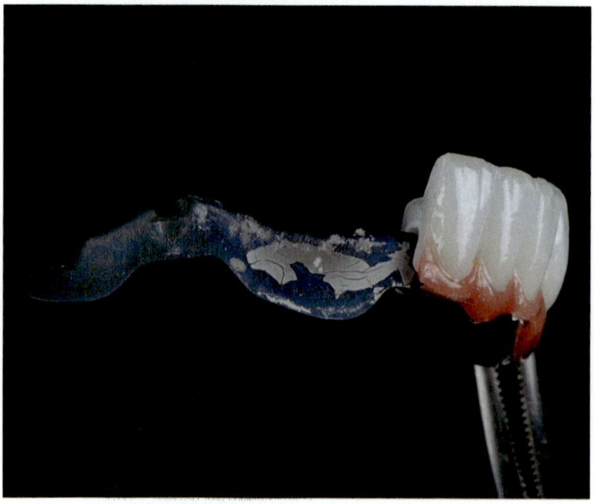

Fig. 17.56 Illustration of space between zirconia and titanium

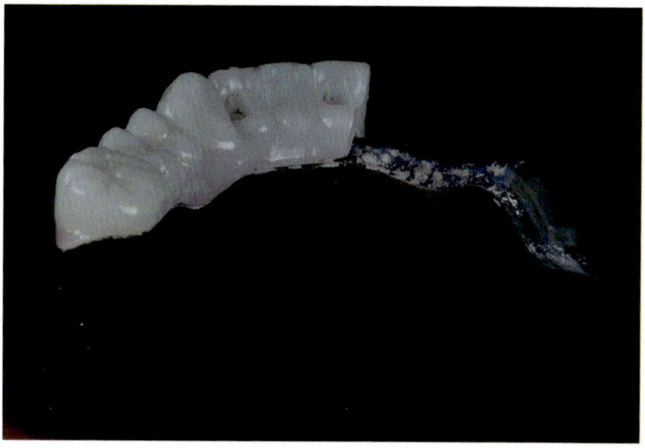

Fig. 17.57 Inadequate dimensions of titanium substructure

17.15 Conclusion

It is readily evident that material selection for full arch implant-supported restorations is multifactorial with a wide range of considerations for clinical success. Design of frameworks, manufacturing processes utilized, and clinical parameters are just a few of these considerations, and this chapter attempts to give guidelines to aid in making relevant decisions for these prostheses. While some basic parameters have been stated, further studies need to be conducted to look into specific areas in greater detail to be able to make more predictable decisions with respect to these therapies.

References

1. Rojas-Vizcaya F. Full zirconia fixed detachable implant-retained restorations manufactured from monolithic zirconia: clinical report after two years in service. J Prosthodont. 2011;20:570–6.
2. Chee W, Felton D, Johnson P, Sullivan D. Cemented versus screw-retained implant prostheses: which is better? Int J Oral Maxillofac Implants. 1999;14(1):137.
3. Chee W, Jivraj S. Screw versus cemented implant supported restorations. In: Treatment planning in implant dentistry. Lowestoft, Suffolk, British Dental Journal; 2007. p. 81–7.
4. Sailer I, Muhlemann S, Zwahlen M, Hammerle CH, Schneider D. Cemented and screw-retained implant reconstructions: a systematic review of the survival and complication rates. Clin Oral Implants Res. 2012;23(Suppl 6):163–201.
5. Jivraj S, Chee WWL, Corrado P. Treatment planning of the edentulous maxilla. Br Dent J. 2006;201(5):699.
6. Wicks RA. A systematic approach to definitive planning for osseointegrated implant prostheses. J Prosthodont. 1994;3:237–42.
7. Jacobs R, Van Steenberghe D. Comparative evaluation of the oral tactile function by means of teeth or implant supported prostheses. Clin Oral Implants Res. 1991;2:75–80.
8. Davis DM, Packer ME, Watson RM. Maintenance requirements of implant supported fixed prosthesis opposed by implant supported fixed prosthesis, natural teeth, or complete dentures. A five year retrospective study. Int J Prosthodont. 2003;16:521–3.

9. Yip KH, Smales RJ, Kaidonis JA. Differential wear of teeth and restorative materials: clinical implications. Int J Prosthodont. 2004;17(3):350–6.
10. Jung YS, Lee JW, Choi YJ, et al. A study on the in-vitro wear of the natural tooth structure by opposing zirconia or dental porcelain. J Adv Prosthodont. 2010;2:111–5.
11. Chang PC, Henegbarth EA, Lang LA. Maxillary zirconia implant fixed partial dentures opposing an acrylic resin implant fixed complete denture. A 2 year clinical report. J Prosthet Dent. 2007;97(6):321–30.
12. Heffernan MJ, Aquilino SA, Diaz-Arnold AM, Haselton DR, Stanford CM, Vargas MA. Relative translucency of six all-ceramic systems. Part I: Core materials. J Prosthet Dent. 2002;88(1):4–9.
13. Larsson C, Wennerberg A. The clinical success of zirconia-based crowns: a systematic review. Int J Prosthodont. 2014;27(1):33–43.
14. Goodacre C, et al. Clinical complications in fixed prosthodontics. J Prosthet Dent. 2003;90: 31–41.
15. Chong KK, Palamara J, Wong RH, Judge RB. Fracture force of cantilevered zirconia frameworks an in vitro study. J Prosthet Dent. 2014;1112:849–56.
16. Zarb GA, Jansson T. Laboratory procedures and protocol. In: Branemark PI, Zarb G, Albrektsson T, editors. Tissue integrated prostheses: osseointegration in clinical dentistry. Chicago: Quintessence; 1985. p. 303.
17. Jemt T. Three-dimensional distortion of gold alloy castings and welded titanium frameworks. Measurements of the precision of fit between completed implant prostheses and the master casts in routine edentulous situations. J Oral Rehabil. 1995;22:557–64.
18. Korsch M, Walther W. Peri-implantitis associated with type of cement: a retrospective analysis of different types of cement and their clinical correlation to the peri-implant tissue. Clin Implant Dent Relat Res. 2014; https://doi.org/10.1111/cid.12265.
19. Voitik AJ. The Kulzer abutment luting; Kal technique. A direct assembly framework method for osseointegrated implant prostheses. Implant Soc. 1991;2(1):11–4.
20. Almasri R, Drago C, Siegel S, et al. Volumetric misfit in CAD/CAM and cast implant frameworks: a university laboratory study. J Prosthodont. 2011;20:267–74.
21. Drago C, Howell K. Concepts for designing and fabricating metal implant frameworks for hybrid implant prostheses. J Prosthodont. 2012;21(5):413–24. https://doi.org/10.1111/j.1532-849X.2012.00835.x. Epub 2012 Mar 13.
22. Drago C. Ratios of cantilever lengths and anterior-posterior spreads of definitive hybrid full-arch, screw-retained prostheses: results of a clinical study. J Prosthodont. 2016; https://doi.org/10.1111/jopr.12519.
23. Kattadiyil MT, Goodacre CJ, Baba NZ. CAD/CAM complete dentures: a review of two commercial fabrication systems. Calif Dent Assoc. 2013;41(6):407–16.
24. Najeeb S, Zafar MS, Khurshid Z, Siddiqui F. Applications of polyetheretherketone (PEEK) in oral implantology and prosthodontics. J Prosthodont Res. 2016;60(1):12–9. https://doi.org/10.1016/j.jpor.2015.10.001.
25. Sereno N, Rosentritt M, Jarman-smith M, Lang R, Kolbeck C. In-vitro performance evaluation of polyetheretherketone (PEEK) implant prosthetics with a cantilever design. Clin Oral Implants Res. 2015;26(S12):296.
26. Tipton P, Siewert B. High performance polymers part 3. Private Dentistry UK; 2016.
27. Siewert B, Parra M. A new group of material in dentistry. PEEK as a framework material used in 12-piece implant-supported bridges. Z Zahnärztl Implantol. 2013;29:148–59.
28. Moura Guedes C. New possibilities for high performance polymers in the MALO clinic protocol. British Association of Restorative Dentistry Conference. 4–6 Jun 2016.
29. Abduo J. Fit of CADCAM implant frameworks: a comprehensive review. J Oral Implantol. 2014;40:758–66.
30. Larsson C, Vult Von Steyern P. Implant supported full arch zirconia based mandibular fixed dental prostheses. Eight year results from a clinical pilot study. Acta Odontol Scand. 2013;71:1118–22.

31. Puri S, Parciak EC, Kattadiyil MT. Complete mouth reconstruction with implant supported fixed partial dental prosthesis fabricated with zirconia frameworks: a 4 year clinical follow up. J Prosthet Dent. 2014;112:397–401.
32. Cheng CW, Chien CH, Chen CJ, Papaspyridakos P. Complete mouth rehabilitation with modified monolithic zirconia implant supported fixed dental prosthesis and an immediate loading protocol: a clinical report. J Prosthet Dent. 2013;109:347–52.
33. Guess PC, Bonfante EA, Silva NR, Coelho PG, Thompson VP. Effect of core design and veneering technique on damage and reliability of Y-TZP-supported crowns. Dent Mater. 2013;29:307–16.
34. Miyazaki T, Nakamura T, Matsumura H, Ban S, Kobayashi T. Current status of zirconia restorations. J Prosthodont Res. 2013;57(4):236–61. https://doi.org/10.1016/j.jpor.2013.09.001. Epub 2013 Oct 18.
35. Preis V, Letsch C, Handel G, Behr M, Schneider-Feyrer S, Rosentritt M. Influence of substructure design, veneer application technique, and firing regime on the in vitro performance of molar zirconia crowns. Dent Mater. 2013;29:e113–21.
36. Mosharraf R, Rismanchian M, Savabi O, Ashtiani AH. Influence of surface modification techniques on shear bond strength between different zirconia cores and veneering ceramics. J Adv Prosthodont. 2011;3(4):221–8. https://doi.org/10.4047/jap.2011.3.4.221.
37. Kim JS, Raigrodski AJ, Flinn BD, Rubenstein JE, Chung KH, Mancl LA. In vitro assessment of three types of zirconia implant abutments under static load. J Prosthet Dent. 2013;109(4):255–63. https://doi.org/10.1016/S0022-3913(13)60054-2.
38. Pozzi A, Tallarico M, Barlattani A. Monolithic lithium disilicate full contour crowns bonded on CADCAM zirconia complete arch implant bridges with 3–5 years of follow up. J Oral Implantol. 2015;41(4):450–8.

An Interdisciplinary Approach to Treatment Planning in Implant Dentistry

18

Saj Jivraj and Winston Chee

18.1 Aesthetic Implant Dentistry: An Interdisciplinary Approach

In recent years, implant dentistry has been increasingly influenced by esthetic considerations [1]. The primary reason for this is the patients demand for naturally appearing restorations.

The goal of modern implant dentistry is no longer represented solely by successful osseointegration. In order to claim success, the definitive restorations must be surrounded by a soft and hard tissue environment in harmony with the existing dentition [2]. Talented ceramists can fabricate restorations that mimic the adjacent teeth; however, if reconstruction of the surrounding tissue is not realized, the end result will not be aesthetically pleasing. It remains the responsibility of the implant team to consider all the variables that can influence the final outcome prior to embarking upon treatment [3].

With the elevated expectations of patients and increased experience and knowledge of clinicians, there is no doubt that an interdisciplinary approach that integrates the knowledge, skills, and experience of all the disciplines of dentistry into a comprehensive treatment plan can yield better results.

Well executed implant-supported restorations can offer exceptional satisfaction to both the patient and dentist. It can transform an unhealthy, unattractive dentition to one which is esthetically pleasing to the patient. In addition, implant-supported restorations can improve comfort and function. The longevity of implants is well documented, and in many situations where posterior support is lacking,

S. Jivraj (✉)
Private Practice, Anacapa Dental Art Institute, Oxnard, CA, USA

W. Chee
Advanced Prosthodontics, Herman Ostrow School of Dentistry, University of Southern California, Los Angeles, CA, USA

W. Chee, S. Jivraj (eds.), *Treatment Planning In Implant Dentistry*, BDJ Clinician's Guides, https://doi.org/10.1007/978-3-031-68726-6_18

implant-supported restorations are the only method of predictably providing this support for occlusion in the long term.

To obtain optimal results, meticulous attention must be paid to a myriad of details. The process starts with the patient interview and meticulous treatment planning, then continues through to active treatment and culminates in regular planned follow-up care.

The objectives are to improve oral health, to establish proper occlusal function, and to create the most ideal esthetic result possible. It is only through an organized and systematic approach that appropriate diagnoses can be made and based on these diagnoses, functional and aesthetic problems can be addressed predictably.

Interdisciplinary therapy involves the combination of diagnostic, treatment planning, and therapeutic procedures. It is imperative that the team leader appropriately selects a team of practitioners. The selection process can either have a positive or a negative impact on the overall treatment. Each provider on the team must have an optimal level of skill in his or her area of expertise to be a positive factor [4].

The complex nature of dentofacial problems necessitates a highly organized method of communication between the team members, so that all aspects of treatment can be equally voiced. It is through this communication that an interdisciplinary treatment plan can be formulated prior to generation of a joint treatment letter. This treatment letter should include a discussion of aspects of treatment that will be provided by each team member, time frame of the proposed treatment, inherent risks involved, informed consent, and financial responsibilities of the patient. It can be said that the quality of treatment is dependent upon the quality of the communication. It is critical that the team leader maintains communication between the specialists both during treatment and once it has been completed. It is only through this approach that optimal care can be delivered and regular planned follow-up care can be implemented.

The purpose of this chapter is to outline the blueprint for a comprehensive interdisciplinary treatment philosophy, designed for developing the foundation for optimal esthetics in implant dentistry. Some cases will be presented to illustrate the utility of interdisciplinary treatment where allied specialists are recruited to enhance and improve the existing presentations of the patients both for function and esthetics.

18.2 Patient 1

A 36-year-old male was seeking replacement of his current removable partial denture with fixed restorations. His specific complaint was the instability and aesthetics of the removable restorations (Figs. 18.1, 18.2, 18.3 and 18.4).

On clinical and radiographic examination, some problems were presented. Periodontally, the molars on the maxillary left were deemed to have a poor prognosis. The mandibular molars were tilted mesially and there was insufficient space between the posterior teeth to provide the patient with fixed partial dentures that would satisfy his aesthetic requirements (Figs. 18.5, 18.6, 18.7 and 18.8).

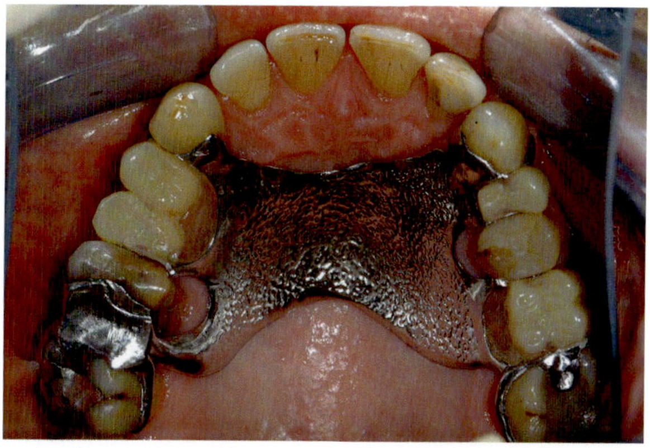

Fig. 18.1 Maxillary occlusal view illustrating removable partial denture in situ

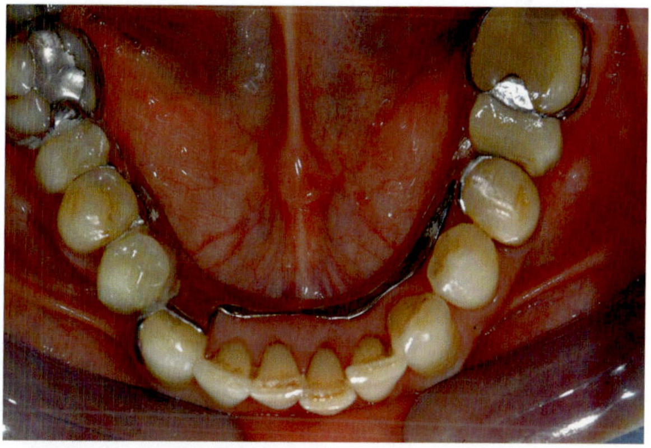

Fig. 18.2 Mandibular occlusal view illustrating mandibular removable partial denture in situ

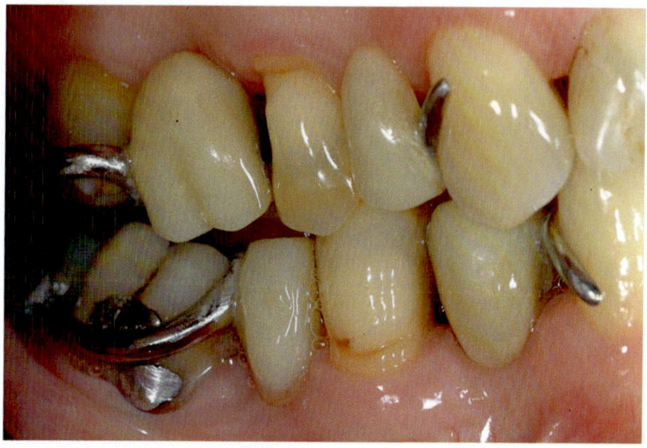

Fig. 18.3 Right lateral view with removable partial denture

The objectives of treatment included creating space between the posterior teeth so that implant-supported restorations could be provided, extracting teeth which were deemed to have poor prognosis and to provide restorations for the patient that would fulfill his esthetic and functional desires.

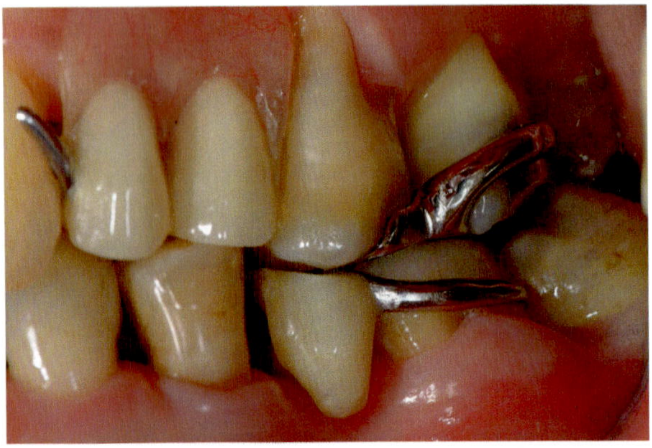

Fig. 18.4 Left lateral view with removable partial denture

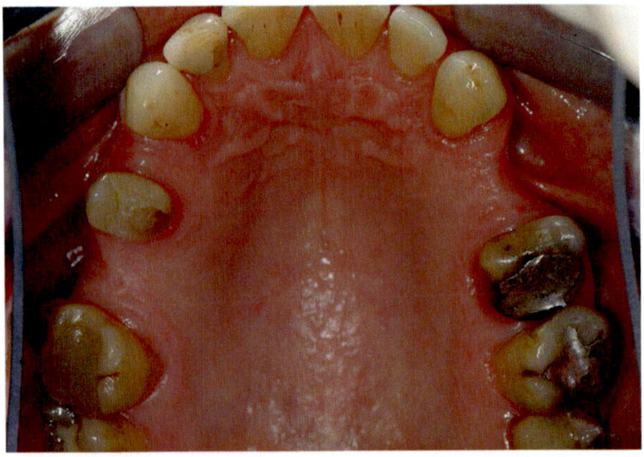

Fig. 18.5 Maxillary occlusal view illustrating inadequate space between teeth for implant placement

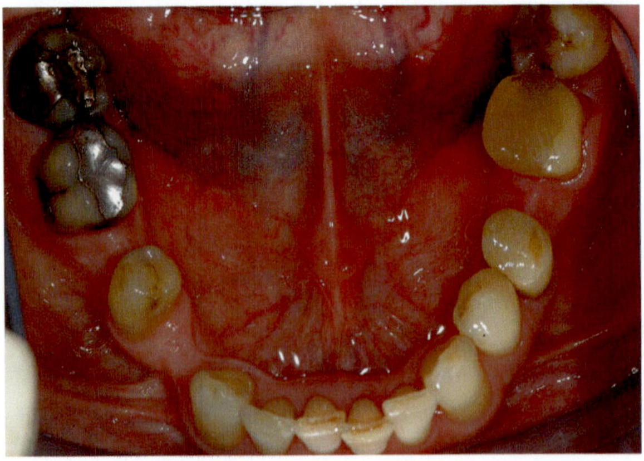

Fig. 18.6 Mandibular occlusal view illustrating inadequate space between teeth for implant placement

Orthodontics can serve as a valuable adjunct to treatment planning in restorative dentistry. When significant numbers of teeth are missing, the implants can also be used to effect the desired tooth movement. The literature has shown that dental

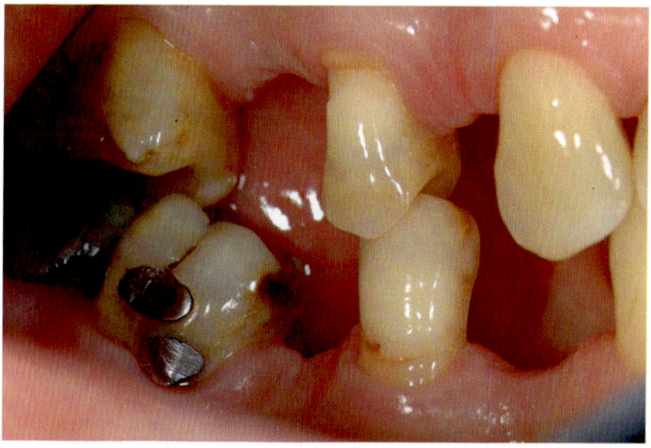

Fig. 18.7 Right lateral view illustrating inadequate mesiodistal space for implant placement

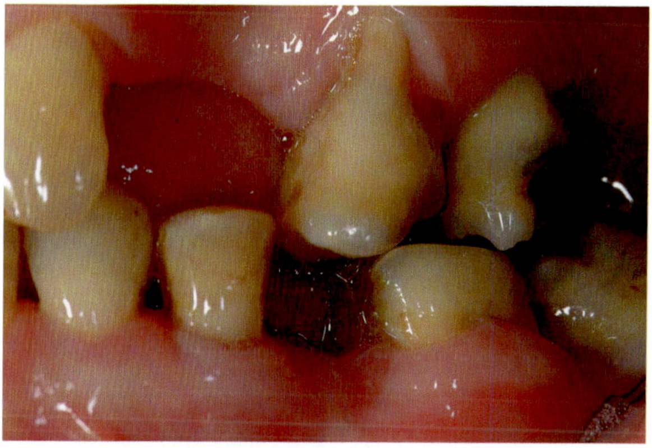

Fig. 18.8 Left lateral view illustrating inadequate mesiodistal space for implant placement

implants can be used as anchors for both orthodontic and orthopaedic movement [5–7]. It can also serve to create space between teeth, so that implants can be placed.

With these objectives in mind, a treatment plan was formulated which required communication between the surgeon, orthodontist, and prosthodontist.

The first stage was to complete extraction of mandibular third molars and maxillary molars on the maxillary left side.

An orthodontic setup was completed on the cast to determine the post-orthodontic position of the teeth (Figs. 18.9, 18.10, 18.11, 18.12 and 18.13). This set up was used to communicate the ideal tooth positions required to the orthodontist. Sufficient space would be required to allow the implants to be placed at least 1.5 mm away from the roots of the adjacent teeth and to allow appropriate coronal space for aesthetic contouring of the restorations. Brackets were placed, and the appropriate tooth movements were made (Figs. 18.14, 18.15, 18.16 and 18.17). During the orthodontic phase, a sinus lift was performed in the maxillary left area and bone was harvested from the chin for augmentation.

Once the appropriate tooth positions had been achieved, impressions were made for casts on which a diagnostic wax up was completed. This diagnostic wax up was used to fabricate provisional restorations which would be used to stabilize the

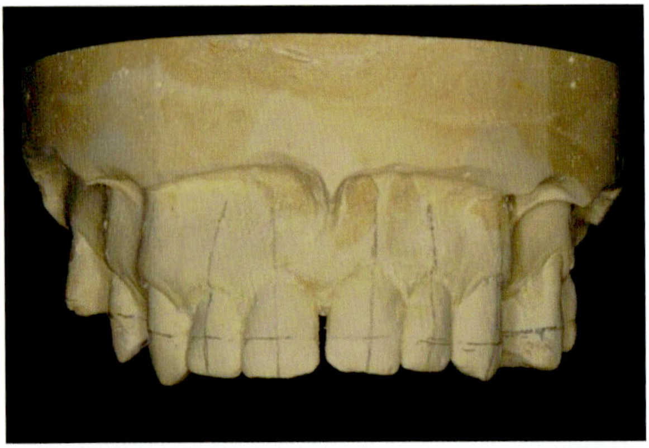

Fig. 18.9 Maxillary diagnostic cast with lines marked for orthodontic repositioning

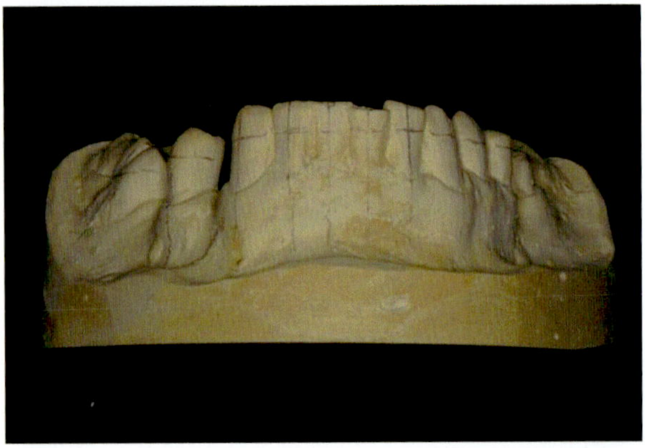

Fig. 18.10 Mandibular diagnostic cast with lines marked for orthodontic repositioning

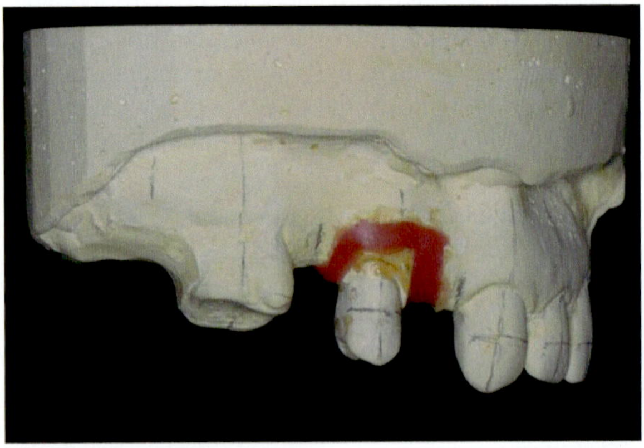

Fig. 18.11 Maxillary cast showing repositioning of teeth

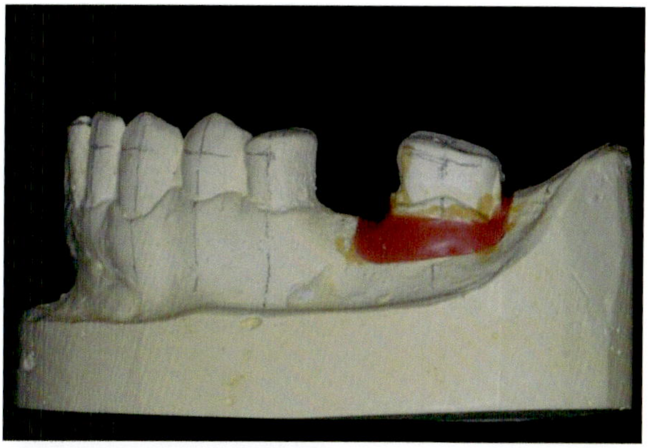

Fig. 18.12 Mandibular cast showing repositioning of teeth on left

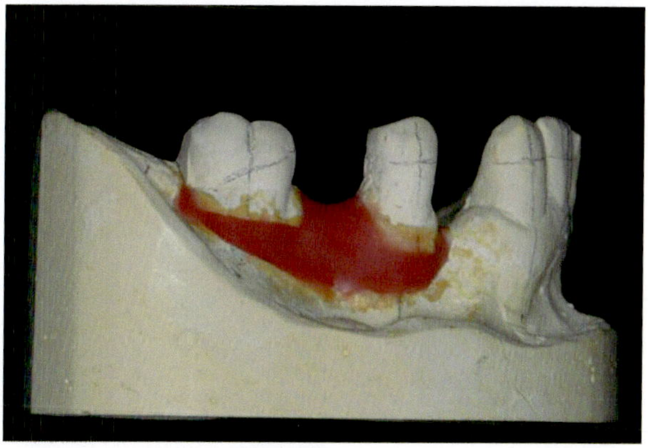

Fig. 18.13 Mandibular cast showing repositioning of teeth right

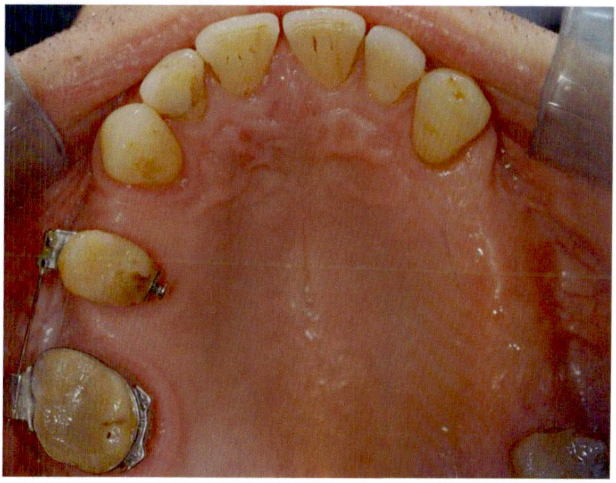

Fig. 18.14 Maxillary occlusal view showing clinical repositioning of teeth

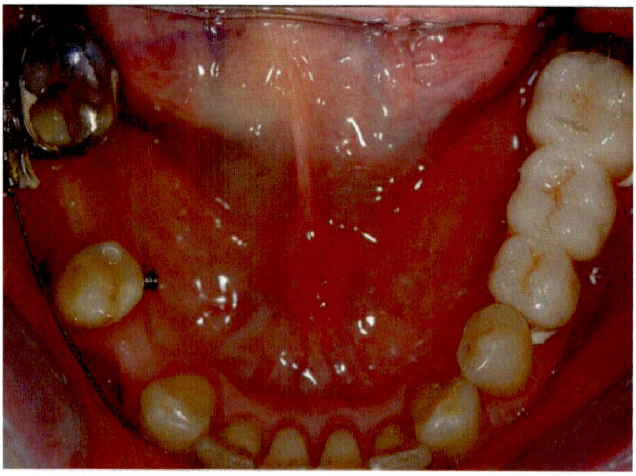

Fig. 18.15 Mandibular occlusal view showing repositioning of teeth

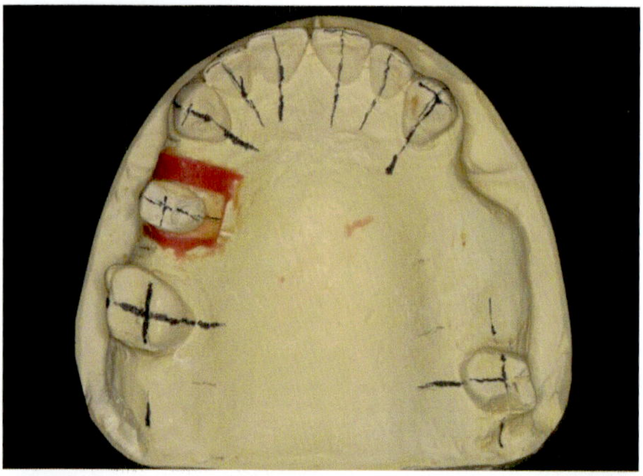

Fig. 18.16 Maxillary occlusal view of diagnostic cast showing repositioning of teeth

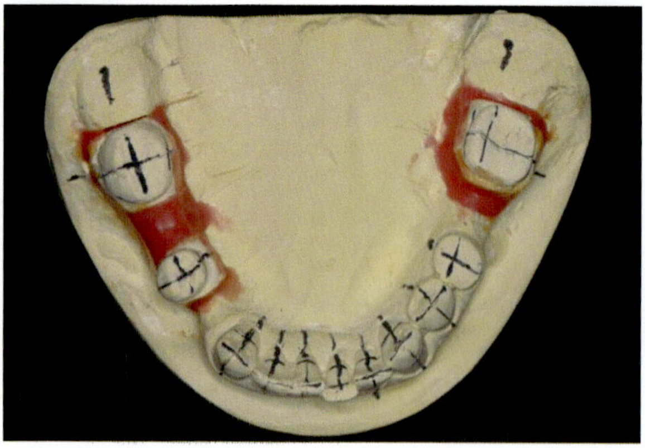

Fig. 18.17 Mandibular occlusal view of diagnostic cast showing repositioning of teeth

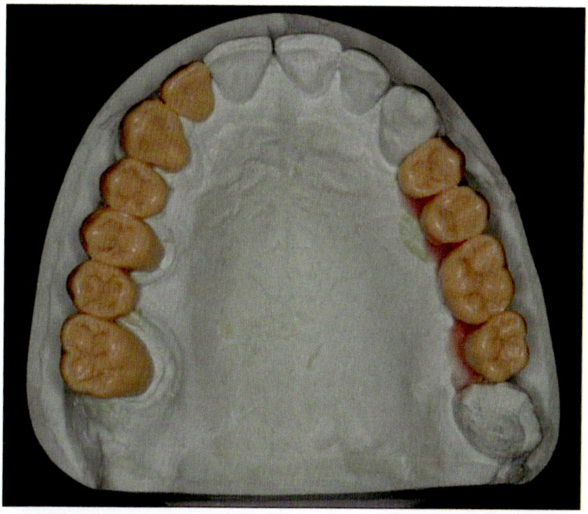

Fig. 18.18 Maxillary diagnostic wax up

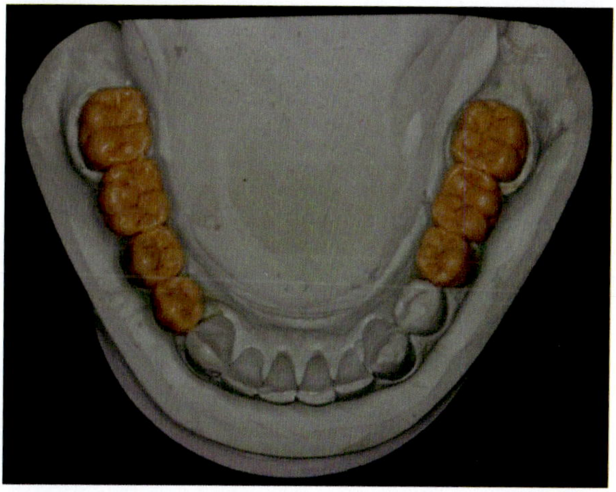

Fig. 18.19 Mandibular diagnostic wax up

post-orthodontic positions of the teeth. These restorations also improved aesthetics, provided posterior support, and served as blueprints for the definitive implant borne restorations (Figs. 18.18, 18.19, 18.20 and 18.21) [8, 9]. Once the patient accepted the esthetics of the provisional restorations, these were duplicated to provide surgical guides for implant placement and implants were placed taking care to position them appropriately from the adjacent teeth (Fig. 18.22).

Following osseointegration, a second set of provisionals were provided to re-confirm the patient's acceptance of esthetics and function. The maxillary right canine and lateral; incisor were prepared for metal ceramic restorations and a final impression was taken for the definitive prosthesis. All final restorations were planned as single units except for the maxillary left area where the premolars were cemented due to implant angulations and the molars were splinted to improve biomechanical outcomes (Figs. 18.23, 18.24, 18.25, 18.26, 18.27, 18.28, 18.29, 18.30 and 18.31).

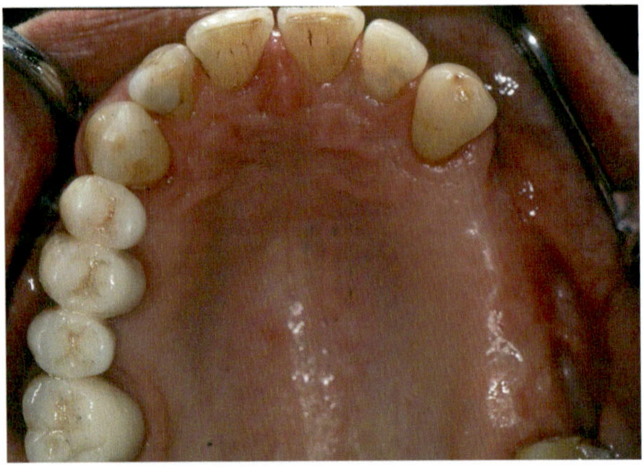

Fig. 18.20 Maxillary provisional restorations

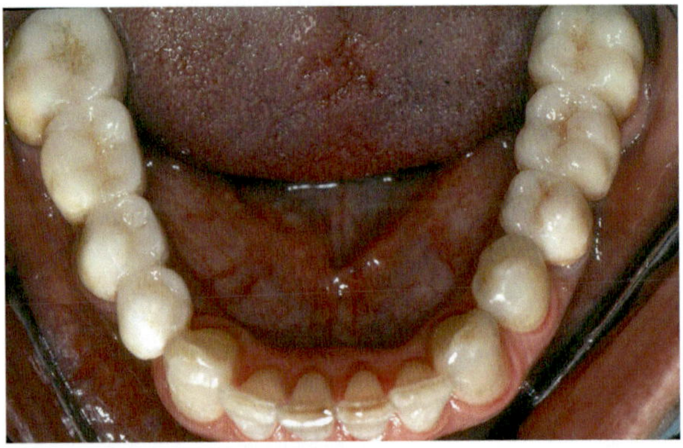

Fig. 18.21 Mandibular provisional restorations

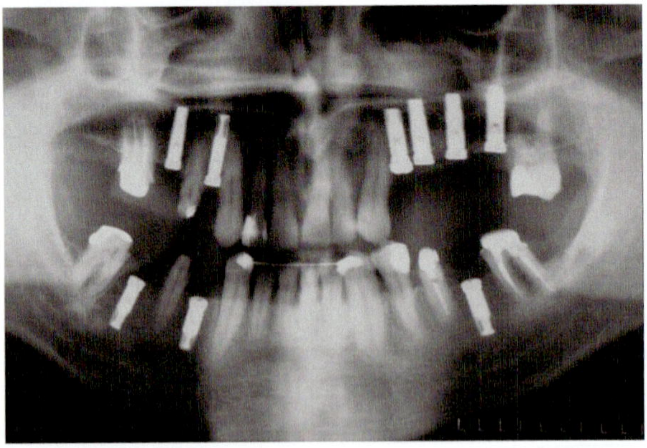

Fig. 18.22 Panoramic radiograph illustrating implant placement

Communication between the allied specialists is essential to achieve optimal results. Without adequate communication, the treatment provided irregardless of the initial planning will fall short of the desired results. A systematic planned and executed treatment protocol will meet the desired goals and inevitably will result in a satisfied patient.

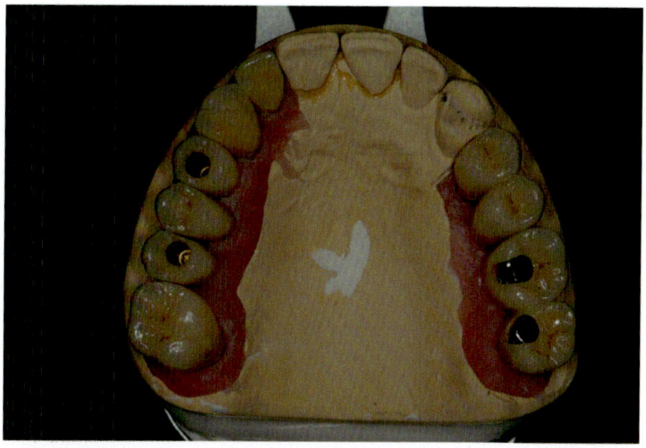

Fig. 18.23 Maxillary view of master cast showing definitive restorations

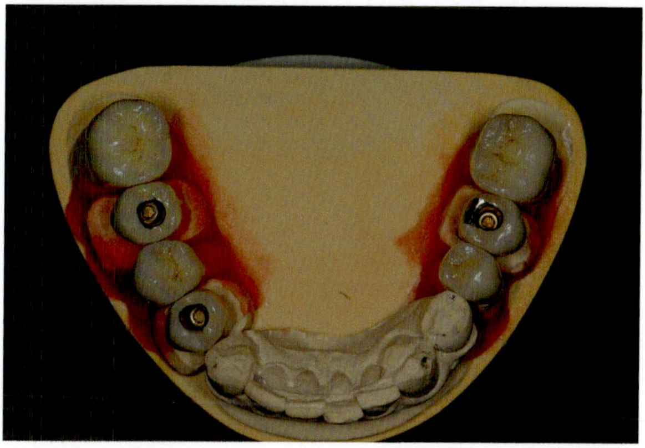

Fig. 18.24 Mandibular occlusal view of master cast showing definitive restorations

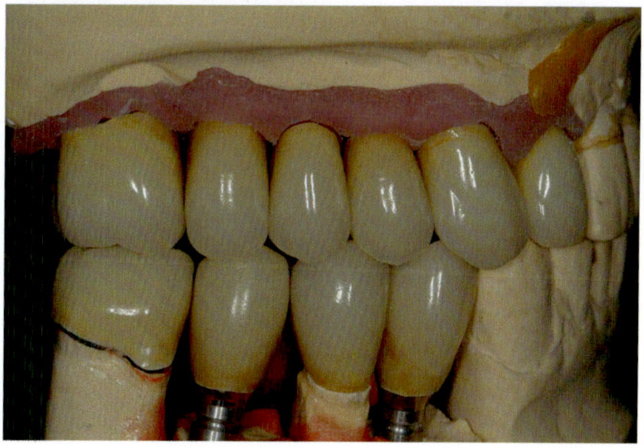

Fig. 18.25 Right lateral view of definitive restorations on master cast

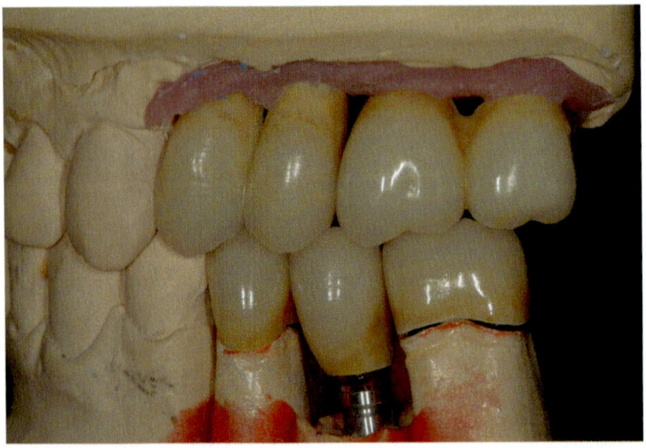

Fig. 18.26 Left lateral view of definitive restorations on master cast

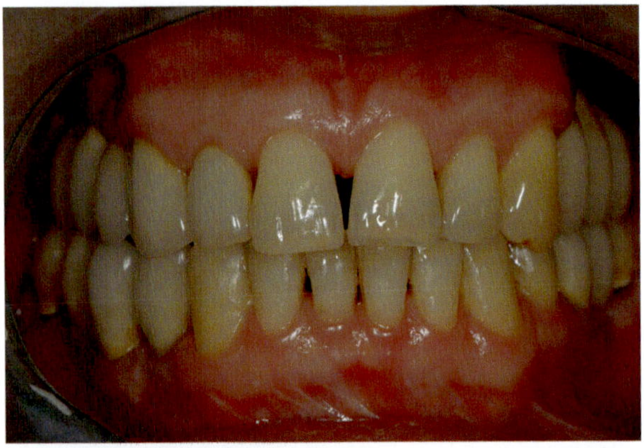

Fig. 18.27 Frontal view of definitive restorations in the mouth

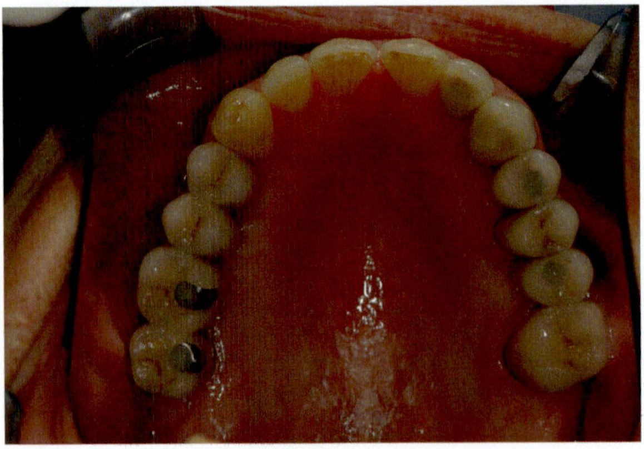

Fig. 18.28 Maxillary occlusal view of definitive restorations

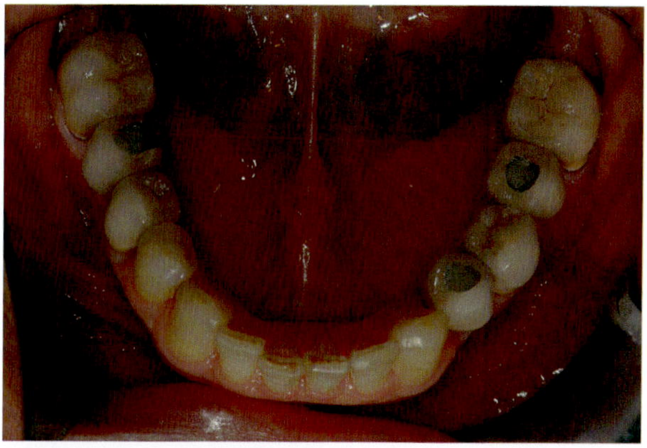

Fig. 18.29 Mandibular occlusal view of definitive restorations

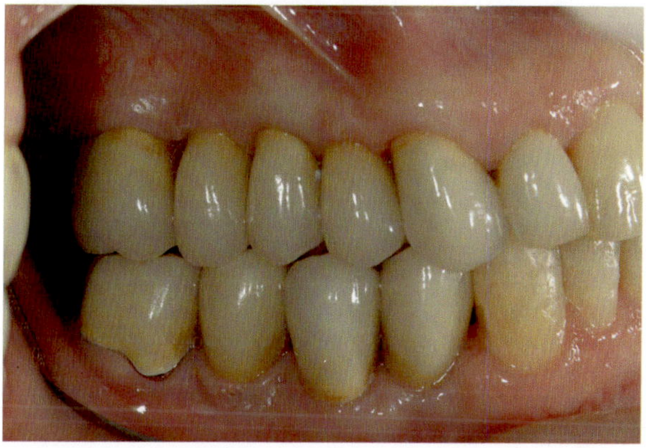

Fig. 18.30 Right lateral view of definitive restorations

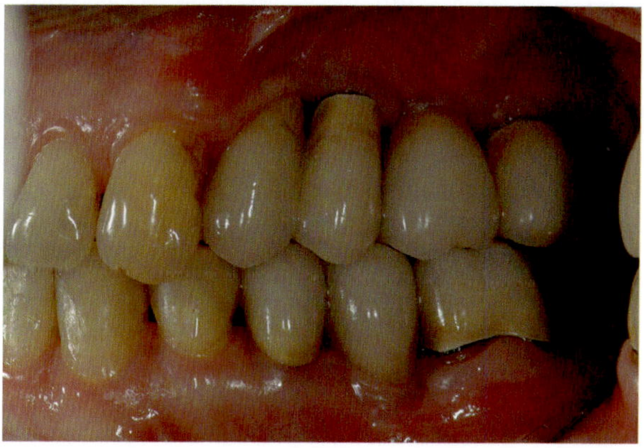

Fig. 18.31 Left lateral view of final restorations

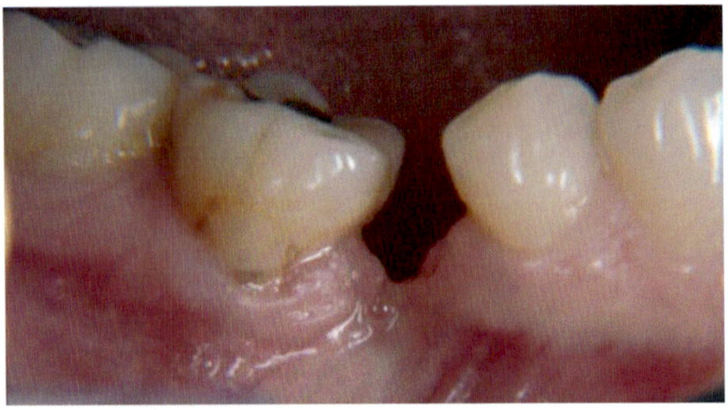

Fig. 18.32 Lateral view of mandibular right region illustrating mesial drift of first molar and inadequate mesiodistal space for implant placement

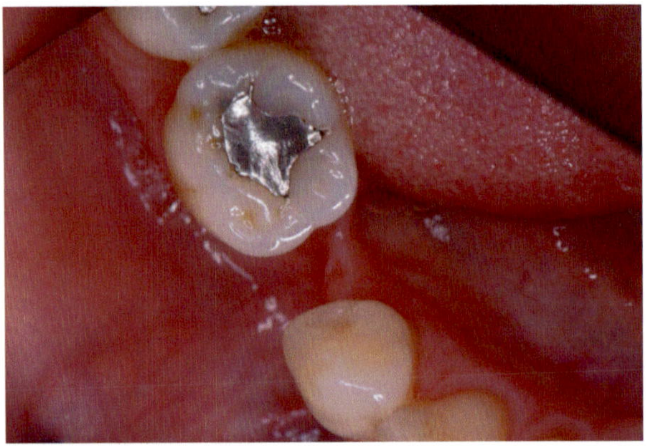

Fig. 18.33 Occlusal view illustrating inadequate buccolingual osseous volume for implant placement

18.3 Patient 2

A 34-year-old female presented with the desire to have implant therapy for her missing lower right second premolar. This particular tooth had been extracted 10 years ago. Clinical examination revealed mesial drift of the first molar (Fig. 18.32). There was also inadequate buccolingual bone for ideal placement of an implant (Fig. 18.33). The patient was made aware of the complex nature of the therapy and on approval, an interdisciplinary approach was initiated. The first and second molars were orthodontically up righted (Fig. 18.34) until sufficient mesiodistal space was created to allow fabrication of a restoration which mimicked the dimensions of the contralateral side. Following up righting, autogenous bone was harvested from the mandibular symphysis to augment buccolingual width so that an implant could be placed (Fig. 18.35). Following healing, a surgical guide was fabricated to allow implant placement in the ideal position. The implant was subsequently placed and restored to ideal form and function (Fig. 18.36).

This interdisciplinary treatment allowed the patient to have implants placed and conserve the adjacent teeth, without communication between the specialties, this type of treatment would not have been possible.

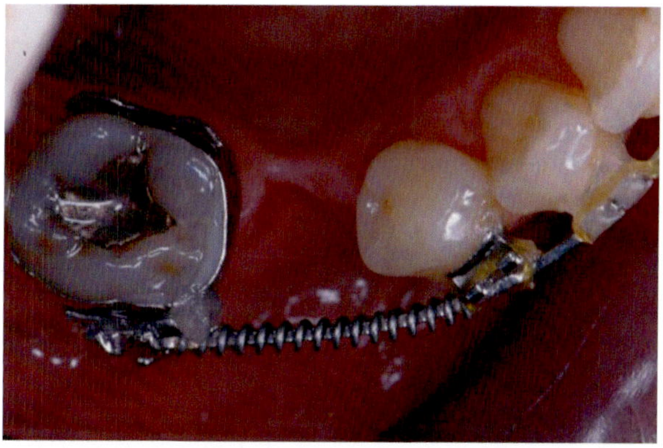

Fig. 18.34 Orthodontic up righting of molar

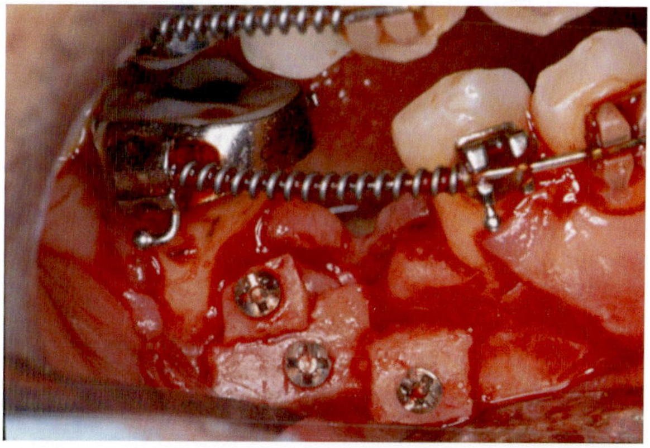

Fig. 18.35 Autogenous bone graft to augment buccolingual volume

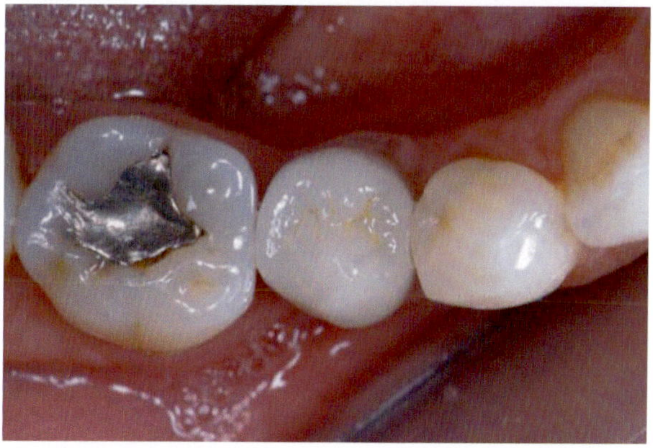

Fig. 18.36 Occlusal view of definitive implant supported restoration

18.4 Patient 3

A 64-year-old male presented seeking a functional and esthetic solution to manage and treat tooth surface loss. His specific concerns were the deep vertical overlap of the anterior teeth and the position of the maxillary anterior teeth (Figs. 18.37 and 18.38). The anterior teeth were in a Cl 2 division 2 presentation.

On clinical and radiographic examination, the following were observed:

1. Deep vertical overlap
2. Severe palatal attrition of the maxillary anterior teeth
3. Attrition and loss of tooth structure of the mandibular anterior teeth
4. The mandibular incisors had over-erupted into the palatal mucosa
5. The maxillary anterior teeth had drifted downwards and on enunciating the "F" sound, there was a strong contact between the incisal edges and the vermillion border of the lower lip
6. Irregular occlusal plane
7. Intact posterior teeth
8. The patient had a restricted envelope of function due to the Cl 2 Div 2 anterior tooth relationship (Figs. 18.39 and 18.40)

Management of patients to provide restorative solutions that have been compromised by spatial considerations requires an interdisciplinary approach. The practitioner must have a clear understanding and visualize the end result prior to

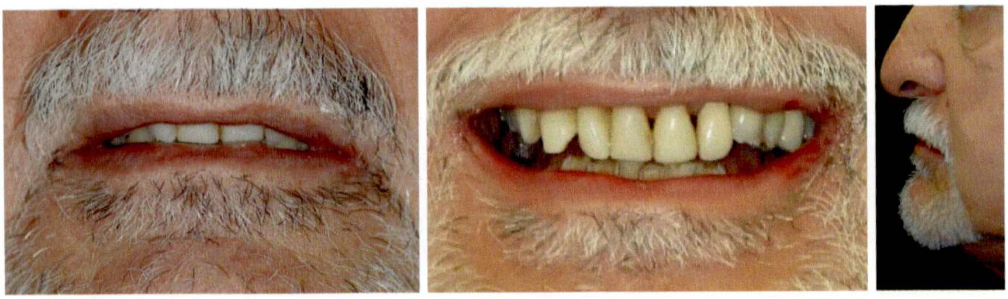

Fig. 18.37 Anterior view of tooth display at rest, patient unhappy with incisal edge overly long. Profile of lip support is shown

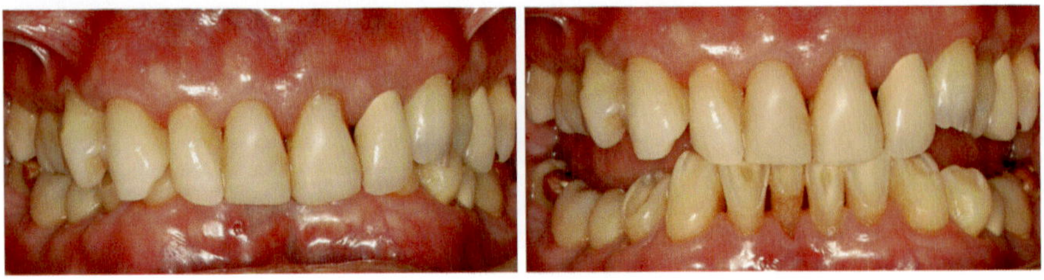

Fig. 18.38 Intraoral retracted view from anterior to the maxillary anterior teeth vertically overlap 100% of the mandibular incisors, both maxillary and mandibular incisors are over-erupted

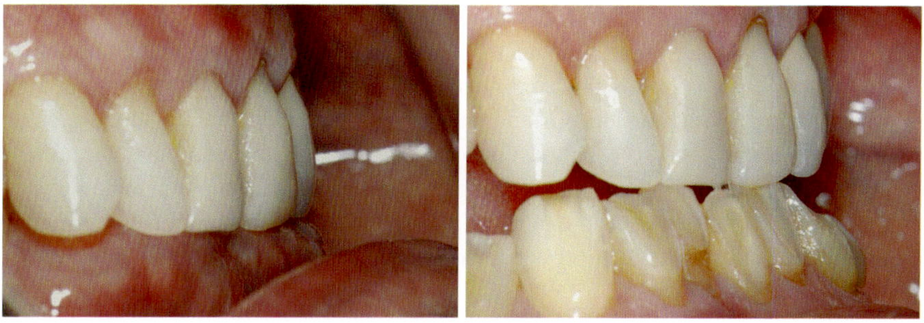

Fig. 18.39 A 45° view shows the deep vertical overlap and the wear on the facial surfaces of the mandibular anterior teeth

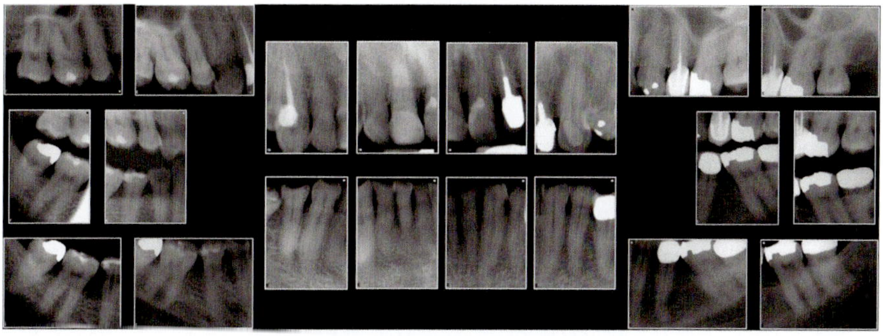

Fig. 18.40 Radiographs show periodontal attachment levels are healthy, and no decay is detected

embarking upon extensive therapy. Considerations must be given the amount of vertical and horizontal restorative space that is needed for different types of restoration, amount of tooth structure that will need to be removed and how the space will be created. Failure to design a prosthetic construction without considering space issues can result in rehabilitation with diminished stability, poor esthetics, and inadequate contours. Therefore, available restorative volume must be computed before initiating therapy to ensure proper prosthesis design. One of the most difficult factors is that the posterior teeth are intact and their intercuspal relationship would be maintained—no changes in vertical dimension will take place.

Space management in restorative dentistry can encompass some or all the treatment modalities listed below.

1. Orthodontic movement
2. Extraction and/or ostectomy
3. Endodontic therapy
4. Tooth preparation for partial or full coverage restorations
5. Implant placement

On evaluating the patient, the following decisions influenced treatment planning:

1. The patient had intact posterior teeth contact at a vertical dimension that he was comfortable with. In this instance, there was no indication to increasing/restoring the vertical dimension. Often practitioners observe anterior tooth surface loss and assume that vertical dimension may have been compromised and full mouth reconstruction is completed. When posterior teeth are intact, and the anterior teeth exhibit severe tooth surface loss the astute practitioner must consider solutions that minimize tooth structure removal and maintain the integrity of the teeth.
2. The maxillary anterior teeth had over-erupted and were in the incorrect position. Consideration must be given to orthodontic therapy to reposition the teeth.
3. The root length, amount of tooth structure remaining and anticipated occlusal forces may influence the clinician's judgement on whether to keep or remove teeth.
4. The clinician must anticipate the amount of tooth structure removal required to receive a full coverage restoration.

The following steps towards a treatment plan were considered after a thorough diagnostic evaluation.

1. Casts were evaluated to determine the incisal edges for maxilla and mandible.
2. After modifying the casts, both maxilla and mandible have a proper occlusal plane and incisor positions (Figs. 18.41, 18.42 and 18.43).
3. Decisions were made to have the maxillary anterior teeth intruded and flared to alter the proclination, intrusion, and widening the arch form. The proclination will allow tooth preparation to be minimal due to the tooth wear. A lesser tooth reduction mesiodistally is also accommodated due to the widening of the arch form (Figs. 18.44, 18.45 and 18.46).
4. For the mandible, the incisors would have to undergo too many procedures and much of the tooth structure has been removed. Implants will be placed to support restorations of the four incisors, and crown lengthening and endodontic treatments will be needed to restore the first premolars and cuspids (Figs. 18.47, 18.48 and 18.49).
5. Post-orthodontics diagnostic waxing to determine positioning of teeth (Figs. 18.50 and 18.51).

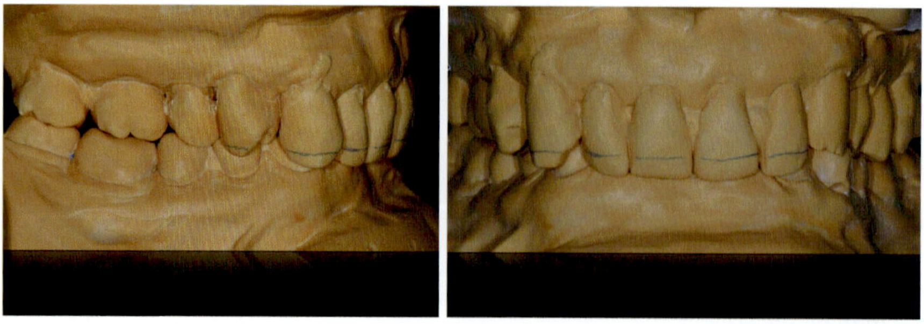

Fig. 18.41 Casts of the arches are mounted, and a pencil line is drawn to shorten the incisal edges

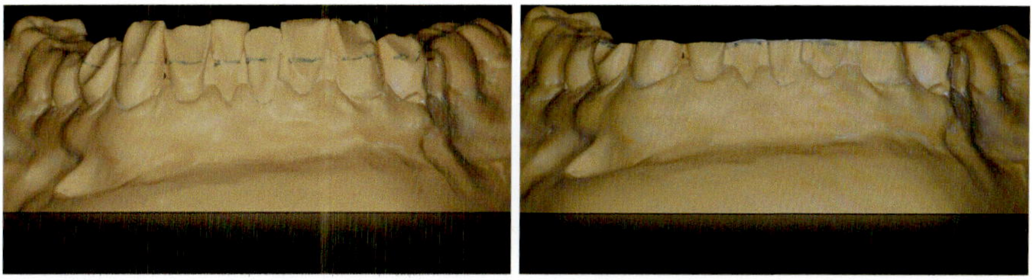

Fig. 18.42 The mandibular cast is also drawing a line to level out the occlusal plane, this provides much information

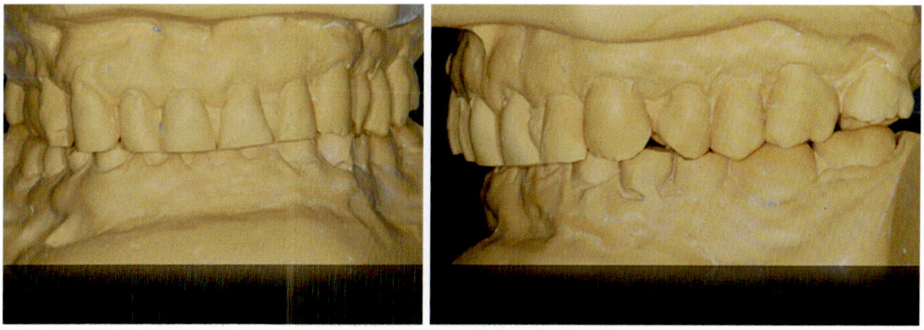

Fig. 18.43 The casts are mounted to show the occlusal planes of both arches and the overlap of the incisors, the mandibular incisors are significantly over-erupted

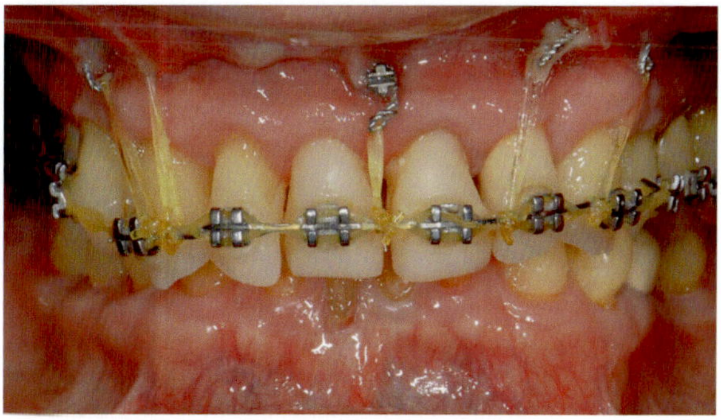

Fig. 18.44 Orthodontics is proceeding with temporary anchorage devices intruding and flaring the teeth, this will procline the teeth to provide palatal space to accommodate full coverage restorations, as teeth flare diastema will present and less tooth structure will be removed palatally and mesiodistally

6. Provisional fabrication to verify esthetics phonetics and function, often patients require modifications and a second set of provisional is required (Figs. 18.52, 18.53, 18.54 and 18.55).
7. Final impressions and fabrication of definitive metal ceramic restorations. Patients often request changes from the original provisional restorations. It is

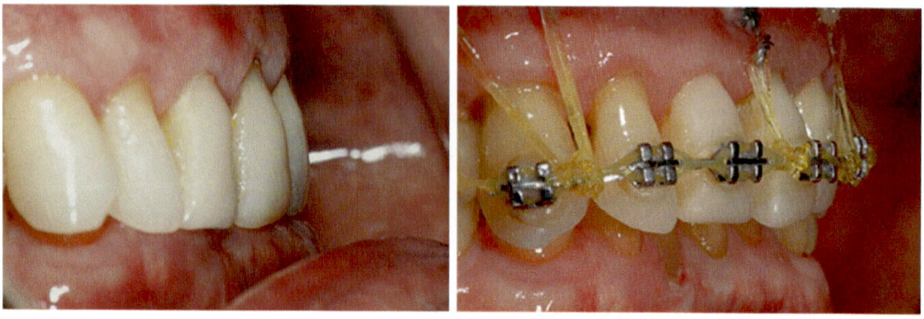

Fig. 18.45 The comparison of beginning and end of the orthodontic of tooth intrusion and flaring can be observed

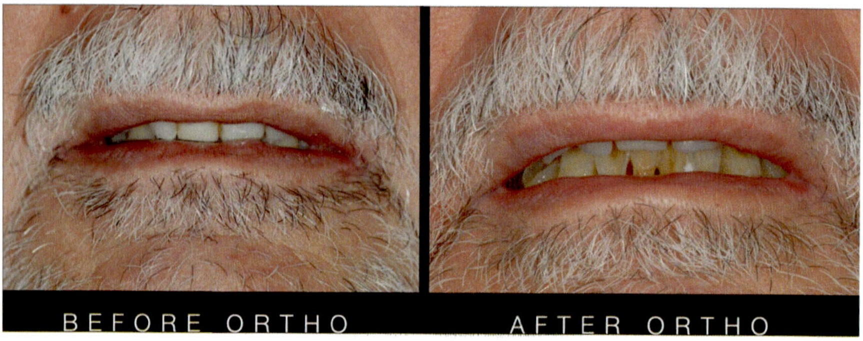

Fig. 18.46 Incisal edge display can be seen reduced before and after orthodontic movement

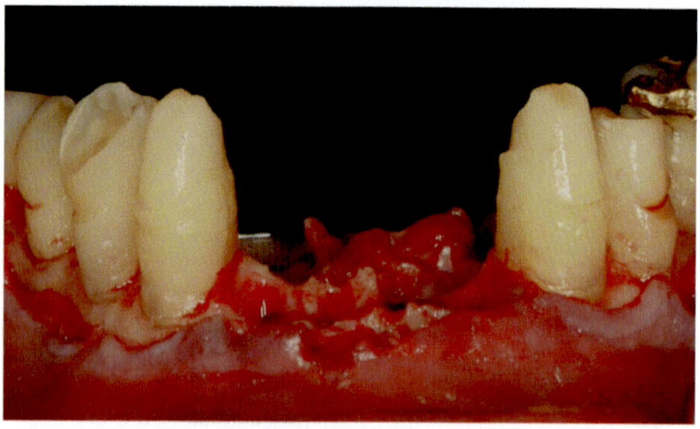

Fig. 18.47 In the mandibular arch, the incisors are extracted, crown lengthening has taken place

prudent to accomplish the patient's objectives in an additional set of provisional restorations prior to completing the definitive metal ceramic restorations (Figs. 18.56, 18.57, 18.58, 18.59, 18.60, 18.61, 18.62, 18.63 and 18.64).

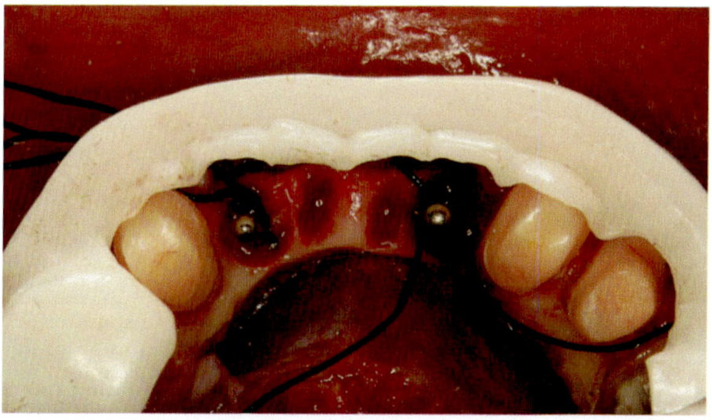

Fig. 18.48 Surgical guide is in place, and the implants are placed in position of the lateral incisors with proper trajectories to facilitate screw retained restorations

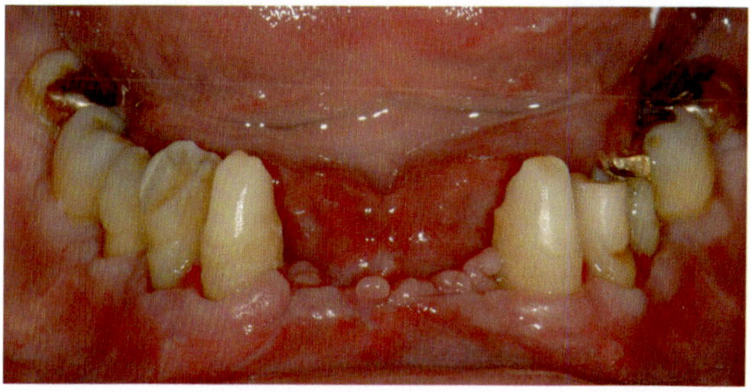

Fig. 18.49 Soft tissue is healing, the canines and premolars will be reduced to accommodate the occlusal plane and they will require elective endodontic treatment

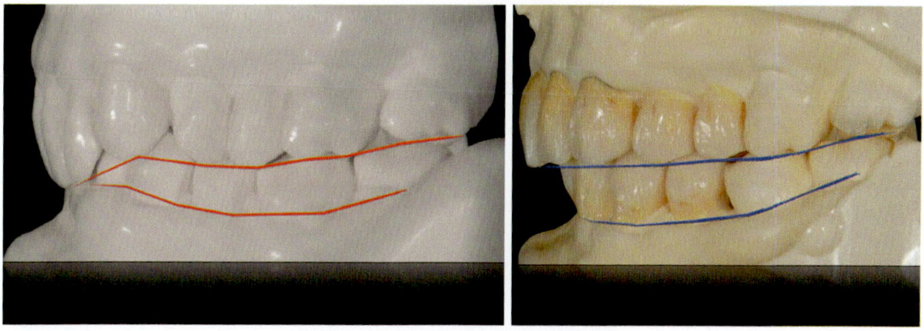

Fig. 18.50 A wax up on the right is the goal compared to the left pre-operative cast

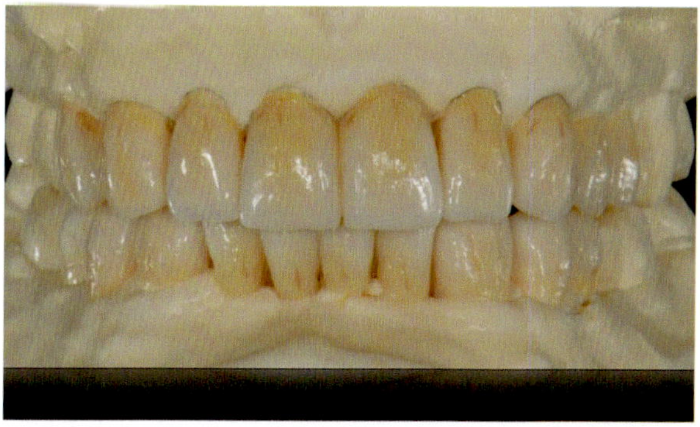

Fig. 18.51 The anterior view will be the template for provisional restorations to be fabricated

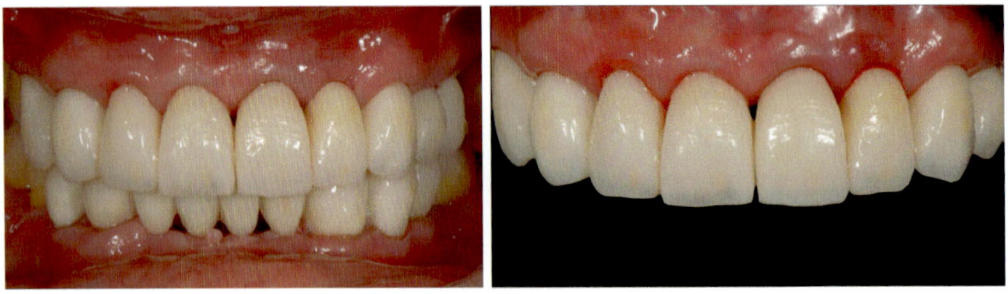

Fig. 18.52 The provisional restorations are inserted over the tooth preparations

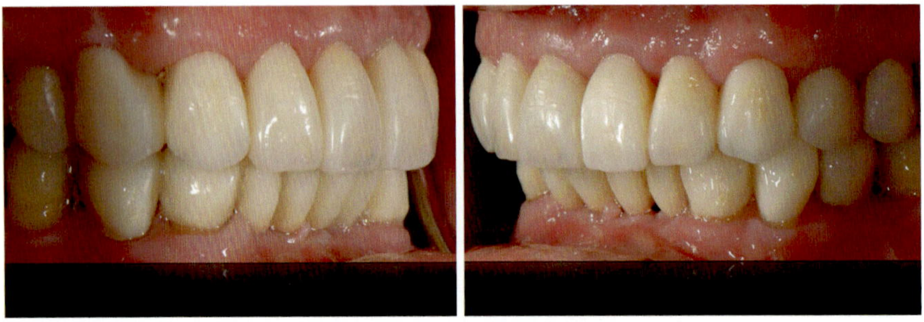

Fig. 18.53 The lateral views after 2 weeks show very healthy gingiva and well-fitting provisional restorations

Fig. 18.54 Anterior view of maxillary and mandibular provisional restorations

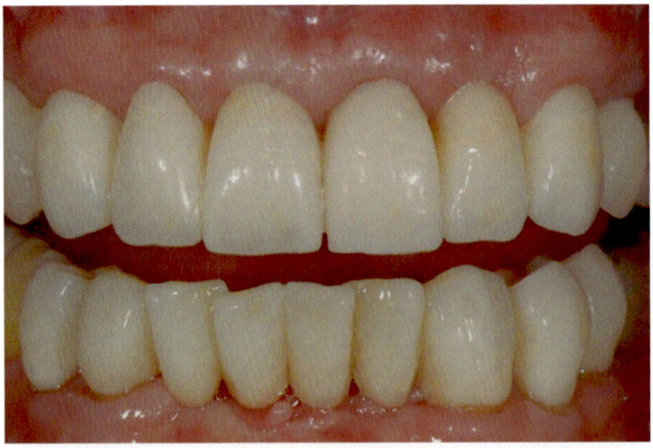

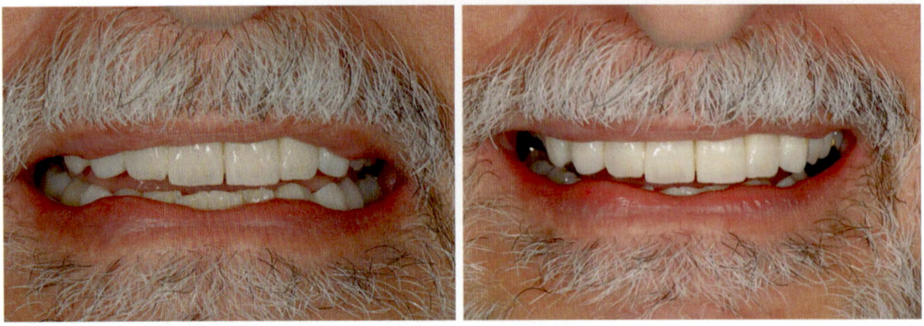

Fig. 18.55 Anterior views of provisional restorations with differing lip postures

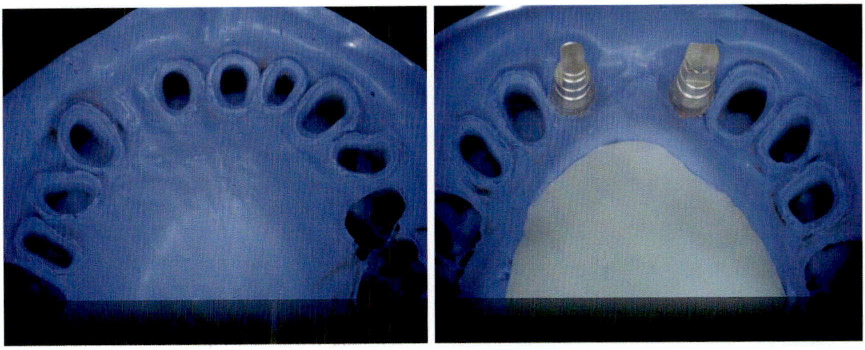

Fig. 18.56 Impressions are taken of the maxilla and mandible

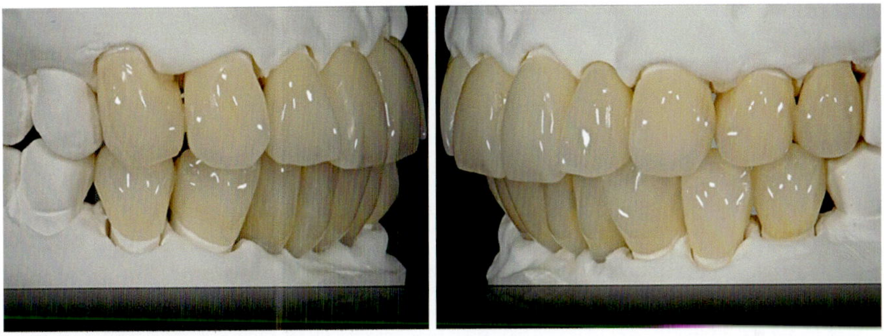

Fig. 18.57 Another set of provisional restorations are made directly on tooth preparations replicated on master casts

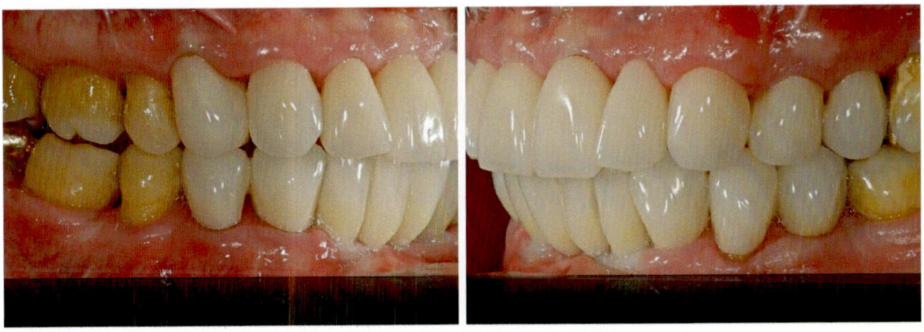

Fig. 18.58 The provisional restorations are placed for patients acceptance of aesthetics and function

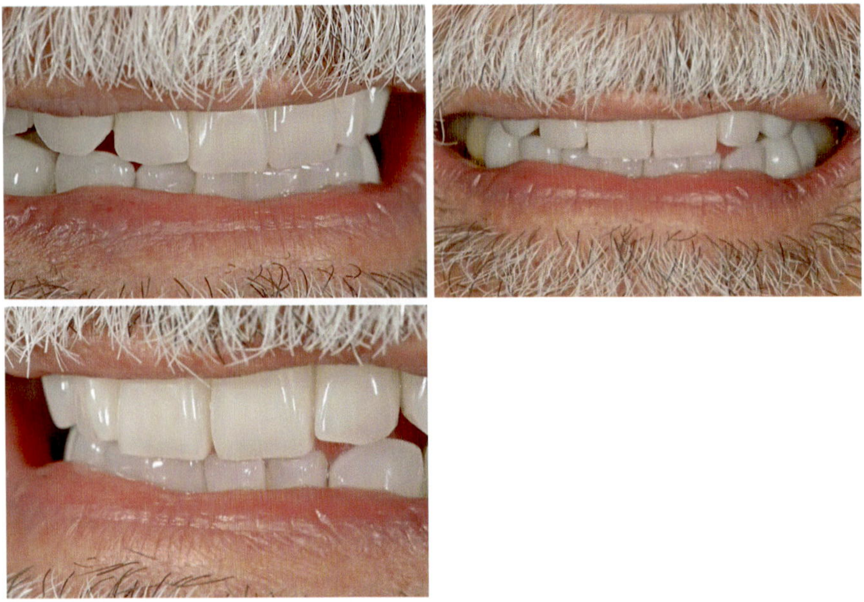

Fig. 18.59 Extra oral views taken the patient are satisfied

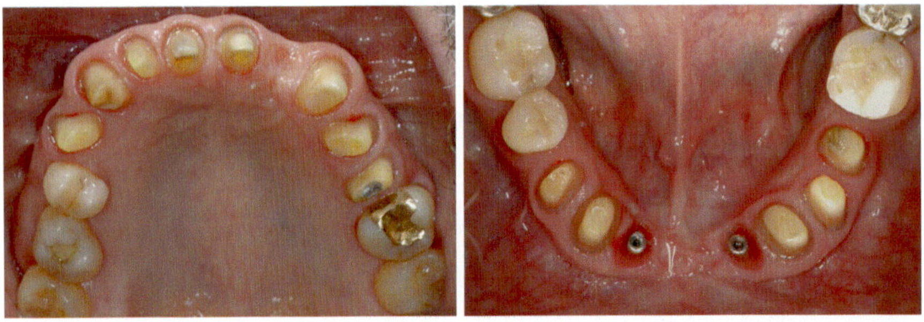

Fig. 18.60 The tooth preparations are visualized, the soft tissues are also in good health, the implants are well placed with well-formed submucosal contours

Fig. 18.61 Intra oral anterior view of definitive restorations in occlusion

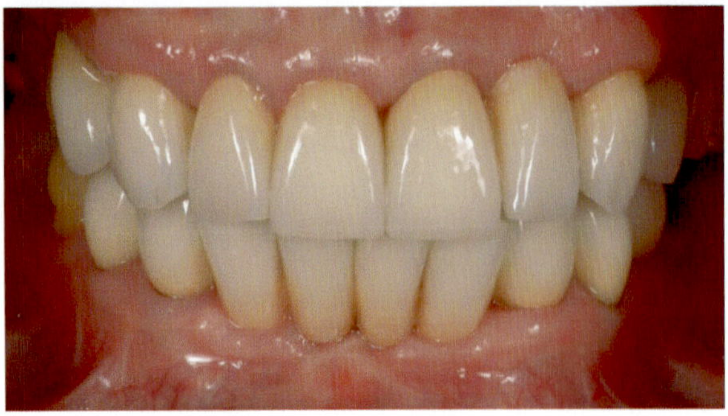

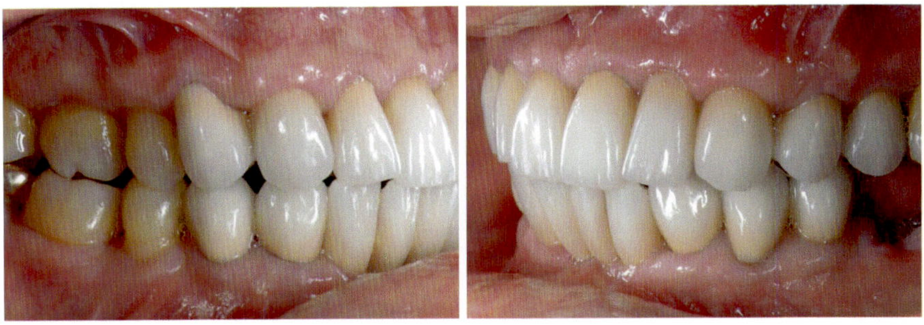

Fig. 18.62 Lateral views of restorations placed

Fig. 18.63 Intra oral view of teeth separated

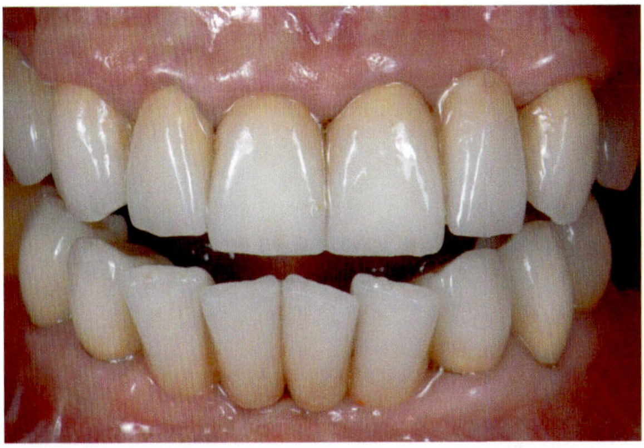

18.5 Patient 4

A 20-year-old male presented with trauma to his maxilla, he was hit with a baseball that caused his maxillary left central #9 and lateral #10 to become avulsed. The two teeth were re-inserted into their sockets after which both teeth had endodontic treatment.

After 3 years, the patient began orthodontic treatment, and the orthodontist was informed of the prior accident and warned the patient about the possibility of root resorption. Towards the end of treatment, radiographs showed external root resorption of both teeth with the severity of the resorption caused the central incisor to be removed. The lateral incisor had endodontic therapy to try stopping further resorption and the central incisor was extracted as the resorption was severe (Fig. 18.64). The tooth fragment was attached to the orthodontic wire as a provisional restoration (Fig. 18.65).

Figure 18.66 was another radiograph taken to evaluate any progression of the resorption on the distal portion of the lateral incisor at this time the resorption on the lateral did not progress.

An implant was placed after bone healing, and a healing cap was attached (Fig. 18.67). The definitive restoration was delivered, soft tissues appeared normal

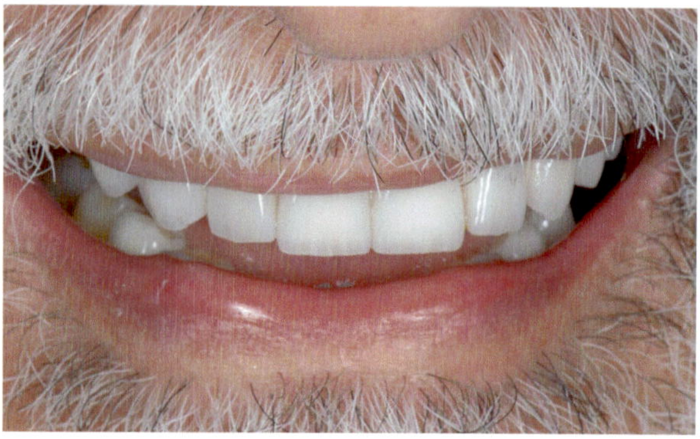

Fig. 18.64 Image of patient's smile

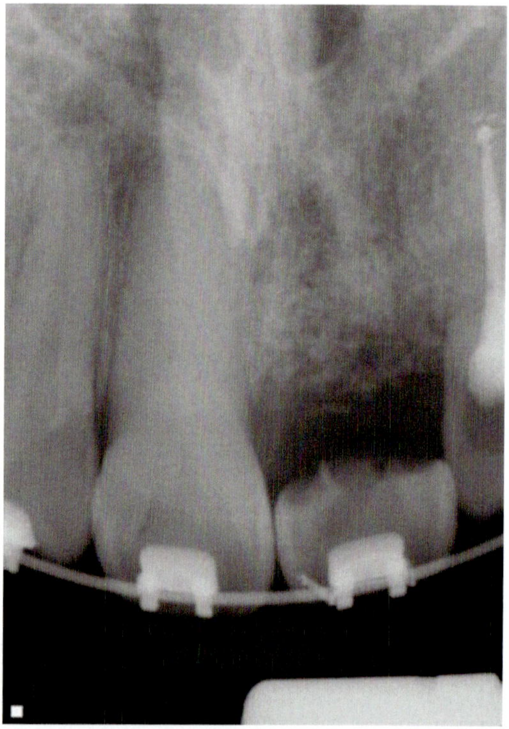

Fig. 18.65 Radiograph of tooth with root resorption is extracted

with no inflammation on the mucosal margin #9 or gingival margin #10, and the patient was satisfied with the outcome (Fig. 18.68).

Another 5 years later on a regular recall, visit the gingiva on the distal appeared inflamed, the area was explored with a periodontal probe, and the probe penetration clarified that the external root resorption progressed (Figs. 18.69, 18.70 and 18.71).

It was decided among the periodontist, orthodontist, and prosthodontist to erupt the lateral incisor at a rapid pace to have the resorptive lesion above the level of the bone, then had the tooth stabilized (Figs. 18.72, 18.73 and 18.74). The prosthodontist removed the existing restoration on the central incisor and delivered a

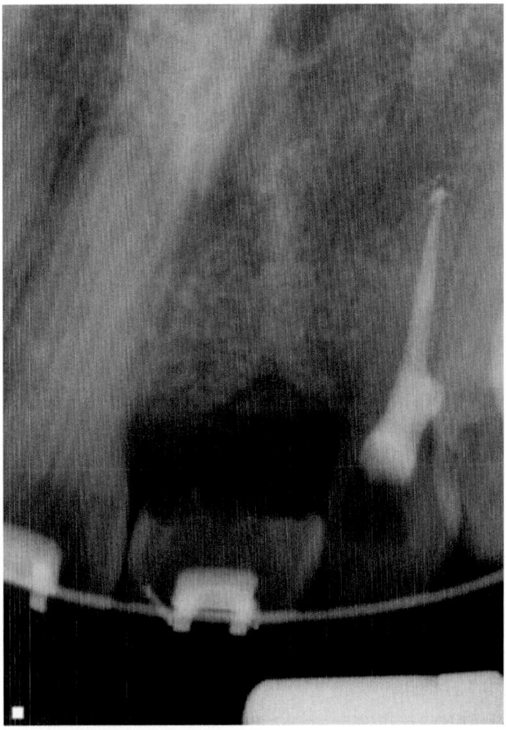

Fig. 18.66 Radiograph of lateral incisor adjacent to extraction site

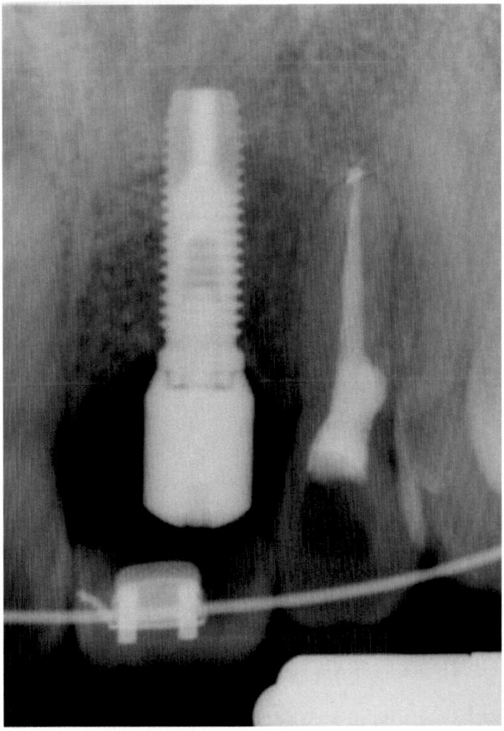

Fig. 18.67 Radiograph of implant in place of extracted central incisor note the lateral root is intact without progressing root resorption

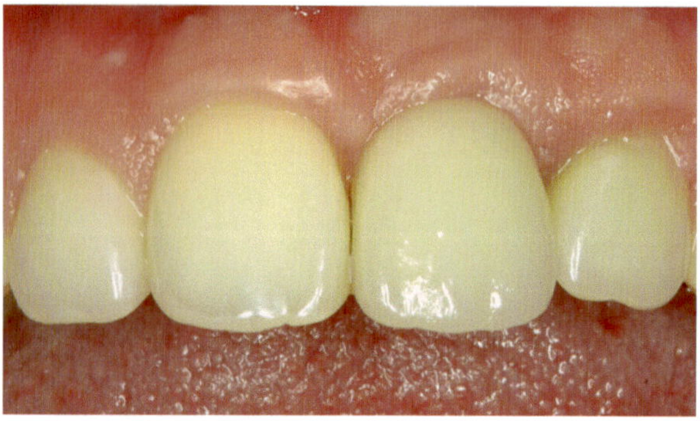

Fig. 18.68 The maxillary left central incisor definitive implant-supported restoration note the healthy gingival tissue around the left lateral incisor

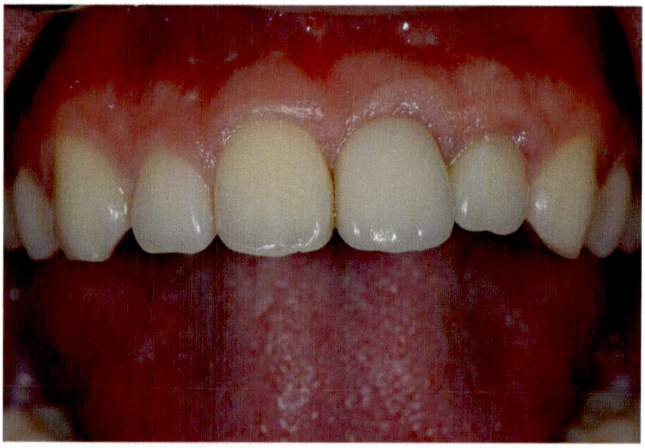

Fig. 18.69 The patient presents after 5 years and the tissues around the gingival margin and around the left lateral incisor appear inflamed especially in the distal area

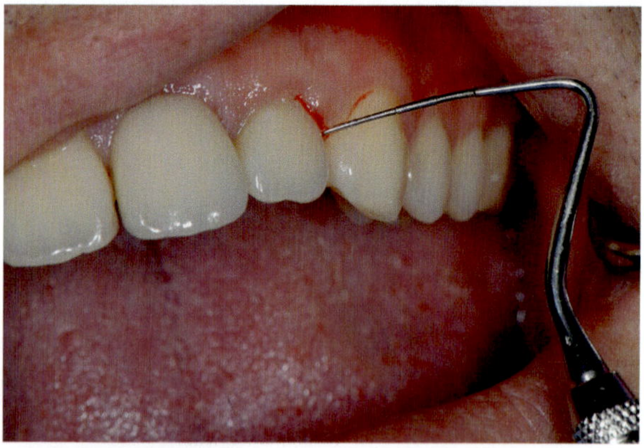

Fig. 18.70 A periodontal probe is place in the area, note the bleeding

provisional restoration with a pontic, the crown of the lateral was removed, and the resorptive lesion was visible, and the patient was sent to the periodontist (Fig. 18.75). The periodontist removed the provisional restoration, then cut the lateral root diagonally to remove the resorption lesion in the distal part of the root. The diagonal cut did not cause a flattened papilla between the lateral and canine as the papilla would

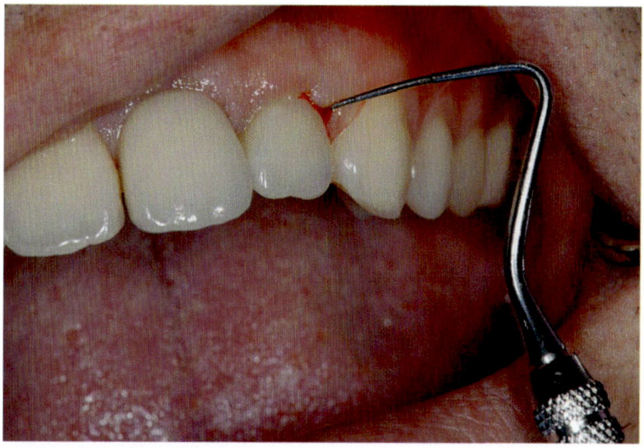

Fig. 18.71 The periodontal probe is inserted into the root—the root resorption has progressed over time

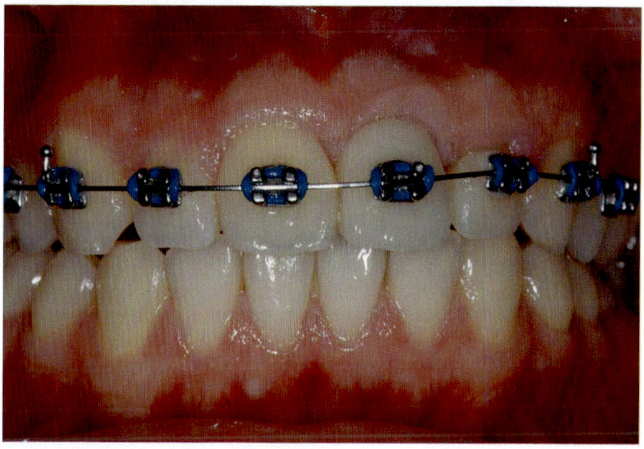

Fig. 18.72 The orthodontic brackets and wire are placed to rapidly erupt the left lateral incisor to have the resorption shifted above the bone

be maintained by the attachment level of the adjacent canine and similarly the mesial part of the lateral root would maintain the papilla between the central and lateral with the attachment level of the periodontium supporting the papilla (Figs. 18.76, 18.77 and 18.78).

The patient was sent back to the prosthodontist who recontoured the submucosal part of the pontic to support the soft tissue contours and have sufficient distance from the bone to have the mucosa covered over the root (Figs. 18.79 and 18.80).

The lateral root being banked, and the papilla between the central and lateral was maintained to have symmetry between the central and lateral papillae on the left and right (Fig. 18.81).

This is an example of interdisciplinary treatment that allows a good outcome when different skillsets are co-operative and understanding.

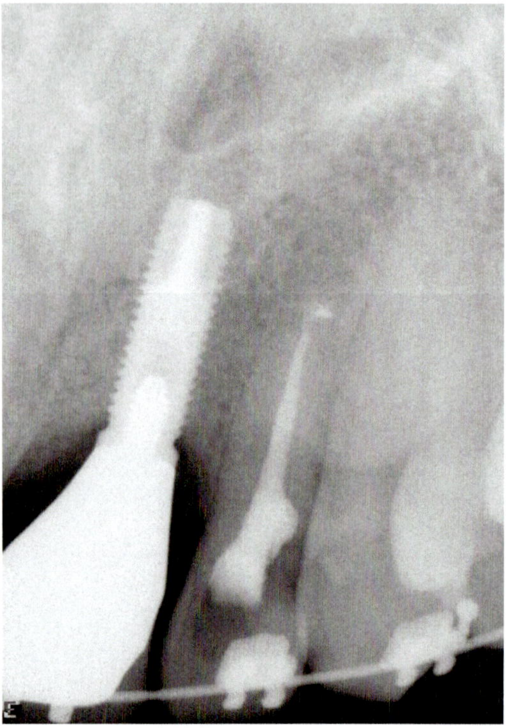

Fig. 18.73 Radiograph shows the distal resorption shifted coronally and above the bone

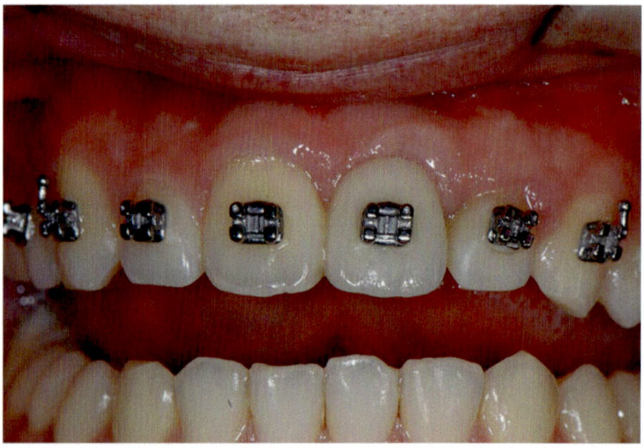

Fig. 18.74 The wire is removed after stabilizing the lateral incisor and ready to bank the tooth root

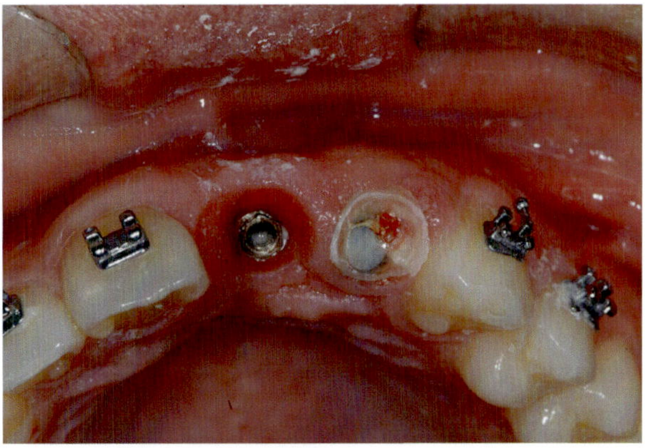

Fig. 18.75 The restoration on the central incisor is removed, the clinical crown of the lateral incisor is removed, note the resorption of the root is above the bone level, the provisional restoration will be delivered with the cantilevered pontic

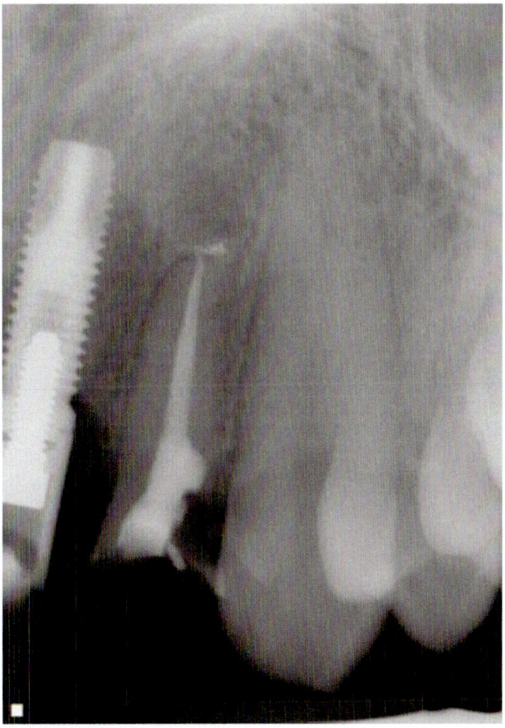

Fig. 18.76 Radiograph is ready to be cut diagonally to shift the root resorption above the bone

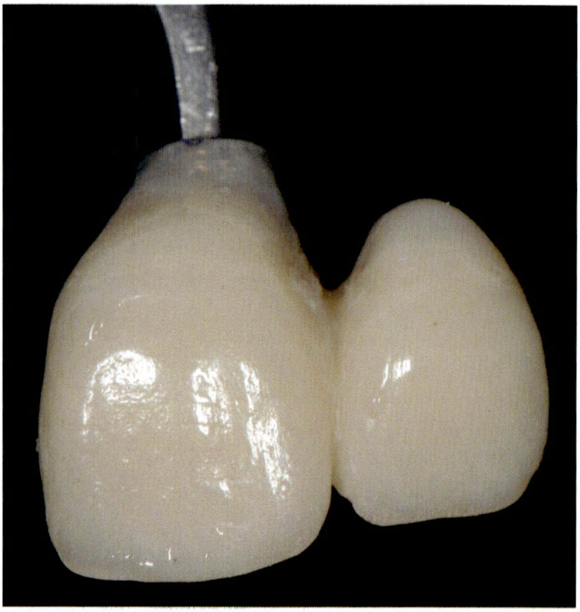

Fig. 18.77 The provisional with the lateral cantilevered, and the pontic apical end is shaped to emerge from the alveolus

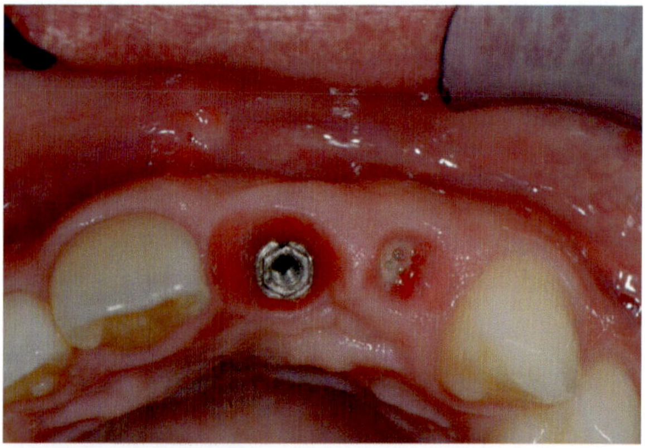

Fig. 18.78 Occlusal image of root cut at an angle to have mesial part of the root supporting the papilla between the central and lateral, the apical contour of the provisional restoration is adjusted to facilitate mucosal closure over the root

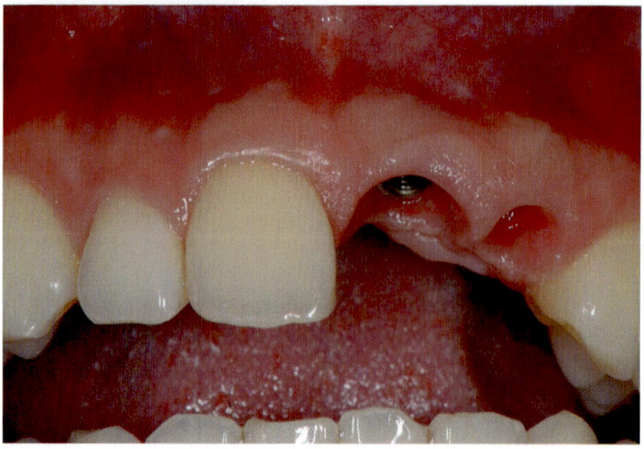

Fig. 18.79 Intraoral image of the restoration removed with submucosal contours of the implant and pontic with a well-developed papilla

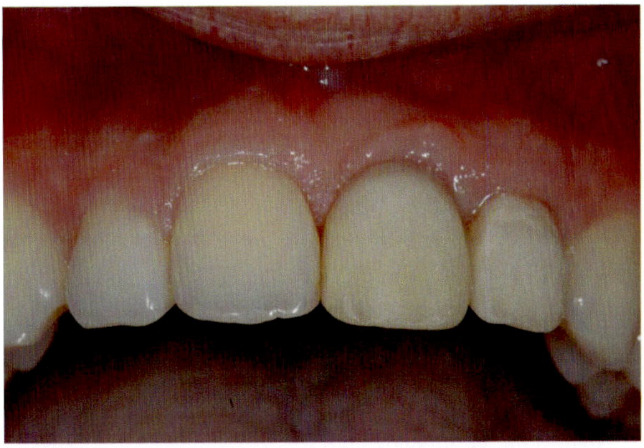

Fig. 18.80 Intra oral view of provisional restoration in place with adequate soft tissues around the implant supported restoration and pontic

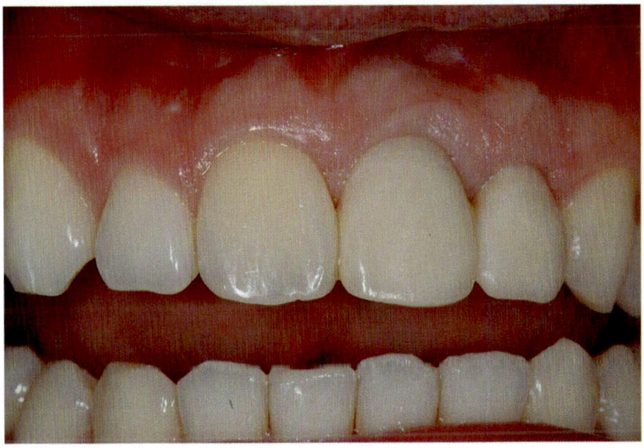

Fig. 18.81 Intra oral view of definitive restoration

18.6 Summary

This article illustrates the advantages of an interdisciplinary approach to the management of patients who require implant dentistry. Treatment planning must begin through visualization of the end result. By paying attention to details and systematically analysing each factor that affects the esthetic result, recognizing inadequacies in osseous and gingival contour, the restorative dentist can take advantage of the benefits of orthodontic and periodontal treatment to enhance the esthetic and functional outcomes. Without an interdisciplinary approach, final outcomes can be compromised. With a team approach to the management of patients who require implant dentistry treatment, fewer compromises will occur and more ideal restorations can be developed.

Acknowledgments Patient in case 1 was treated by Dr. Paolo Corrado D.D.S.
Patient in case 3 was treated by Dr. Anas Aloum D.D.S, FACP.

References

1. Rufenacht CR. Fundamentals of esthetics. Chicago, IL: Quintessence Publishing; 1990.
2. Phillips K, Kois JC. Aesthetic peri-implant site development. The restorative connection, vol. 42. Dent Clin North Am; 1998. p. 57–70.
3. Schincaglia GP, Nowzari H. Surgical treatment planning for the single-unit implant in aesthetic areas. Periodontology. 2000;27:162–82.
4. Roblee RD. Interdisciplinary dentofacial therapy. A comprehensive approach to optimal patient care. Chicago, IL: Quintessence Publishing; 1994. p. 17–43.
5. Smalley W, et al. Osseointegrated titanium implants for maxillofacial protraction in monkeys. Am J Orthod Dentofacial Orthop. 1988;94:285–95.
6. Douglas J, Killinay D. Dental implants used as orthodontic anchorage. J Oral Implantol. 1988;13:28–38.
7. Kokitch V. Managing complex orthodontic problems. The use of implants for anchorage. Semin Orthod. 1996;2:153–60.
8. Smalley WM. Implants for tooth movement. Determining implant location and orientation. J Esthet Dent. 1995;7:62–72.
9. Smalley WM. Implants for tooth movement. A fabrication and placement technique for provisional restorations. J Esthet Dent. 1995;7:150–4.

Implant Maintenance

19

Satish Kumar and Husain Mohammad

19.1 Peri-implant Health

The tissue surrounding dental implants comprising the soft tissue (peri-implant mucosa) and hard tissue (bone) components are referred to as the peri-implant tissues. The soft tissue creates the peri-implant mucosa which protects the underlying bone surrounding the implant. Osseointegration defined as "*a direct functional and structural connection between living bone and the surface of a load-carrying implant*" occurs following the placement of implant [4]. It is important to understand the differences in the peri-implant tissues compared to the periodontium around natural teeth. Peri-implant tissues, unlike natural teeth, lack cementum and periodontal ligament. Hence, inserting fibres from the connective tissue into the implant surface are not present. In addition, vascularization between the bone crest and the junctional epithelium is reduced. Peri-implant mucosa is about 3–4 mm high with 2 mm of epithelium [5]. The importance of this mucosa, especially keratinized mucosa, plays an important role in the maintenance of peri-implant health. It helps with plaque removal and patient comfort. In contrast, lack of or reduced keratinized tissue width could lead to plaque accumulation, tissue inflammation, mucosal recession, and marginal bone loss eventually leading to peri-implantitis [6].

The American Academy of Periodontology and the European Federation of Periodontology jointly published a series of reviews and consensus manuscripts including defining peri-implant health and peri-implant diseases in 2017 [2, 5, 7–10].

A diagnosis of peri-implant health is made when there is

S. Kumar (✉)
Professor & Director (Pre-Doctoral Director & Chair), Periodontics, Arizona School of Dentistry and Oral Health, A. T. Still University, Mesa, AZ, USA

H. Mohammad
Department of Periodontics, Ministry of Health, Kuwait, Kuwait

W. Chee, S. Jivraj (eds.), *Treatment Planning In Implant Dentistry*, BDJ Clinician's Guides, https://doi.org/10.1007/978-3-031-68726-6_19

- *Absence of clinical signs of inflammation.*
- *Absence of bleeding and/or suppuration on gentle probing.*
- *No increase in probing depth compared to previous examinations.*
- *Absence of bone loss beyond crestal bone level changes resulting from initial bone remodeling* [5].

A healthy peri-implant tissue is clinically identical to healthy periodontal tissue (Fig. 19.1). A main clinical point to note is that there are no range of healthy probing depths indicative of peri-implant health around dental implants. Probing depths are generally deeper at implant sites as it depends on the soft tissue height at the location of the implant. In addition, even in implants that have reduced bone support due to early bone loss, peri-implant health can be established and maintained [10].

The peri-implant health status should be assessed at each clinical examination. Experts recommend peri-implant probing to assess the presence of bleeding on probing and and to monitor changes in probing depth and in the mucosal margin level. They also advise the following:

1. *Baseline probing within 3 months of prosthesis delivery.*
2. *Re-probe at every clinical examination.*
3. *Use a probe with a 0.5-mm diameter tip and a light probing force (0.2 N).*
4. *Record peri-implant probing depths circumferentially (ideally at 6 sites) and bleeding on probing.*
5. *Assess and record the width of keratinized attached peri-implant mucosa.*

In addition, they recommend a baseline intra-oral radiograph be taken after the physiological remodeling occurs to record the marginal bone levels. At subsequent visits, if there is an increase in probing depth in conjunction with bleeding on probing or suppuration, they recommend an intra-oral radiograph to assess the marginal bone levels [10, 11].

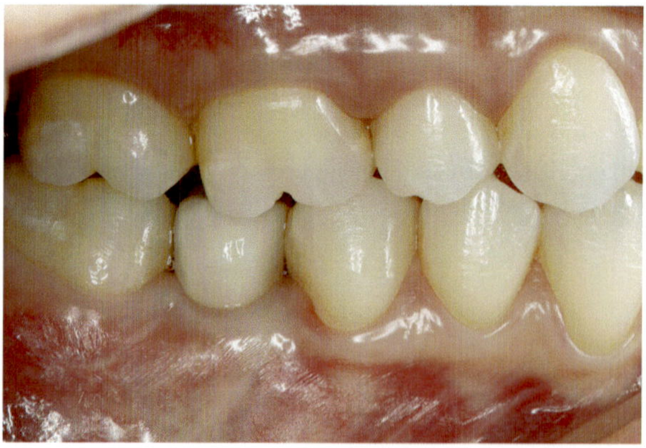

Fig. 19.1 Peri-implant health. Clinical photograph showing an implant in the position of mandibular right first molar demonstrating clinical signs of peri-implant health. Notice the thick band of keratinized tissue and absence of clinical signs of inflammation. There were also no signs of bleeding on probing, suppuration, and probing depths remained stable compared to previous clinical examinations

19.2 Peri-implant Diseases (Peri-implant Mucositis and Peri-implantitis)

Peri-implant diseases are primarily inflammatory conditions caused by peri-implant plaque biofilms. Two distinct peri-implant diseases that affect the peri-implant tissues are peri-implant mucositis and peri-implantitis [10, 11]. When the host–microbial homeostasis at the implant–mucosa interface is disturbed, it leads to peri-implant mucositis which is a reversible condition.

A diagnosis of peri-implant mucositis is made when there is

- *Presence of bleeding and/or suppuration on gentle probing with or without increased probing depth compared to previous examinations.*
- *Absence of bone loss beyond crestal bone level changes resulting from initial bone remodeling* [2].

A diagnosis of peri-implantitis is made when there is

1. *Presence of bleeding and/or suppuration on gentle probing.*
2. *Increased probing depth compared to previous examinations.*
3. *Presence of bone loss beyond crestal bone level changes resulting from initial bone remodeling* [7].

However, previous clinical and radiographic examination may not be available to make a diagnosis especially when implants have been placed by other clinicians. In these situations, the diagnosis of peri-implantitis is based on:

- *Presence of bleeding and/or suppuration on gentle probing.*
- *Probing depths of ≥6 mm.*
- *Bone levels ≥3 mm apical of the most coronal portion of the intraosseous part of the implant* [7].

The incidence of peri-implant mucositis has been estimated to be 70.8% [3]. The incidence of peri-implantitis has been estimated to be 37.5% [3]. In another study, the prevalence of peri-implantitis was estimated to be 19.53% and 12.53% at the patient level, and at the implant level, respectively [12]. The prevalence of peri-implant mucositis and peri-implantitis in patients rehabilitated with full-arch, implant-supported restorations was reported to be between 1.5% and 29.7% at the patient level and between 2.1% and 20.3% at the implant level [13]. Hence, there is a wide-ranging prevalence rates, mostly because of varying definitions. In addition, an alternate view that challenges the microbial etiology has contributed to the differing prevalence rates. Bone remodeling around dental implants being influenced by the immune system and also immune rejection causing progressive bone loss is the alternate view which attributes minimal role to the biofilms [14, 15].

There are several risk factors that have been identified to be associated with peri-implant diseases. They include medical conditions such as diabetes, age-related cognitive decline and loss of dexterity, medications such as immunosuppressants and antiresorptive therapy, lack of oral hygiene, previous history of periodontitis, existing periodontal disease, and smoking [16–18]. Clinicians should not only educate the patients about these risk factors but should take measures to mitigate these risk factors to prevent implant complications. When patients are educated that periodontal disease and poor oral hygiene affect the implants, they would be willing to follow implant maintenance protocols including maintaining good oral hygiene. In the case of smoking, >10 cigarettes/day smokers have been reported to have a higher incidence of marginal bone loss than those patients who smoked <10 cigarettes/day. Clinicians should use this fact to discuss deleterious effect of smoking on wound healing and implant failure with the patient and encourage patients to consider quitting smoking or consider enrolling in smoking cessation program [19]. With growing ageing population and increase in life expectancy, age-related cognitive decline and associated loss of dexterity would affect oral health. Personalized oral hygiene instructions and aids should be considered for these patients to maintain peri-implant health. With reported unsatisfactory compliance with the supportive periodontal and peri-implant maintenance therapy, clinicians should educate and motivate patients to follow oral hygiene at-home as well as keep up with the dental appointments [20]. Prosthetic factors such as presence of submucosal cement and surgical factors such as malpositioning of implants preventing oral hygiene may increase the risk of peri-implant diseases [10]. However, it should be noted that there is currently no evidence that occlusal overload is a risk factor for peri-implantitis [7].

To reduce the risk of prosthetic factors, treatment planning for three-dimensional implant positioning is recommended to ensure certain conditions:

- *Adequate buccal and lingual bone thickness to allow the implant to be placed in a prosthetically guided position with good primary stability and surrounded circumferentially by bone.*
- *Adequate mesio-distal distance between an implant and adjacent tooth or implant to allow adequate space for prosthetic components and access for oral hygiene aids.*
- *Appropriate apical-coronal position of the implant platform (shoulder) to allow adequate space for prosthetic components and to avoid an excessively deep mucosal sulcus ("tunnel")* [11].

In addition, prosthetic treatment planning is recommended to facilitate optimal plaque control around implants and to prevent peri-implant diseases as follows:

- *Good access for oral hygiene aids used by the patient to remove plaque.*
- *Good access for professional monitoring (peri-implant probing) and professional mechanical plaque removal.*
- *A prosthesis contour with a favourable emergence angle and profile to facilitate optimal plaque control* [11].

19.3 Peri-implant Hard and Soft Tissue Deficiencies

Long-term peri-implant health and stability rely on healthy hard and soft tissue around the implants. During treatment planning for implants, deficient hard tissue and soft tissue should be addressed before or during implant placement surgery with bone augmentation surgeries (Figs. 19.2 and 19.3). Adequate bone volume allows accurate placement of implants in the ideal restorative position which in turn leads to long-term success of the implant and prosthesis [7].

When implants are placed in sites with thin buccal bone and/or lack of keratinized tissue, this could lead to recession of the peri-implant mucosa (Fig. 19.4). At times, malpositioning of implant leads to the same unfavourable outcome and implant removal and further management may be necessary (Fig. 19.5). Receded gingival tissue could favour plaque accumulation and initiate peri-implant inflammation. If implants are deemed functional with no major prosthetic issues, soft tissue augmentation procedures such as free gingival graft, connective tissue graft, or allografts and xenografts tissue can be used to improve the peri-implant recession [21]. Autogenous grafts such as free gingival grafts and connective tissue grafts are usually more effective in gaining keratinized tissue width compared to soft tissue substitutes. However, to avoid a second surgical site of donor tissue, soft tissue substitutes could be used as an alternative to enhance peri-implant soft tissue coverage [22, 23].

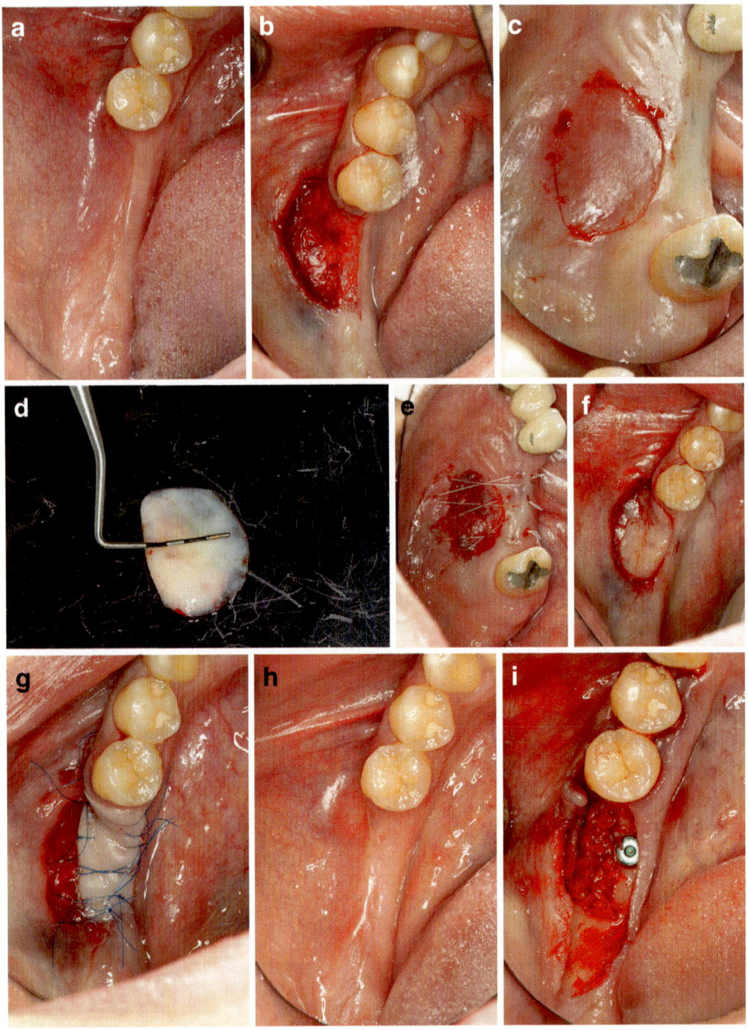

Fig. 19.2 Peri-implant soft tissue (free gingival graft) and hard tissue augmentation. (**a**) Mandibular left posterior edentulous region planned for implant placement showing lack of keratinized attached tissue on the buccal side as well as deficient hard tissue. This indicates that the future implants placed in the site would be at risk for peri-implant diseases. (**b**) Free gingival graft is planned for the site before implant placement. The graft recipient site is prepared by partial thickness flap. (**c**) Donor site is hard palate. The required size of graft is measured, and incision is made according to the measurement. (**d**) Harvested free gingiva graft. (**e**) Donor site is sutured well, and haemostasis is achieved. (**f**) Harvested graft is placed in the recipient site. (**g**) Multiple sutures including periosteal sutures placed to secure the graft in site. (**h**) Healed site showing increased keratinized width. (**i**) Implant is placed in the mandibular left first molar site along with and particulate bone on the buccal side to augment the hard tissue portion surrounding the implant. (**j**) Flap reflected to place healing abutment on the implant. Note the augmented bone well healed and surrounding the implant. (**k**) Soft tissue closure with sutures around the healing apartment. Note the thick band of keratinized tissue surrounding the implant. (**l**) Periapical radiograph showing the implant placed in position with healing abutment. (**m**) Clinical photograph showing the final restoration. (**n**) Periapical radiograph showing the implant with the final restoration

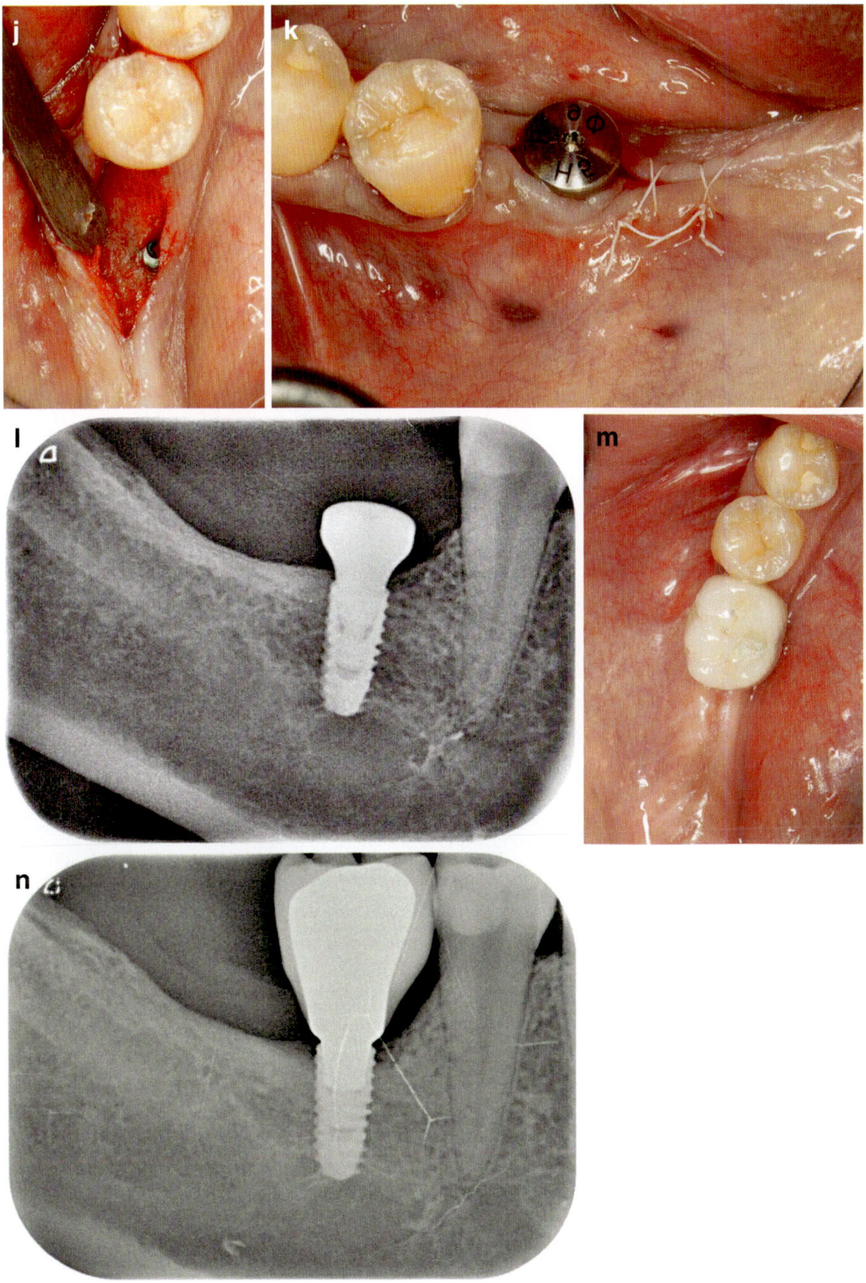

Fig. 19.2 (continued)

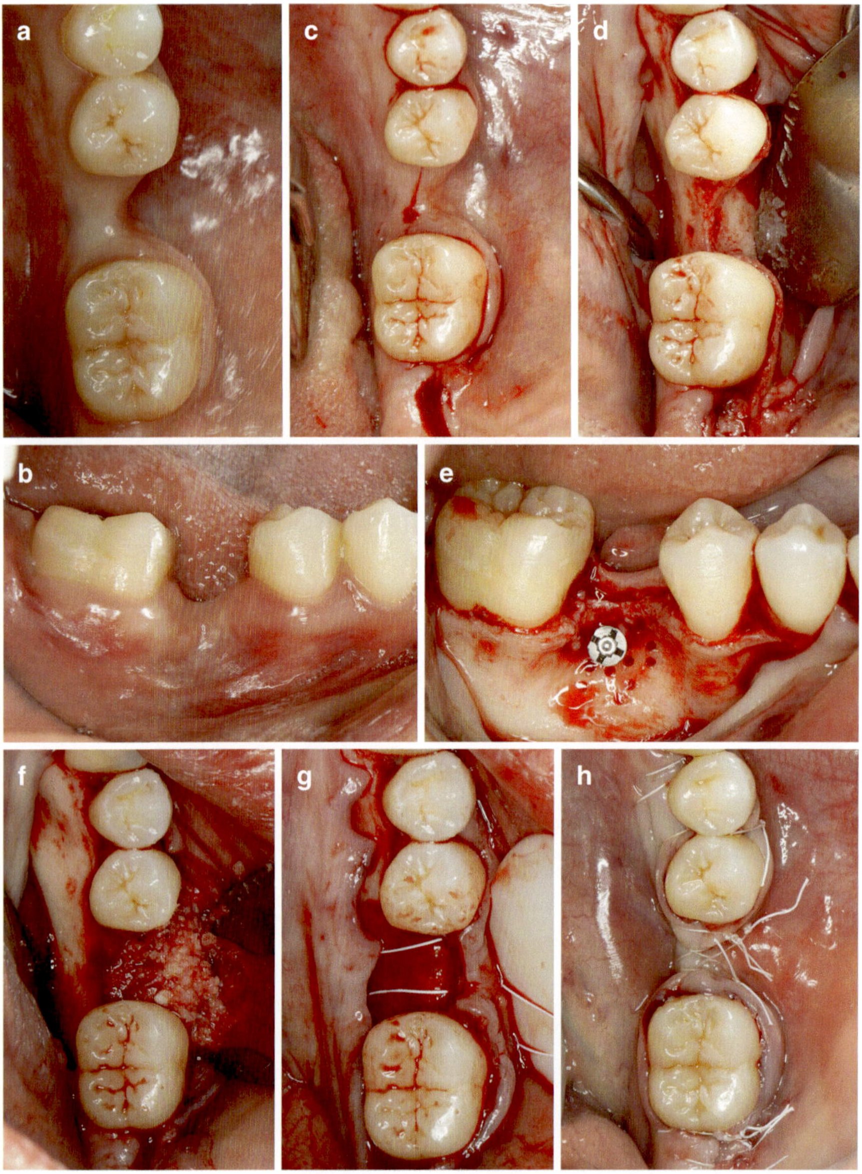
a
c
d
b
e
f
g
h

Fig. 19.3 Peri-implant soft tissue (connective tissue graft) and hard tissue augmentation. (**a**) Clinical photograph showing the occlusal view of the significant hard tissue deficiency in the area of mandibular right first molar region treatment planned for implant placement. (**b**) Buccal view of the same defect. Notice the limited keratinized tissue in the buccal aspect. (**c**) Hard tissue augmentation using guided bone regeneration technique is treatment planned for this region. A crestal incision is made in the surgical site. (**d**) Full thickness flap in the region reveals the deficient buccal bone. (**e**) A tenting screw is placed for support along with several corticotomies made to increase vascular supply for the bone to be grafted. (**f**) Allograft and resorbable barrier membrane are placed. (**g**) Periosteal sutures placed to stabilize the bone graft in place. (**h**) Primary closure is obtained with multiple sutures. (**i**) Re-entry into the area after 8 months shows bone graft has healed well. (**j**) Dental implant is placed within the alveolar housing including the regenerated bone. However, the buccal bone is still deficient and may not be adequate to maintain peri-implant health long term. (**k**) A barrier membrane is placed to support bone allograft. (**l**) Allograft bone is placed to augment the buccal bone. (**m**) Primary closure is obtained with multiple sutures. (**n**) Re-entry into the area after 4 months with a crestal incision. Soft tissue augmentation with connective tissue graft is also planned at the time of second-stage surgery. (**o**) Dental implant has osseointegrated well, and the augmented bone has healed well. (**p**) Connective tissue graft is harvested from maxillary tuberosity region. (**q**) Clinical photo of the harvested connective tissue graft. (**r**) Connective tissue graft is secured on the buccal aspect of the flap after placement of the healing abutment. (**s**) Connective tissue graft is secured under the flap with multiple sutures. (**t**) After 4 weeks, buccal view shows that the connective tissue graft has healed well. (**u**) Lingual view shows the presence of healthy tissue as well. (**v**) Occlusal view shows the implant in ideal position with adequate, healthy hard and soft tissue surrounding the implant. (**w**) Buccal view after 19 months post restoration and loading of the implant. Notice the thick band of keratinized tissue. (**x**) Lingual view showing healthy tissue surrounding the implant. (**y**) Occlusal view showing the restored implant in ideal position with adequate, healthy hard and soft tissue surrounding the implant. (**z**) Periapical radiograph showing healthy crestal bone around the implant

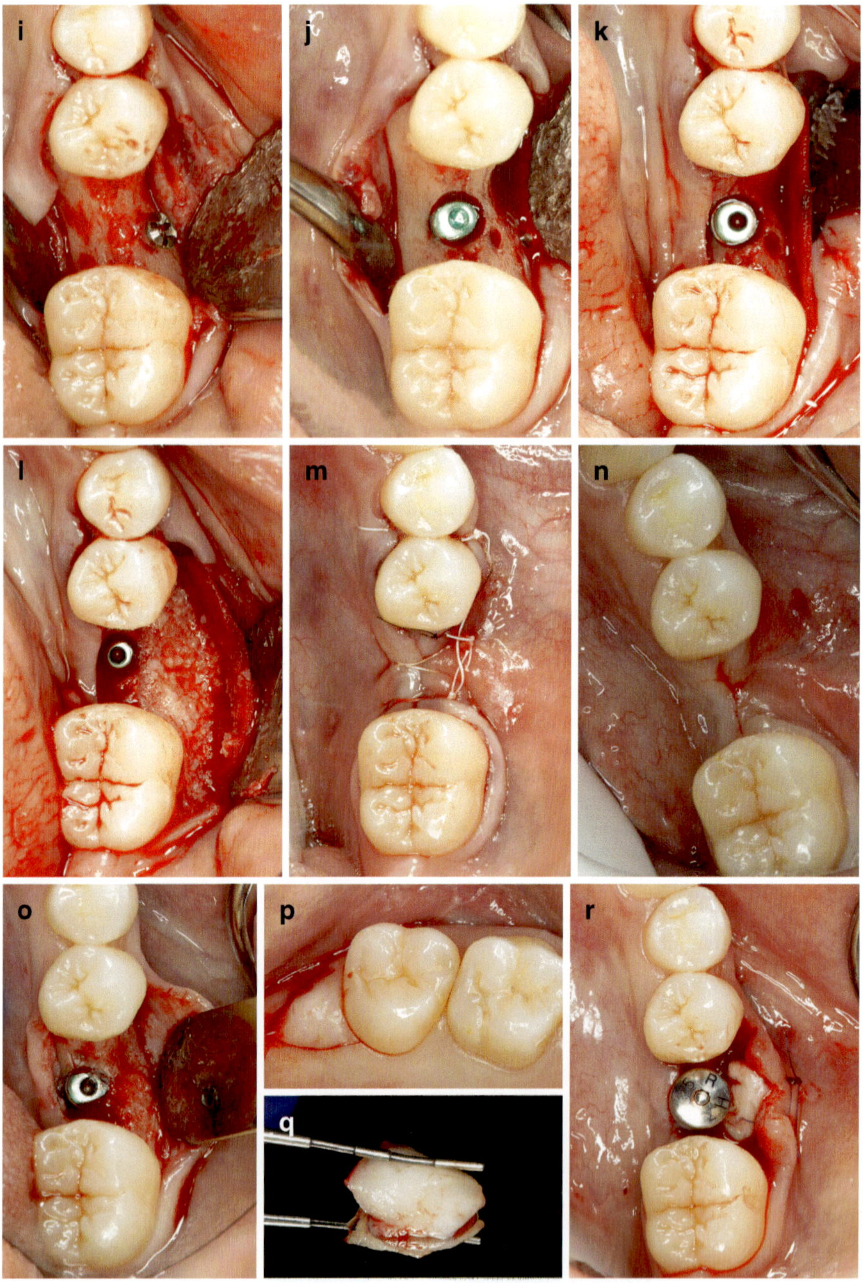

Fig. 19.3 (continued)

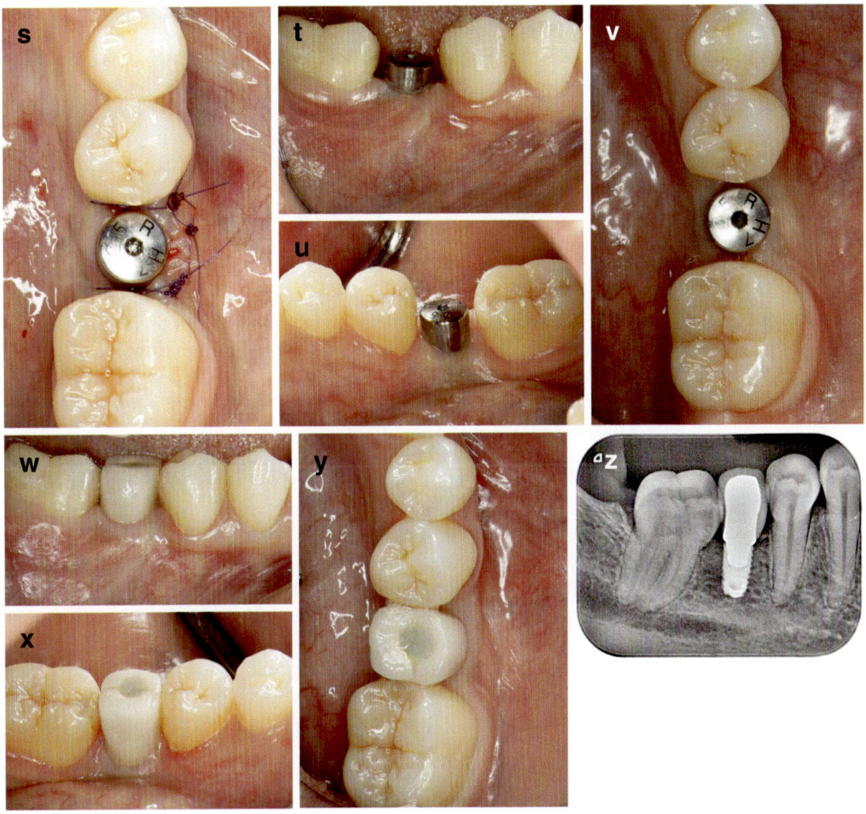

Fig. 19.3 (continued)

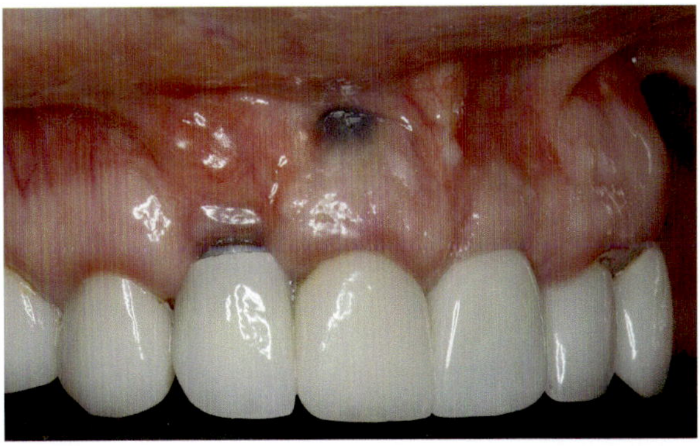

Fig. 19.4 Peri-implant recession. Clinical photograph showing peri-implant recession in the implant placed at the maxillary right lateral incisor site. Also, note the lack of adequate keratinized tissue on the facial surface of the implant. This is a complication usually occurring from malpositioning the implant in buccal position

Fig. 19.5 Implant malposition and management. (**a**) CBCT showing the implant in maxillary right second premolar position positioned entirely outside the alveolar housing buccally. An implant was also in place in maxillary right first molar position. The patient had not followed up for more than 2 years after implant placement for restoration of these two implants. Maxillary right second molar tooth had mesially drifted significantly making restoring of implant in the maxillary right first molar position impossible. A decision was made to extract the maxillary right second molar after management of malpositioned implant in maxillary right second premolar position. (**b**) Clinical photograph showing the edentulous space in the maxillary right posterior quadrant what two implants in place under the healed soft tissue. (**c**) After flap reflection, the implant in the maxillary right second premolar position is noted to be entirely outside the alveolar housing buccally. Also note the appropriately placed implant in the maxillary right first molar position along with the mesial drift of maxillary right second molar tooth. (**d**) The malpositioned implant in the maxillary right second premolar position is surgically removed. (**e**) The defect from the removal of the implant is managed with guided bone regeneration. A tenting screw is placed initially. (**f**) A barrier membrane is placed with a membrane tack. (**g**) Allograft bone is placed under the membrane covering the defect. (**h**) Primary closure is obtained with multiple sutures. (**i**) The surgical site is well healed. (**j**) With the flap reflected for implant placement, the regenerated bone is clearly visible. (**k**) The tenting screw and membrane tack are removed. (**l**) A new implant is placed in the maxillary right second premolar site. (**m**) Primary closure is obtained using multiple sutures. (**n**) Periapical radiograph showing placement of implant in the maxillary right second premolar site. (**o**) Clinical image with final restoration in place after 1 year—buccal view; (**p**) palatal view; (**q**) occlusal view. (**r**) Periapical radiograph with final restoration in place after 1 year. Note the maxillary right second molar had been extracted and site has healed completely. (**s**) Bitewing radiograph with final restoration in place after 1 year. (**t**) Clinical image with final restoration in place after 4 years—buccal view; (**u**) palatal view; (**v**) occlusal view. (**w**) Periapical radiograph with final restoration in place after 4 years. (**x**) Bitewing radiograph with final restoration in place after 4 years

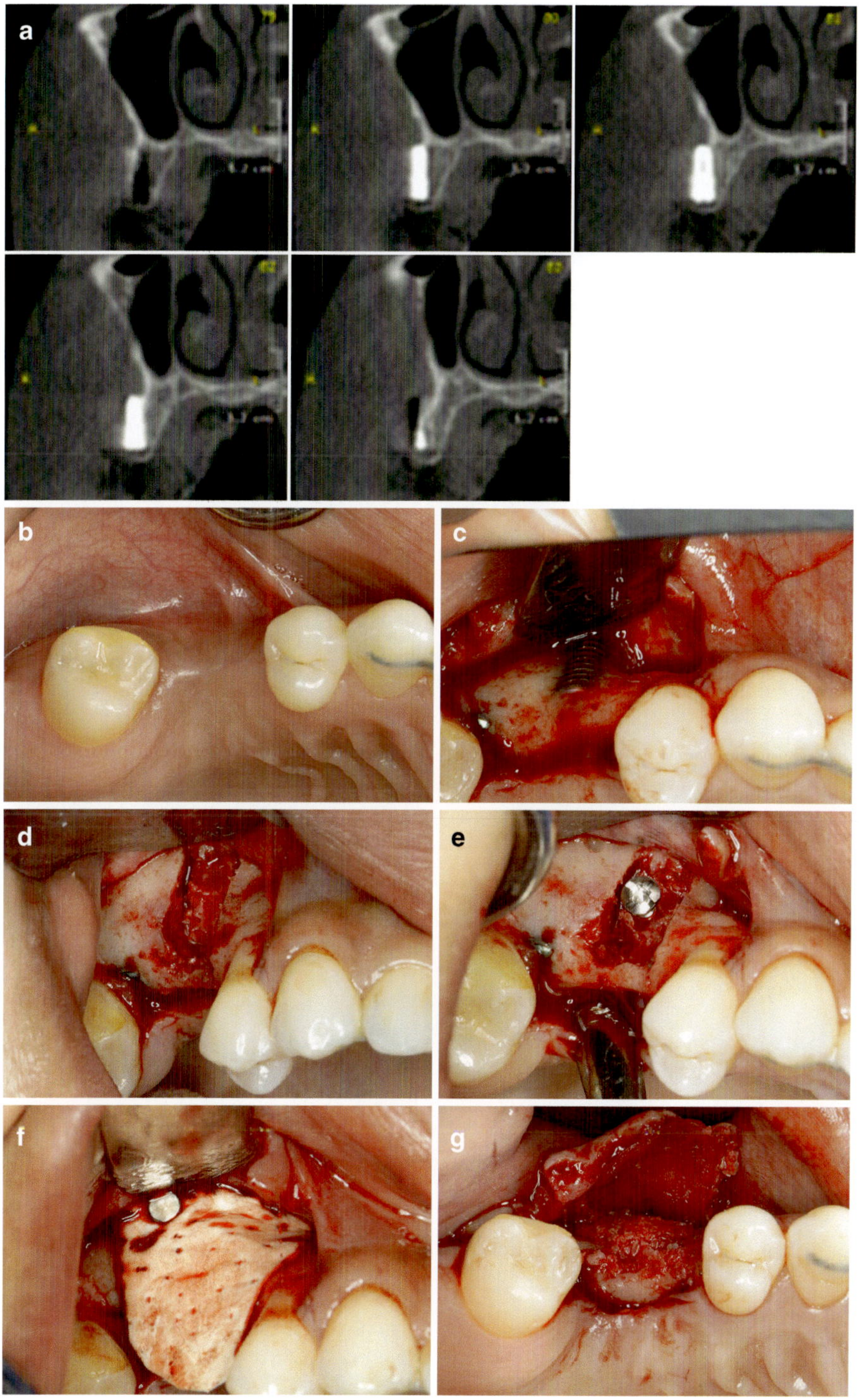

(continued)

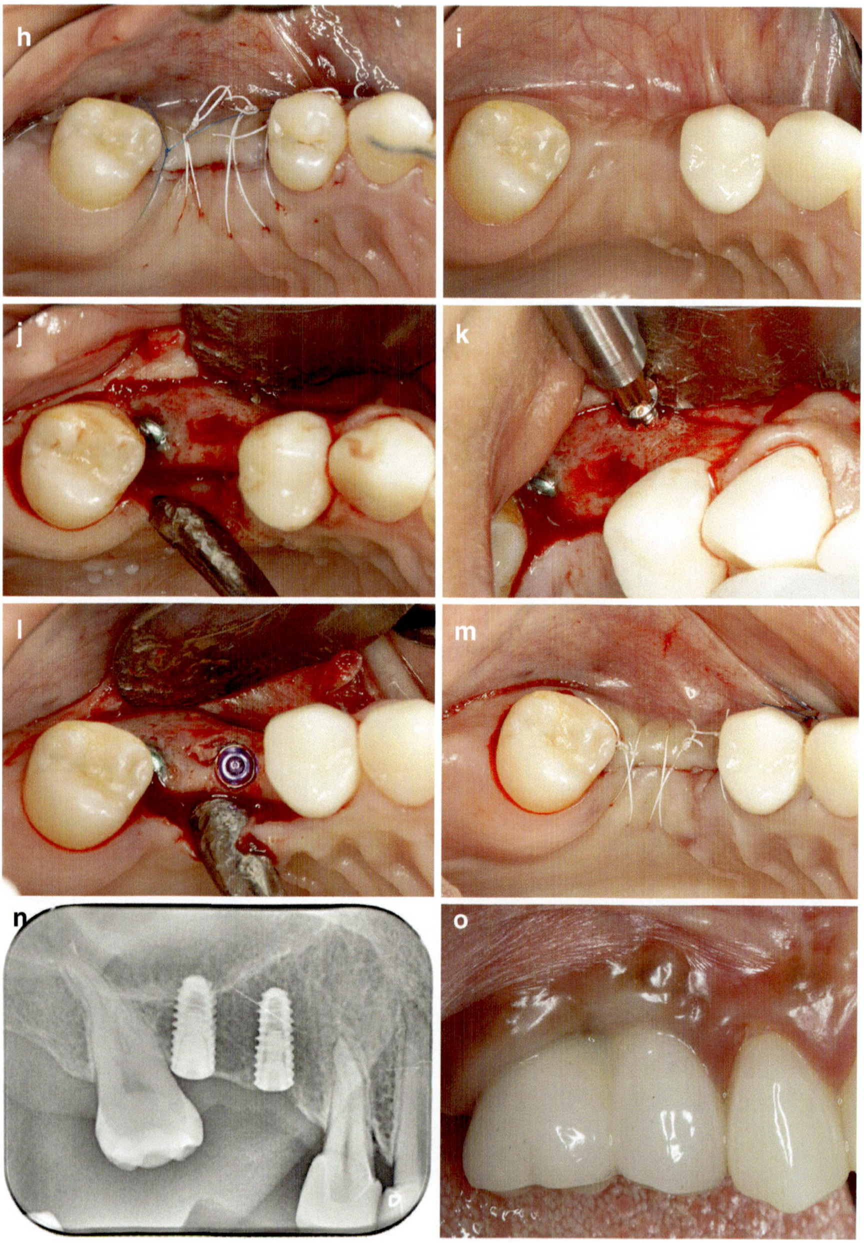

Fig. 19.5 (continued)

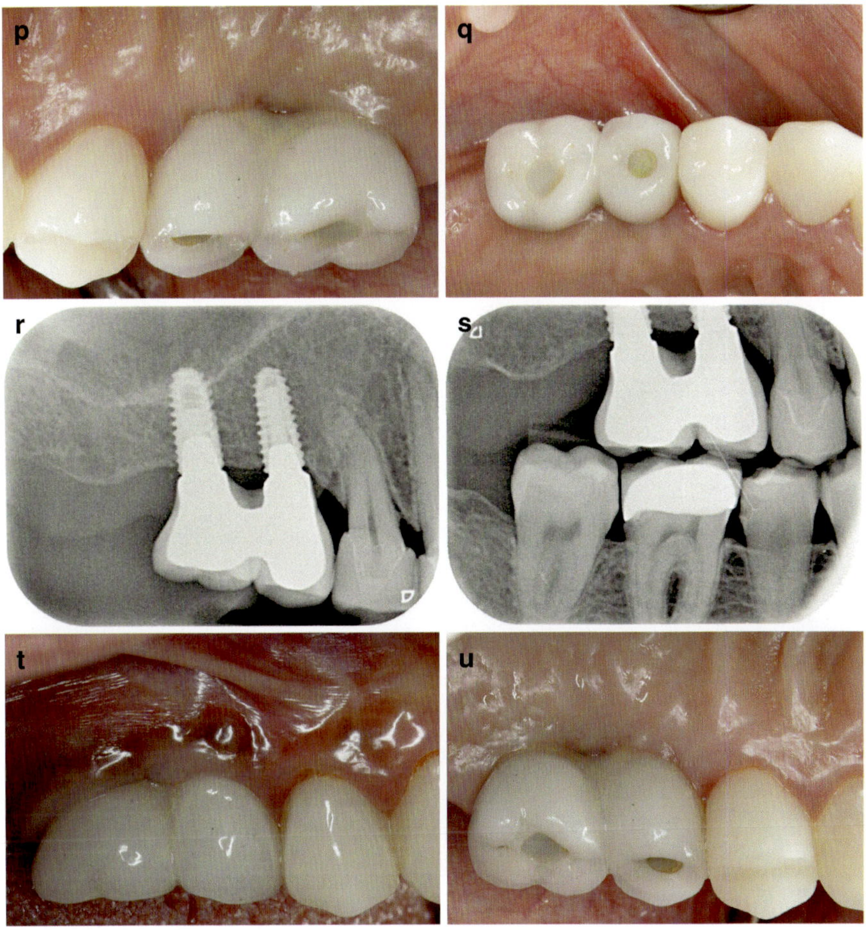

Fig. 19.5 (continued)

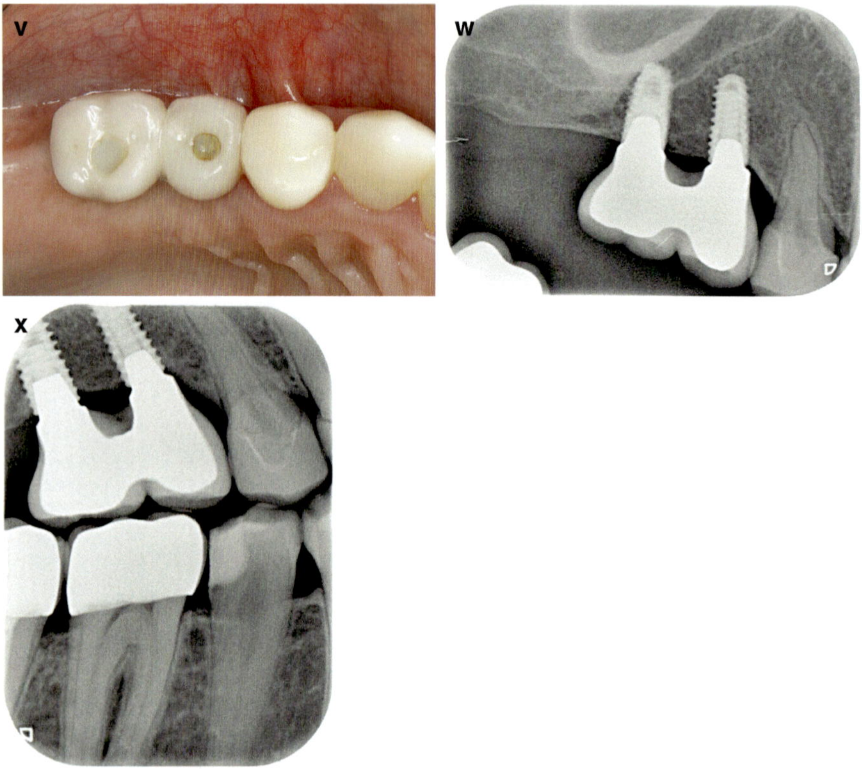

Fig. 19.5 (continued)

19.4 Supportive Periodontal and Peri-implant Therapy

Supportive peri-implant therapy improves peri-implant health and hence survival rate and reduced incidence of peri-implantitis and peri-implant mucositis [24]. In addition, in patients receiving supportive peri-implant therapy compared to those who did not, peri-implant marginal bone loss is significantly reduced [25]. This is because regular maintenance of implants will facilitate early detection of peri-implant complications and help with early intervention. Peri-implant diseases are best prevented than managed. Prevention starts from identifying population who are planned to receive dental implants but have risk factors such as poor oral hygiene. They are then targeted for risk factor avoidance and health behaviour adoption such as good oral hygiene. This is referred to as *primordial prevention*. Other behaviour or interventions to reduce peri-implant diseases in patients awaiting dental implant placement include:

- *Educating the patient about the importance of their adherence to supportive peri-implant care visits and home care.*
- *Improving glycemic control in diabetic patients.*
- *Smoking cessation (including e-cigarettes) or reducing smoking habit.*

- *Participation in regular supportive periodontal care programs.*
- *Improving oral hygiene.*
- *Reducing bruxing and/or parafunctional habits.*
- *Periodontal therapy to eliminate gingival inflammation and achieve periodontal stability* [11].

In patients who have dental implants with healthy per-implant tissue but also have risk factors, preventive measures should be directed towards control of risk factors. Advising personalized oral hygiene measures around implant-supported restoration is an example. This is referred to as *primary prevention.* In patients who already have peri-implant diseases, prevention of recurrence is key with regular peri-implant supportive care. This is referred to as *secondary prevention.* At times, peri-implant disease becomes chronic, and implant is still in function. Preventive measures to slow down the disease progression and complications and to avoid implant loss are referred to as *tertiary prevention* [26].

The success of primary prevention of peri-implantitis is dependent on regular supportive periodontal care. This includes professional supra- and sub-marginal plaque biofilm removal, oral hygiene motivation and coaching, and early detection of peri-implant pathological conditions and prosthetic issues [11]. For example, in diabetes patients receiving dental implant therapy, management of diabetes and glycemic control is essential for primary prevention of peri-implantitis. In patients with minimal to no keratinized mucosa around dental implants, increasing the peri-implant keratinized mucosa would aid in maintaining peri-implant health [26].

The appropriate protocol for supportive peri-implant care provision includes the following:

- *Interview (medical, social and oral history update, risk assessment, patient feedback).*
- *Assessment of oral, including peri-implant tissue health, prosthetic components, and patient competence, to undertake oral hygiene.*
- *Reinforce risk factor control such as smoking, oral dryness, glycemic control.*
- *Professional intervention: individualized oral healthcare plan, including oral hygiene coaching, professional mechanical plaque removal (PMPR) to include entire dentition/implants.*
- *Determination of next recall interval tailored according to patient-, implant- and restoration-based risk factors* [11, 26, 27].

Mechanical/physical sub-marginal instrumentation performed by clinicians along with home care by patients remains the mainstay of supportive periodontal and peri-implant care. These are typically performed using titanium or stainless-steel curettes, ultrasonics or sonic instruments, rubber cups, brushes, air-polishing devices with glycine powder, or erythritol alone or in combination (Fig. 19.6) [27]. Scalers made with plastic or nylon tips with the intention to prevent damage to abutment surfaces are usually ineffective [28]. Other methods include using lasers, but their benefits have not been distinctly demonstrated [29, 30]. Home care aids include oral irrigator devices, interdental brushes, and floss threaders which reduce peri-implant mucosal inflammation and mechanical biofilm control (Fig. 19.7) [31]. In

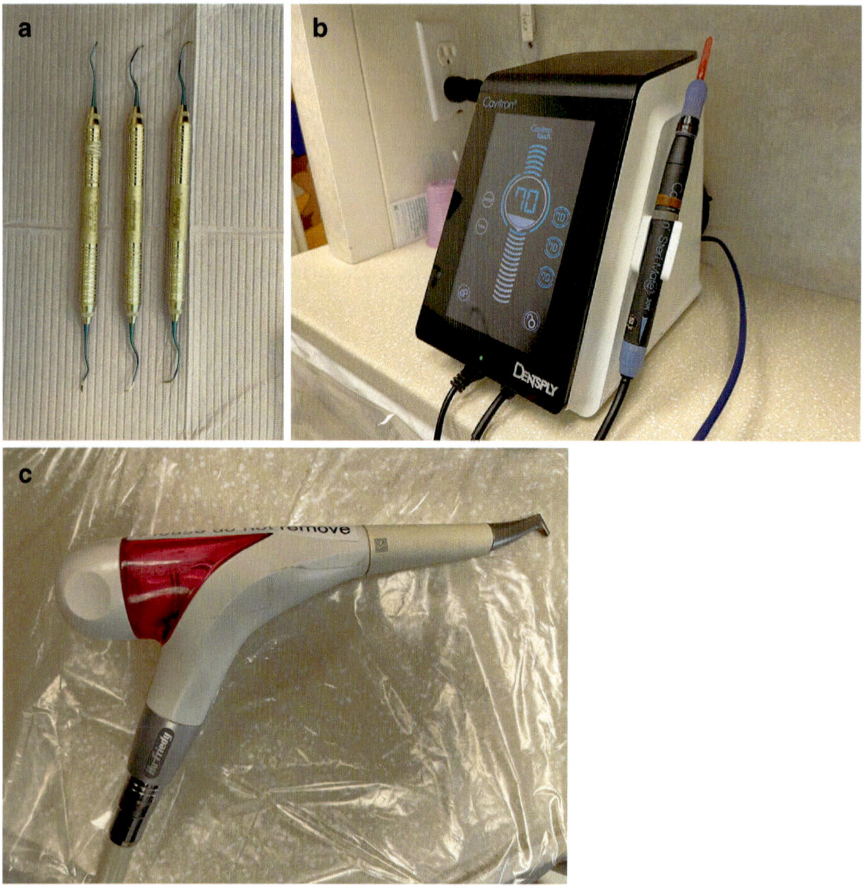

Fig. 19.6 Professional devices for implant maintenance. (**a**) Titanium curettes. (**b**) Ultrasonic device. (**c**) Airflow device

addition, systemically administered probiotics and antibiotics, and antiseptic mouth rinses, have been shown to reduce biofilms and provide clinically beneficial effect for up to 3 months when used as an adjunct to sub-marginal instrumentation [31]. However, adjunctive application of antimicrobial photodynamic therapy (aPDT), 0.95% NaOCl (sodium hypochlorite), or 0.12% CHX (chlorhexidine) has not been shown to improve bleeding on probing and/or probing depths compared to sub-marginal instrumentation alone [32]. Some studies have shown that adjunctive use of chlorhexidine may provide short-term benefits in reducing the inflammation when used with mechanical debridement. However, chlorhexidine is not recommended for long-term use as it could cause discoloration and taste disturbances. In patients with dry mouth, over-the-counter mouth rinses without alcohol is recommended [33]. With rising antibiotic resistance, clinicians should use clinical judgement and prescribe antibiotics and antiseptics only when the benefits clearly outweigh the risk of antibiotic resistance [31].

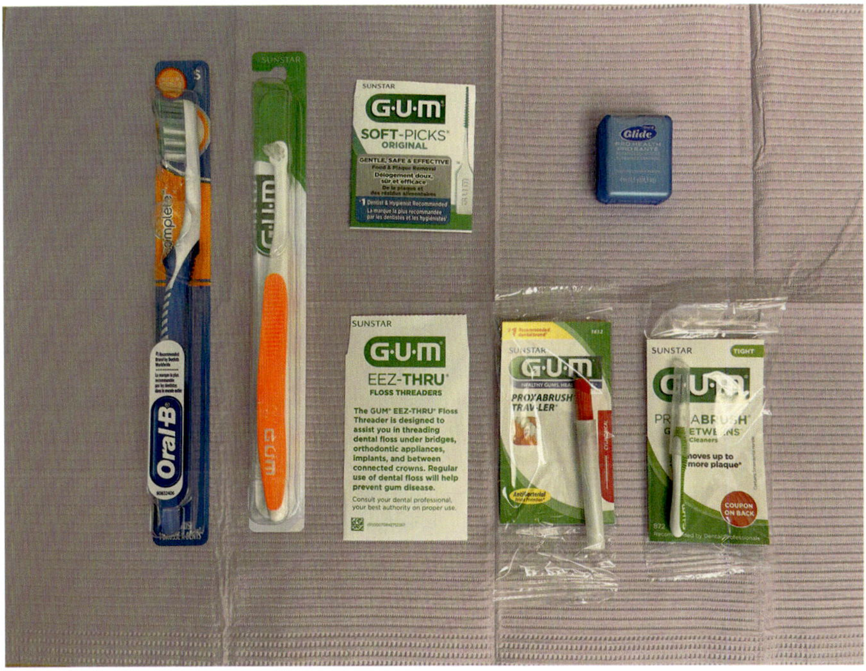

Fig. 19.7 Home care—oral hygiene aids. Toothbrush, interdental brushes, floss, and floss threaders

If patients with peri-implant mucositis do not return to peri-implant health status within 3 months, professional mechanical plaque removal along with oral hygiene instructions should be provided. With a lack of evidence on the efficacy of recall intervals, expert consensus and reviews have mostly recommended recall intervals between 3 and 6 months as a lifelong regimen [34]. The recall maintenance frequency of every 3–6 months should be adjusted to suit the risk factor profile of the patient such as oral hygiene compliance and cleansability of the prosthesis [29]. During the maintenance visits of patients with peri-implant diseases, it is recommended to clean or remove or modify the prosthesis where the implant-supported prosthesis does not allow for proper self-performed and/or professional cleansability [11, 35].

In patients with peri-implantitis, the first line of treatment to consider would be to retain a functional implant/prosthesis. Non-surgical therapy is usually attempted first to reduce inflammation followed by supportive peri-implant care and re-evaluation. If anticipated outcomes are not achieved, surgical therapy is provided [30, 36, 37].

As part of the non-surgical step of peri-implantitis, the following steps are recommended [30, 36, 37]:

- *Oral hygiene instructions and motivation.*
- *Risk factor control.*

- *Prosthesis cleaning/removal/modification including controlling biofilm retentive factors and evaluation of the components of the prosthesis, whenever needed and feasible.*
- *Supramarginal and sub-marginal instrumentation.*

It is recommended to perform re-evaluation and evaluate the outcome of the non-surgical step of therapy after 6–12 weeks, but some cases may need frequent monitoring during healing. The end points of the non-surgical step of peri-implantitis treatment are, at implant level, residual probing depths ≤5 mm with no bleeding on probing at more than one point and no suppuration. During recall visits after initial treatment, it is critical to monitor residual inflammation or suppuration and probing depths. Patient satisfaction, compliance with good oral hygiene, and cleansability of prosthesis should also be checked. Additional treatment should be considered if therapeutic endpoints are not met [30, 36, 37].

Surgical therapy is chosen when bone loss around implants is moderate to severe, but implants are still functional and not mobile. Access flap and pocket elimination surgery procedures have been shown to be effective in reducing probing depths and bleeding on probing in peri-implantitis. However, disease recurrence is common, leading to implant loss when followed up for an observation period of 1–5 years [38]. When the peri-implant defect is conducive for regeneration, for example, with intrabony components a depth of ≥3 mm and intact bony walls present within the defect morphology, reconstructive surgery is ideal with bone grafts and with or without barrier membranes. Positive results have been documented on the benefit of reconstructive surgery (Fig. 19.8). Similar to the access flap surgery without regenerative approaches, resolution of peri-implantitis is difficult to achieve regardless of the surgical approach and biomaterial used. Disease recurrence is common leading to additional surgeries or eventual implant loss [39].

Standard mechanical debridement procedure with or without saline is usually adequate during peri-implant surgical procedures [40]. Titanium brushes, if available and used, have been shown to be beneficial in reducing inflammation. Air-polishing or Er:YAG laser for implant surface decontamination during surgical treatment of peri-implantitis is not recommended, and there is no sufficient evidence to support the use of implantoplasty [41]. Adjunctive use of local antibiotics, chlorhexidine, and photodynamic therapy for surface decontamination during surgery of peri-implantitis have not been shown to superior to standard debridement with or without saline [40]. The adjunctive use of the systemic or local antimicrobials in peri-implantitis surgical therapy has not been reported to improve clinical outcomes when compared to surgical therapy alone [42]. As mentioned before, clinicians should use clinical judgement before prescribing antibiotics, keeping in mind the risk of antibiotic resistance. Once again, supportive peri-implant care is extremely critical to achieve peri-implant tissue stability after peri-implantitis treatment [27].

When performing surgical treatment of peri-implantitis, it is recommended that implant-supported prostheses that prevent access for self-performed oral hygiene be adjusted prior to surgical therapy of peri-implantitis. In addition, implant-supported

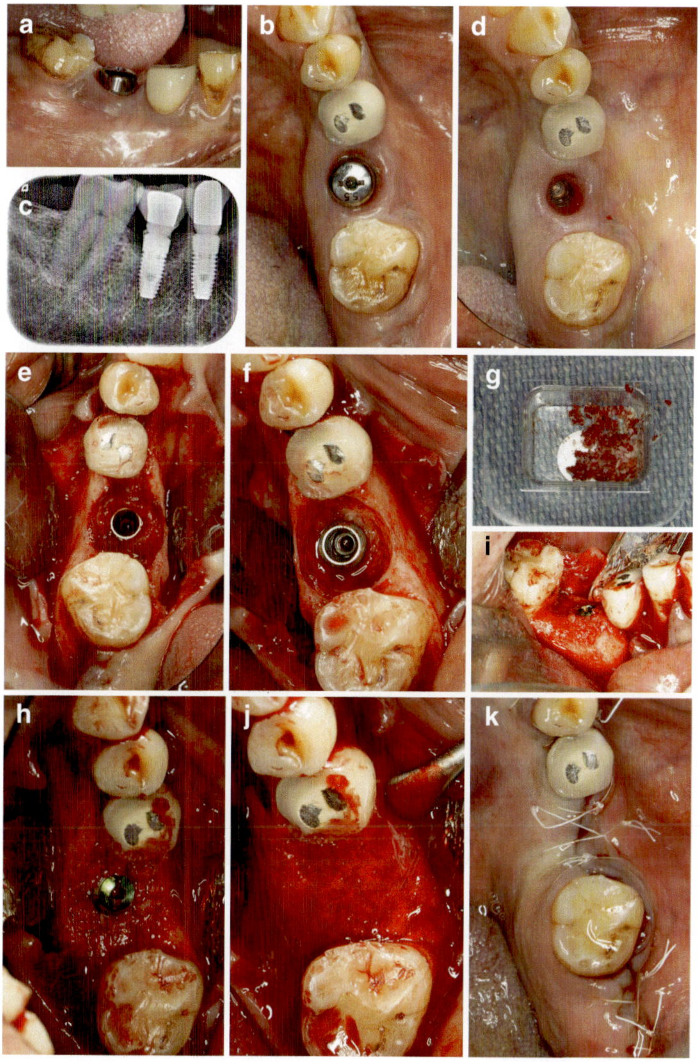

Fig. 19.8 Peri-implantitis and management. (**a**) Dental implant placed in lower right first molar demonstrating plaque biofilm accumulation around the healing abutment and peri-implant inflammation. (**b**) Occlusal view of the same site. (**c**) Periapical radiograph showing crater-like defect around the dental implant. Note the anterior implant in second premolar site shows no evidence of radiographic bone loss. (**d**) Soft tissue inflammation around the implant sulcus after removal of healing abutment. (**e**) Surgical access flap was made, and the implant site reveals significant bone loss and surrounded by granulation tissue. (**f**) Thorough debridement of granulation tissue was performed. (**g**) Bone allograft was made ready to be grafted in the peri-implantitis defect. (**h**) Bone graft material was placed into the defect. (**i**) Lateral view of the defect filled with bone graft. (**j**) Barrier membrane placed over the bone graft. (**k**) Primary closure obtained with sutures. (**l**) Site has healed well in 2 weeks. (**m**) Periapical radiograph shows bone graft in place. (**n**) After 8 months of healing, bone graft has healed completely. (**o**) Lateral view of the healed augmented site. (**p**) Healing abutment placed with sutures in place. (**q**) Lateral view of the site showing healing abutment. (**r**) Periapical radiograph showing the peri-implantitis site completely filled with bone. (**s**) Clinical view of the restored implant. (**t**) Periapical radiograph of the final restoration in place with the health peri-implant site

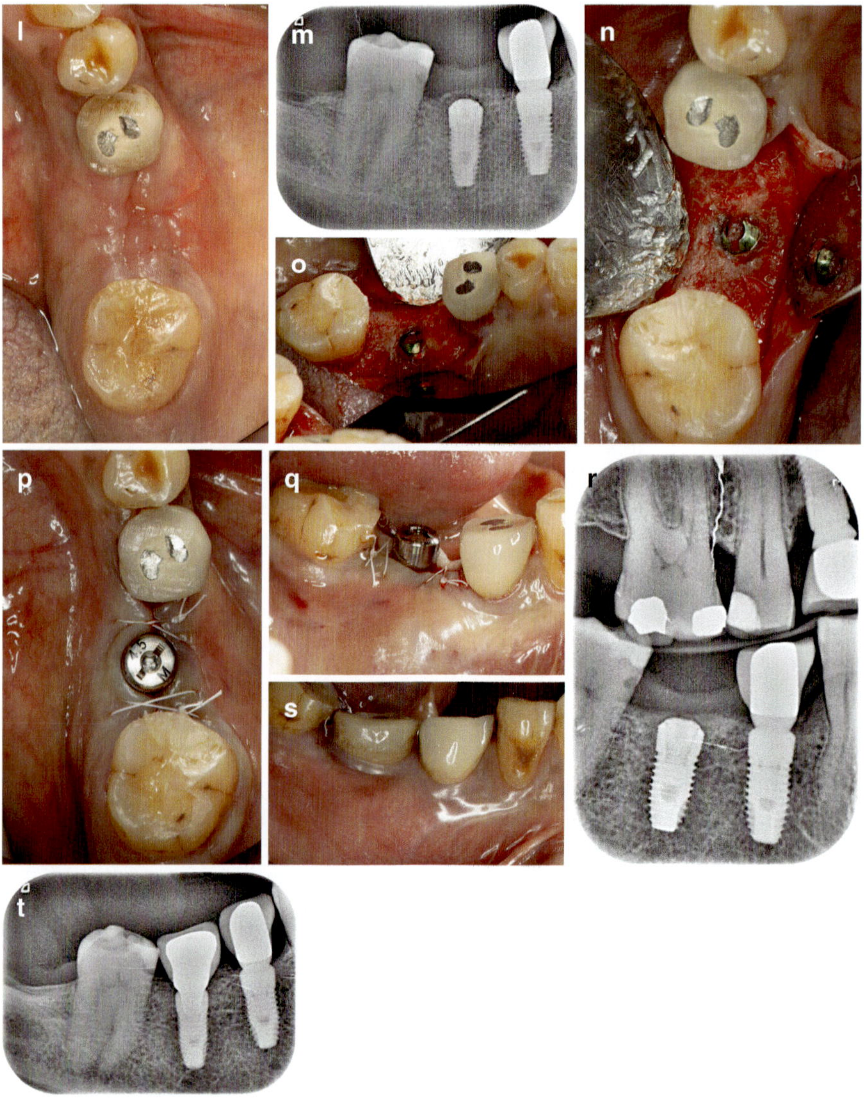

Fig. 19.8 (continued)

prostheses are recommended to be removed during surgical treatment of peri-implantitis to provide surgical access and peri-implant tissue healing [11].

The end points of successful surgical therapy of peri-implantitis are, "*at implant level, ≤1 point of bleeding on probing, absence of suppuration on probing, probing depth ≤5 mm and absence of progressive bone loss compared to pre-treatment bone levels to verify disease resolution.*" It is recommended to document all the clinical parameters 6 months after treatment and then radiographs be taken at 12 months. Long-term evaluation of treatment outcomes should include complication-free survival of the implant and implant-supported prosthesis and patient satisfaction such as esthetics [11]. The recommended frequency of supportive peri-implant care is 3–4 months for the first 12 months, starting 3 months after non-surgical or surgical treatment of peri-implantitis. The frequency thereafter should be tailored according to patient-, implant-, and restoration-based risk factors [27].

There is lack of evidence on which specific oral hygiene method is most effective in reducing the risk of recurrent peri-implantitis. Evidence and expert opinion recommend individually tailored to the patient and prosthesis care including the following:

- *Twice daily brushing of dental implants and teeth using either manual or rechargeable power brushes.*
- *Once daily use of interproximal brushes of an appropriate size.*

Limited use of oral rinse antiseptics (chlorhexidine and herbal-based) adjunctive has been recommended to professional mechanical plaque removal [31]. It is also recommended that oral hygiene methods be demonstrated by the patient to the oral healthcare professional and periodically reinforced [27].

19.5 Professional Full-Arch Fixed and Removable Prosthesis Maintenance

The American College of Prosthodontists, American Dental Association, Academy of General Dentistry, and American Dental Hygienists Association appointed a scientific panel of experts to write clinical practice guidelines on patient recall, biological and mechanical professional maintenance, and at-home maintenance for patients having implant-borne restorations and tooth-borne restorations [43].

Poor implant prostheses design such as concave intaglio surfaces can lead to poor accessibility for removal of plaque and poor function and could lead to complications and failure of implant-supported full-arch prostheses. It has been shown that convex emergence profile of the abutment or prosthesis and >30 angle of emergence leads to from lack of accessibility for oral hygiene which in turn leads to peri-implantitis [44]. Mechanical professional maintenance guidelines are given below [43]:

- *Perform detailed examination of the prosthesis, prosthetic components, and patient education about complications.*
- *Recommend and perform adjustment, repair, replacement, or remake of any or all parts of the prosthesis and prosthetic components that could impair patient's optimal function.*
- *Consider using new prosthetic screws when an implant-borne restoration is removed and replaced for professional mechanical maintenance and fabricate an occlusal device whenever indicated such as in patients with clenching and bruxism.*

- *Educate the patient to wear the occlusal device during sleep.*
- *Hygiene instructions, detailed examination of the occlusal device, and patient education about problems with the occlusal device.*
- *The occlusal device should be professionally cleaned extra-orally using professionally accepted mechanical and chemical methods.*

References

1. Ali Z, Baker SR, Shahrbaf S, et al. Oral health-related quality of life after prosthodontic treatment for patients with partial edentulism: a systematic review and meta-analysis. J Prosthet Dent. 2019;121(1):59–68.e3.
2. Heitz-Mayfield LJA, Salvi GE. Peri-implant mucositis. J Clin Periodontol. 2018;45(Suppl 20):S237–45.
3. Costa FO, Costa AM, Ferreira SD, et al. Long-term impact of patients' compliance to peri-implant maintenance therapy on the incidence of peri-implant diseases: an 11-year prospective follow-up clinical study. Clin Implant Dent Relat Res. 2023;25(2):303–12.
4. Albrektsson T, Sennerby L. State of the art in oral implants. J Clin Periodontol. 1991;18:474–81.
5. Araujo MG, Lindhe J. Peri-implant health. J Clin Periodontol. 2018;45(Suppl 20):S230–6.
6. Ramanauskaite A, Schwarz F, Sader R. Influence of width of keratinized tissue on the prevalence of peri-implant diseases: a systematic review and meta-analysis. Clin Oral Implants Res. 2022;33(Suppl 23):8–31.
7. Schwarz F, Derks J, Monje A, et al. Peri-implantitis. J Clin Periodontol. 2018;45(Suppl 20):S246–66.
8. Hämmerle CHF, Tarnow D. The etiology of hard- and soft-tissue deficiencies in dental implants: a narrative review. J Periodontol. 2018;89(Suppl 1):S291–303.
9. Renvert S, Persson GR, Pirih FQ, et al. Peri-implant health, peri-implant mucositis, and peri-implantitis: case definitions and diagnostic considerations. J Periodontol. 2018;89(Suppl 1):S304–12.
10. Berglundh T, Armitage G, Araujo MG, et al. Peri-implant diseases and conditions: consensus report of workgroup 4 of the 2017 World Workshop on the Classification of Periodontal and Peri-Implant Diseases and Conditions. J Periodontol. 2018;89(Suppl 1):S313–8.
11. Herrera D, Berglundh T, Schwarz F, et al; EFP workshop participants and methodological consultant. Prevention and treatment of peri-implant diseases—the EFP S3 level clinical practice guideline. J Clin Periodontol. 2023;50(Suppl 26):4–76.
12. Diaz P, Gonzalo E, Villagra LJG, et al. What is the prevalence of peri-implantitis? A systematic review and meta-analysis. BMC Oral Health. 2022;22(1):449.
13. Ramanauskaite A, Galarraga-Vinueza ME, Obreja K, et al. Prevalence of peri-implant diseases in patients with full-arch implant-supported restorations: a systematic review. Int J Prosthodont. 2021;34:s27–45.
14. Albrektsson T, Becker W, Coli P, et al. Bone loss around oral and orthopedic implants: an immunologically based condition. Clin Implant Dent Relat Res. 2019;21(4):786–95.
15. Albrektsson T, Tengvall P, Amengual-Peñafiel L, et al. Implications of considering peri-implant bone loss a disease, a narrative review. Clin Implant Dent Relat Res. 2022;24(4):532–43.
16. Dreyer H, Grischke J, Tiede C, et al. Epidemiology and risk factors of peri-implantitis: a systematic review. J Periodontal Res. 2018;53(5):657–81.
17. Lagunov VL, Sun J, George R. Evaluation of biologic implant success parameters in type 2 diabetic glycemic control patients versus health patients: a meta-analysis. J Investig Clin Dent. 2019;10(4):e12478.
18. Lin CY, Chen Z, Pan WL, et al. Is history of periodontal disease still a negative risk indicator for peri-implant health under supportive post-implant treatment coverage? A systematic review and meta-analysis. Int J Oral Maxillofac Implants. 2020;35(1):52–62.

19. Afshari Z, Yaghini J, Naseri R. Levels of smoking and peri-implant marginal bone loss: a systematic review and meta-analysis. J Evid Based Dent Pract. 2022;22(3):101721.
20. Amerio E, Mainas G, Petrova D, et al. Compliance with supportive periodontal/peri-implant therapy: a systematic review. J Clin Periodontol. 2020;47(1):81–100.
21. Giannobile WV, Jung RE, Schwarz F, Groups of the 2nd Osteology Foundation Consensus Meeting. Evidence-based knowledge on the aesthetics and maintenance of peri-implant soft tissues: Osteology Foundation Consensus Report Part 1—Effects of soft tissue augmentation procedures on the maintenance of peri-implant soft tissue health. Clin Oral Implants Res. 2018;29(Suppl 15):7–10.
22. Montero E, Molina A, Matesanz P, et al. Efficacy of soft tissue substitutes, in comparison with autogenous grafts, in surgical procedures aiming to increase the peri-implant keratinized mucosa: a systematic review. Clin Oral Implants Res. 2022;33(Suppl 23):32–46.
23. Cairo F, Barbato L, Selvaggi F, et al. Surgical procedures for soft tissue augmentation at implant sites. A systematic review and meta-analysis of randomized controlled trials. Clin Implant Dent Relat Res. 2019;21(6):1262–70.
24. Lin CY, Chen Z, Pan WL, et al. The effect of supportive care in preventing peri-implant diseases and implant loss: a systematic review and meta-analysis. Clin Oral Implants Res. 2019;30(8):714–24.
25. Atieh MA, AlAli F, Alsabeeha NHM. Outcome of supportive peri-implant therapy on the rates of peri-implant diseases and marginal bone loss: a systematic review and meta-analysis. Quintessence Int. 2021;52(2):122–31.
26. Carra MC, Blanc-Sylvestre N, Courtet A, et al. Primordial and primary prevention of peri-implant diseases: a systematic review and meta-analysis. J Clin Periodontol. 2023;50(Suppl 26):77–112.
27. Stiesch M, Grischke J, Schaefer P, Heitz-Mayfield LJA. Supportive care for the prevention of disease recurrence/progression following peri-implantitis treatment: a systematic review. J Clin Periodontol. 2023;50(Suppl 26):113–34.
28. Greenstein G, Eskow R. High prevalence rates of peri-implant mucositis and peri-implantitis post dental implantations dictate need for continuous peri-implant maintenance. Compend Contin Educ Dent. 2022;43(4):206–13; quiz 214.
29. Verket A, Koldsland OC, Bunaes D, et al. Non-surgical therapy of peri-implant mucositis—mechanical/physical approaches: a systematic review. J Clin Periodontol. 2023;50(Suppl 26):135–45.
30. Cosgarea R, Roccuzzo A, Jepsen K, et al. Efficacy of mechanical/physical approaches for implant surface decontamination in non-surgical submarginal instrumentation of peri-implantitis. A systematic review. J Clin Periodontol. 2023;50(Suppl 26):188–211.
31. Gennai S, Bollain J, Ambrosio N. Efficacy of adjunctive measures in peri-implant mucositis. A systematic review and meta-analysis. J Clin Periodontol. 2023;50(Suppl 26):161–87.
32. Dommisch H, Hoedke D, Valles C, et al. Efficacy of professionally administered chemical agents as an adjunctive treatment to sub-marginal instrumentation during the therapy of peri-implant mucositis. J Clin Periodontol. 2023;50(Suppl 26):146–60.
33. Zhao R, Liu S, Liu Y, et al. Adjunctive use of active compounds such as chlorhexidine in the nonsurgical treatment of peri-implant mucositis for oral health: a systematic review and meta-analysis. Oxidative Med Cell Longev. 2022;2022:2312784.
34. Bidra AS, Daubert DM, Garcia LT, et al. A systematic review of recall regimen and maintenance regimen of patients with dental restorations. Part 2: Implant-borne restorations. J Prosthodont. 2016;25(Suppl 1):S16–31.
35. de Tapia B, Bonnin M, Valles C, et al. Clinical outcomes and associated factors in the treatment of peri-implant mucositis, combining mechanical debridement and prosthesis modification: a 30-month follow-up prospective case series. J Clin Periodontol. 2022;49(12):1357–65.
36. de Waal YCM, Winning L, Stavropoulos A, et al. Efficacy of chemical approaches for implant surface decontamination in conjunction with sub-marginal instrumentation, in the non-surgical treatment of peri-implantitis: a systematic review. J Clin Periodontol. 2023;50(Suppl 26):212–23.

37. Liñares A, Sanz-Sánchez I, Dopico J, et al. Efficacy of adjunctive measures in the non-surgical treatment of peri-implantitis: a systematic review. J Clin Periodontol. 2023;50(Suppl 26):224–43.
38. Karlsson K, Trullenque-Eriksson A, Tomasi C, et al. Efficacy of access flap and pocket elimination procedures in the management of peri-implantitis: a systematic review and meta-analysis. J Clin Periodontol. 2023;50(Suppl 26):244–84.
39. Donos N, Calciolari E, Ghuman M, et al. The efficacy of bone reconstructive therapies in the management of peri-implantitis. A systematic review and meta-analysis. J Clin Periodontol. 2023;50(Suppl 26):285–316.
40. Wilensky A, Shapira L, Limones A, et al. The efficacy of implant surface decontamination using chemicals during surgical treatment of peri-implantitis: a systematic review and meta-analysis. J Clin Periodontol. 2023;50(Suppl 26):336–58.
41. Ramanauskaite A, Schwarz F, Cafferata EA, et al. Photo/mechanical and physical implant surface decontamination approaches in conjunction with surgical peri-implantitis treatment: a systematic review. J Clin Periodontol. 2023;50(Suppl 26):317–35.
42. Teughels W, Seyssens L, Christiaens V, et al. Adjunctive locally and systemically delivered antimicrobials during surgical treatment of peri-implantitis: a systematic review. J Clin Periodontol. 2023;50(Suppl 26):359–72.
43. Bidra AS, Daubert DM, Garcia LT, et al. Clinical practice guidelines for recall and maintenance of patients with tooth-borne and implant-borne dental restorations. J Prosthodont. 2016;25(Suppl 1):S32–40.
44. Schwarz F, Alcoforado G, Guerrero A, et al. Peri-implantitis: summary and consensus statements of group 3. The 6th EAO Consensus Conference 2021. Clin Oral Implants Res. 2021;32(Suppl 21):245–53.

20 Failures in Implant Dentistry

Saj Jivraj and Winston Chee

20.1 Loss of Integration

This is an infrequent occurrence with multicentre studies and several meta-analyses indicating average 93% survival rates of dental implants [1–4]. In general, there are higher implant integration rates in mandibular arches compared to maxillary arches, in addition, it has also been shown that implants are more successful when placed into host bone compared to grafted bone [5, 6]. Though it is disappointing for the patient and provider to experience an implant failing to integrate, the morbidity of failure is low when cylindrical implants are employed (Figs. 20.1, 20.2, 20.3 and 20.4). This mode of failure usually presents before a definitive restoration is delivered, in this example of the implant failing to integrate was an attempt to load the implant immediately with a provisional restoration, it is likely that the primary stability was not sufficient to allow bone-to-implant integration could take place without micro movement. With early implant failure, fewer resources will be spent on fabricating the definitive restorations but the major clinical concern would be delay of completion of treatment and patient management due to the time factor and added procedures.

Often a re-attempt at implant placement with larger diameters or lengths to provide better primary stability may facilitate a successful implant integration; however, it has been documented that there are issues of patient-related factors such as smoking, poor oral hygiene, health status, implant site characteristics for replacement and time of loading when implants are placed [27].

In other aspects of failures, there are components of iatrogenic treatment by some providers, patients can present for second opinions after implant placement. At times intervention due to procedures that have not followed the covention that

S. Jivraj
Private Practice, Anacapa Dental Art Institute, Oxnard, CA, USA

W. Chee (✉)
Advanced Prosthodontics, Herman Ostrow School of Dentistry, University of Southern California, Los Angeles, CA, USA

W. Chee, S. Jivraj (eds.), *Treatment Planning In Implant Dentistry*, BDJ Clinician's Guides, https://doi.org/10.1007/978-3-031-68726-6_20

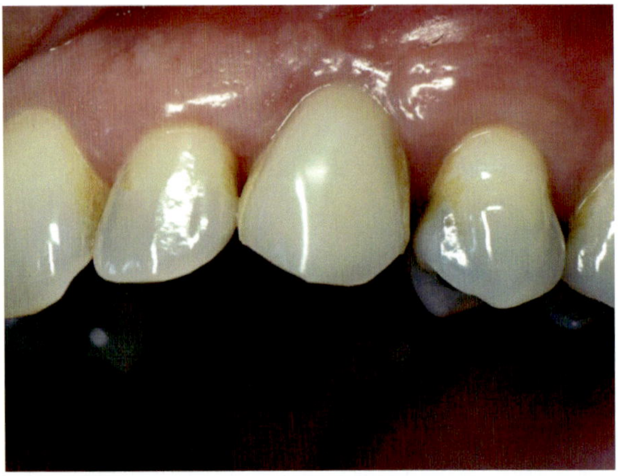

Fig. 20.1 Lateral image of maxillary left cuspid provisional restoration

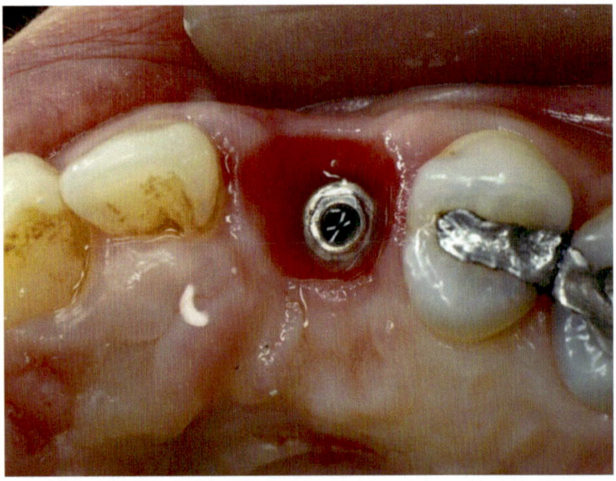

Fig. 20.2 The restoration is removed soft tissues appear healthy

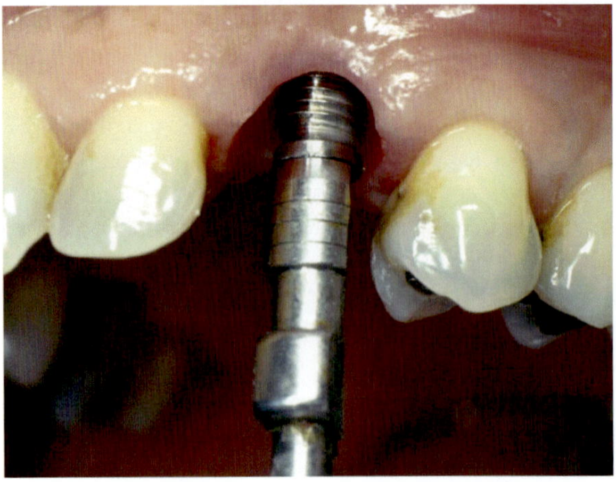

Fig. 20.3 The implant is loose and after attaching an impression, coping the implant was removed with a counterclockwise rotation

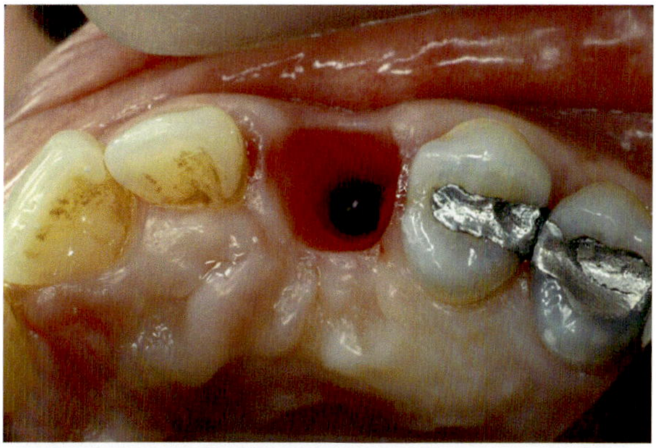

Fig. 20.4 The socket is without the implant with little bleeding, the socket will be curetted to remove any granulation tissue and encourage bleeding

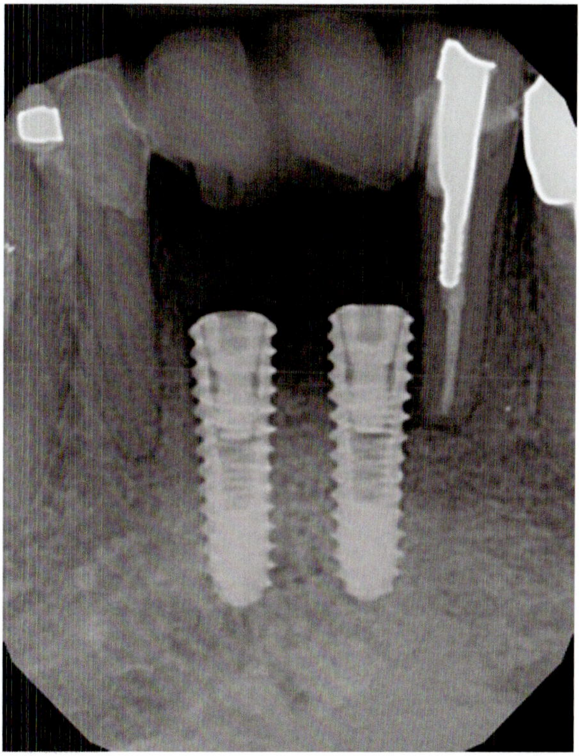

Fig. 20.5 Periapical radiograph that shows two implants placed and they appear to be adequately placed

led to a successful treatment proceduure. Especially when a flapless technique is used, some examples of iatrogenic treatment would be implants that are placed in positions that are "out of the bone" [7]. Figures 20.5 and 20.6 would illustrate the severity of an implant position that would appear to be well placed when viewing a periapical radiographic image (Fig. 20.5), then when viewed with a three-dimensional radiograph, the implants are placed almost entirely buccally placed anterior

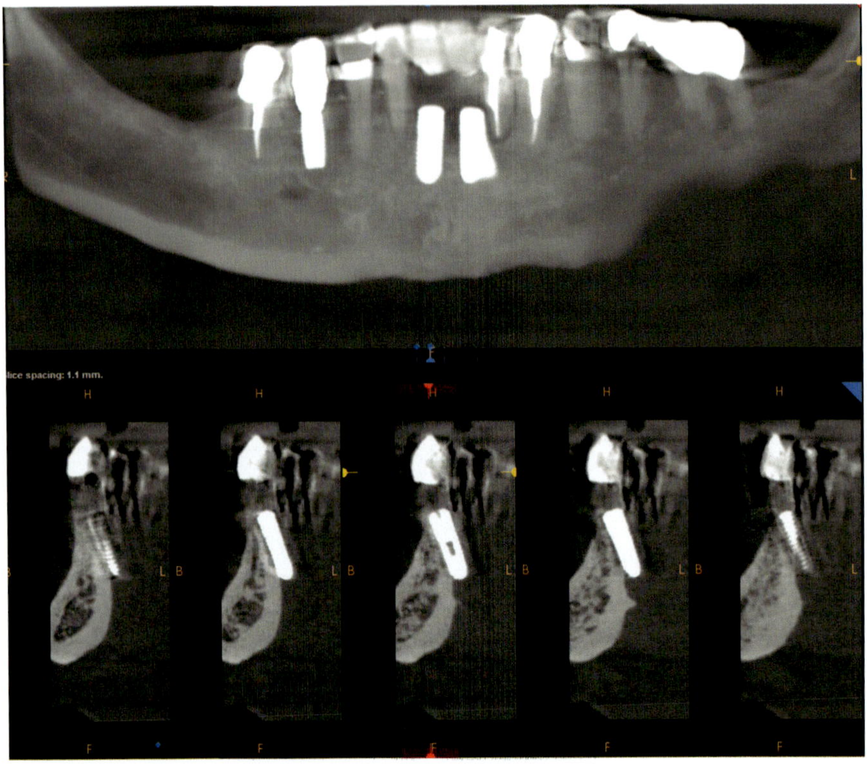

Fig. 20.6 The CBCT scan that shows the implants are placed out of the bony anatomy and it is likely that the implants were placed flapless

to the bone (Fig. 20.6). Figures 20.7 and 20.8 illustrate another example in the maxilla.

Another example when implants are placed in bony anatomy that is too narrow it will cause dehiscence when implants are placed, or implants are placed too facially, the implant can be stable however there will be no bone encasing the implant and discolouration of the soft tissues will be evident and the soft tissues not attached to the implant body (Fig. 20.9). A periapical radiograph is taken, and it shows bone loss in the mesio-distal aspects (Fig. 20.10). When the flap is opened to evaluate the implant, the facial dehiscence of the implant can sometimes cause bone loss as seen on the periapical radiograph (Figs. 20.10 and 20.11).

A more difficult problem to manage is bone loss occurring around an integrated implant where definitive restorations have been delivered. The issue is best described as peri-implant bone loss because there can be many different reasons where peri-implant bone loss presents [8–11]. One of the major causes of bone loss would be peri-implantitis which has similar aspects to periodontitis, the chapters in this book will describe in detail prevention and treatment of peri-implantitis [12–14] (see Chaps. 10 and 19). Other causes can be failure of a bone graft, history of smoking, uncontrolled diabetes, medications, and as described less than ideally placed implant positions.

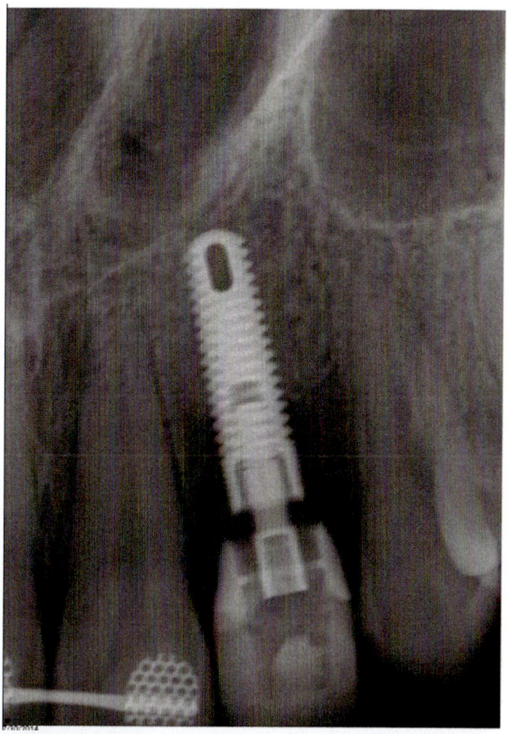

Fig. 20.7 Periapical radiograph shows that implant is adequately placed

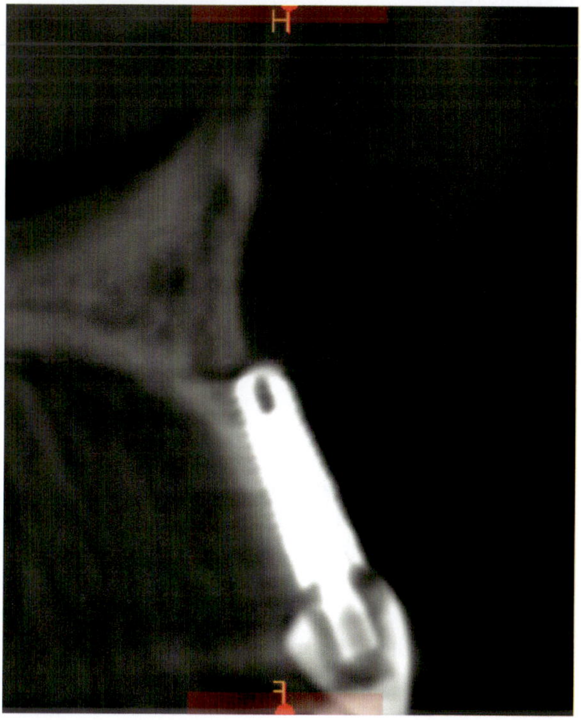

Fig. 20.8 CBCT scan shows that the implant is placed out of bone, and in this situation, the ridge is more narrower than the implant in the bucco lingual dimension

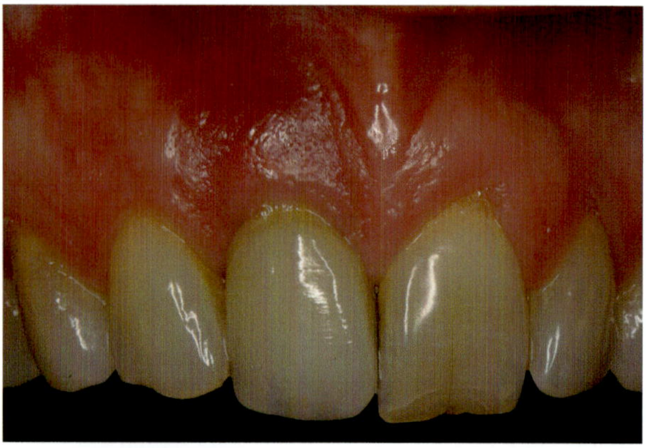

Fig. 20.9 Anterior view of an implant-supported restoration #8 (maxillary right central incisor), the grayish tinge is seen in the mucosa labial to the implant

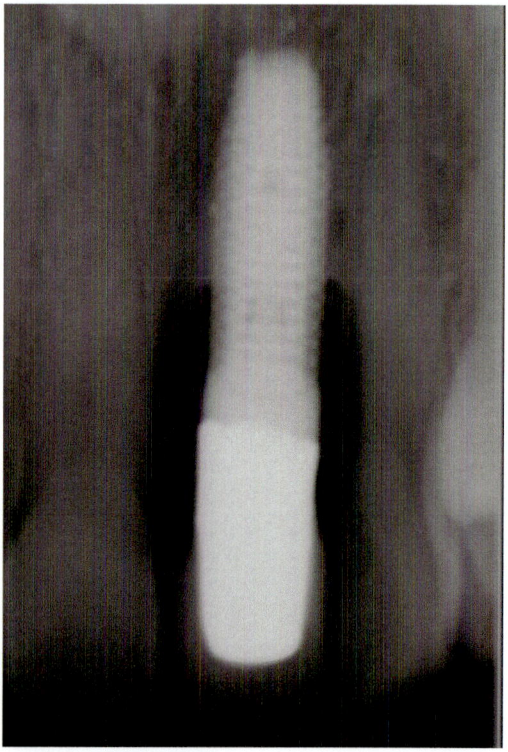

Fig. 20.10 The periapical radiograph shows bone loss mesial and distal of the implant

Many patients with implants in place and present with bone loss around the implants, many causes can be considered, it would not be correct to make a diagnosis of peri-implantitis without a history of the implant placement procedures. Some examples will illustrate other occurrences of peri implant bone loss may not be due to peri-implantitis. Figure 20.12 is a lateral view of an implant-supported fixed partial denture on the mandibular right sextant, on examination with some probing some bleeding was seen, a radiograph was taken, it shows significant bone loss on

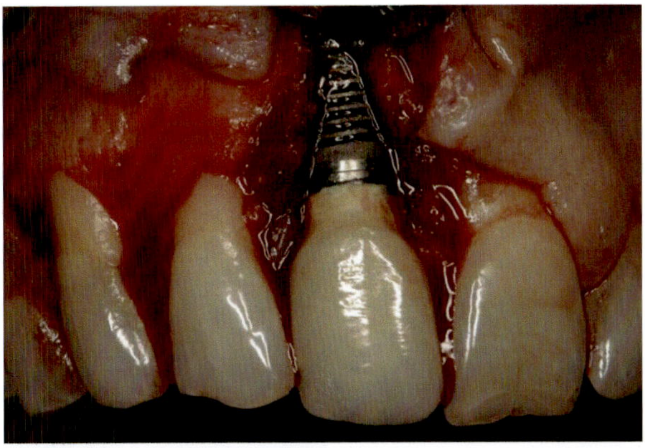

Fig. 20.11 With the flap raised, the implant is placed with large dehiscence on the buccal surface

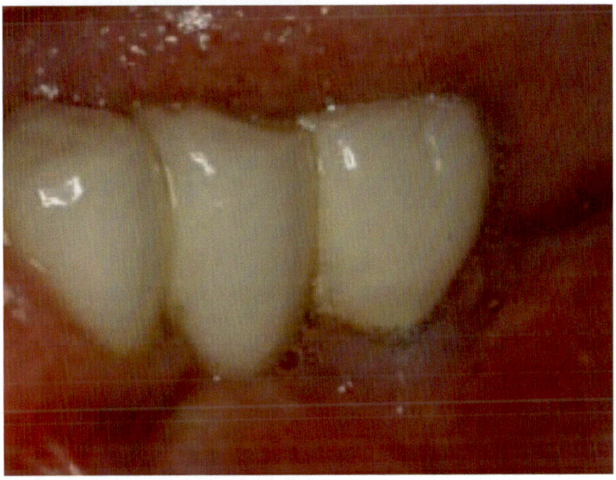

Fig. 20.12 Lateral view of an implant-supported FPD the tissue on the molar is discoloured

the distal implant, the mesial implant presents no bone loss and the adjacent tooth shows that there is no attachment loss or periodontitis on the tooth mesial to the implant-supported restorations—in this situation to immediately diagnose peri-implantitis might not be correct (Fig. 20.13).

A patient presented with an implant that had purulence and deep probing, the implant was stable with a history of a bone graft, then when removed, the tip of the implant was integrated to bone and most of the implant was not integrated (Fig. 20.14). In another example, the patient reported that the implant was in function for more than 10 years but was reported that the restoration was loose, a radiograph was taken, and a radiolucence was found in peri-implant. The restoration and implant were removed without much effort; both teeth adjacent to the implant were healthy with no attachment loss. The implant had no bone attached, and the patient did not experience any pain or discomfort (Figs. 20.15, 20.16, 20.17 and 20.18).

Without a history of the placement of an implant, it would be difficult to make a diagnosis of peri-implantitis. Patients who suffer periodontitis and are restored with implants will need to have regular visits to hygienists or dentists, if there is any

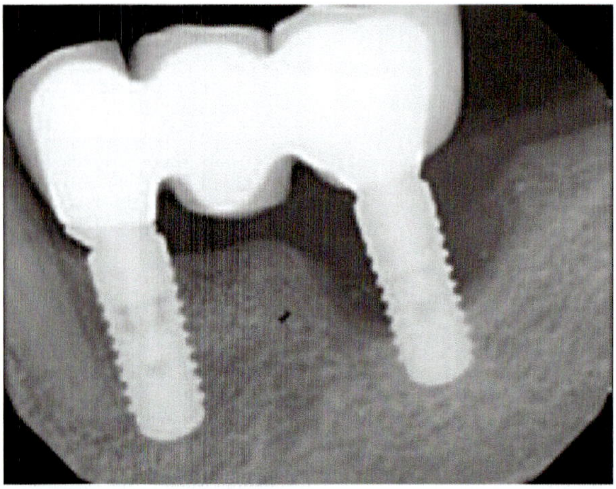

Fig. 20.13 A radiograph of the FPD shows severe bone loss on one implant and no bone loss on another, some remnants of grafting material are visible, and the graft may have failed

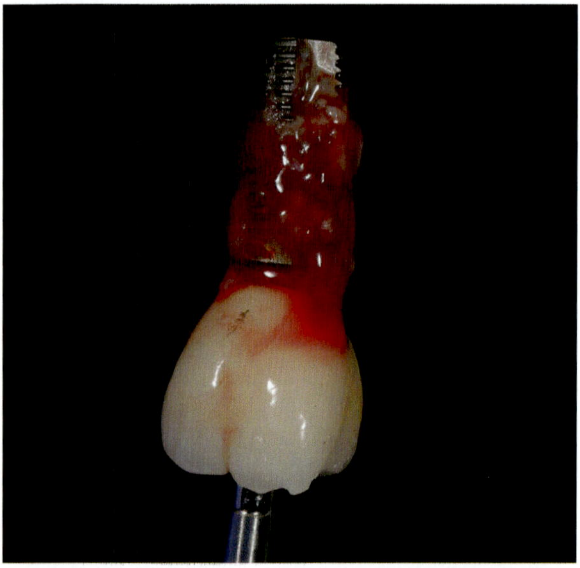

Fig. 20.14 An implant with only the apical tip integrated and the rest of the implant coated with granulation tissue, and purulence and deep probings were found clinically

bleeding on probing, exudates or purulence, radiographs would be required to evaluate any bone loss which would then be diagnosed with peri-implantitis. It is well known that the bone loss would proceed more quickly than teeth with periodontitis.

A patient with severe periodontal disease presented with some discomfort in her posterior right sextant, in Fig. 20.19, purulence can be seen on #2 (maxillary right second molar) and a radiograph taken illustrates severe bone loss around the roots of #2 and #4 (maxillary right first premolar) (Fig. 20.20). After extractions, implant placement and restorations were delivered (Figs. 20.21 and 20.22), the patient did not follow up with regular visits and had less than ideal homecare, and the patient also did not discontinue smoking. After a 6-year hiatus, the patient presented with significant peri-implantitis (Fig. 20.23). A radiograph shows the progress of

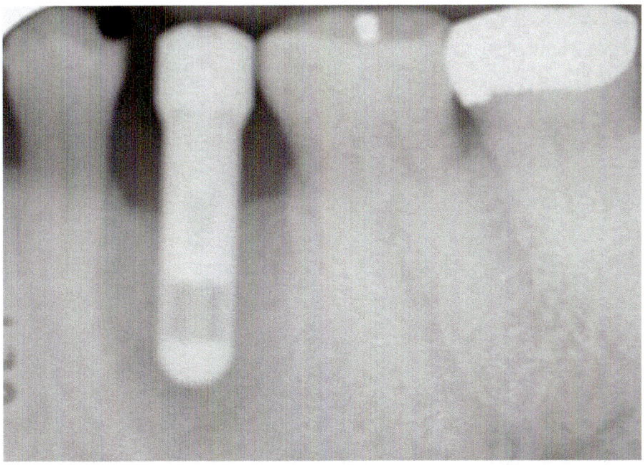

Fig. 20.15 Radiograph of bone loss around implant with no connection to bone

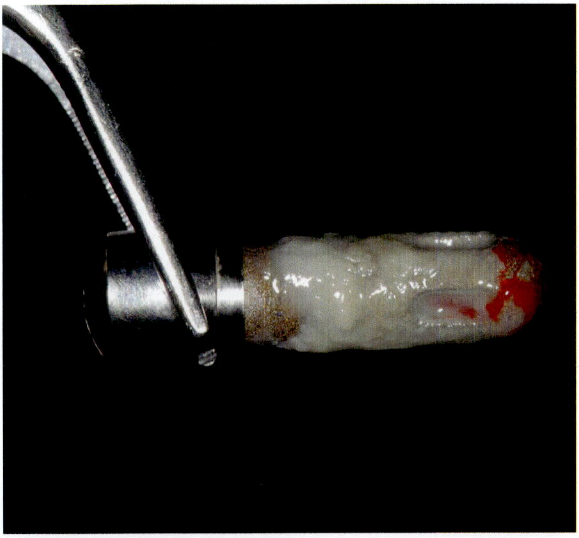

Fig. 20.16 The implant entirely coated with granulation tissue

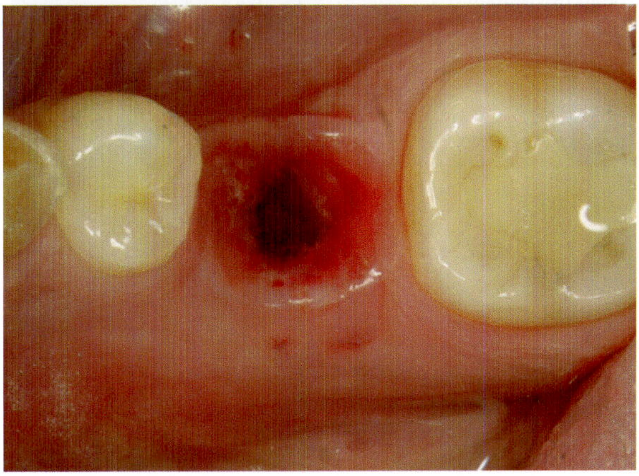

Fig. 20.17 An intra oral occlusal view shows no bleeding

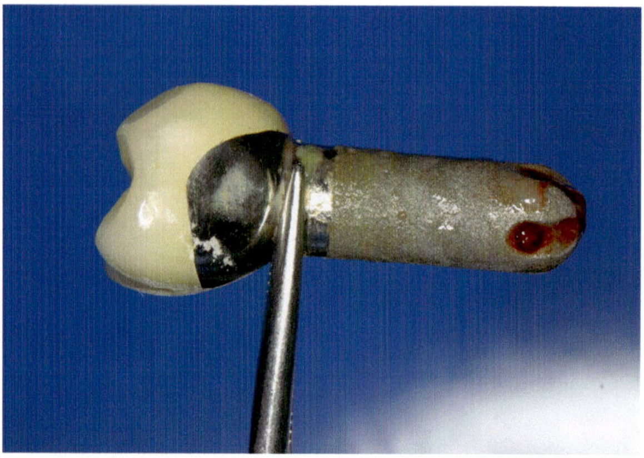

Fig. 20.18 Image of implant and restoration after granulation tissue is removed

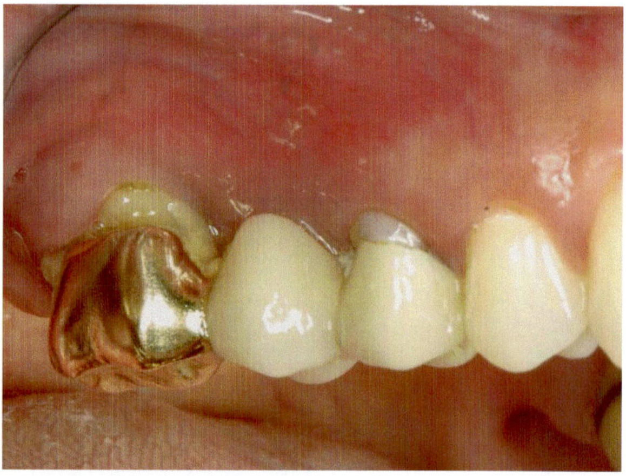

Fig. 20.19 Lateral view of maxillary right sextant, purulence is visible on the distal molar

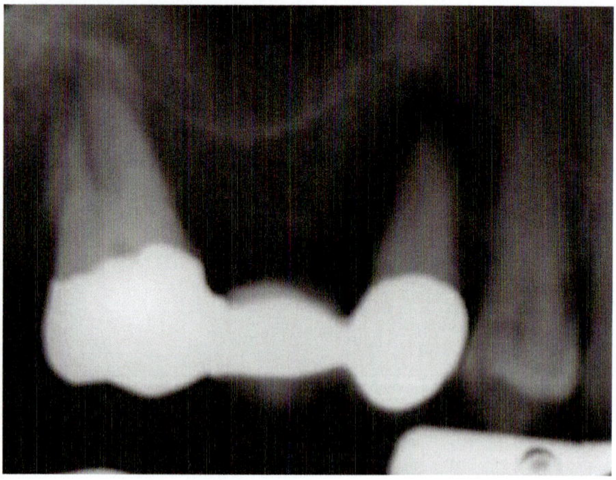

Fig. 20.20 Radiograph of Fig. 20.20 shows significant attachment loss due to periimplantitis

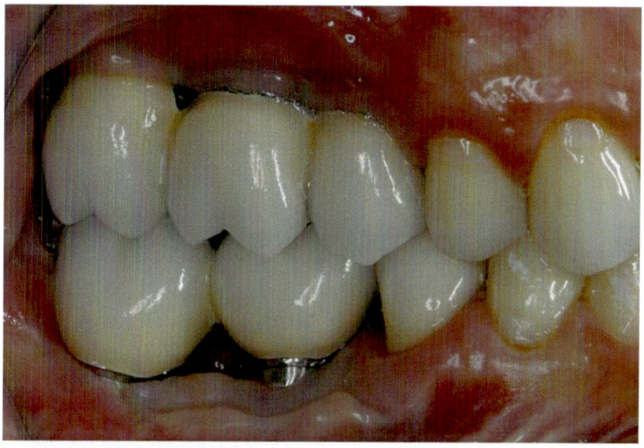

Fig. 20.21 Implants and restorations are delivered

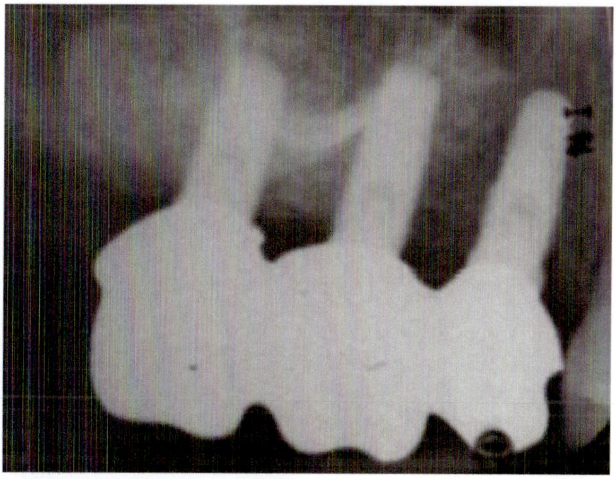

Fig. 20.22 Radiograph of implants and restorations from Fig. 20.21

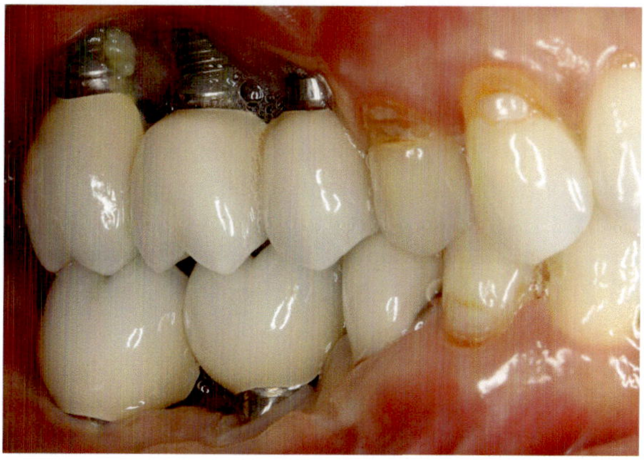

Fig. 20.23 Lateral view of restorations after 6 years

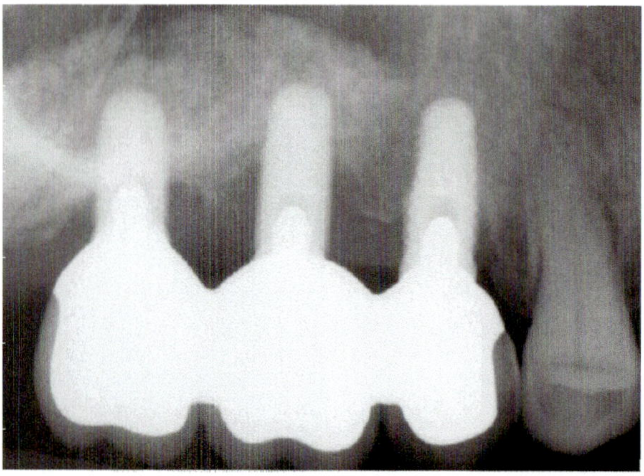

Fig. 20.24 Radiograph of Fig. 20.23

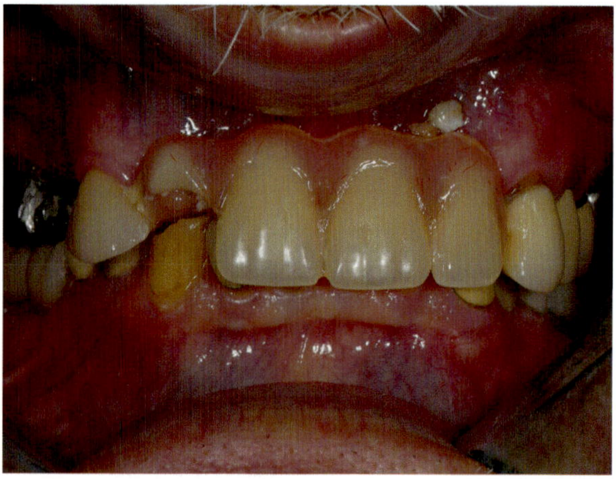

Fig. 20.25 Intra oral frontal view of fractured restoration, a deep vertical overlap of anterior teeth is visible

peri-implantitis (Fig. 20.24). With a history, a definite diagnosis of peri-implantitis can be made.

There is no definitive method to treat progressive peri-implant bone loss, several methods have been proposed: (1) antibiotic therapy, (2) resective treatment, (3) bone grafting, and (4) removal of the implants.

20.2 Positional Failure

The most common cause of positional failure is poor treatment planning and/or poor surgical execution. It should be the restoration that will dictate ideal implant positioning which will serve both esthetics and function [15] (please refer to Chaps. 12–14). In this chapter, some examples of non-ideal implant positions will be presented.

A patient presented with a fractured #7 (right lateral incisor) which was part of an implant-supported restoration (Fig. 20.25), Fig. 20.26 shows the

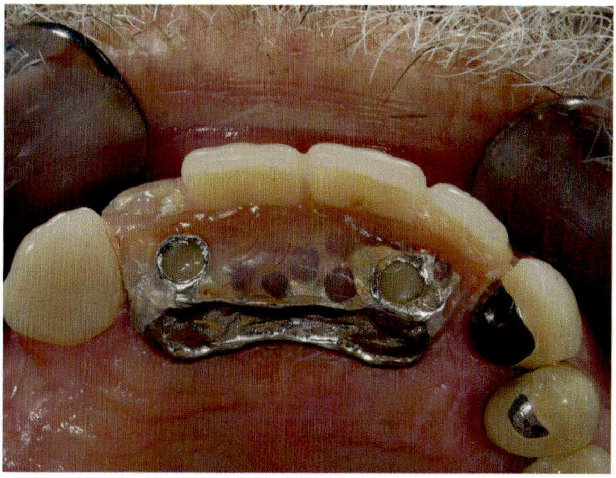

Fig. 20.26 Occlusal aspect of Fig. 20.25

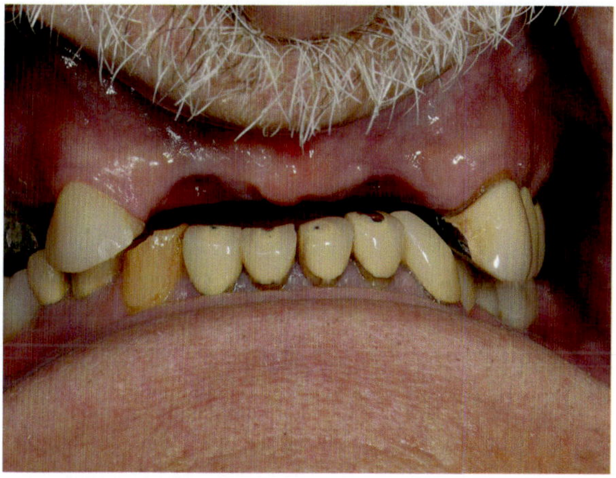

Fig. 20.27 Frontal view without restoration illustrates an insufficient restorative space

restoration from the occlusal aspect, the restoration covers part of the maxilla, and on Fig. 20.25 it shows the coverage of the ridge with a flange. In the periphery of the flange, debris can be seen and the mucosa appears inflamed. On removal of the prostheses, it is evident that the restorative space is insufficient, hence the form of the prostheses (Fig. 20.27). In areas covered by the prosthesis, debris was found to be trapped and some soft tissue inflammation and hypertrophy were seen (Fig. 20.28). Images of the underside of the prostheses when removed illustrate much debris trapped under the prostheses, the other image of the prosthesis demonstrates the poorly placed implant positions and the ridge lap which caused the trapping of debris and soft tissue inflammation (Figs. 20.29 and 20.30). With the restoration removed, the mucosa healed and tissues were healthy (Fig. 20.31). It is clear that the implants integrated well; however, the treatment planning and poor placement of implants did not lead to hygienic contours of the restoration [15].

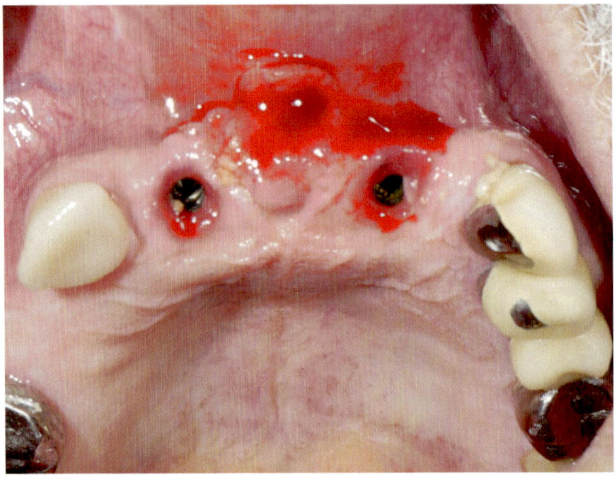

Fig. 20.28 Occlusal view after removing restoration shows inflammation of soft tissue

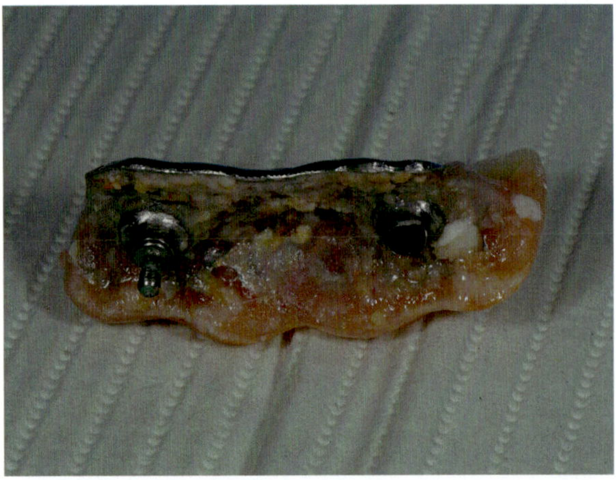

Fig. 20.29 Image of restoration when removed retained debris is evident

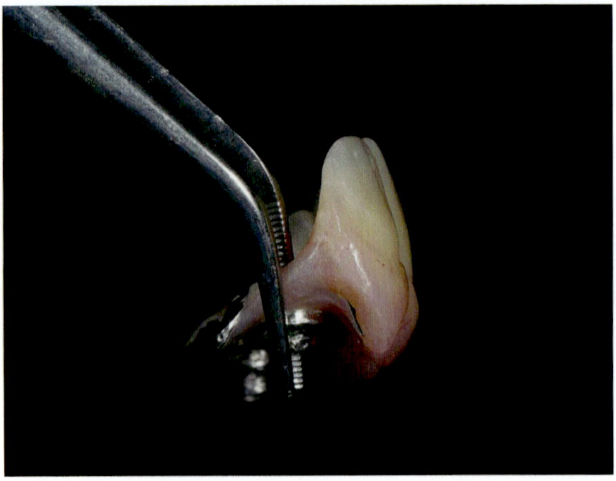

Fig. 20.30 Image of the restoration from sagittal view note the ridge lap and coronal and palatal position of the implants

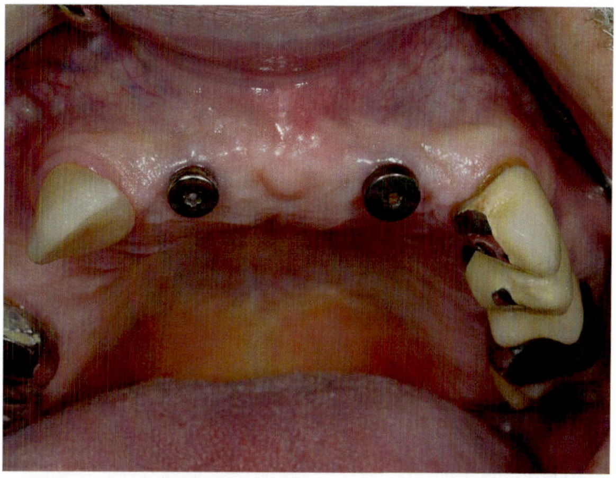

Fig. 20.31 Occlusal image showing healthy soft tissues with restoration removed

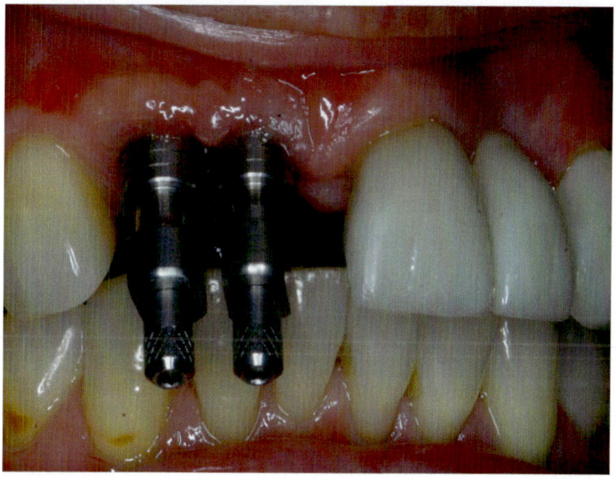

Fig. 20.32 Anterior view of two impression copings close together, both have a labial trajectory

Another issue that needs to be addressed is a suitable distance from implant to implant, a 3 mm or more separation from the edges of implants would be ideal. When implants are in close proximity, there can be bone loss in the interproximal areas that would affect aesthetics and, in some situations, can also cause implant failure [16]. Figure 20.32 illustrates implants being too closely placed. Figure 20.33 shows restorations of #7 and #8 (maxillary right lateral and central incisors) being restored with no papilla in between and at a risk of bone loss in between if care is not taken for home and professional care. In an extreme example, two implants were placed closely leading to bone loss and implant failure Fig. 20.34 a radiograph shows bone loss and Fig. 20.35 is the image of the restoration that was exfoliated with no integration to the bone.

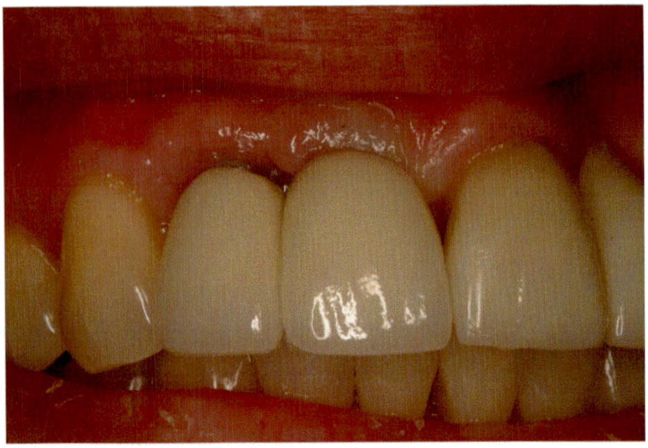

Fig. 20.33 Completed restoration with no papilla and the zenith of the right central incisor to emerge distally

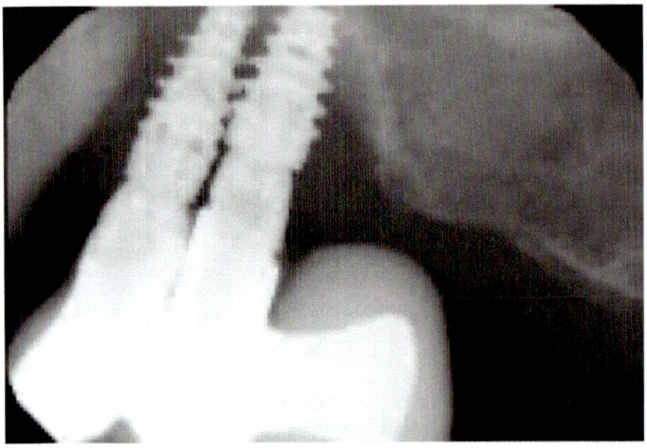

Fig. 20.34 Radiograph of severe bone loss of two implants placed in contact

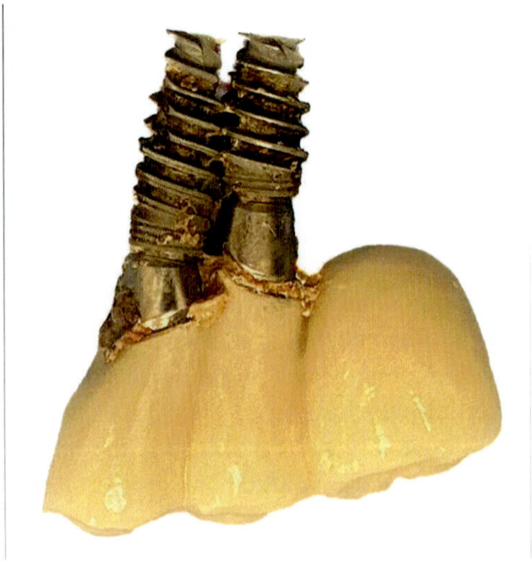

Fig. 20.35 Restoration removed with two implants in contact

20.3 Biomechanical Failures

Biomechanical failures occur when forces overcome weak points of implant components and restorations. Forces that are directed laterally and distance from pivot points can increase forces to weak points, and single implants are most vulnerable to breakage or screw loosening. Forces that are applied for implant fractures are due more commonly to occlusal forces in posterior areas of the oral cavity. Ideally wider implants can be placed if sufficient width of the bone will accommodate the implant; however, when a narrower ridge cannot receive a wide implant, then an implant that is placed flares from a regular-sized implant to a wider platform, it facilitates gradual contours from the widened implant platform. A radiograph of the completed restoration in Fig. 20.36 it can show the flared implant and a relatively deeply placed implant, a width and height of the restoration can be seen. It can also be seen that due to a wider platform on the implant, lateral forces can cause stress to implant, and the screw will clamp the restoration to the implant with the preload affected by the screw (Fig. 20.37). However the weaker point may be the implant body itself where the valleys of the implant are thinner, and a fracture can be seen in Fig. 20.38 and the radiograph in Fig. 20.39. Other examples of implant fractures can also be seen with intra coronal connections, the forces caused are similar to the prior case with large occlusal platforms that lead to lateral forces and damage to the implant (Figs. 20.40, 20.41, 20.42 and 20.43) [17, 18].

Components other than the implant or screw can also fail, again it is forces that will cause the weakest link to fail, in this example with an internal connection implant, the components need to fit within the implant and accommodate the abutment and the screw, Fig. 20.44 shows #30 (mandibular right first molar) with an implant placed distally and requires the mesial portion of the restoration to contact the anterior tooth, that will create a cantilever that will cause lateral forces to be applied. Figures 20.45, 20.46 and 20.47 will illustrate the mesial cantilever. Figure 20.48 shows the fractured ti-base within the restoration, and Fig. 20.49

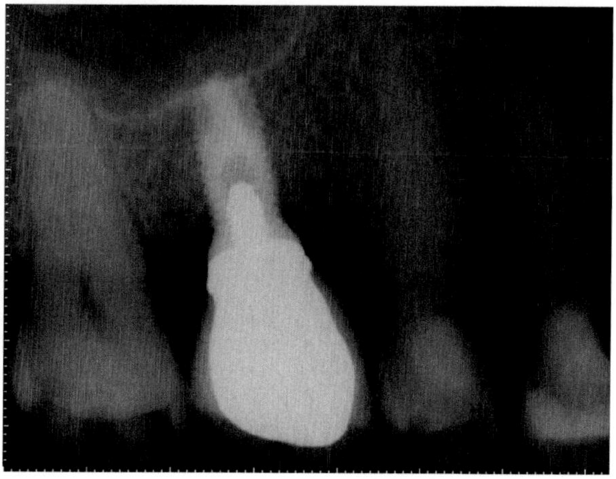

Fig. 20.36 Radiograph of a molar restoration and an implant with a flared platform, a widened platform facilitated a gradual contour

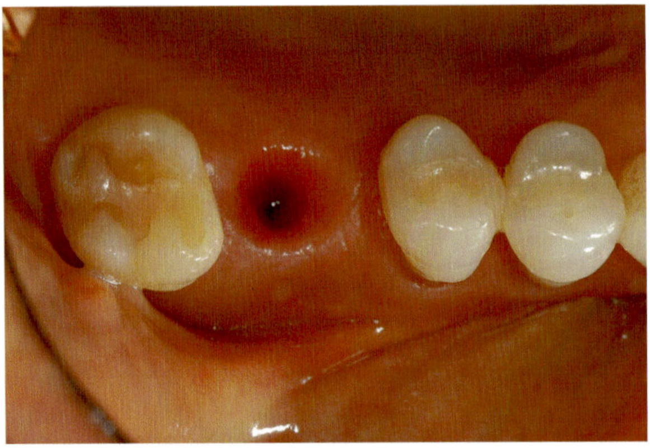

Fig. 20.37 An occlusal image of Fig. 20.36 shows the fractured portion of the implant removed

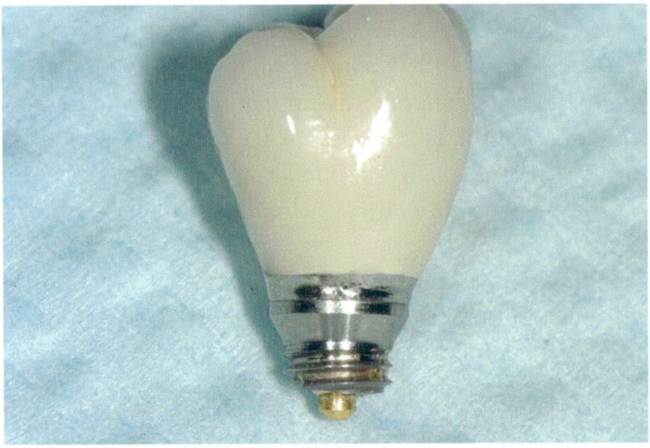

Fig. 20.38 The fractured implant and restoration are removed, note the widened platform

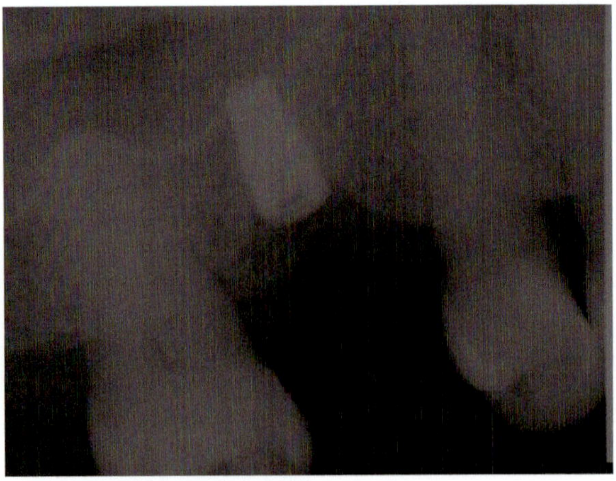

Fig. 20.39 Radiograph of the integrated fragment of the implant

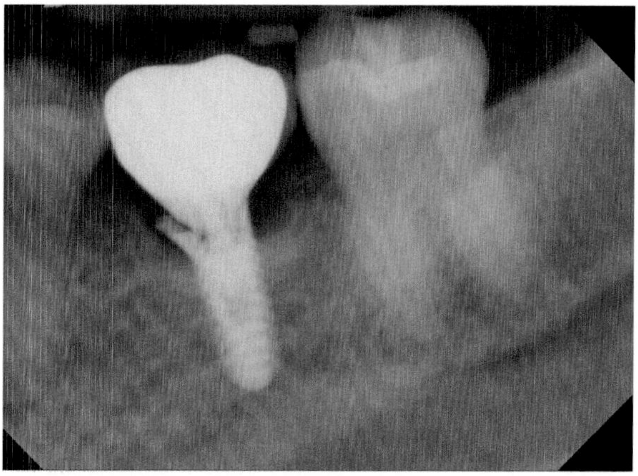

Fig. 20.40 Fractured wall of the internal connection implant, the molar restoration magnifies the occlusal forces with the occlusal table much larger than the implant platform

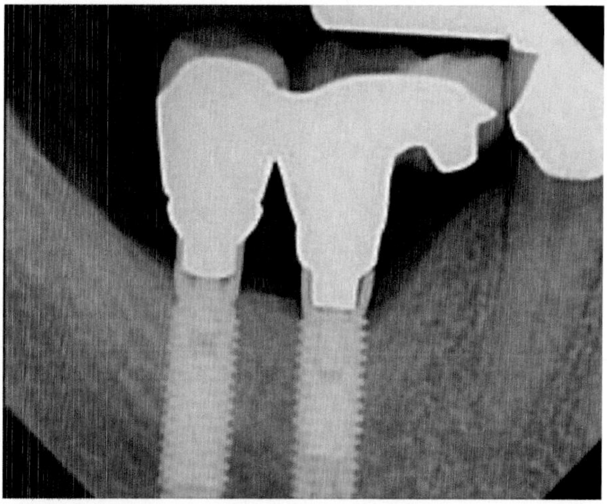

Fig. 20.41 Radiograph of two implants with a cantilevered pontic

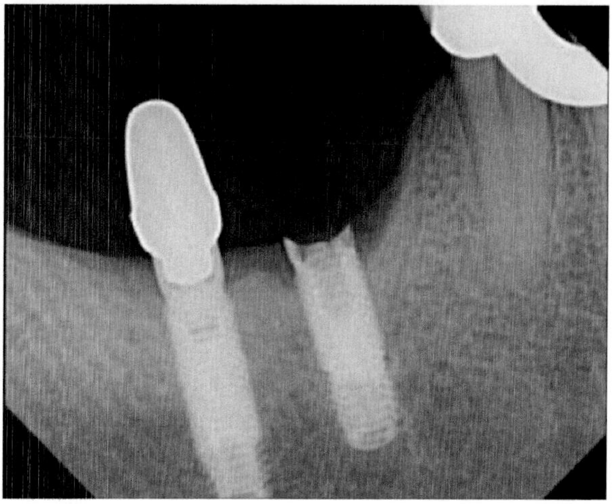

Fig. 20.42 Radiograph of the implant wall fractured

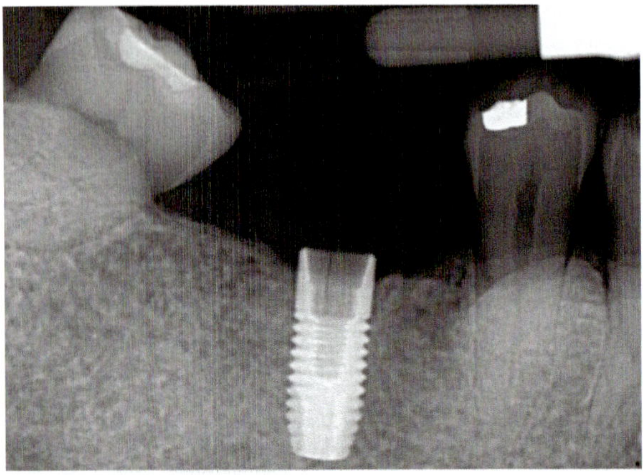

Fig. 20.43 Radiograph of an implant with a large mesio-distal span with fracture in the wall of the implant

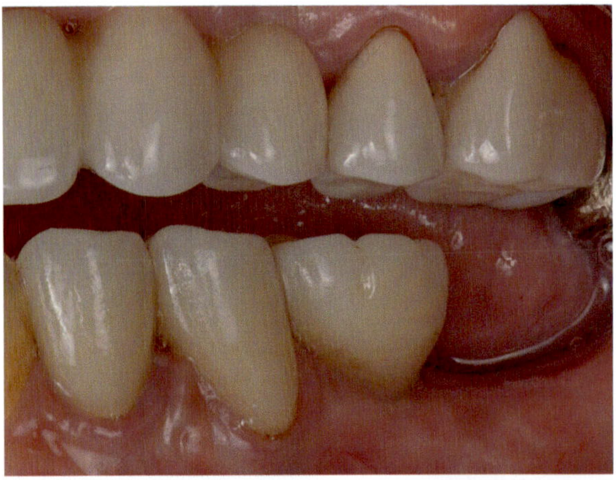

Fig. 20.44 Lateral intra oral view of mandibular left first molar

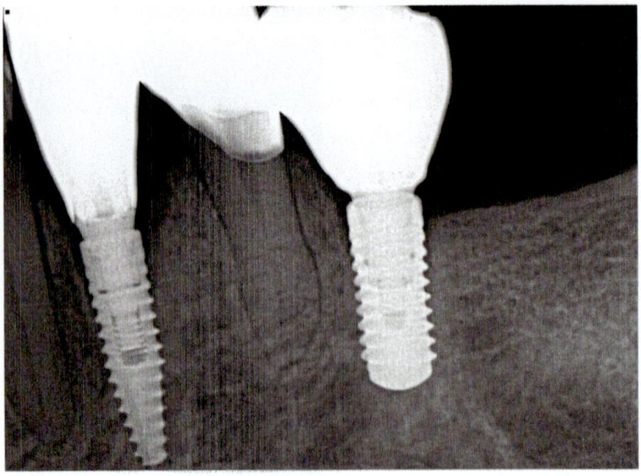

Fig. 20.45 Radiograph of implant and restoration of Fig. 20.44

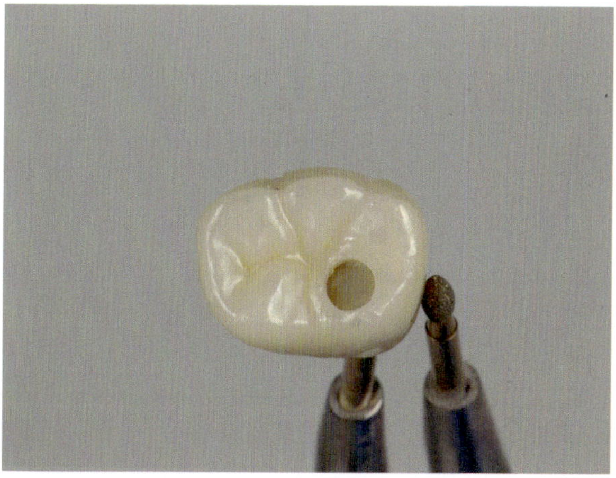

Fig. 20.46 The restoration presents a mesial cantilever

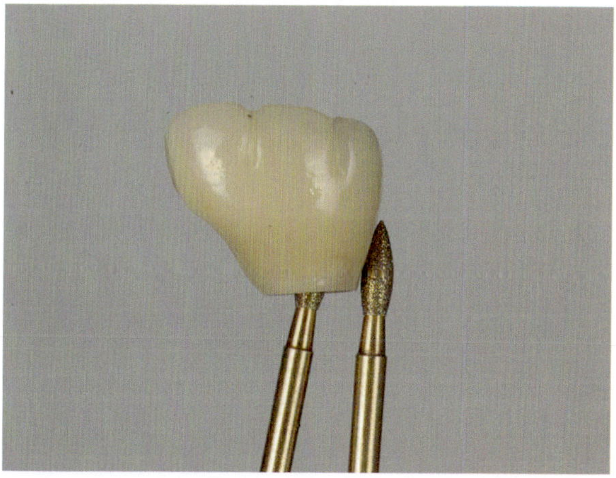

Fig. 20.47 The lateral view presents a similar lever

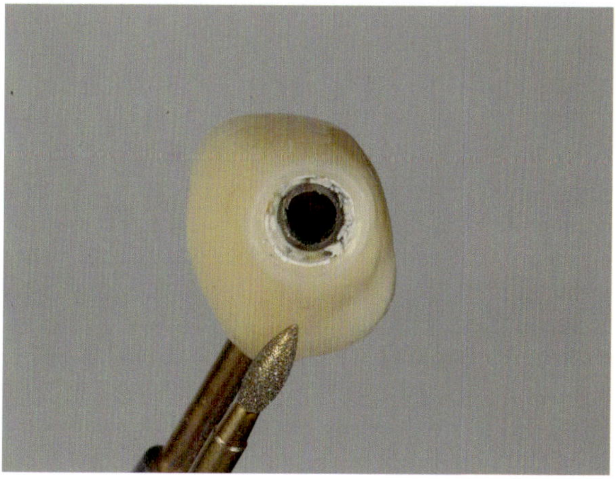

Fig. 20.48 The view from the restoration shows the fractured ti-base that was cemented to the zirconia restoration

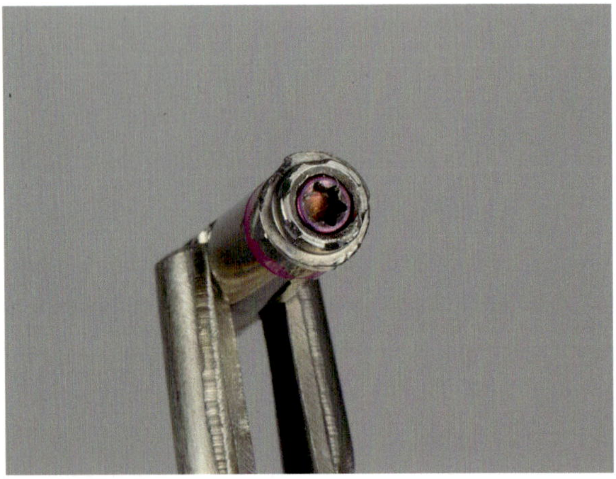

Fig. 20.49 An image of the fractured ti-base with the screw in place on an analog

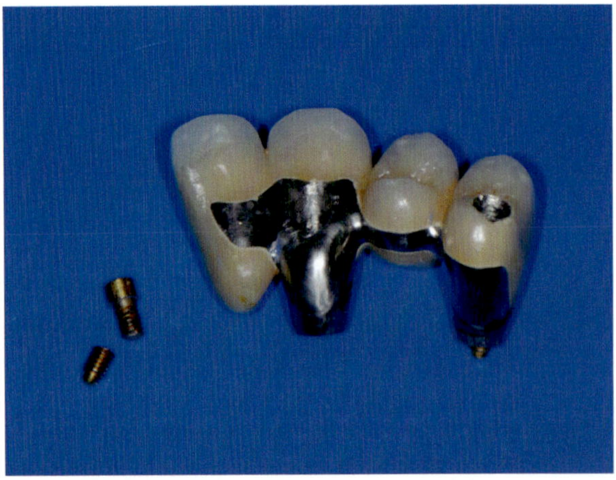

Fig. 20.50 A patient chronically presents with a loosened restoration or fractured screw, a tall restoration is noted and also a cantilevered pontic

shows the remnant of the ti-base that is held into the analog as it was intra-orally with the fracture.

Single tooth implants are exposed to forces in all directions, and when two implants are splinted, they are still vulnerable to lateral forces directed to an axis. When patients have strong occlusal forces and the restorations have tall restorations where lateral forces are amplified, screws are stressed and can lead to fracture. Figures 20.50 and 20.51 show one of the screws that is fractured and within the implant, it is likely that the posterior implant had a screw loosened followed by the restoration being dislodged [19–21]. This patient presented several times with the loosened restoration and twice with fractured screws. Each time a patient comes with loosened screws, new screws should be placed as with the lateral forces overcoming the preload of the screws, the screws may have been stretched beyond their elastic limits. For this patient, it was recommended to add an implant to have more stability by eliminating all axes of rotation (Figs. 20.52 and 20.53). The completed restoration is in place and over the years has not had the restoration dislodged again.

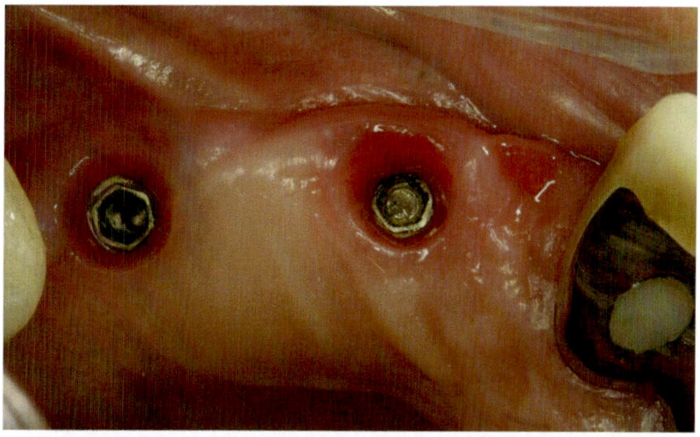

Fig. 20.51 An occlusal view of the implants of Fig. 20.50 with a fractured screw within the mesial implant

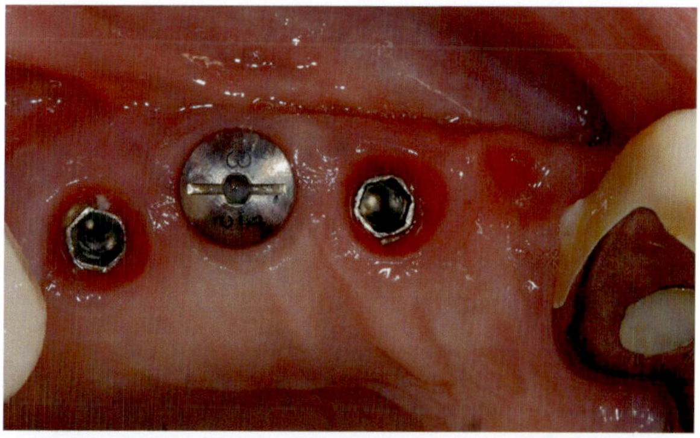

Fig. 20.52 An implant was placed in between the two existing implants to form a tripod to have more stability of the restoration

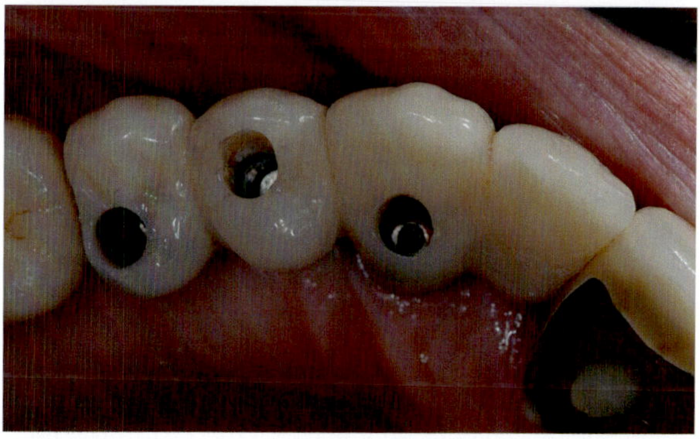

Fig. 20.53 The newer restoration in place with the additional implant, and the patient has not presented with loosened or fractured screws

Immediate placement and immediate loading of dental implants with full arch fixed implant-supported prostheses have repeatedly been shown to be a successful treatment modality [22–26]. Today, it is becoming a standard treatment approach that provides an incredible service to patients by streamlining the transition from a terminal dentition to a fixed prosthesis, eliminating the need for an interim removable denture and reducing overall treatment time [28–30]. However, obtaining and maintaining a successful treatment outcome with this therapy can be challenging.

From a prosthodontic standpoint, complications can be numerous and arise during the different phases of the treatment process.

Failures will be categorized under the following headings:

1. Diagnosis and treatment planning failures
2. Failures related to inadequate treatment execution
3. Biological failures
4. Mechanical failures
5. Material failures

20.3.1 Diagnosis and Treatment Planning Failures

The importance of this phase cannot be overemphasized. It entails carefully examining the patient and gathering a series of detailed records, including photos and mounted casts, to facilitate the key decisions that will impact the final prosthodontic result.

Complications arising from this phase are iatrogenic in nature. They will lead to a suboptimal prosthesis from either a mechanical or aesthetic perspective.

Complications do arise when time is not spent on diagnosis. Careful evaluation of the patient is key, and presentation of a treatment plan that is based on a sound scientific foundation is imperative.

From a diagnostic perspective, several parameters need to be evaluated before deciding upon the type of prosthesis that is most appropriate for the patient. The following considerations pertain to restorative treatment planning:

1. Positioning of the maxillary and mandibular incisal edge
2. Restorative space, choice of material and number of implants
3. Lip support, smile line, and lip length
4. Contours and emergence
5. Tissue contact
6. Occlusion

20.3.1.1 Position of the Maxillary and Mandibular Incisal Edge

The maxillary incisal edge position is determined utilizing the principles of aesthetics and phonetics. Traditional guidelines tell us when the patient makes the "F" sound, the incisal edge should touch the vermillion border of the lower lip. Once the incisal edge position has been established, the length for the central incisors is determined.

Often this is not realized in restorative treatment planning. Implant dentistry is a restorative driven discipline and if the maxillary central incisor is incorrectly positioned in the patients face, the implants also will not be placed to correct depth. This has repercussions on aesthetics and function. This will be illustrated in the following patient presentation. Patient presented with existing integrated implants and an implant and mucosa supported full mouth restorations. Her existing complaints included:

1. Unhappy with aesthetics.
2. The patient felt the maxillary incisal edge was touching the lower lip with too much intensity.
3. Too much support for the lip.
4. The patient reported excessive contact of her teeth at rest.
5. She had requested a fixed restoration from her previous dentist and was provided with a removable.

On clinical evaluation, implants were found to be integrated. Maxillary incisal edge was deemed to be in the incorrect position. The patient's lip was over supported, and the patient had been restored at an excessive occlusal vertical dimension. The implants had been placed at an inadequate depth and were encroaching upon restorative space (Figs. 20.54 and 20.55).

The following factors needed to be addressed in the treatment plan.

1. Positioning the maxillary incisal edge appropriately
2. Correction of the excessive lip support
3. Closure of the excessive vertical dimension
4. Creation of restorative space for a fixed restoration
5. Improvement of aesthetics

Impressions were made, and a wax tooth try-in was performed to evaluate the incisal edge position and overall aesthetics (Fig. 20.56). On approval of the try-in, a flangeless tooth try-in was performed to ensure the patient was a candidate for fixed implant-supported restorations (Fig. 20.57). It was deemed that the existing implants were in the incorrect position and required removal. Although not an optimal choice, the patient must understand why implant removal is required and the risks involved.

The treatment plan and sequence involved the following:

1. Data collection including required imaging.
2. Removal of the existing implants, required alveolectomy to create restorative space and placement of implants at correct depths and angulations (Fig. 20.58).

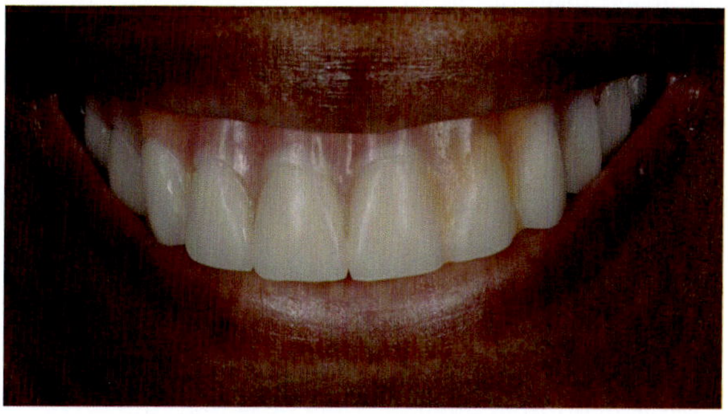

Fig. 20.54 Patient presentation with excessive display of pink acrylic and maxillary incisal edges in incorrect position

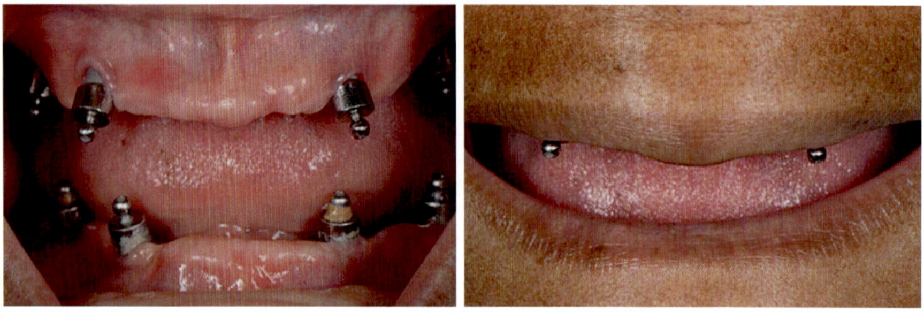

Fig. 20.55 Incorrect implant position. Implants placed too shallow compromising restorative space

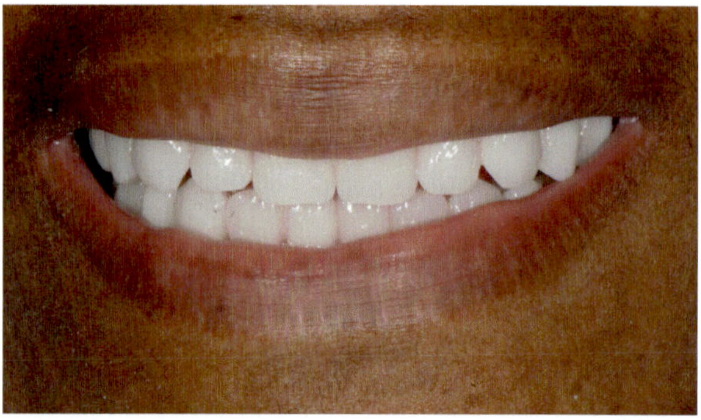

Fig. 20.56 Wax try-in to evaluate occlusal plane and esthetics

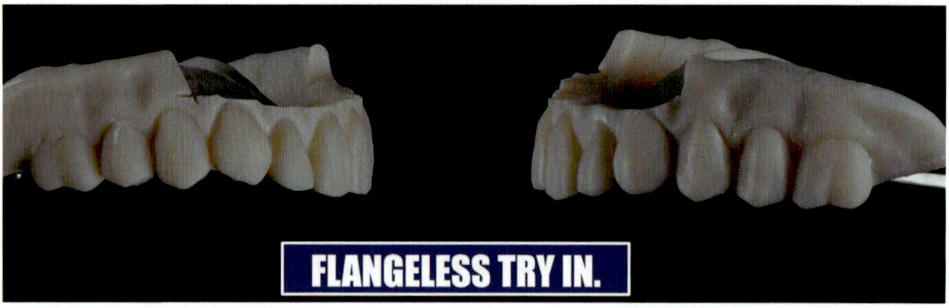

Fig. 20.57 Flangeless try-in

3. Immediate loading of the implants and fabrication of a transitional restoration at the required occlusal vertical dimension (Fig. 20.59).
4. Evaluation of aesthetics, phonetics, and occlusal vertical dimension during the healing phase and appropriate adjustments made (Figs. 20.60 and 20.61).
5. Fabrication of the definitive restoration (Figs. 20.62, 20.63 and 20.64).

The clinician's objective when treating failures is to objectively assess all the diagnostic criteria and evaluate how each one can be addressed. With a systematic approach, optimal outcomes can be achieved.

Fig. 20.58 Implant removal, alveolectomy, and implant placement. (Paltop Dynamic Implants Keystone Dental Group)

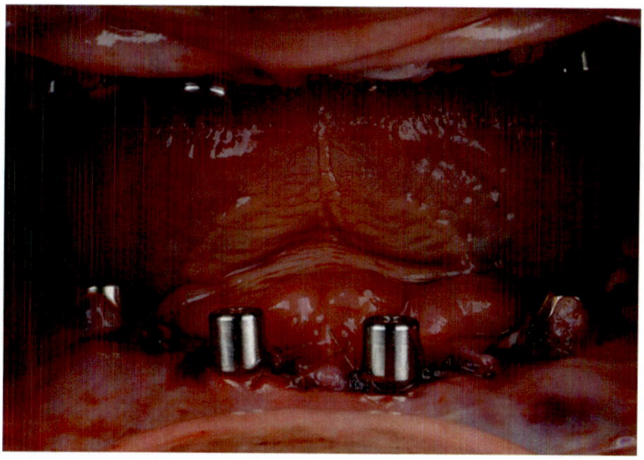

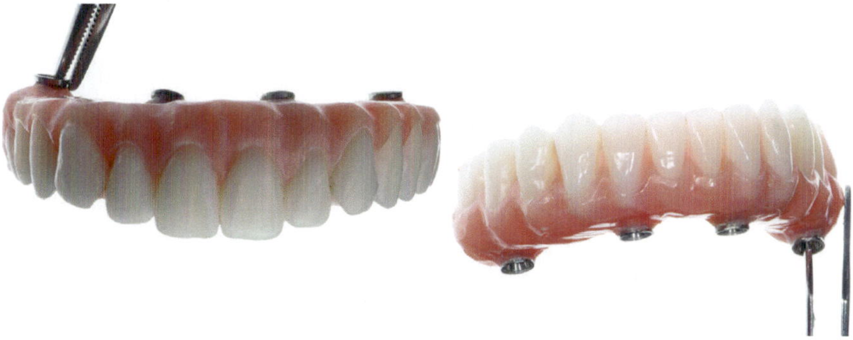

Fig. 20.59 Maxillary and mandibular immediate load provisional restorations

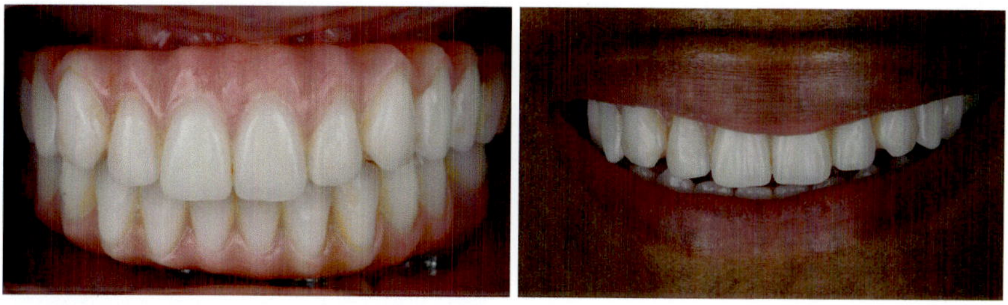

Fig. 20.60 Immediate load provisionals in situ

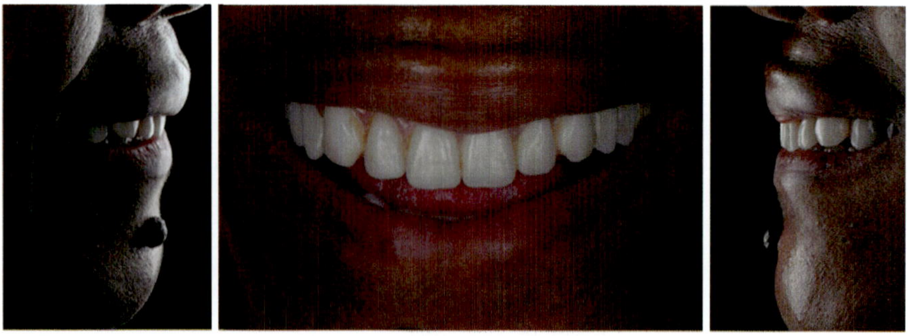

Fig. 20.61 Frontal and profile view of provisional restorations

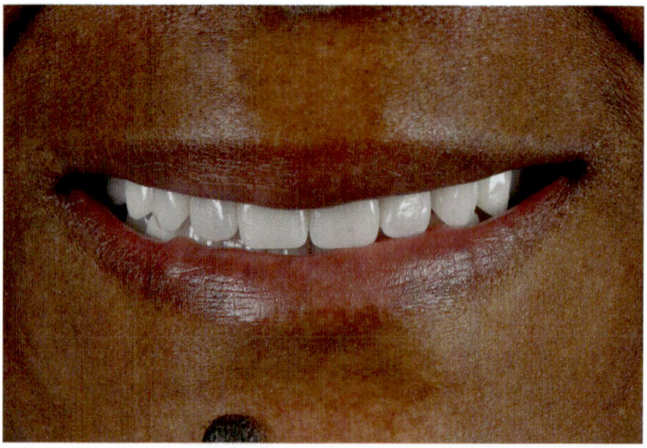

Fig. 20.62 Frontal view of definitive restoration in situ

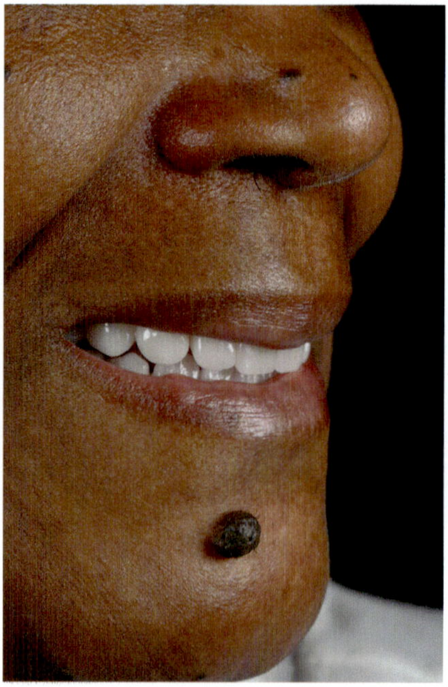

Fig. 20.63 Profile view of definitive restoration in place

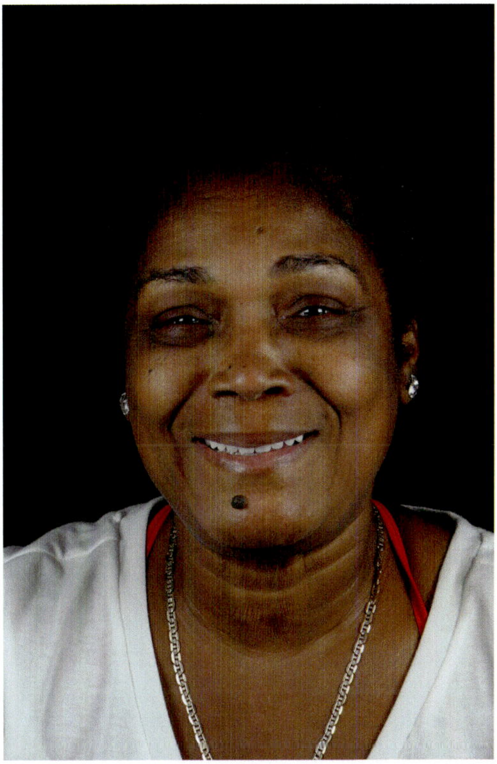

Fig. 20.64 Facial view of definitive restoration in place

20.3.1.2 Failures Pertaining to Restorative Space, Choice of Restorative Material and Number of Implants

1. Lack of restorative space is one of the most common occurrences that can compromise a restoration.

Inadequate restorative space will result in two scenarios:

(a) Restorative complications such as material failure leading to repair or replacement of the veneering materials or complete framework fracture leading to failure of the entire prosthetic restoration.

(b) Changing the treatment plan from one restoration type to another to accommodate the space requirements.

2. Incorrect choice of material may also be detrimental. Selecting a material that requires additional bone reduction for restorative space is questionable. It is the authors' opinion that materials should be chosen which requires minimal bone reduction. The restoration should be biomechanically sound and maximize aesthetics.
3. Number of implants

Unfortunately, the All-on-4™ concept has been used as a panacea for full arch implant reconstruction and often patients are treated dogmatically with this treatment protocol [22–25]. Often bone is removed needlessly to satisfy a certain treatment philosophy [25, 26]. The All-on-4™ concept has been proposed for specific clinical situations. It has a specific surgical, prosthetic, and maintenance protocol. It should not be a treatment solution for all edentulous or soon to be edentulous patients [28, 29].

Minimally invasive full arch implant dentistry adheres to concept of preserving and keeping bone. Bone reduction is virtually eliminated, and the patient maintains their own gingiva. Although four implants are considered standard, the placement of additional implants is considered advantageous. As a practicing clinician, implant failure should always be a consideration. If additional implants have been placed, the clinician can still transition the patient in a fixed restoration. These additional implants also help in distributing stress over a wider area. Treatment planning based on the diagnostic factors will dictate how much bone will need to be removed. The goal should always be bone preservation and over-engineering to ensure a long-term successful outcome.

In many clinical situations, there is an abundance of bone where more than four implants can be placed, and bone reduction may not be required.

In the authors' opinion, more than four implants are required when

1. There is an abundance of bone and biomechanically cantilevers can be avoided.
2. The patient presents with a dentition that exhibits signs and symptoms of excessive force.
3. Patient has uncontrolled metabolic disease which compromises healing.
4. Poor quality bone.

The advantage and considerations of placing more implants and preserving bone include the following:

1. There is the ability to segment the prosthesis, and complication management becomes easier for the clinician.
2. If in the future an implant were to fail, there are enough implants, where the patient may not have to undergo surgery again.
3. The thought process that making an impression on four implants is easier than making an impression on 5 or 6 does not hold merit. Today with advancements in digital technologies, analogue impression making may soon become obsolete at multi-unit abutment level.

When placing implants, the clinician must begin with the end in mind visualizing the definitive restoration. Zirconia requires specific connector dimensions and the implants not be placed too close together. Zirconia also requires specific thickness so the implants together with the multi-unit abutments must be positioned to allow for this.

4. Maintenance of bone in between the implants can be obtained by banking roots.
5. If a catastrophic failure was to occur and all the implants were lost, then we still have the opportunity to retreat the patient.

The following patient presentation will illustrate a restorative failure encompassing all the points discussed above.

Patient presented with severe tooth wear seeking a solution to his terminal dentition. His desire was to have fixed restorations throughout the whole treatment process.

On clinical evaluation, the following were found:

1. Inadequate restorative space.
2. Lack of tooth structure for predictable tooth replacement (Fig. 20.65).
3. Patient exhibited signs of bruxism.
4. Over-eruption of teeth as a compensatory mechanism to the wear which resulted in excess bone (Fig. 20.66).

Often clinicians are faced with decisions pertaining to the occlusal vertical dimension. Should the vertical be restored or not in a full mouth implant rehabilitation? Will opening the vertical cause additional issues from a biomechanical perspective. Rather than focus on the occlusal vertical dimension, the clinician should be more concerned about restorative space and how to obtain it.

Space for full mouth rehabilitation on implants can be obtained through.

1. Restoring occlusal vertical dimension if required.
2. Reduction of bone strategically.
3. Combination of the above.

The patient was diagnosed as having a terminal dentition. Evaluation of the vertical dimension of occlusion revealed the patient having 6 mm of interocclusal distance. This does not necessarily mean that the patient has lost vertical dimension of occlusion, but it does provide the clinician with some space to open the vertical should they decide. The patient was also sent for a sleep study to eliminate sleep disordered breathing as a contributory cause of the breakdown.

The following treatment was planned:

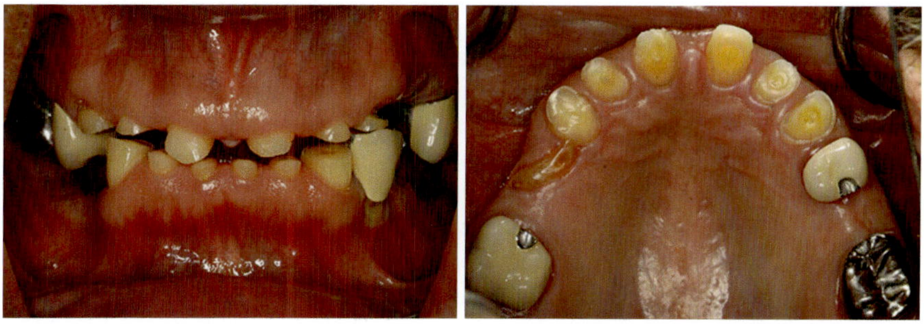

Fig. 20.65 Occlusal and buccal views demonstrating severe tooth surface loss

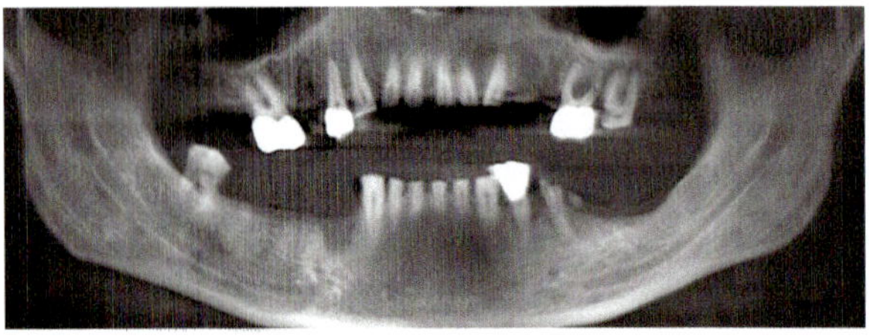

Fig. 20.66 Presenting panoramic radiograph

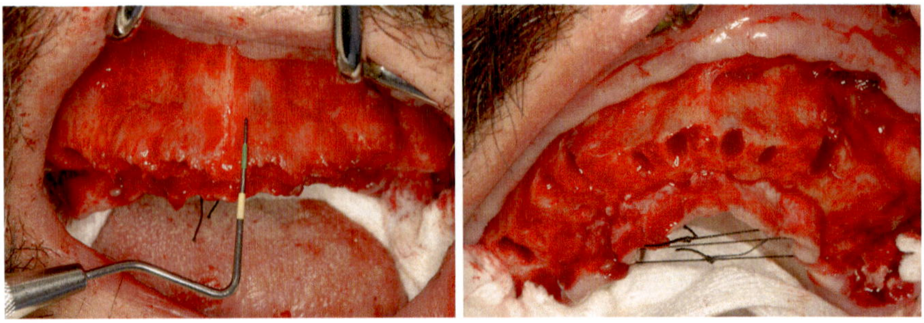

Fig. 20.67 Surgical measurement for alveolectomy

1. Extraction of all remaining teeth.
2. Execution of the All-on-4™ treatment concept.
3. Alveolectomy with four implants placed in the maxilla and four implants in the mandible (Figs. 20.67, 20.68 and 20.69).
4. Immediate loading (Fig. 20.70).
5. Definitive restoration would be an acrylic resin/metal-based restoration with metal occlusal surfaces to minimize wear on the posterior teeth (Figs. 20.71 and 20.72).

Treatment execution went to plan, and the patient was extremely satisfied with the outcome in both the provisional and definitive phase.

On reflecting on the treatment plan, several critical errors were made:

1. The patient presents with an abundance of bone and severe tooth surface loss. This tooth surface loss could be attributed to attrition, abrasion, or erosion. Most likely it would be a combination of them. In patients with an abundance of bone and signs of excessive force, it is the authors opinion that the All-on-4™ treatment concept is not the treatment of choice. In this clinical scenario, additional implants would be indicated to distribute the forces over a wider area. The patient had an abundance of bone and 6–8 or even 10 implants could have been placed based on the clinician's treatment proposal. With the abundance of bone, there is no need to tilt the distal implants and have a cantilever. This can be eliminated with additional implants (Fig. 20.73).
2. The restorative material of choice is incorrect. Despite providing metal occlusal surfaces, acrylic resin/metal-based restorations require a significant amount of space. This space is created by unnecessary alveolectomy. Alveolectomy could

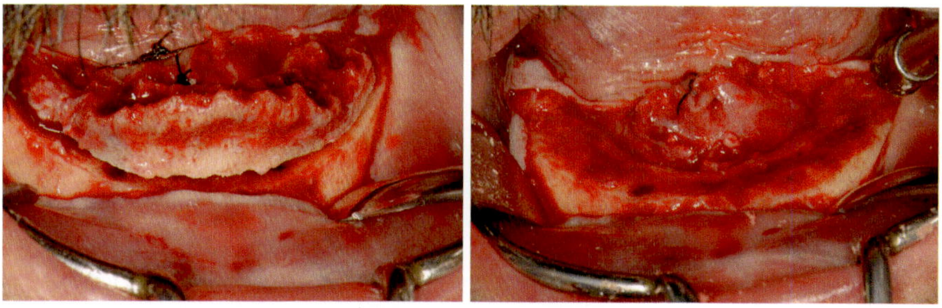

Fig. 20.68 Mandibular alveolectomy

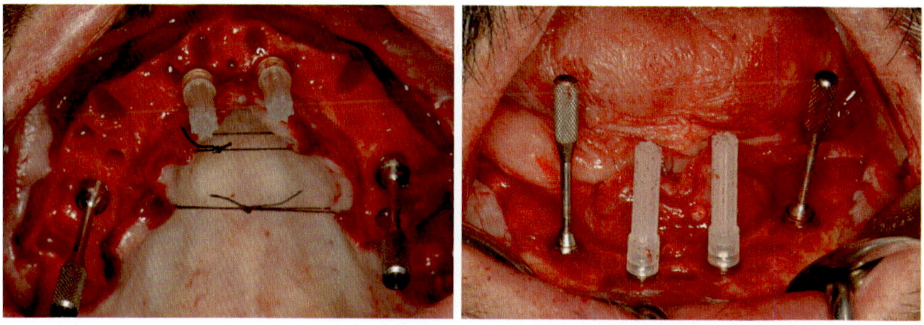

Fig. 20.69 Dental implants placed following the All-on-4™ protocol

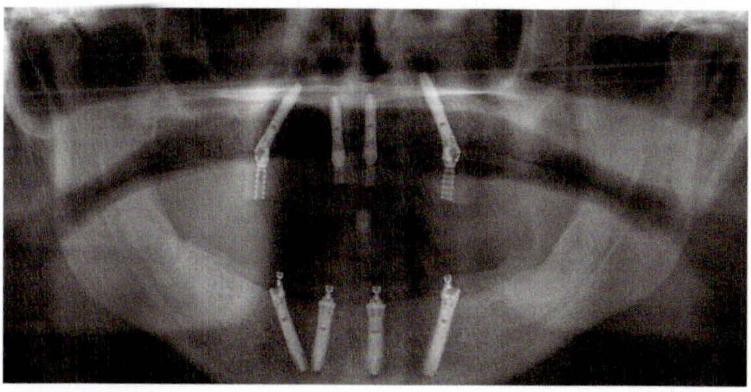

Fig. 20.70 Panoramic view of implant placement

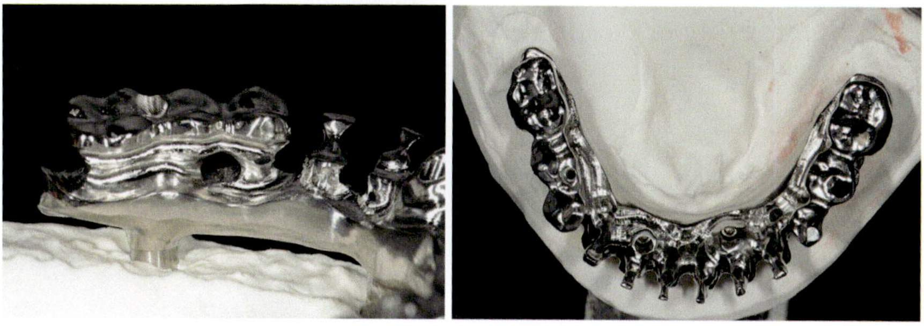

Fig. 20.71 Framework design with metal occlusal surface

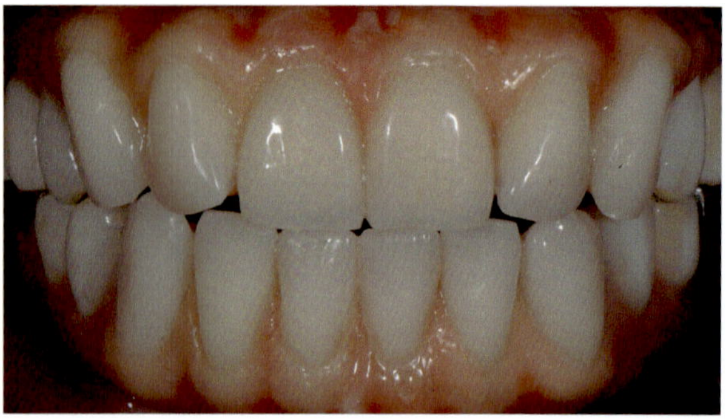

Fig. 20.72 Acrylic resin metal-based restoration

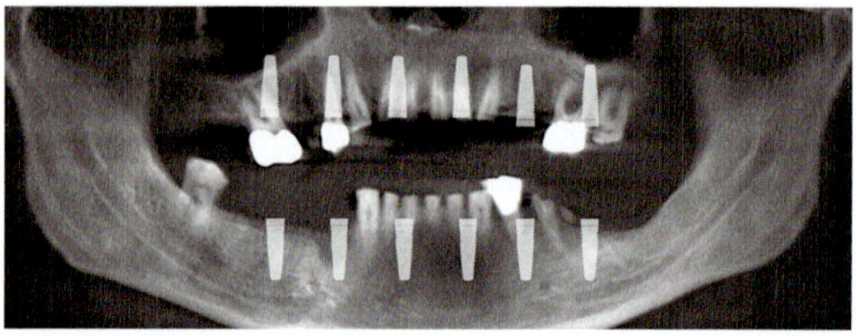

Fig. 20.73 Panoramic illustrating abundance of bone and the possibility of placing additional implants

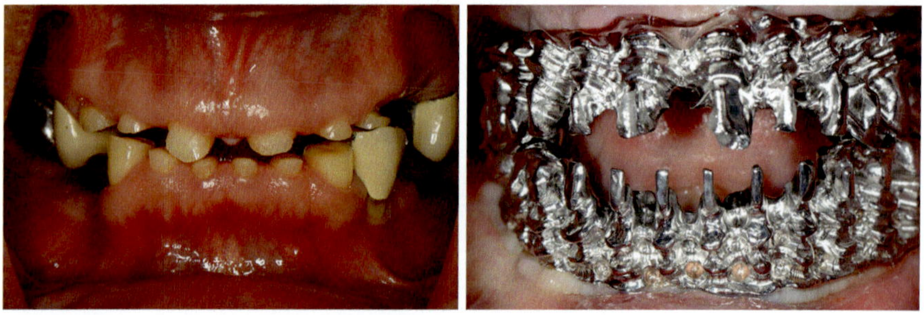

Fig. 20.74 Bone reduction done to accommodate restorative materials

be avoided by choosing a more conservative restorative option (Figs. 20.74 and 20.75).

3. Failure of the acrylic resin restoration by over-engineering the metal framework. The clinician must be cognizant of the space requirement for materials. Acrylic resin requires at least 3 mm of thickness over the framework to be biomechanically sound.

Despite the above errors, the restoration has been in situ for 13 years (Figs. 20.76 and 20.77). Repairs are readily done due to the restoration being screw retained and retrievable.

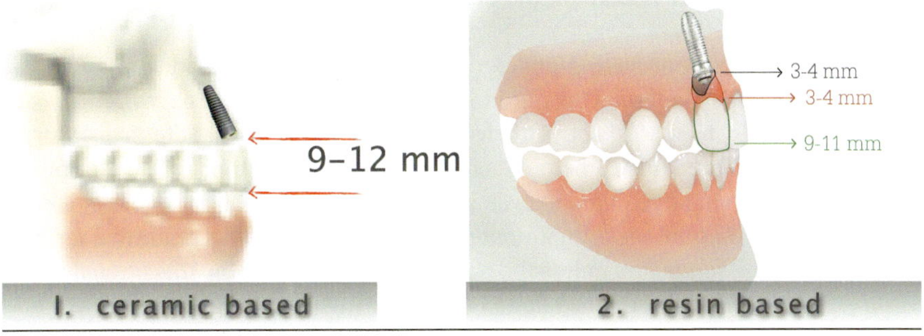

Fig. 20.75 Restorative space required for ceramic- and acrylic-based restorations

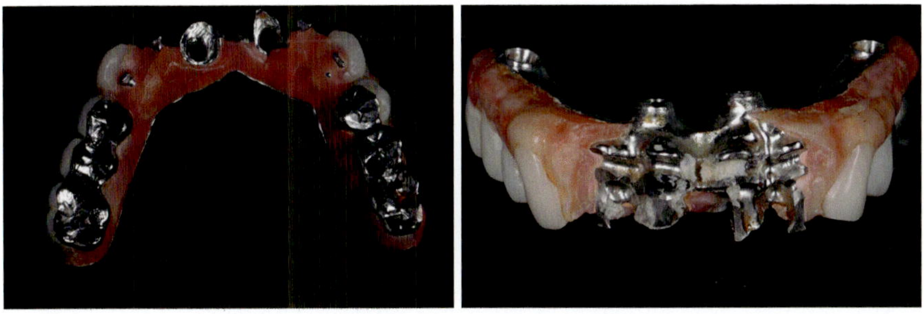

Fig. 20.76 Biomechanical failure. Acrylic resin delaminated from metal

Fig. 20.77 Restoration has been in situ for 13 years

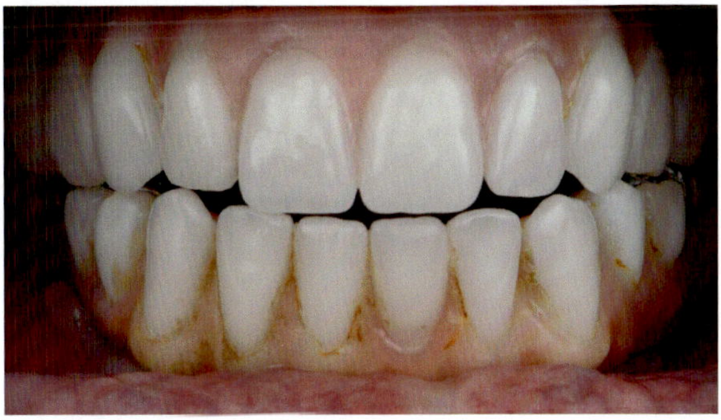

20.3.1.3 Failures Related to Lip Support and Smile Line

The movement of the upper lip during speech and smiling should be evaluated. Assessment of the patient's facial and lip support in frontal view and in profile needs to be made so the clinician can determine which type of prostheses would be more suitable. Often patients present with a removable denture seeking a fixed solution. Patients that have had removable prostheses for an extended period often required a buccal flange to provide lip support for aesthetics. Fixed prostheses cannot have a buccal flange because a concave intaglio surface would collect plaque and food debris, thereby preventing access for proper hygiene.

The clinician must evaluate all the diagnostic factors (Chap. 1), to determine if this is feasible.

Patients often present having undergone treatment and being unhappy with the result [31, 32]. It's important to question the patient to determine what they are unhappy with and which aspect of their smile they would like addressed. Prior to embarking upon retreatment, the clinician must explain to the patient that a provisional prosthesis will be required to evaluate aesthetics and function. The provisional must be presented as the most important phase of treatment and a definitive restoration should not be fabricated unless the patient is satisfied with the transitional restoration [33, 34]. This will be illustrated in the following patient presentation.

The patient presented with the following concerns that she would like addressed. She had previous had implants supported restorations in another office and was not satisfied with them.

Her concerns included the following:

1. Excessive gingival display.
2. In adequate lip support.
3. Discrepancy in the proportions of then teeth.

On clinical examination, the following were found:

1. Closed vertical dimension.
2. Excessive display of pink on smiling (Figs. 20.78 and 20.79).
3. Poor tooth proportions.
4. Failing implants in the maxilla.
5. Space beneath restorations causing a food trap.

The following treatment plan was implemented.

The maxillary implants were to be removed, and bone recontouring done in the maxilla to lift the occlusal plane apically. Four implants were placed in each arch, and a provisional prosthesis was fabricated for both maxilla and mandible.

The objectives of the provisional were to

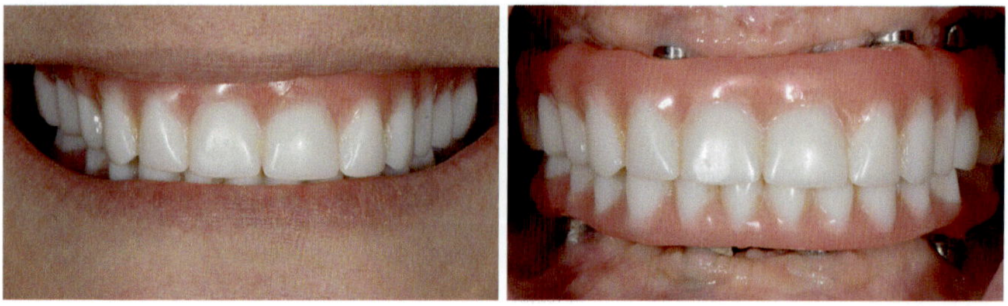

Fig. 20.78 Patient presented with existing restorations. Patient unhappy with contours and esthetics

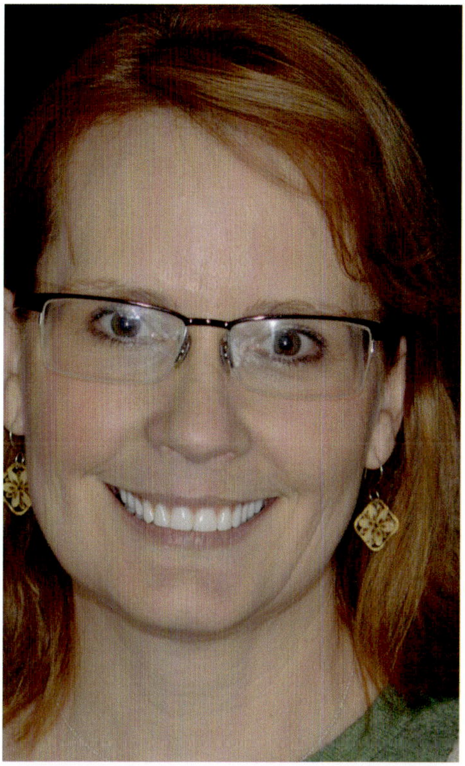

Fig. 20.79 Smile view demonstrating excessive display of pink acrylic

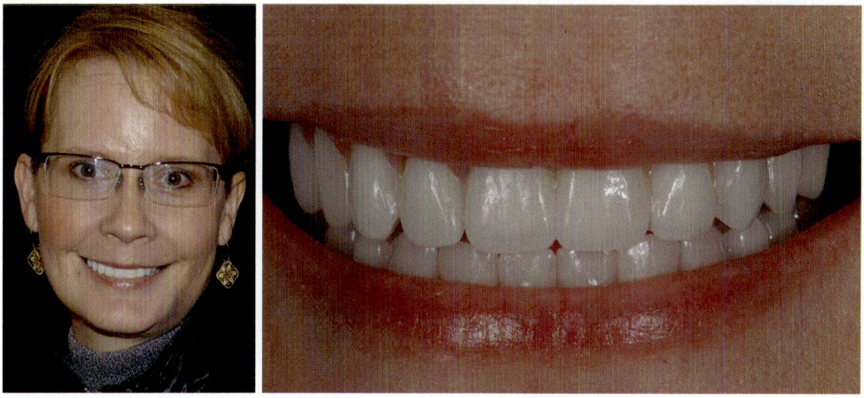

Fig. 20.80 Frontal and smile view of new transitional restorations demonstrating correct position of teeth and gingiva

1. Decrease gingival display (Fig. 20.80).
2. Improve tooth proportions (Fig. 20.81).
3. Restore the height of the lower third of the face.
4. Eliminate food entrapment.

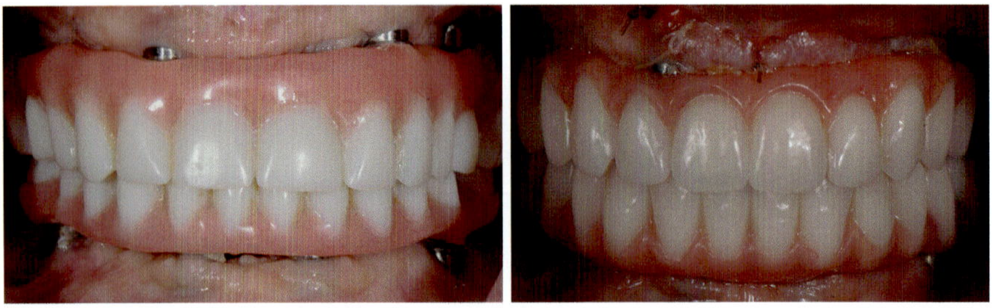

Fig. 20.81 Pre and post op views

Fig. 20.82 Concave undersurface of restoration. Patient is unable to keep it clean

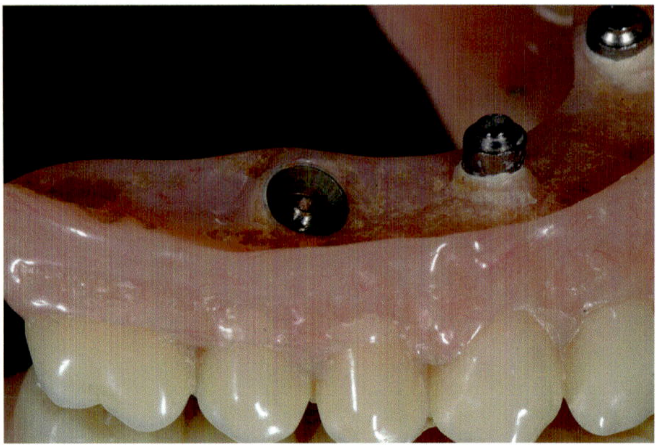

All of the above objectives must be achieved in the provisional restoration prior to embarking upon fabrication of the definitive prosthesis.

20.3.1.4 Failures Related to Emergence and Contours

The contours of the restorations must be planned from the outset. The emergence profile of the restorations should be straight as it exits the gingival margin [35, 36]. Often this requires alveolectomy to create sufficient space.

One misconception about graft less protocols is that they always require a significant amount of bone reduction. Bone reduction must have a rationale, and the minimum bone reduction must be done to satisfy the requirements of implant placement and fabrication of a biomechanically sound restoration.

Contours and emergence are related to implant placement in relation to the maxillary incisal edge position. Often errors result from inadequate implant placement and dental technicians compensate for that by ridge lapping the tissue. A concave undersurface is not cleansable (Figs. 20.82 and 20.83). Patients often want a fixed restoration over a removable. In patients with severe resorption and severe lack of lip support, this is not always possible, and the advantages of a removable implant-supported restoration with a buccal flange should be considered. If fixed restorations are provided, these often result in speech impediments and contours that cannot be cleaned (Fig. 20.84).

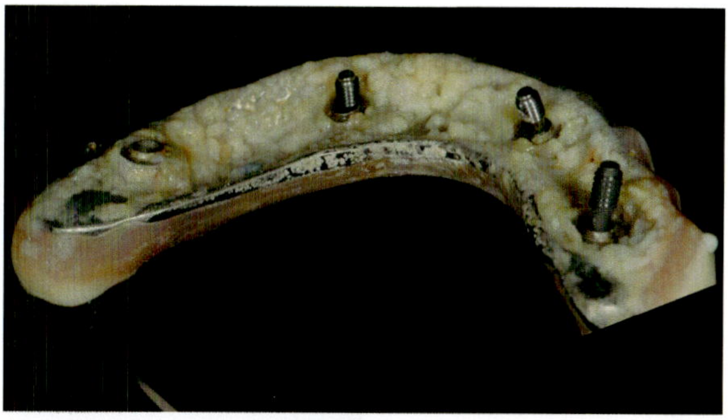

Fig. 20.83 Plaque accumulation within the intaglio of the restoration

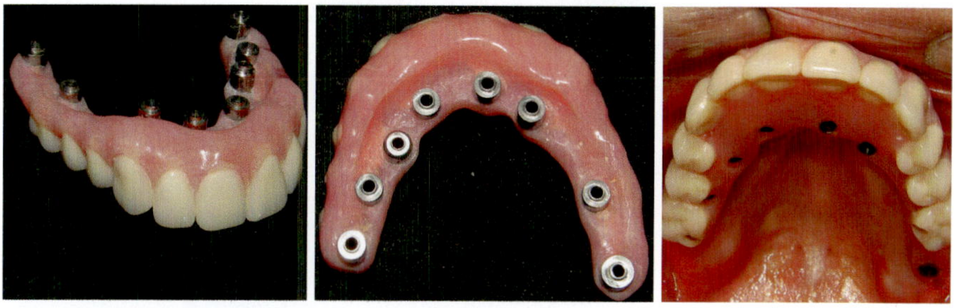

Fig. 20.84 Concave undersurface and bulky contours of restoration

20.3.1.5 Failures Related to Tissue Surface

The provisional and definitive restoration should satisfy the following criteria.

1. Reduce food entrapment—Following 3 months of healing, the acrylic provisional should be relined so that it compresses the tissue surface and creates a concave tissue surface allowing a convex restoration surface.
2. Provide cleansable contours by developing the tissue as outlined above.
3. Eliminate speech impairment. The t and d sounds relate to the palatal aspects of the maxillary prosthesis, and this area can be adjusted to accommodate for that. The "S" sound is developed utilizing the closest speaking space, and this should also be corrected in the provisional prior to proceeding to the definitive restoration.
4. The tissue contact should be intimate, but accessible to oral hygiene procedures.
5. The tissue surface should be highly polished.

Patients often present with the complaint of bleeding from the undersurface of the prosthesis. Bleeding is usually related to inflammation of the tissue surface. Inflammation can be caused by poor hygiene or an undersurface that is concave and not highly polished (Figs. 20.85 and 20.86).

Correction of this issue may require replacement of the restoration if it is zirconia based or relining and repolishing of the restoration if it is acrylic based (Fig. 20.87). The undersurface of the restoration should be convex and highly

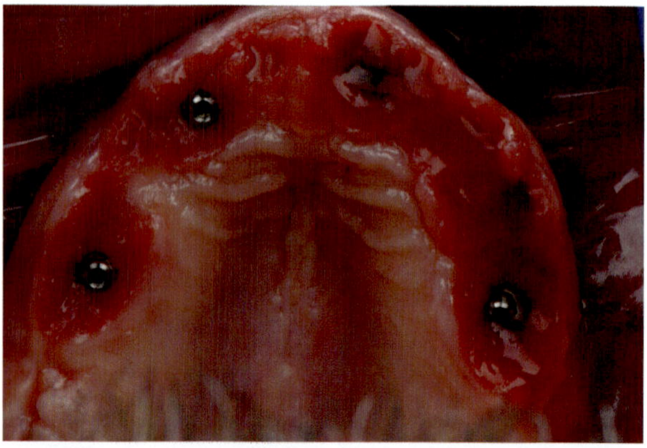

Fig. 20.85 Tissue inflammation as a result of poor contours and polish

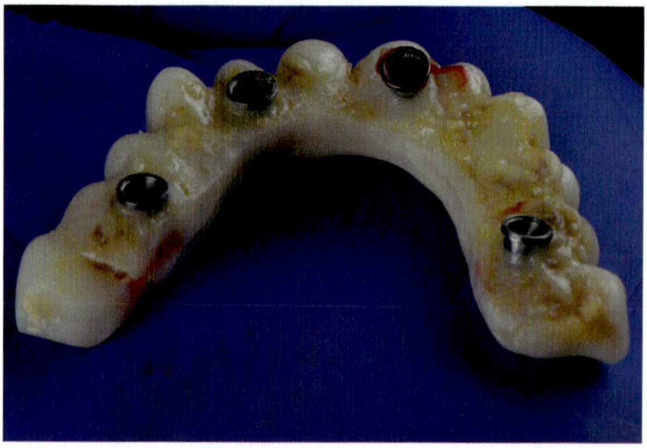

Fig. 20.86 Undersurface of restoration demonstrating excessive plaque build up

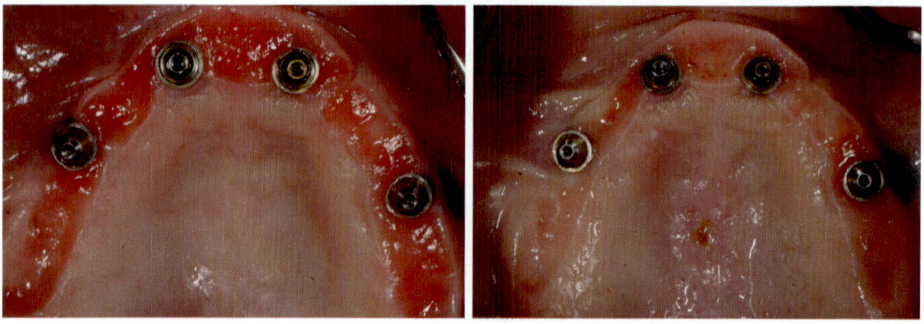

Fig. 20.87 Pre and post op view of tissue after undersurface is corrected

polished (Fig. 20.88). The area adjacent to the implants should allow passage of an interproximal oral hygiene cleaning aid.

20.3.1.6 Failures Related to Occlusion

Most of the patients seeking treatment with full arch fixed prostheses have a terminal dentition that forces them to develop a modified jaw position in order to masticate their food. Therefore, capturing the patient's jaw relationship in this habitual

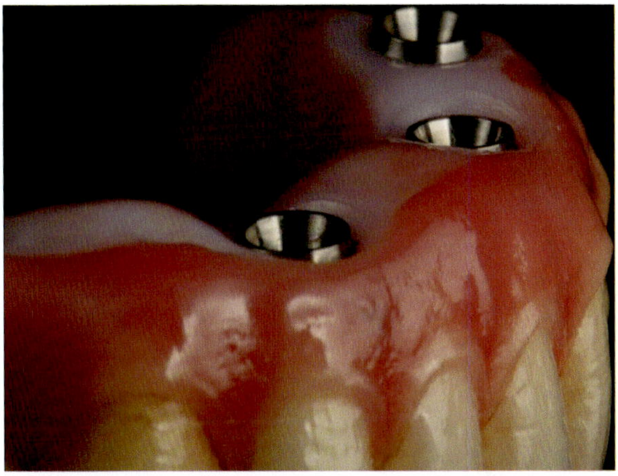

Fig. 20.88 Undersurface restoration should be well polished and convex

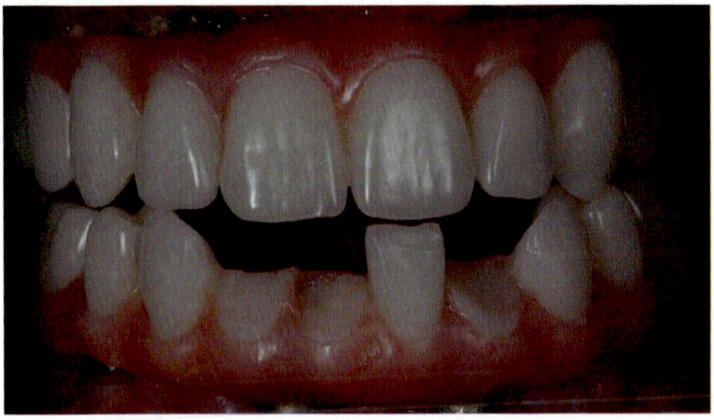

Fig. 20.89 Fracture of restoration

position is likely to be inaccurate and result in transitional fixed prostheses that do not occlude with an even force distribution. As a result, the interim prostheses are much more prone to fracture (Fig. 20.89). Thankfully, this is an aspect that can be corrected from the transitional phase to the definitive phase. In order to avoid this scenario, clinicians should capture interocclusal record in centric relation, which is the most predictable position available.

The design of the occlusal relationship and occlusal scheme really is dependent upon the restorations that are being fabricated. If both the maxilla and mandible are being restored simultaneously, it would be recommended that the restorative materials be compatible. It is also recommended that any full mouth rehabilitation supported by implants patients be given an occlusal device to wear especially at night to minimize the potential for fracture of the restorative materials. When both arches have fixed implant restorations, the basic occlusal principles are to be followed such as mutually protected occlusion's that allow for anterior guidance. The goal of the restorative dentist should be two place the final restoration or restorations into a position that is coincident with condylar position and repeatable. In excursive movements, the posterior teeth should disclude. This is based on mechanics rather than science. Implant-supported restorations lack proprioception [37]. Patients many times will present with fracture or severe wear of the restorative material (Fig. 20.90).

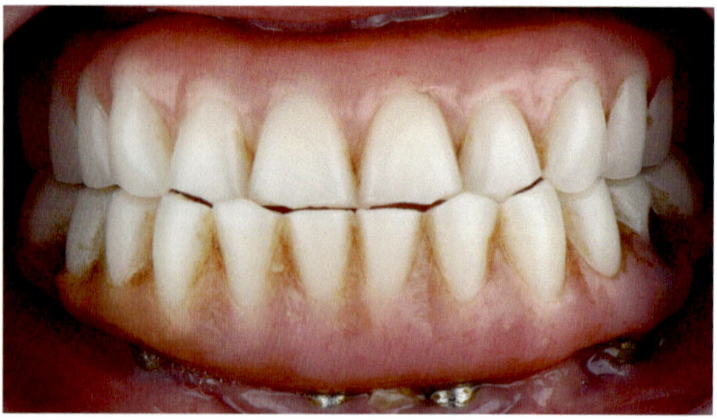

Fig. 20.90 Severe wear of acrylic-based restorations

It is advisable that flatter cusps and wider fossas be used to allow for some freedom of movement.

20.3.2 Failure Resulting from Inadequate Treatment Execution

Full arch implant-supported restorations are more complex to fabricate than single or multiple units on implants. There are numerous variables that must be recognized and managed.

Every stage of the treatment procedure, from making impressions to delivery of the definitive restorations, is susceptible to errors. Many companies promote digital technology as a strategy to simplify treatment protocols. Companies also negate the importance of diagnosis and treatment planning. Digital technology must be seen as an adjunct to sound analogue principles. Digital technology will not compensate for inadequate understanding of the steps required. The clinician has a responsibility to understand the workflow and be cognizant of what can go wrong in each step.

For the inexperienced clinician, the immediate load process during surgery poses a substantial challenge. This is typically delegated to the laboratory technician. It is the duty of the clinician to comprehend the prerequisites, the process that must be followed, and the intended result of the provisional restoration. Digital technologies such as scanning, 3D printing are also utilized to simplify the process. As stated, before the clinician must have a sound understanding of analogues principles before embarking upon extensive implant therapy.

The objectives of the immediate load should be

1. Aesthetics.
2. Adequate vertical dimension.
3. Adequate occlusal management.
4. A passive restoration as possible.
5. Appropriate contours for cleansability.

The most significant complication is for the immediate provisional not to fit. If this is the case, the offending temporary cylinder must be removed from the provisional and re-attached at chairside (Figs. 20.91 and 20.92). It is not common for the provisional prosthesis to apply pressure through the soft tissue over the residual ridge. In many instances, this is a result of post-surgical swelling and will resolve itself once the healing phase is firmly underway. If the patient demonstrates sub-prosthesis ulcerations after a 2-week period of healing, the prosthesis should be carefully removed, and the intaglio surface adjusted.

20.3.2.1 Impression Making and Cast Verification

The impression dictates fit of the definitive restoration. Significant experience and time are required at this step. Assessing fit of a restoration is based on clinical judgment, and this varies from practitioner to practitioner. It is a modality that cannot be taught objectively. Various techniques exist for impression making including, splinting, non-splinting and scanning. Outcome of each technique appears to be operator dependent [38]. Once the impression is made, it must be poured very carefully in low expansion die stone and the master cast verified for accuracy. Most laboratories provide a verification jig. These verification jigs can be made of different materials that range from acrylic resin to impression plaster. Each material has its advantages and disadvantages. A material that is non-forgiving such as impression plaster for the verification jig is the authors' preference. If the framework does not fit, this will necessitate additional impressions and verifications (Fig. 20.93).

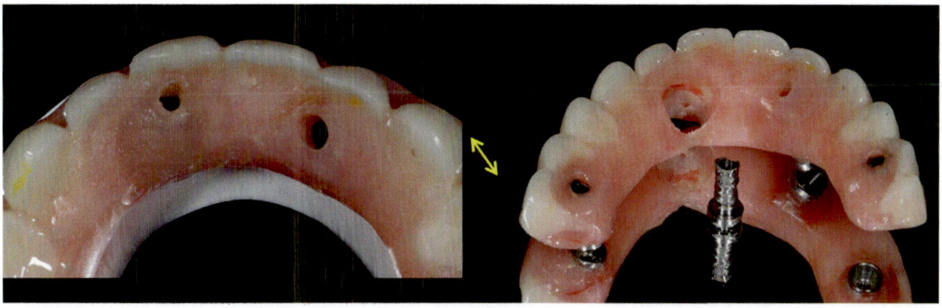

Fig. 20.91 Lack of fit may require detaching offending temporary cylinder and chairside pick up

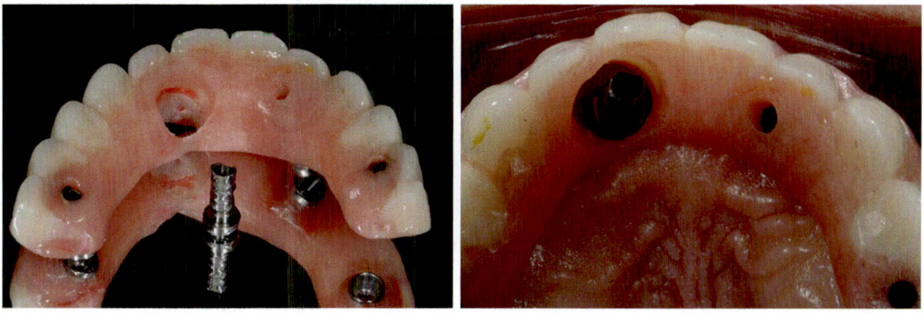

Fig. 20.92 Chairside pick up

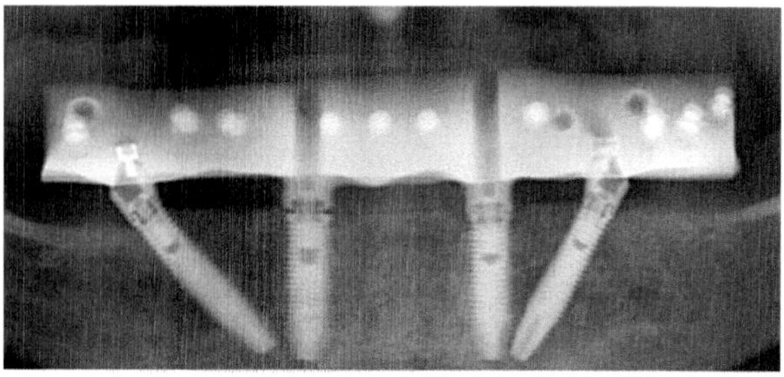

Fig. 20.93 Framework misfit

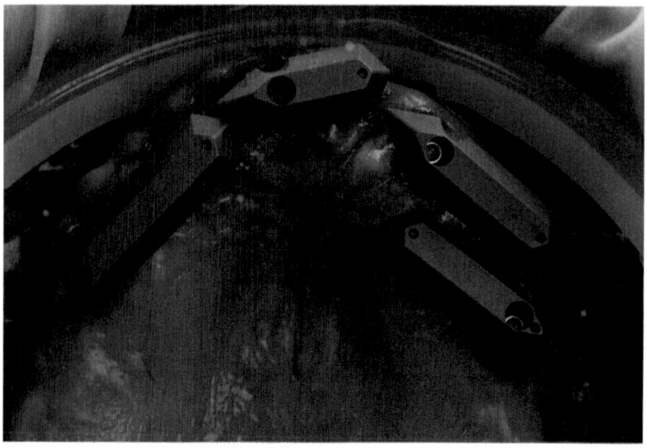

Fig. 20.94 Scan gauges in situ designed to allow accuracy in full arch scanning. (Osteon medical technologies)

With the advent of scan gauges, clinicians may be able to scan a full arch and expect to receive a restoration that will have a passive fit intra-orally. The scanning process does require a learning curve but ultimately decreases the time to the definitive restoration. This requires additional study to be fully recommended for routine use, and manufacturer advertising claims should not be accepted without caution (Fig. 20.94).

20.3.2.2 Complications/Considerations with the Definitive Restorations

Insertion

All the objectives of the definitive restorations should have been accomplished in the provisional. If this is done well, insertion should be seamless. Most insertion issues are usually the result of either not accurately recording soft tissue relationships and therefore having the patient experiencing discomfort upon insertion of the final restoration or not seating the final restoration due to an inaccurate recording of the implant positions [38]. Inadequate recording of jaw relations can also result in excessive occlusal adjustment at time of delivery which is undesirable.

If these have been done correctly and laboratory fabrication has followed the suggested recommendations of the manufacturer of the materials, one should experience a predictable appointment.

The initial placement of the prosthesis can result in blanching because of the pressure from the intaglio surface of the prosthesis. If the contour and position of the prostheses are correct, this is transitory and readily dissipates in 5–10 min. The clinician needs to be aware that soft tissue can act as an impediment to the prostheses not seating. If this is the case, the intaglio surface will need to be adjusted. The patient should not be feeling acute pain during the insertion appointment, some minor discomfort or pressure is normal. The clinician should use a sequential protocol for tightening abutment and/or prosthetic screws and monitor the soft tissue colour in addition to the patient feedback. Radiographic confirmation is a valuable tool to ensure that the soft tissue is not preventing the full arch prosthesis from engaging either the implant or abutment.

A frequent question in a full arch restoration retained by multiple prosthetic screws or abutment screws is what is the sequence by which the screws are tightened. There is no hard and fast rule, but it is probably advised to tighten screws by hand that are directly across from each other and work your way around the prosthesis. Every effort should be made to engage all the screws by gently hand tightening them. At that point, the patient should be left for a few minutes to allow for relaxation of the engaged screws and some possible compression of soft tissue end seating of the full prosthesis. The practitioner can then go back and secure the screws one more time. It is not recommended that the screws be torqued to the manufacturer's recommendation on the initial insertion. For numerous reasons, the prosthesis may need to be removed for soft tissue adjustments or be returned to the laboratory if the patient is not satisfied with the aesthetic results. It would be advisable to torque the screws once the patient is completely satisfied, the occlusion has been stabilized and there are no soft tissue issues and the period that the patient is wearing the permanent restoration has been uneventful. This varies by patient.

20.3.3 Biological Failures

Biologic complications can occur from a myriad of events and can be divided into early intermediate and late. In the early or immediate stage, they are a result of the surgical event and/or the immediate load prosthesis, if that was placed. Strictly speaking complications of the surgical event will either be one or a combination of bleeding, pain, swelling, altered sensation, or paresthesia and must be handled immediately by the surgeon.

20.3.4 Mechanical Failures

Mechanical failures are related to the implant, abutment screw, and prosthetic screw. When there is screw loosening of the prosthetic screw or abutment screw, this is a complication that needs to be dealt with immediately [39–42]. Any mobility of the prosthesis may result in fracture of the restorative material or prosthetic retaining screw (Figs. 20.95 and 20.96).

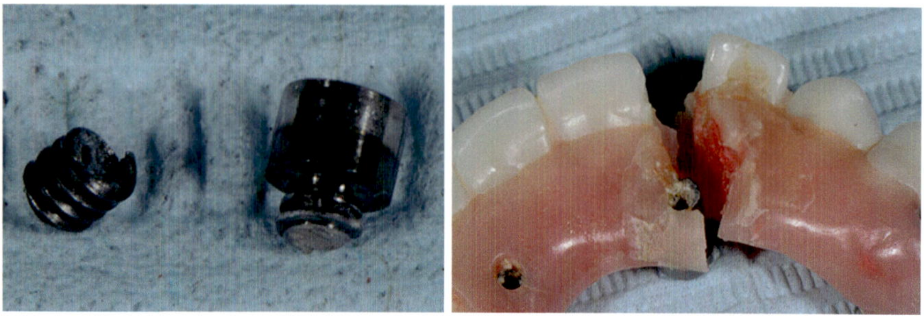

Fig. 20.95 Screw fracture and interim restoration fracture

Fig. 20.96 Clinical screw fracture

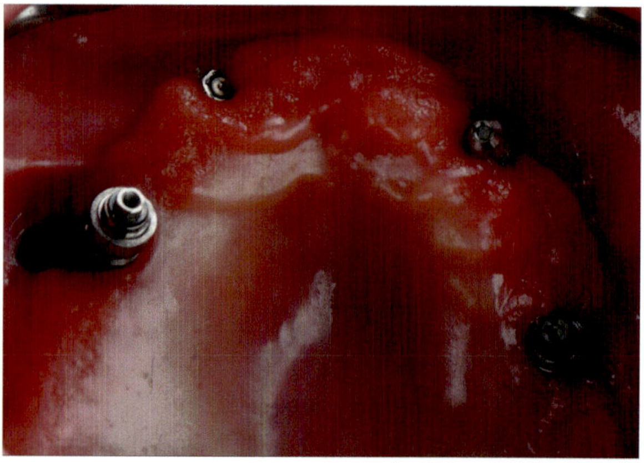

The diagnosis of screw loosening must be undertaken. This can occur as a result of

1. Misfit
2. Excessive force
3. Inadequate torque

Should the screw fracture and screw removal can be a laborious process. If the screw is not distorted within the abutment or implants, they are relatively easy to remove. Screw removal can be facilitated with an explorer moved in a counterclockwise direction or an ultrasonic unit with fine tip. If the screw is not retrievable, especially the abutment screw one option is to turn the screw as far apical as it can go either with an explorer or other instrument and make enough threads accessible for another abutment screw. When the prosthetic screw is not retrievable, this sometimes requires cutting through the abutment and removing the abutment itself so that you can replace it.

There are few studies to guide clinicians on length of cantilever in the maxilla especially when utilizing the more contemporary materials such as zirconia [43]. Length of cantilever has a significant effect on failure of these types of restorations, and length of cantilever can be more significant than the number of implants [44, 45] (Fig. 20.97). Deflection of the cantilever is related to its length; so minute increases in length have a significant impact on the fracture complications of restorations. Lab-based studies on zirconia have shown that

1. The longer the cantilever the lower the load to failure (Fig. 20.98).
2. The smaller the connector size the less load to failure.
3. Failure usually occurred in the distal abutment wall.

Recommendations for cantilever include the following:

1. Limit distal cantilever.
2. Limit buccal cantilever.
3. Increase thickness of the framework in the cantilever section distal to the most distal implant.
4. Limit occlusion on the cantilever.

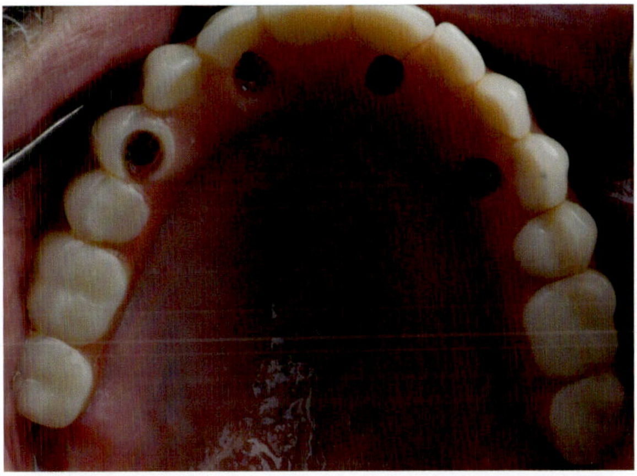

Fig. 20.97 Restoration demonstrating excessive cantilever

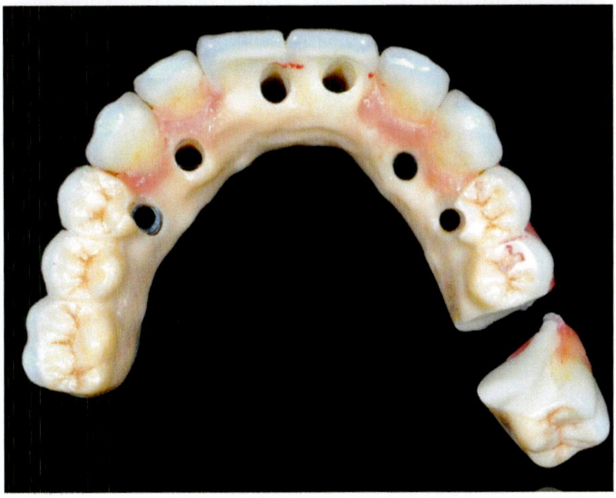

Fig. 20.98 Cantilever fracture in zirconia restoration

20.3.5 Material Failures

Today there are various materials to choose from when designing full arch fixed implant-supported restorations. Unfortunately, when looking at the literature for guidance, it is not supportive of a true evidence base in terms of an ideal material to utilize. There is no evidence to show one design is superior to another or one combination of materials is superior to another. Most articles are case reports, which follow a limited number of patients over a limited period of time.

As in all dental restorations, the choice of material comes with potential complications and these are similar to those seen in tooth borne restoration [45].

Material failure can be grouped into the failure of the tooth component and/or the substructure. Acrylic/metal restorations are much more accommodating in managing failures. One must realize that acrylic resin was not designed for implants but used as it was one of the only materials available at the time. Wear or breakage of acrylic resin-based restorations should not be seen as a complication but rather a consequence of the restorative material. This must be explained to the patient prior to embarking upon extensive treatment so disappointments can be avoided at a later date.

The loss of a denture tooth can be dealt with simply by replacing it and re-attaching it to the prosthesis (Fig. 20.99).

Large scale fracture of the alveolar component, such as acrylic, can also be repaired intra-orally under certain circumstances. If that is not possible, the prosthesis should be removed very carefully, and the separated components re-attached with acrylic resin. Often this requires the restoration to be sent to the laboratory for definitive repair (Figs. 20.100 and 20.101). Large scale delamination of acrylic is a result of inadequate framework design or inadequate processing.

Failures in zirconia-based restorations are much more difficult to manage. If it is a simple ceramic fracture, the restoration can be removed from the mouth and sent to the laboratory for definitive repair (Fig. 20.102).

When designing zirconia-based implant frameworks, the following should be considered:

Fig. 20.99 Acrylic tooth fracture

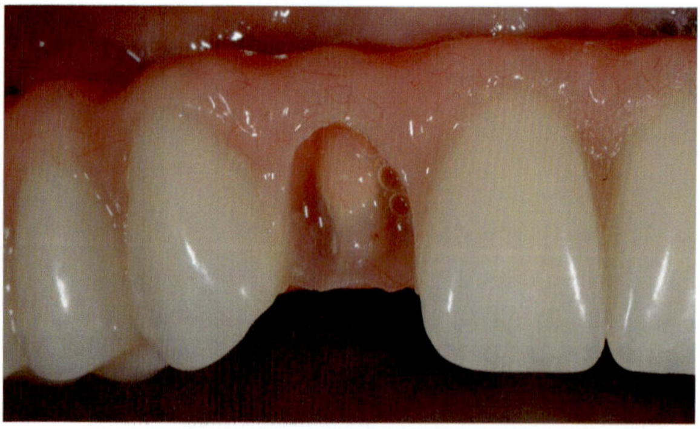

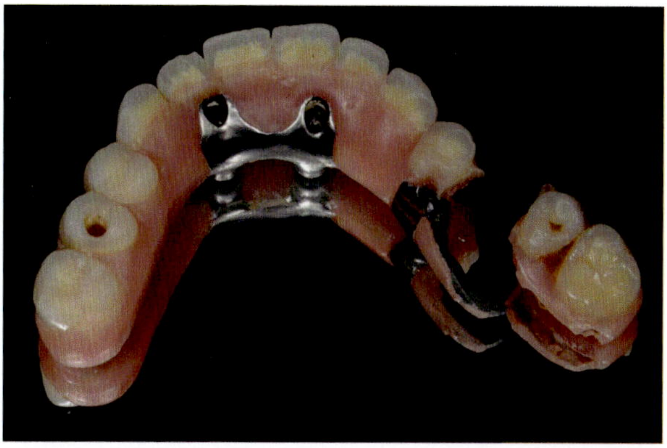

Fig. 20.100 Fracture of acrylic from framework. Could be a result of inadequate framework design

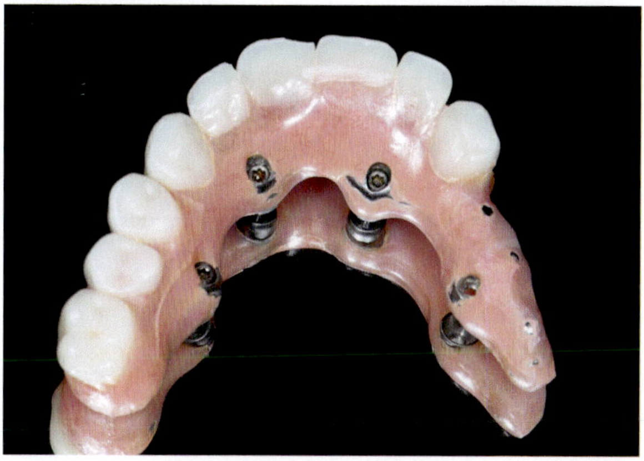

Fig. 20.101 Delamination of section of acrylic resin from substructure

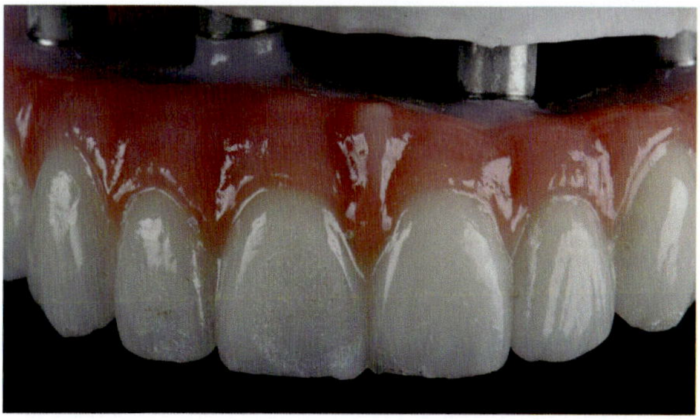

Fig. 20.102 Fracture of ceramic from zirconia framework

1. Maximize connector dimensions, buccal-lingually and occlusal-gingivally.
2. Minimize distal cantilever length.
3. Minimize buccal cantilever.
4. Ensure very light occlusal contacts in the cantilever region.
5. Thicken the chimney around the most distal implant and thicken the buccal and lingual walls around the chimney of the implant.

6. Ensure monolithic zirconia is well polished. Studies have shown it to be kind to the opposing occlusion.
7. Minimal post-sintering adjustment. This will also help with preserving the strength of the material and avoiding accelerated ageing failures in the presence of saliva.
8. Design for retrievability. This allows simple detachment of the appliance and the chance to service the restoration or treat any implant-related problems. With proper implant placement, this can be achieved in most situations when treating the edentulous arch.

20.4 Conclusion

Successful treatment with implant support requires substantial amounts of planning and skilled execution. Many prosthetic complications can occur when rendering treatment, but many of these are avoidable and highly manageable. Efforts should be made to prevent these complications and plan for the challenges that will inevitably occur over the years after treatment.

References

1. Lindh T, Gunne J, Tillberg A, Molin M. A meta-analysis of implants in partial edentulism. Clin Oral Implants Res. 1998;9(2):80–90.
2. Howe MS, Keys W, Richards D. Long-term (10-year) dental implant survival: a systematic review and sensitivity meta-analysis. J Dent. 2019;84:9–21.
3. Gallucci GO, Hamilton A, Zhou W, Buser D, Chen S. Implant placement and loading protocols in partially edentulous patients: a systematic review. Clin Oral Implants Res. 2018;29(Suppl 16):106–34.
4. Goodacre CJ, Bernal G, Rungcharassaeng K, Kan JY. Clinical complications with implants and implant prostheses. J Prosthet Dent. 2003;90(2):121–32.
5. Becktor JP, Isaksson S, Sennerby L. Survival analysis of endosseous implants in grafted and nongrafted edentulous maxillae. Int J Oral Maxillofac Implants. 2004;19(1):107–15.
6. Zhou W, Wang F, Monje A, Elnayef B, Huang W, Wu Y. Feasibility of dental implant replacement in failed sites: a systematic review. Int J Oral Maxillofac Implants. 2016;31(3):535–45.
7. Carr BR, Rekawek P, Gulko JA, Coburn JF, Boggess WJ, Chuang SK, Panchal N, Ford BP. Does implant placement using a minimally invasive technique increase early failures among trainees at an academic center? Oral Maxillofac Surg. 2023;27(2):245–50.
8. Albrektsson T, Canullo L, Cochran D, De Bruyn H. "Peri-implantitis": a complication of a foreign body or a man-made "disease". Facts and fiction. Clin Implant Dent Relat Res. 2016;18(4):840–9.
9. Albrektsson T, Jemt T, Mölne J, Tengvall P, Wennerberg A. On inflammation-immunological balance theory—a critical apprehension of disease concepts around implants: mucositis and marginal bone loss may represent normal conditions and not necessarily a state of disease. Clin Implant Dent Relat Res. 2019;21:183–9.
10. Wilson TG Jr. The positive relationship between excess cement and peri-implant disease: a prospective clinical endoscopic study. J Periodontol. 2009;80(9):1388–92.
11. Wilson TG Jr, Valderrama P, Burbano M, Blansett J, Levine R, Kessler H, Rodrigues DC. Foreign bodies associated with peri-implantitis human biopsies. J Periodontol. 2015;86(1):9–15.

12. Chapple ILC, Mealey BL, Van Dyke TE, et al. Periodontal health and gingival diseases and conditions on an intact and a reduced periodontium: consensus report of workgroup 1 of the 2017 World Workshop on the Classification of Periodontal and Peri-Implant Diseases and Conditions. J Clin Periodontol. 2018;45(Suppl 20):S68–77.
13. Berglundh T, Armitage G, Araujo MG, et al. Peri-implant diseases and conditions: consensus report of workgroup 4 of the 2017 World Workshop on the Classification of Periodontal and Peri-Implant Diseases and Conditions. J Clin Periodontol. 2018;45(Suppl 20):S286–91.
14. Lindhe J, Berglundh T, Ericsson I, Liljenberg B, Marinello C. Experimental breakdown of peri-implant and periodontal tissues. A study in the beagle dog. Clin Oral Implants Res. 1992;3:9–16.
15. Jivraj S, Chee W. Treatment planning of implants in the aesthetic zone. Br Dent J. 2006;201(2):77–89.
16. Tarnow DP, Cho SC, Wallace SS. The effect of inter-implant distance on the height of inter-implant bone crest. J Periodontol. 2000;71(4):546–9.
17. Eckert SE, Meraw SJ, Cal E, Ow RK. Analysis of incidence and associated factors with fractured implants: a retrospective study. Int J Oral Maxillofac Implants. 2000;15:662–7.
18. Jin SY, Kim SG, Oh JS, You JS, Jeong MA. Incidence and management of fractured dental implants: case reports. Implant Dent. 2017;26(5):802–6.
19. Winkler S, Ring K, Ring JD, Boberick KG. Implant screw mechanics and the settling effect: overview. J Oral Implantol. 2003;29:242–5.
20. Khraisat A, Abu-Hammad O, Dar-Odeh N, Al-Kayed AM. Abutment screw loosening and bending resistance of external hexagon implant system after lateral cyclic loading. Clin Implant Dent Relat Res. 2004;6:157–64.
21. Jivraj SA, Chee WW. Use of a removable partial denture in the management of chronic screw loosening. J Prosthet Dent. 2005;93:13–6.
22. Malo P, de Araújo Nobre M, Lopes A, Moss SM, Molina GJ. A longitudinal study of the survival of All-on-4 implants in the mandible with up to 10 years of follow-up. J Am Dent Assoc. 2011;142(3):310–20.
23. Maló P, de Araújo Nobre M, Lopes A, Francischone C, Rigolizzo M. "All-on-4" immediate-function concept for completely edentulous maxillae: a clinical report on the medium (3 years) and long-term (5 years) outcomes. Clin Implant Dent Relat Res. 2012;14(s1):e139–e50.
24. Maló P, Araújo Nobre M, Lopes A, Ferro A, Gravito I. All-on-4® treatment concept for the rehabilitation of the completely edentulous mandible: a 7-year clinical and 5-year radiographic retrospective case series with risk assessment for implant failure and marginal bone level. Clin Implant Dent Relat Res. 2015;17(S2):e531–e41.
25. Maló P, Lopes A. The rehabilitation of completely edentulous maxillae with different degrees of resorption with four or more immediately loaded implants: a 5-year retrospective study and a new classification. Eur J Oral Implantol. 2011;4(3):227.
26. Patzelt S, Bahat O, Reynolds MA, Strub JR. The all-on-four treatment concept: a systematic review. Clin Implant Dent Relat Res. 2014;16(6):836–55.
27. Afrashtehfar KI. The all-on-four concept may be a viable treatment option for edentulous rehabilitation. Evid Based Dent. 2016;17(2):56–7.
28. Felton DA. Complete edentulism and comorbid diseases: an update. J Prosthodont. 2016;25(1):5–20.
29. Douglass CW, Shih A, Ostry L. Will there be a need for complete dentures in the United States in 2020? J Prosthet Dent. 2002;87(1):5–8.
30. Hazem A, Bissada NF, Demko C, Paes A, Lang LA. Comparison of preprosthetic implant complications and failures between obese and nonobese patients. Int J Oral Maxillofac Implants. 2016;31(5):1093–9.
31. Fortin Y, Sullivan RM. Terminal posterior tilted implants planned as a sinus graft alternative for fixed full-arch implant-supported maxillary restoration: a case series with 10- to 19-year results on 44 consecutive patients presenting for routine maintenance. Clin Implant Dent Relat Res. 2017;19(1):56–68.

32. Daudt Polido W, Aghaloo T, Emmett TW, Taylor TD, Morton D. Number of implants placed for complete-arch fixed prostheses: a systematic review and meta-analysis. Clin Oral Implants Res. 2018;29(Suppl 16):154–83. https://doi.org/10.1111/clr.13312.
33. Tuminelli FJ, Neugarten J, Ayvazian EG. Clinical report on restoration of patient with immediate loaded maxillary restoration supported by zygomatic/endosseous implants and mandibular prothesis utilizing three-implant solution. N Y State Dent J. 2022;88:4.
34. Ramezanzadwe S, Yates J, Tuminelli F, Keyhan SO, Yousefi P, Lopez-Lopez J. Zygomatic implants placed in atrophic maxilla: an overview of current systematic reviews and meta-analysis. Maxillofac Plast Reconstr Surg. 2021;43(1):1.
35. Tuminelli FJ. Contributor to edentulous treatment guidelines. Lucerne, Foundation for Oral Rehabilitation, Author of 20+ modules on single tooth implant restorations. 2016. FOR.org. https://www.for.org/en/treatment-guidelines.
36. Goodacre CJ, Goldstein G, Tuminelli FJ. Implant fixed complete dentures. In: Implant dentistry DVD. School of Dentistry, Loma Linda University; 2007.
37. Sheets CG, Earthman JC. Tooth intrusion in implant-assisted prostheses. J Prosthet Dent. 1997;77(1):39–45.
38. Baig MR. Accuracy of impressions of multiple implants in the edentulous arch: a systematic review. Int J Oral Maxillofac Implants. 2014;29(4):869–80.
39. Wittneben JG, Millen C, Brägger U. Clinical performance of screw- versus cement-retained fixed implant-supported reconstructions—a systematic review. Int J Oral Maxillofac Implants. 2014;29(Suppl):84–98.
40. Pjetursson BE, Thoma D, Jung R, Zwahlen M, Zembic A. A systematic review of the survival and complication rates of implant-supported fixed dental prostheses (FDPs) after a mean observation period of at least 5 years. Clin Oral Implants Res. 2012;23(Suppl 6):22–38.
41. Wadhwani C, Hess T, Faber T, Piñeyro A, Chen CSK. A descriptive study of the radiographic density of implant restorative cements. J Prosthet Dent. 2010;103(5):295–302.
42. Zeno HA, Buitrago RL, Sternberger SS, Patt ME, Tovar N, Coelho P, Kurtz KS, Tuminelli FJ. The effect of gingival entrapment on screw loosening at the implant abutment interface. Part 1—An in vitro study. J Prosthodont. 2016;25(3):216–23.
43. Walter L, Greenstein G. Utility of measuring anterior-posterior spread to determine distal cantilever length off a fixed implant-supported full-arch prosthesis: a review of the literature. J Am Dent Assoc. 2020;151(10):790–5.
44. Jemt T. Implant survival in the partially edentulous jaw—30 years of experience. Part 1: A retro-prospective multivariate regression analysis of overall implant failures in 4,585 consecutively treated arches. Int J Prosthodont. 2018;31:425–35.
45. Jemt T. Implant survival in the partially edentulous jaw—30 years of experience. Part III: A retro-prospective multivariate regression analysis of overall implant failures in 2915 consecutively treated arches. Int J Prosthodont. 2019;32:36–43.